IMMUNOLOGY AND IMMUNE SYSTEM DISORDERS

AUTOIMMUNE DISEASES: SYMPTOMS, DIAGNOSIS AND TREATMENT

IMMUNOLOGY AND IMMUNE SYSTEM DISORDERS

Additional books in this series can be found on Nova's website under the Series tab.

Additional E-books in this series can be found on Nova's website under the E-books tab.

IMMUNOLOGY AND IMMUNE SYSTEM DISORDERS

AUTOIMMUNE DISEASES: SYMPTOMS, DIAGNOSIS AND TREATMENT

KYLE J. BRENNER
EDITOR

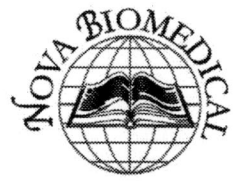

Nova Science Publishers, Inc.
New York

Copyright © 2010 by Nova Science Publishers, Inc.

All rights reserved. No part of this book may be reproduced, stored in a retrieval system or transmitted in any form or by any means: electronic, electrostatic, magnetic, tape, mechanical photocopying, recording or otherwise without the written permission of the Publisher.

For permission to use material from this book please contact us:
Telephone 631-231-7269; Fax 631-231-8175
Web Site: http://www.novapublishers.com

NOTICE TO THE READER

The Publisher has taken reasonable care in the preparation of this book, but makes no expressed or implied warranty of any kind and assumes no responsibility for any errors or omissions. No liability is assumed for incidental or consequential damages in connection with or arising out of information contained in this book. The Publisher shall not be liable for any special, consequential, or exemplary damages resulting, in whole or in part, from the readers' use of, or reliance upon, this material.

Independent verification should be sought for any data, advice or recommendations contained in this book. In addition, no responsibility is assumed by the publisher for any injury and/or damage to persons or property arising from any methods, products, instructions, ideas or otherwise contained in this publication.

This publication is designed to provide accurate and authoritative information with regard to the subject matter covered herein. It is sold with the clear understanding that the Publisher is not engaged in rendering legal or any other professional services. If legal or any other expert assistance is required, the services of a competent person should be sought. FROM A DECLARATION OF PARTICIPANTS JOINTLY ADOPTED BY A COMMITTEE OF THE AMERICAN BAR ASSOCIATION AND A COMMITTEE OF PUBLISHERS.

Additional color graphics may be available in the e-book version of this book.

LIBRARY OF CONGRESS CATALOGING-IN-PUBLICATION DATA

Autoimmune diseases : symptoms, diagnosis, and treatment / editor, Kyle J. Brenner.
   p. ; cm.
   Includes bibliographical references and index.
   ISBN 978-1-61668-007-7 (hardcover)
   1.Autoimmune diseases. I. Brenner, Kyle J.
   [DNLM: 1. Autoimmune Diseases--diagnosis. 2. Autoimmune Diseases--therapy. WD 305 A9379 2010]
   RC600.A835 2010
   616.97'8--dc22
   2010001738

Published by Nova Science Publishers, Inc. ✢ *New York*

CONTENTS

Preface		vii
Chapter 1	Natural Catalytic Antibodies in Norm and in Autoimmune Diseases *G. A. Nevinsky*	1
Chapter 2	Lupus Nephritis: Frontiers and Challenges: A Comprehensive Overview *Hussein Sheashaa, Tarek Abbas, Fatma Moustafa, Khaled Mahmoud, Amgad el-Agroudy, Anil Chandraker, Nidyanandh Vadivel, Rashad Hassan, Ashraf Bakr, Mohamed Zedan, Noha Tharwat, Wael Elkady and Mohamed Sobh*	107
Chapter 3	From Immunobiology to Genetics: In Search of a Cure for Autoimmunity *Sylvie Lesage, Erin E. Hillhouse, Véronique Dugas, Geneviève Chabot-Roy, Adam-Nicolas Pelletier, Marie Vilquin and Fanny Guimont-Desrochers*	167
Chapter 4	Central Nervous System Manifestations in Systemic Lupus Erythematosus: Diagnosis to Treatment *Simone Appenzeller and Mariana Postal*	209
Chapter 5	Emerging Methods in Type 1 Diabetes Immunomodulation: Beyond the Conventional *Brett E. Phillips and Nick Giannoukakis*	233
Chapter 6	Lupus Nephritis: from Diagnosis to Treatment *Nailú Angélica Sinicato, Mariana Postal and Simone Appenzeller*	251
Chapter 7	Clinical Features of Axonal Guillain–Barré Syndrome *Akiyuki Hiraga, Masahiro Mori and Satoshi Kuwabara*	265
Chapter 8	Removal [Blockage] of Hyperproduced Cytokines - A New Approach to the Treatment of Autoimmune Conditions *Simon V. Skurkovich*	277

Chapter 9	Revolutionary Bone Marrow Transplantation Method for Stem Cell Disorders *Susumu Ikehara*	289
Chapter 10	Immunological Control of Adult Neural Stem Cells *Oscar Gonzalez-Perez, Alfredo Quiñones-Hinojosa and Jose Manuel Garcia-Verdugo*	303
Chapter 11	Temporomandibular Joint Disorders and Systemic Lupus Erythematosus *L F Andre Costa and Simone Appenzeller*	317
Chapter 12	Fatigue in Guillain-Barré Syndrome: Activity-Dependent Conduction Block *Hiroyuki Nodera and Atsuko Nodera*	329
Chapter 13	Could Computerized Devices for Optic Nerve Head Analysis Find out Loss of Ganglion Cells in Not-Glaucomatous Damage? *Michele Iester, Marina Papadia and Alessandro Bagnis*	341
Chapter 14	Structural Biology Insights into the Autoantigens of the Myelin Sheath *Petri Kursula*	349
Chapter 15	Autoimmune Initiation of Multiple Sclerosis: Molecular Aspects *C. Fred Westall*	369
Chapter 16	Genetic Control of T Cell Tolerance and Susceptibility to Autoimmune Disease *Lydia Makaroff, Michelle Linterman and Adrian Liston*	403
Index		437

PREFACE

Autoimmune diseases arise from an overactive immune response of the body against substances and tissues normally present in the body. The immune system mistakes some part of the body as a pathogen and attacks it. The treatment of autoimmune diseases is typically with immunosuppression—medication which decreases the immune response. This book presents and reviews important data gathered on autoimmune diseases and related topics such as: systemic lupus erythematosus and nephritis, their diagnosis and management; emerging methods in Type 1 diabetes immunomodulation; blockage of hyperproduced cytokines as a new approach for the treatment of autoimmune conditions; bone marrow transplantation methods for autoimmune/stem cell disorders; the autoimmune attack on myelin proteins which initiate Multiple Sclerosis; and others.

Chapter 1 - In patients with autoimmune (AI) diseases autoantibodies (Abs) directed to polysaccharides, nucleic acids, proteins, peptides, nucleoprotein complexes, and enzymes with different catalytic functions may be induced spontaneously by primary antigens and can have characteristics of the primary antigen, including the catalytic activity of idiotypic and/or antiidiotypic Abs. The discovery of IgG specifically hydrolyzing intestinal vasoactive peptide in the sera of asthma patients (Paul S., 1989) stimulated of the studies of natural catalytic antibodies (abzymes). Detection of abzymes (Abzs) was shown to be the earliest indicator of development of different autoimmune diseases (AD). At the early stages of ADs, the repertoire of Abzs is usually relatively small but it greatly increases with the progress of the disease, leading to the generation of catalytically diverse abzymes with different activities and functions. Some Abzs are cytotoxic and can play an important negative role in the pathogenesis of AI pathologies, while positive roles have been proposed for other abzymes.

During the spontaneous development of profound SLE-like pathology in mice, a specific reorganization of the immune system leads to conditions associated with production of Abzs with low catalytic activities (conditionally pre-diseased mice). A significant increase in the relative Abz activities associated with a transition from pre-diseased to diseased mice is correlated with additional changes in the differentiation and proliferation of bone marrow hematopoietic stem cells and lymphocyte proliferation in different organs. Different mechanisms of Abzs production are observed for healthy mice immunized externally and for autoimmune mice during the spontaneous development of pathology.

In this chapter, new data concerning Abzs with different catalytic activities in various ADs, possible reasons of their catalytic heterogeneity, possible roles of abzymes and their exceptional multiplicity in the pathogenesis of different ADs, and possible uses of the abzyme activity for diagnostic of AI diseases are discussed.

Chapter 2 - Lupus nephritis (LN) is a major cause of morbidity and mortality, affecting over half of systemic lupus erythematosis (SLE) patients. It affects adult and pediatric patients. Kidney biopsy remains the cornerstone of LN diagnosis, and there are new International Society of Nephrology/Renal Pathology Society classifications of LN. Although prognosis of LN has improved with the combined use of cytotoxic and steroid therapy, up to 20% of these patients progress to renal failure. Moreover, toxicity of the current regimens remains a major concern. The accelerating advances in molecular and cellular immunology have paved the way for development biologic agents that target specific pathways that contribute to the inflammatory response, but there is no strong evidence of their safety and efficacy. Moreover, the increased risk of renal allograft thrombosis and recurrence of lupus nephritis constitute a substantial risk that should be thoroughly explored. The aim of this chapter is to explore all these aspects in a comprehensive manner. In addition,the major advances that necessitate the evolution of basic and clinical research to explore the magic management of this syndrome dilemma will be explored.

Chapter 3 - The Human Genome Project has facilitated the identification of various genetic regions associated with disease susceptibility. This identification step is important as it yields clues into the pathways implicated in defining disease susceptibility and may uncover important therapeutic targets. Indeed, by performing genome-wide scans, one can identify many genetic loci associated with autoimmune disease susceptibility. However, the odds ratio of each locus is relatively low. Therefore, the limitation of these studies is in the biological translation of the data. This raises the question of how one validates the contribution of all of these genetic variations to human disease.

An alternative strategy for the identification of various genetic regions associated with disease susceptibility is to compare genetically resistant and susceptible individuals for biological variations. The subsequent challenge is then to demonstrate that the biological variations are causal to disease. For instance, autoimmune diseases are thought to arise as a consequence of disturbances in self-tolerance. Herein, the various mechanisms of self-tolerance, with particular emphasis on the defects potentially contributing to the onset of autoimmune diabetes, will be described. Specifically, this chapter will focus on the contribution of the acquired immune system and the innate immune system, including T and B cell tolerance, dendritic cells, macrophages and NK cells, as well as the potential interplay between these distinct phenotypes in defining the genetic predisposition to autoimmune diseases.

Chapter 4 - Systemic lupus erythematosus (SLE) is an autoimmune disease with central nervous system (CNS) involvement occurring in up to 75% of the patients. However the frequency of these manifestations in SLE studies varies widely, depending on the type of manifestations included and the method used for evaluation. CNS involvement may be considered primary if directly related to SLE activity in the CNS or secondary when related to treatment, infections, metabolic abnormalities or other systemic manifestations such as uremia and hypertension. The involvement may vary from subtle signs such as headache and mood disorders to severe, and life threatening conditions, such as stroke, myelopathy and acute confusionalstate. Any part of the peripheral or CNS may be affected by the disease. The diagnosis of primary CNS involvement by SLE is often difficult, as both focal and diffuse manifestations may occur and there is no gold standard for diagnosis. In this chapter a review of the main clinical manifestations of CNS in SLE, possible etiological mechanisms and neuroimaging features associated with these manifestations are explored. Further analysis of the most important tools that can help bedside diagnosis and discuss current treatment options take place in this chapter.

Chapter 5 - Type 1 diabetes is an autoimmune disease likely initiated by stress on insulin-producing pancreatic beta cells which eventually leads to beta cell-specific pathogenic T-cell activation and the eventual eradication of significant beta cell mass. The absence of insulin therefore leads to hyperglycemia that requires replacement of the hormone for normal glucohomeostasis. Exogenous insulin replacement alone, however, is insufficient in preventing diabetes-associated complications because it is unable to match the tight metabolic control the body is able to marshal with the endogenous production of insulin. Therefore, the aim of type 1 diabetes therapy is the return of insulin production to levels that achieve normal glucose homeostasis with an abrogation of the underlying autoimmunity. Therapies that modulate and restore proper immune function before loss of the beta cell mass are key in the development of a true cure for type 1 diabetes. These immunoregulatory therapies will be discussed along with methods of early disease diagnosis.

Chapter 6 - Systemic lupus erythematosus (SLE) is a complex, multisystem autoimmune disorder, which often involves referral to multiple medical specialists. Lupus nephritis (LN) occurs in approximately 35% of adults with SLE and predicts poor survival. The 2003 joint International Society of Nephrology and Renal Pathology Society (ISN/RPS) histological classification improved the characterization of the biopsies of patients with lupus nephritis, to provide additional prognostic information and enhance guidance for therapy. Understanding of the value of partial remission, and the prognosis for certain socio economic and ethnic groups in lupus nephritis has also improved. Despite this progress, however, therapy is still not optimal. Although effective immunosuppressive therapies are available for many patients with SLE, some patients do not respond to initial treatment, and others have a relapsing course of disease after remission. The optimal maintenance immunosuppressive treatment and the duration of therapy for patients with lupus nephritis are not entirely clear. Immunosuppressive regimens for severe lupus nephritis can also be associated with a variety of major adverse effects, which include an increased risk of infection, infertility, bone damage, bladder lesions, and cosmetic changes (such as cushingoid appearance or alopecia).These adverse reactions harm patients and limit the potential for future therapy. In this chapter a review tales place of clinical manifestations, histology correlation, and treatment options in SLE nephritis.

Chapter 7 - Guillain–Barré syndrome is currently classified into 2 major forms based on pathologic and electrophysiologic criteria: (1) acute inflammatory demyelinating polyneuropathy (AIDP), by far the most common form in western countries; and (2) acute motor axonal neuropathy (AMAN), which is more prevalent in East Asia (China and Japan). AMAN is characterized by electrophysiologic and pathologic evidence of axonal degeneration of the motor nerves as well as functional conduction failure or other pathophysiology. It is possibly associated with anti-ganglioside antibodies; in particular, IgG antibodies to the gangliosides GM1, GM1b, GD1a and GalNAc-GD1a, which may be induced by particular infectious agents such as *Campylobacter jejuni* or *Haemophilus influenza*. Although AMAN appears to be similar to AIDP, there are important clinical differences. AMAN is a pure motor syndrome, with infrequent and mild involvement of the autonomic nervous system. When sensory fibres are also affected, this axonal subtype is called acute motor and sensory axonal neuropathy. Patients with AMAN often show hyperreflexia in the recovery phase. AMAN has a rapid progression in its early stage and has an earlier nadir than AIDP. AMAN has 2 patterns of clinical recovery, rapid and prolonged, in contrast to the relatively uniform recovery seen in AIDP. Electrophysiologic evidence of axonal degeneration is thought to be an indicator of poor prognosis. However, the most severely disabled AMAN patients are able to walk independently within a few years, indicating that electrodiagnosis of AMAN is not always a marker of poor recovery. This review provides an update on the clinical features, recovery pattern and long-term prognosis in AMAN patients.

Chapter 8 - Treatment of many autoimmune conditions was for a long period of time based on different preparations that decrease inflammation. Anticytokine therapy, which is a new chapter in immunotherapy, is one of the first pathogenetic approaches to the treatment of autoimmune conditions. Presently, it is clear that normal production of different cytokines in cells is a marker of normal homeostasis and good health. Any hyper-production caused by exogenous or endogenous cytokine inducers can lead to significant pathological changes. Disturbances of cytokine synthesis can affect different organ systems including immune, endocrine, neuro-psychiatric and others. My colleagues and I pioneered anticytokinotherapy in 1972 and 1974 (2). The use of anticytokinotherapy with specific modifications for different autoimmune diseases has had positive results in clinics around the world (more than 1 billion people suffer from autoimmune diseases worldwide).

Anticytokine therapy is currently at the very early stages of development. Most expect that it will be successful in the treatment of such autoimmune diseases as rejection of organ and tissue transplants, multiple sclerosis, schizophrenia, Parkinson's disease, and others. It is not excluded that disturbance of cytokine synthesis can be very important in pathogenesis of atherosclerosis. Removal of some hyperproductive cytokines and their receptors together with the use of antibodies to LDL will be a crucial factor in the treatment of atherosclerosis. According to the editorial of The New England Journal of Medicine (US) anticytokine therapy is a new era in the treatment of autoimmune diseases especially rheumatoid arthritis (44).

Chapter 9 – It was previously proposed that autoimmune diseases are hemopoietic stem cell (HSC) disorders (Proc. Natl. Acad. Sci. USA 87:8341-8344, 1990).

In this review article, evidence is provided that most age-associated diseases such as osteoporosis are mesenchymal stem cell (MSC) disorders and, based on this evidence, a new concept of "stem cell disorders" (SCDs) is proposed that includes HSC and MSC disorders.

To treat SCDs, a recent new strategy has been developed (intra-bone marrow-bone marrow transplantation: IBM-BMT) for replacing the abnormal stem cells of recipients with donor-derived normal stem cells (both HSCs and MSCs).

This strategy heralds a revolution in the field of transplantation (BMT and organ transplantation) and regeneration therapy.

Chapter 10 - Adult neurogenesis occurs only in discrete regions of adult central nervous system: the subventricular zone and the subgranular zone. These areas are populated by adult neural stem cells (**aNSC**) that are regulated by a number of molecules and signaling pathways, which control their cell fate choices, survival and proliferation rates. For a long time, it was believed that the immune system did not exert any control on neural proliferative niches. However, it has been observed that many pathological and inflammatory conditions significantly affect NSC niches. Even more, increasing evidence indicates that chemokines and cytokines play an important role in regulating proliferation, cell fate choices, migration and survival of NSCs under physiological conditions. Hence, the immune system is emerging is an important regulator of neurogenic niches in the adult brain, which may have clinical relevance in several brain diseases.

Chapter 11 - Temporomandibular joint disorder (TMD) is the most common cause of orofacial pain and has multifactorial etiologies. Commonly, temporomandibular joint (TMJ) is often a forgotten joint in rheumatologic evaluation, but well known affected in several diseases, including systemic lupus erythematosus (SLE). It is important for clinicians and rheumatologists to be able to recognize symptoms of TMD. TMD involvement may be secondary to systemic inflammation and arthritis or a clinical manifestation of an independent pathology, such as infections, degeneration and osteonecrosis. Since there are overlapping signs and symptoms, the diagnosis can be confusing. It is therefore important for clinicians and rheumatologists to be able to recognize symptoms of TMD. Imaging may help to establish diagnosis. Several imaging modalities are available, including X-rays, tomography and magnetic resonance imaging. Since TMD may lead to severe disabilities, early diagnosis, as well as timely and appropriate management is warranted.

In this chapter, most frequent TMD associated with SLE is described and provide an overview of the evaluation of the common TMJ in a simplified version that will help to identify the clinical findings and imaging patterns.

Chapter 12 - Fatigue is commonly reported by patients with Guillain-Barré syndrome (GBS), even long after the patients "recover" from the weakness and when no apparent weakness by brief muscle strength testing is present. Fatigue may be a major limiting factor for GBS survivors in social life. The causes for the fatigue are multifactorial, including dysfunction of central and peripheral nervous systems, including depression and other mental conditions. However, the objective analysis of fatigue in GBS may not be straightforward, since many patients with such condition show unremarkable results of conventional nerve conduction studies. The authors discuss little known concept of activity-dependent conduction block (ADCB), a conduction characterized by nerve conduction failure induced by high frequency nerve transmission as occurring in prolonged muscle contraction. The mechanism behind this is transient hyperpolarization of axon membrane by activation of Na^+-K^+-ATP pump, which is triggered by axonal depolarization when impulse transmission and influx of Na^+ occur. Neurophysiologic techniques to identify ADCB include recording of compound muscle action potentials (CMAP) serially before and after supramaximal voluntary muscle contraction. In ADCB there is temporary conduction block after muscle contraction, demonstrated as lower CMAP amplitudes, prolongation of CMAP durations, and lower conduction velocities. Better recognition of fatigue in GBS by appropriate tests and potential therapeutic intervention based on the pathophysiology is important.

Chapter 13 -Multiple sclerosis (MS) is a chronic neurological autoimmune disease that can affect vision. Visual complaints might be one of the first signs of MS and the ophthalmologist can be the first physician consulted, therefore familiarity with the pathology and appropriate diagnosis are of great importance. This pathology typically occurs in young people (mean age between 20 and 40 years) and the incidence is higher in women. The aetiopathology is still unknown, but seems to be multifactorial. The environment seems to play an important role and migration studies showed that people moving before age 15 have the same risk level as the native population of the nation they move in. Genetics has an important role too: the association with HLA-DR2 antigen is proved, and the association of

MS susceptibility with two or more genes is suspected. First degree family members of MS patients have approximately 10 times greater chance to develop the pathology compared to controls. Another etiological theory is that the infection of a virus in childhood might cause in genetically predisposed patients the activation of the immune system after years of latency. Demyelination of the optic nerve caused by the autoimmune attack leads to ganglion cell loss and subsequent nerve atrophy [1]. The tissue damage often involves the prechiasmatic visual pathways. With the progession of the disease, demyelination is associated with mononuclear cell infiltration and removal of myelin by macrophages. At the end stage of the pathology common findings are gliotic lesions ("plaques") that derive from astrocytic proliferation with production of glial fibrils.

Chapter 14 - The fast 'saltatory' conduction of nerve impulses is mandatory for vertebrates, and the normal functioning of the nervous system requires a coordinated interplay between neurons and glia. One specific region of intercellular interactions is the myelin sheath, a tightly packed multilayered membrane structure, which is formed around myelinated axons in both the central (CNS) and peripheral nervous systems (PNS). Defective myelin in inherited or autoimmune disease causes severe neurological disorders, affecting both CNS and PNS. In addition, axonal regeneration in the adult CNS after neuronal injury is limited by myelin proteins interacting with the axonal surface. Myelin contains a specific set of proteins, which have unique properties and interact closely with membranes; several of them are also implicated as autoantigens. When structural and functional data on these molecules are obtained, functions of myelin and the ways, explain a better understanding in which its deficiencies may lead to disease. In this chapter, the current knowledge about myelin protein 3-dimensional structure and the interactions of myelin proteins with their ligands will be discussed, with specific emphasis on the implications for understanding autoimmune diseases of the nervous system, such as multiple sclerosis and Guillain-Barré syndrome.

Chapter 15 - Multiple sclerosis (MS) is considered to be initiated by an autoimmune attack on myelin proteins by a mimic within a protein from some unidentified microorganism. Experimental allergic encephalomyelitis (EAE) is the model for MS. Different peptides from four myelin proteins are potent known EAE immunogens. The contribution of particular amino acids to encephalitogenicity within several immunogens and the minimum adjuvant requirements have been ascertained. Thus, the EAE initiation process at a molecular level is known. Using this EAE molecular information with known aspects of clinical MS, e.g. patient's age, variable histology, clinical immunological data, epidemiology, etc., the molecular initiation process of the autoimmune aspects of MS is defined. This definition includes: a.) type of organism providing the mimic, b.) estimation of single versus multiple immunogens, c.) location of the mimic, d.) involvement of adjuvant molecules and other inflammatory agents, e.) elucidation of magnetic resonance imaging (MRI) data, f.) dissection of confusing cellular immunology data, and g.) explanation of variable histological lesion locations. With this information various therapeutic options are discussed.

Chapter 16 - The majority of human autoimmune diseases have a complex aetiology with strong genetic and environmental components. The genetic component of disease susceptibility is generally highly polygenic, with multiple loci acting synergistically, and genetically heterogenous, with diverse sets of polymorphic loci capable of driving the same autoimmune reaction. The genetics of autoimmunity is further complicated by the division of genetic susceptibility into general autoimmune propensity polymorphisms and disease-specific polymorphisms. Despite the complexity of autoimmune genetics at the locus level, it appears that a limited number of conserved mechanistic pathways are affected by genetic polymorphisms. The conserved tolerance pathways subverted by autoimmune polymorphisms are being unravelled by the analysis of mouse models of autoimmunity. These models have identified three key fragile links in the T cell tolerance pathway - antigen presentation and the apoptotic response in the thymus, cis- and trans-acting peripheral suppression of autoreactive T cells, and the target organ response to autoimmunity.

Chapter 1

NATURAL CATALYTIC ANTIBODIES IN NORM AND IN AUTOIMMUNE DISEASES

G. A. Nevinsky[*]

Institute of Chemical Biology and Fundamental Medicine of Siberian Division of Russian Academy of Sciences, Novosibirsk, 630090, prosp. M.A. Larentieva, 8, Russia

In patients with autoimmune (AI) diseases autoantibodies (Abs) directed to polysaccharides, nucleic acids, proteins, peptides, nucleoprotein complexes, and enzymes with different catalytic functions may be induced spontaneously by primary antigens and can have characteristics of the primary antigen, including the catalytic activity of idiotypic and/or antiidiotypic Abs. The discovery of IgG specifically hydrolyzing intestinal vasoactive peptide in the sera of asthma patients (Paul S., 1989) stimulated of the studies of natural catalytic antibodies (abzymes). Detection of abzymes (Abzs) was shown to be the earliest indicator of development of different autoimmune diseases (AD). At the early stages of ADs, the repertoire of Abzs is usually relatively small but it greatly increases with the progress of the disease, leading to the generation of catalytically diverse abzymes with different activities and functions. Some Abzs are cytotoxic and can play an important negative role in the pathogenesis of AI pathologies, while positive roles have been proposed for other abzymes.

During the spontaneous development of profound SLE-like pathology in mice, a specific reorganization of the immune system leads to conditions associated with production of Abzs with low catalytic activities (conditionally pre-diseased mice). A significant increase in the relative Abz activities associated with a transition from pre-diseased to diseased mice is correlated with additional changes in the differentiation and proliferation of bone marrow hematopoietic stem cells and lymphocyte proliferation in different organs. Different mechanisms of Abzs production are observed for healthy mice immunized externally and for autoimmune mice during the spontaneous development of pathology.

In this chapter, new data concerning Abzs with different catalytic activities in various ADs, possible reasons of their catalytic heterogeneity, possible roles of abzymes and their

---

[*] Corresponsing autor: Tel.: 007-3832-356226, Fax: 007-3832-333677, E-mail: nevinsky@niboch.nsc.ru

exceptional multiplicity in the pathogenesis of different ADs, and possible uses of the abzyme activity for diagnostic of AI diseases are discussed.

1. INTRODUCTION

Classically, antibodies (Abs) have been characterized as proteins produced by the immune system, which have the sole function of binding other molecules, called antigens, with the goal of eliciting an immune response. In this classical concept, Abs function similarly to enzymes in specifically binding other molecules, but are distinct from enzymes in that they do not have the ability to catalyze chemical conversions of the bound molecules. For the vast majority of Abs, this observation is correct. In 1946, Linus Pauling noted similarities between the mechanisms of antibody-antigen recognition and the interaction of transition states of catalytic reactions with enzymes and suggested a principal possibility of the induction of catalytic Abs [1]. This idea led Jencks in 1969 to observe that Abs generated in an anti-hapten immune response have their binding site configuration determined by the choice of hapten, therefore, Ab-derived enzymes could potentially be produced by making Abs against a chemically stable analog of the transition state of a reaction of interest [2].

In 1985, a general method for generating catalytic monoclonal Abzs against transition state analogs, and a way to use those Abs to accelerate chemical reactions, was first described [3]. One year later, two groups were able to produce the first monoclonal Abs with catalytic properties, which were generated against hapten analogs of the transition states for p-nitrophenylphosphorylcholine [4] or for monoaryl phosphonate esters [5, 6].

These catalytic Abs were termed abzymes (derived from antibody enzyme) [7-16]. The first example of a natural Abz was an IgG found in bronchial asthma patients, which hydrolyzes intestinal vasoactive peptide (VIP) [17], the second was an IgG with DNase activity in SLE [18], and the third was an IgG with RNase activity in SLE [19]. Later, different natural catalytic IgG and/or IgA, IgM hydrolyzing DNA, RNA, nucleotides, and polysaccharides were detected in the sera of patients with several autoimmune (AI) and viral pathologies, and Abzs with these and other different activities were discovered in healthy human milk (for review see [20-27]). AI and viral diseases were also found to stimulate production of IgG and/or IgM and IgA abzymes hydrolyzing different peptides and proteins, such as thymoglobulin (Hashimoto's thyroiditis and rheumatoid arthritis) [28], prothrombin (multiple myeloma) [29], protein factor VIII (hemophilia A) [30], basic myelin protein (multiple sclerosis) [31-33], viral reverse transcriptase and integrase (HIV-infected patients) [34-35].

In this chapter, for simplicity and in order to distinguish natural catalytic Abs from those against transition-state analogs, the latter will be termed "artificial abzymes". Artificial Abzs against transition states of reactions catalyzing more than 100 distinct chemical reactions are novel biological catalysts that attracted much interest in the past years (for review see [7-16]). Some artificial Abzs have been described that require cofactors for activity, similar to canonical enzymes [36]. The field of artificial Abzs has been amply reviewed (see [7-16] and refs therein for more detailed description of the relevant reactions).

The evolution of the technology of artificial Abzs during the past two decades has led not only to the rapid development of direct approaches for the generation of Abs with specified properties, but also to the creation of strategies to revise the targeting specificity of individual Abzs ([11, 16, 37-41] and references therein). Such modifications of antigen binding specificity can be achieved genetically *in vitro*, by application of the site-directed mutagenesis, or genetic selection or screening (using approaches such as phage display outlined below). Alternatively, modification can be induced directly in purified antibodies *via* selective chemical modification by direct introduction of catalytic groups into the antigen-binding site. The employment of these approaches have demonstrated that the substrate specificity (and/or the specific activity) of some artificial Abzs is comparable to or even higher than that of enzymes with the same catalytic activity [42-44]. The mechanistic basis for the activity of such Abzs is presently well understood [16, 45].

Abz-mediated catalysis is usually characterized by relatively low reaction rates and it is therefore important to prove that catalytic activities are not due to contaminating enzymes, but there are few studies concerning human monoclonal Abs. In contrast, natural Abzs from the sera of patients with different AI diseases are usually polyclonal in origin and are products of different immuno-competent cells ([22-27] and refs therein). Their purification is one of the most complicated aspects of natural polyclonal Abzs studies. Different methods of purification of electrophoretically and immunologically homogeneous natural polyclonal Abzs were developed and discussed in detail earlier in several reviews [23-27].

The second problem in the studies of natural Abzs is providing strong evidence that the enzymatic activity is an intrinsic property of Abs derived from sera of diseased humans and animals and is not due to traces of copurifying enzymes. The first natural Abz was reported in the mid-60s when Slobin [46] demonstrated the hydrolysis of p-nitrophenyl acetate by an IgG; Kullberg et al. [47] found proteolytic activity in highly purified rabbit Abs. But although these Abs were isolated by affinity chromatography on an antigen sorbent, the authors could not exclude that the catalytic activity was due to contaminating enzymes. In 1989, the application of several strict criteria allowed Paul et al. [17] to conclude that the VIP-hydrolyzing activity is an intrinsic property of IgGs from the sera of asthma patients. The most important of these criteria are: **1**, electrophoretic homogeneity of the IgG as visualized by silver staining; **2**, catalytic activity of the F(ab) fragments of the Ab; **3**, complete adsorption of the activity on anti-IgG Sepharose and its elution with a low-pH buffer; **4**, precipitation of the activity by anti-IgG Abs; **5**, presence of the activity only in IgG of patients with asthma and not in healthy donors; **6**, retention of the activity upon gel-filtration of IgG under the conditions of "acid shock" and co-elution of the activity exactly with 150-kDa IgG; **7**, the K_M value for hydrolysis of VIP (38 nM) suggesting high affinity for the substrate comparable to the K_d of antigen-Ab complexes; and **8**, differences between the substrate specificity of VIP hydrolysis by Abs and other known proteases [17].

This finding has strongly stimulated studies of natural Abzs in AI diseases and led to development of several additional criteria to the above list, including: **9**, thermal stability of Abs as compared with canonical enzymes; **10**, affinity modification of different Abz by chemically reactive analogs of substrates; **11**, analysis of the activity of isolated L- and H-subunits of Igs after their separation by affinity chromatography under mild dissociating conditions; **12**, detection of catalytic activity of Ab, its F(ab) fragments, and isolated L- and H-subunits *in situ* after SDS-PAGE under non-reducing or reducing conditions in a gel containing its substrate (RNA, DNA, ATP, proteins, etc.), and some other useful criteria. All these criteria have been discussed in details in several reviews [23-27].

The development of new modern techniques of purification, analysis, and characterization of natural catalytic Abzs led to a new view of possible biological roles of this subset of Abs in the development and pathogenesis of some AI diseases and pathologies caused by different viral and bacterial infections ([23-27, 30-35, 48-49]. The phenomenon of catalysis by auto-Abzs is extremely interesting and potentially applicable in many different fields including new types of efficient catalysts, new generation of drugs, and evaluation of the functional roles of Abzs in innate and adaptive immunity, and understanding of certain aspects of self-tolerance and of the destructive or positive responses in AI diseases. Some aspects concerning different natural Abzs covered in several earlier reviews include the theory of proteolytic Ab occurrence and mechanism and functional role of protease Ab catalysis [50-52], potential therapeutic application of Abzs [53-59], prothrombin-cleaving Ab [60], catalytic Abs to amyloid beta peptide [61, 62], Abs with hydrolytic activity towards factor VIII [63-67], Abs destroying H. pylori urease [68], Ab-catalyzed water oxidation [69], and cytotoxic effects of DNA-hydrolyzing Abs [70].

In this chapter we collate the data concerning the features of the immune status of patients with various AI diseases, the origin of auto-Abs and natural Abzs, association of different auto-Abs and Abzs formation with changes in the differentiation and proliferation of bone marrow hematopoietic stem cells, possible reasons of extreme diversity of AI Abzs and increase in repertoire of Abzs with development of pronounced AI pathologies, and differences between Abzs from healthy donors and AI patients. In addition, a possible nature and biological role of natural abzymes and some major current themes are discussed as well as potential applications of natural Abzs in scientific, medical and biotechnological fields.

2. FEATURES OF THE IMMUNE STATUS OF PATIENTS WITH VARIOUS AUTOIMMUNE DISEASES

A special feature of ADs is high concentrations of auto-Abs (Abs to many different endogenous antigens) [71, 72]. The development of ADs is characterized by spontaneous generation of primary Abs to proteins, nucleic acids and their complexes, polysaccharides, nucleotides etc. [73-75]. Later the secondary idiotypic and then antiidiotypic Abs to the primary ones are usually generated, etc. Immunization of animals with DNA or RNA and especially their complexes with proteins leads to the production of anti-DNA and anti-RNA Abs [76-79]. Interestingly, the titers of anti-DNA Abs are detectable even in the sera of healthy mammals but there they are low and highly variable [80, 81].

SLE is a systemic AI polyetiologic diffuse disease that is characterized by disorganization of conjunctive tissues with the paramount damage to skin and visceral capillaries [82]. Autoimmune and complex immunologic processes determined by genetic predisposition to an immunoregulation disturbance are important in the pathogenesis of SLE [83]. The polyetiologic and polysyndromic character of SLE shows itself in highly variable manifestations of this disease in terms of the biochemical, immunological, and clinical indices. SLE is usually considered to be related to patient's autoimmunization with DNA, since the sera of such patients usually contain DNA and anti-DNA Abs in high concentrations [72]. The association of damage with auto-Ab profile, age, ethnic origin, sex and disease duration in SLE was studied [84]. It was shown that the development of the disease with age and duration of pathology correlates with Abs against several nuclear antigens, and statistically significant associations were found between the level of anti-Ro Abs and ocular damage and between Abs to nuclear antigens Scl-70 and/or Jo-1 and premature gonadal failure [85]. For 87 Chinese patients with SLE, a positive correlation of Abs to cardiolipin with the severity of the disease and a negative correlation of Abs to cardiolipin with the concentration of C3 complement was shown [85]. In addition, an increase of the titers of IgAs to cardiolipin in SLE patients with thrombosis and titers of IgGs and IgMs to cardiolipin in patients with damage to the central nervous system in comparison with SLE patients without these indices was found.

More than 70 different indices (clinical, biochemical, immunological, analysis of blood cells, etc.) are used in clinical practice for diagnosis and description of SLE development. Recently, the relative titers of auto-Abs to different antigen in the serum blood of 48 SLE patients were analyzed [86]. Most of these SLE patients were characterized by moderate and serious status of disease with definite signs of active nephritis, vasculitis of the central nervous system, lung damage (more often with syndrome of lung hypertension, carditis, and antiphospholipid syndrome in combination with hematological dysfunction). The indices characterizing the immune system of the SLE patients of this group usually demonstrate relative and/or absolute lymphopenia, a relative decrease in differentiated CD3+ T-cells, the ratio of CD4+/CD8+ T-cells, and the relative amount of CD20+ B-cells, as well as an increase in the relative concentration of IgGs, circulating immune complexes, and auto-Abs to native DNA, cardiolipin, microsomal fraction of thyrocytes (MFT), and thyroglobulin [86].

As mentioned above, one of the most prominent indices of SLE patients is an increased titer of Abs to native DNA [23, 72]. In one study, an increased concentration of Abs to DNA in comparison with healthy donors was observed for 29 out of 48 SLE patients [86]. At the same time, it is known that in the active stage of SLE, anti-DNA Abs are increased in 90–99% of SLE patients [87].

Antiphospholipid syndrome associated with an increased concentration of Abs to cardiolipin is a typical attribute of several AI diseases including SLE [88]. In the same group of 48 SLE patients mentioned above, 23 individuals demonstrated increased concentrations of Abs to cardiolipin [86].

Small amounts of auto-Abs to thyroglobulin can usually be detected in the sera of healthy donors. An increase in titers of auto-Abs to thyroglobulin is usually associated with a dysfunction of the thyroid, especially in patients with Hashimoto's thyroiditis [89]. However, an increase in the concentration of anti-thyroglobulin Abs is also often observed for patients with other AI diseases including SLE [89]. In the analyzed group of 48 SLE patients, an increased level of anti-thyroglobulin Abs was observed for 20 patients [86].

A wide repertoire of auto-Abs in SLE patients may result from polyclonal activation of B cells as a consequence of damage to many different organs that reflects polyetiologic, polysyndromic, and multisystemic character of this disease. The increase in the concentration of Abs to MFT most probably can be considered a typical index of many AI diseases including SLE [90]. The blood of 23 out of 48 SLE patients contained Abs to MFT at increased concentrations [86].

The rheumatoid factor is usually indicative of auto-Abs to antigenic determinants of Fc fragments of all types of immunoglobulins (IgM, IgG, IgA, and IgE). Rheumatoid factor (RF) is usually used as a diagnostic criterion for rheumatoid arthritis, but it is not strictly specific for this pathology and can be revealed in many systemic AI diseases and in some infections.

The frequency of RF in SLE varies from 15% to 35% of patients [87]. Abs to RF was revealed for 11 out of 48 analyzed SLE patients [86].

Statistically significant correlation coefficients were observed between the following pairs of auto-Abs: Abs to cardiolipin and to thyroglobulin ($r = 0.37$); cardiolipin and MFT (0.39); thyroglobulin and MFT (0.77) [86]. Titers of Abs to native DNA negatively correlate with titers of IgA (-0.39), while titers of Abs to cardiolipin positively correlate (0.39) with titers of IgMs. Some of these data are summarized in Table 1.

The titers of Abs to DNA correlate with the following parameters: urea concentration ($r = 0.69$), alkaline phosphatase (0.76), creatinine (0.83 for biochemical analysis and 0.71 for Ruberg's test), and uric acid in blood (0.50) [86]. A statistically significant negative correlation was observed between titers of Abs to DNA and the concentration of Ca^{2+} ions in blood ($r = -0.5$). Concentration of Abs to MFT positively correlates with general Fe-binding ability of blood serum ($r = 0.39$). Abs to cardiolipin demonstrated a negative correlation with the concentration of bilirubin ($r = -0.41$), while titers of Abs to thyroglobulin and to rheumatoid factor showed no significant correlation with any of the biochemical characteristics of urine or blood. Some of the reported data are summarized in Table 2.

Table 1. Coefficients of correlation (r) between titers of Abs to DNA, cardiolipin (CL), thyroglobulin (TG) microsomal fractions of thyrocytes (MFT) and rheumatoid factor (RF) in the group of 48 SLE patients and in subgroups obtaining by cluster fragmentation[*] [86]

Abs to	Number of patients	Correlation coefficient				
		DNA	CL	TG	MFT	RF
Abs to CL						
Whole group[**]	48	0.18	1.00	**0.37**[†]	**0.39**	-0.01
Subgroup 1	12	-0.14	1.00	-0.06	-0.30	-0.06
Subgroup 2	16	0.31	1.00	**0.60**	**0.79**	0.03
Abs to TG						
Whole group	45	0.06	**0.37**	1.00	**0.77**	0.00
Subgroup 1	12	0.34	-0.06	1.00	0.29	0.22
Subgroup 2	16	0.26	**0.60**	1.00	**0.93**	-0.22
Abs to MFT						
Whole group	45	0.05	**0.39**	**0.77**	1.00	0.01
Subgroup 1	12	0.29	-0.30	0.29	1.00	-0.47
Subgroup 2	16	0.29	**0.79**	**0.93**	1.00	-0.21

[*]Only the biochemical parameters that demonstrated at least one statistically significant r ($p < 0.05$) are included. Titers of Abs to rheumatoid factor showed no statistically significant r values with other parameters.

[**]Two subgroups containing 12 and 16 patients were defined by cluster analysis, while the remaining 20 individuals did not form clusters with comparable characteristics.

[†]Statistically significant r values are given in boldface.

Table 2. Coefficients of correlation (r) between titers of auto-Abs and some biochemical indexes in the group of 48 SLE patients and in subgroups obtaining by cluster fragmentation*[86]

Biochemical characteristics	Number of patients	General protein	Sorbitol dehydrogenase	Urea	Creatinine	Bilirubin	Aspartate aminotransferase	Alkaline phosphatase	Ca^{2+}	Fe-binding ability	General Fe-binding capacity of the blood serum	Fibrinogen	Uric acid
Abs to DNA**													
Whole group	48	-0.22	-0.08	**0.69**†	**0.83**	-0.14	-0.09	**0.76**	**-0.50**	-0.33	-0.16	0.12	**0.52**
1st subgroup	12	-0.32	-0.27	-0.02	0.07	0.24	**-0.73**	**-0.64**	-0.59	0.10	0.18	0.01	-0.17
2nd subgroup	16	0.36	-0.23	0.39	0.18	0.28	-0.13	0.17	**-0.75**	0.13	0.04	0.27	0.52
Abs to CL													
Whole group	48	0.25	-0.01	-0.13	-0.15	**-0.41**	0.01	0.11	-0.29	0.22	0.26	-0.01	-0.30
1st subgroup	12	0.13	-0.04	-0.05	**-0.78**	0.07	0.08	0.18	-0.02	-0.08	-0.41	-0.25	-0.67
2nd subgroup	16	-0.20	**-0.76**	0.07	0.08	0.16	-0.02	-0.04	-0.70	0.33	**0.80**	-0.29	-0.20
Abs to TG													
Whole group	48	0.12	0.06	-0.31	-0.19	-0.06	0.04	-0.08	-0.16	-0.05	0.37	0.09	-0.06
1st subgroup	12	-0.07	-0.30	0.18	0.47	0.45	-0.61	-0.05	0.10	**-0.68**	0.46	-0.48	-0.21
2nd subgroup	16	-0.60	0.29	-0.55	-0.29	0.38	0.57	-0.12	-0.14	0.05	-0.11	0.12	0.34
Abs to MFT													
Whole group	48	**0.41**	-0.19	-0.20	-0.28	-0.10	-0.10	-0.24	0.03	0.09	**0.39**	-0.26	-0.21
1st subgroup	12	-0.35	**-0.67**	0.38	0.00	0.00	**-0.72**	-0.18	-0.21	-0.47	-0.05	**-0.66**	-0.50
2nd subgroup	16	-0.28	0.43	**-0.93**	**-0.87**	-0.08	-0.11	0.35	-0.09	0.02	0.29	0.36	0.13
Abs to RF													
Whole group	48	0.10	-0.06	-0.16	-0.17	0.12	-0.08	-0.19	-0.03	0.07	0.08	-0.18	-0.14
1st subgroup	12	0.08	-0.17	-0.07	-0.56	0.41	-0.36	0.16	-0.17	-0.39	0.11	-0.41	0.63
2nd subgroup	16	0.42	**1.00**	-0.17	-0.56	-0.30	-0.25	0.25	0.34	-0.62	-0.53	**0.82**	0.03

*Only the biochemical parameters that demonstrated at least one statistically significant r ($p < 0.05$) are included.
**Two subgroups containing 12 and 16 patients were defined by cluster analysis, while the remaining 20 individuals did not form clusters with comparable characteristics.
†Statistically significant r values are given in boldface.

Statistically significant correlations of the titers of Abs to DNA were observed with such blood cell count characteristics in SLE as reticulocytes ($r = 0.5$) and stab neutrophils ($r = 0.46$) [86]. Concentration of Abs to thyroglobulin correlates positively with platelets ($r = +0.4$) and a negative correlation was observed between Abs to MFT and reticulocytes ($r = -0.31$). Some of these data are summarized in Table 3.

Most probably, widening of the repertoire of different auto-Abs in patients with various AI diseases can serve as a specific index of the progress of AI disease. In the group of 48 SLE patients, a simultaneous increase in the titers of Abs to all five above-mentioned antigens (AGs) was observed in 2 individuals, while 9 patients showed an increase in Abs to four AGs, 9, to three AGs, and 10, to two AGs. Six patients demonstrated the concentrations of all five types of auto-Abs comparable with those for healthy donors and blood of the remaining 12 patients contained auto-Abs of only one type [86]. These data indicate that the analyzed group of SLE patients was very heterogeneous with respect to the depth and direction of immune status disturbance. For 48 patients, we have determined 70 different indices used as indicators of SLE development. Analysis of correlation of titers of different auto-Abs with these clinical, biochemical, immunological, and blood cell characteristics may help to find specific relationships between AI reactions in SLE patients and other factors characterizing this pathology.

The titers of five types of auto-Abs were extremely variable in the group of 48 SLE patients (Tables 1-3) [86]. Taking into account different levels of disturbance of immune system in these individuals, the multifactor character of this pathology and possibility of damage to different organs in each patient, we have divided this group into subgroups with similar clinical manifestations using cluster analysis software. The cluster analysis of all auto-Abs data allowed us to define two subgroups containing 12 and 16 patients, while the remaining 20 individuals did not form groups with comparable characteristics. Interestingly, the division of the patients into subgroups led to an increase in statistically significant correlation coefficients in the subgroup of 16 patients for the same Abs pairs that were revealed during the initial analysis of the whole group of 48 patients [86]. The correlation coefficients increased as follows: Abs to cardiolipin and to thyroglobulin ($0.37 \rightarrow 0.6$); Abs to cardiolipin and to MFT ($0.39 \rightarrow 0.79$), Abs to thyroglobulin and to MFT ($0.77 \rightarrow 0.93$) (Table 1). Correlation coefficients for anti-DNA Abs with other auto-Abs also increased in both subgroups but did not become statistically significant. A similar situation was observed for Abs to rheumatoid factor and Abs to other antigens. Interestingly, some of the correlation coefficients in the subgroups of 12 and 16 patients were of the opposite sign, while there were no statistically significant correlations at all in the remaining 20 patients (Table 1). After the subdivision of the group, an increase in the absolute values of r for correlation of auto-Abs with biochemical and blood count characteristics (see above) in different subgroups was observed, but whereas some indices demonstrated positive correlation in one group, they showed negative correlation in another group (Tables 2-3) [86]. Therefore, it is not surprising that there are no strictly consistent dependences or high correlation coefficients between different indices for the complete group of 48 patients.

Table 3. Coefficients of correlation (r) between titers of auto-Abs and some biochemical and cell indexes in the group of 48 SLE patients and in subgroups obtaining by cluster fragmentation[*] [46]

Indexes of blood cells and hemoglobin		Erythrocytes	Hemoglobin	Color index	Reticulocytes	Platelets	Eosinophils	Stab neutrophils
Abs to DNA								
Whole group[**]	48	-0.26	-0.22	0.06	**0.50**[†]	-0.25	-0.05	**0.46**
1st subgroup	16	0.42	0.45	-0.07	0.15	0.28	-0.14	-0.25
2nd subgroup	20	-0.16	0.26	0.31	-0.23	**0.53**	0.31	-0.35
Abs to CL								
Whole group	48	0.19	0.06	-0.15	0.03	0.15	0.04	-0.03
1st subgroup	16	0.22	0.22	-0.03	0.12	0.42	-0.09	-0.30
2nd subgroup	20	0.14	-0.03	-0.12	-0.28	**0.55**	0.26	0.02
Abs to TG								
Whole group	48	0.11	0.08	-0.06	-0.29	**0.40**	0.26	-0.03
1st subgroup	16	-0.21	-0.46	-0.23	-0.48	0.43	0.09	-0.17
2nd subgroup	20	-0.04	0.28	0.25	-0.20	**0.48**	0.38	-0.26
Abs to MFT								
Whole group	46	0.24	0.12	-0.16	**-0.31**	0.27	0.28	-0.17
1st subgroup	16	-0.08	-0.32	-0.25	-0.47	0.39	-0.04	-0.25
2nd subgroup	20	0.20	0.29	0.07	-0.28	0.23	**0.49**	-0.41
Abs to RF								
Whole group	46	0.15	0.15	-0.05	-0.10	-0.04	-0.07	-0.08
1st subgroup	16	**0.52**	0.32	-0.29	-0.18	0.27	-0.09	-0.09
2nd subgroup	20	-0.05	**-0.59**	**-0.50**	0.43	-0.14	0.21	0.00

[*]Only the blood parameters that demonstrated at least one statistically significant r ($p < 0.05$) are included.
[**]Two subgroups containing 16 and 20 patients were defined by cluster analysis, while the remaining 12 individuals did not form clusters with comparable characteristics.
[†]Statistically significant r values are given in boldface.

Overall, the discussed data indicate a complicated mosaic association of the investigated parameters in different subgroups of SLE patients [86]. It should be kept in mind that SLE patients may diverge in the primary cause of pathology development, which can include exposure to a number of chemically active compounds or components of various viruses that can lead to damage of immune system. In each SLE patients, a transient error of the immune system may result from different genetic factors and/or specific environmental challenges. Consequently, SLE pathology in an individual can be characterized by a particular status of his or her immune system, and specific combinations of chronic, viral, inflammatory, AI factors, etc. [86]. Taking this into account, it is obvious that understanding of the relationships between changes in the immunity parameters and clinical, biochemical, immunological and other indices in SLE will require a detailed analysis and integration of all these parameters during the full course of disease development for many individuals.

Compared with healthy donors, concentrations of DNA and anti-DNA Abs are higher not only in patients with SLE (36% of SLE patients), but also in multiple sclerosis (17-18%), primary Sjogren's syndrome (18%), Hashimoto's thyroiditis (23%), myasthenia gravis (6%), rheumatoid arthritis (7%) [80], autoimmune hepatitis [91], and also in lymphoproliferative [92] and some viral diseases (e.g., viral hepatitis and AIDS) [93]. Although viral diseases like AIDS and viral hepatitis are not related to ADs, they significantly disturb the immune status of the patients. For example, the development of both viral hepatitis [94] and AIDS [93, 95] as in the case of many ADs, is accompanied by humoral and cellular AI reactions, with detectable tissue-specific and organ-nonspecific Abs.

Many SLE anti-DNA Abs are directed against histone-DNA nucleosomal complexes appearing as a result of internucleosomal cleavage during apoptosis [96]. Apoptotic cells are the primary source of antigens and immunogens in SLE, and certain features in recognition, processing, and/or presentation of apoptotic auto-antigens by antigen-presenting cells can trigger AI processes [96].

In the sera of patients with several diseases, RNA and anti-RNA Abs were also detected [97-100]. Anti-RNA Abs were revealed in 9.4% patients with SLE by an enzyme-linked immunosorbent assay but other AI rheumatic diseases were not associated with these Abs [98]. Abs were analyzed in the sera of 120 patients with AI diseases by the ribonuclease protection assay using six fragments covering 28S ribosomal RNA as probes [98]. Fifteen of 90 sera from patients with SLE, but none of 30 sera of the other AI diseases, contained a 60-nucleotide fragment corresponding to 28S rRNA. Several unique RNA sequences were also obtained from the random RNA library; the sera of patients with Sjogren's syndrome (52.5%), SLE (19.5%), and rheumatoid arthritis (12.0%) contained TS1-RNA [99]. It has been suggested that anti-TS1-RNA is a novel Ab against sequence-specific RNA in many patients with Sjogren's syndrome. Anti-TS1-RNA antibodies were found in 31.7% of patients with mixed connective tissue disease, the occurrence significantly higher than in SLE [100]. Anti-DNA Abs, antihistone antibodies, anti-RNA-protein complexes and other antinuclear antibodies were revealed in the sera of patients with multisystem connective tissue disease [101].

Multiple sclerosis (MS) is a chronic demyelinating disease of the central nervous system. Its etiology remains unclear, and the most widely accepted theory of MS pathogenesis assigns the main role in the destruction of myelin to the inflammation related to AI reactions [102]. Evidence supports activated CD4+ myelin-reactive T cells as major mediators of MS. Several recent findings imply an important role of B cells and auto-Abs against myelin autoantigens in the pathogenesis of MS [102-104]. Current evidence from animal models and clinical studies suggests that a crucial role in MS immunopathogenesis belongs to auto-Abs against myelin autoantigens which are involved in Ab-mediated demyelination [104], and to auto-Abs against oligodendrocyte progenitor cell surface protein, which could block remyelination by eliminating or impeding these cells [105]. An important dual role of auto-Abs is suggested: they may be harmful in lesion formation but also potentially beneficial in the repair [103]. It is appropriate to mention here that the main targets of both above-mentioned auto-Abs are glycoproteins: myelin oligodendrocyte glycoprotein that is expressed preferentially on the outermost surface of the myelin sheath [106] and progenitor cell-specific surface glycoprotein AN2 [105], respectively. As far as we know, the possibility that carbohydrate groups of those glycoproteins participate in epitope formation have not been investigated yet. Elevated Abs levels and oligoclonal IgG bands in the cerebrospinal fluid (CSF) as well as clonal B cell accumulation in the CSF and lesions of MS patients are among the main lines of evidence of humoral response involvement in demyelination [107].

As in other ADs, poly-specific DNA-binding Abs have also been detected in MS patients [80]. New keys for understanding MS pathogenesis have appeared after cloning the IgG repertoire directly from active plaques and periplaque regions in MS brain and from B-cells recovered from the cerebrospinal fluid of a patient with MS with subacute disease [108]. It was found that high-affinity anti-DNA Abs were a major component of the intrathecal IgG response in the MS patients. Furthermore, DNA-specific monoclonal Abs derived from two individuals with MS as well as a DNA-specific Ab derived from an SLE patient bound efficiently to the surface of neuronal cells and oligodendrocytes. For these Abs, cell-surface recognition was DNA-dependent. The findings indicate that anti-DNA Abs may promote important neuropathologic mechanisms in chronic inflammatory disorders, such as MS and SLE [108].

Relative levels of auto-Abs to native (nat) and denatured (den) DNA in the blood of 49 MS patients and healthy donors were recently compared [109, 110]. The levels of anti-nat-DNA and anti-den-DNA Abs in 18% and 53% of the patients, respectively, were significantly higher than in controls. In contrast to anti-den-DNA Abs for MS and SLE, the level of Abs to nat-DNA in SLE is statistically significantly higher than in MS, with the exception of patients with secondary chronic-progressive type of MS, for which these levels are comparable. The titers of Abs to den-DNA in MS patients are usually higher than to nat-DNA. The coefficients of correlation between titers of Abs to nat-DNA and den-DNA for a complete group (0.88) and its subgroups with remission (0.81), primary progressing (0.88), and secondary chronic-progressive (0.89) state of the disease were estimated [109, 110]. An analysis of correlation between titers of Abs to DNA and 13 different standard clinical parameters including Poser criteria [111] was carried out [109, 110]. For the whole group of MS patients, the absolute values of positive and negative correlation coefficients between titers of anti-DNA Abs and clinical parameters were low (between -0.08 and 0.18), but they significantly increased for three subgroups with remission, primary progressing and secondary chronic-progressive state of this disease (Table 4). Separation of these three subgroups to additional sub-subgroups led to an increase in the statistically significant coefficients of correlations (Table 4) [109-110].

Table 4. Coefficients of correlation (r) between Abs to DNA in the blood of 49 MS patients and in subgroups with remitting (RC), primary progressive (PPC), and secondary progressive course (SPC) of the pathology [109-110]

Number of groups and subgroups	Number of NS patients	Age, years	Age at the onset of MS, years	Duration of disease, years	EDSS**	Rate of progression	fs 1	fs 2	fs 3	fs 4	fs 5	fs 6	fs 7	Sum of indexes
		1	2	3	4	5	6	7	8	9	10	11	12	13
Antibodies to native double-stranded DNA														
Compl.group	49	0.00	-0.05	0.10	0.13	0.03	0.15	-0.08	-0.06	0.09	0.18	0.18	0.01	0.11
RC	16	0.11	-0.09	**0.43***	0.25	**-0.44**	0.18	0.35	**0.52**	0.04	**0.64**	-0.01	-0.38	**0.48**
PPC	7	**-0.89**	-0.62	**-0.65**	**-0.49**	0.34	-0.46	-0.26	**-0.60**	0.45	-0.38	-0.11	**-0.76**	**-0.71**
SPC	26	-0.06	-0.02	-0.08	0.01	0.14	0.16	-0.32	-0.33	-0.02	-0.05	0.23	0.11	-0.06
Antibodies to denatured single-stranded DNA														
Compl.group	49	0.00	0.00	0.04	0.12	0.01	0.11	-0.08	-0.05	-0.06	0.18	0.15	-0.04	0.06
RC	16	-0.06	-0.19	0.19	-0.07	-0.40	-0.02	0.16	**0.36**	-0.19	**0.53**	0.12	**-0.41**	**0.24**
PPC	7	**-0.68**	**-0.56**	-0.37	-0.10	0.12	-0.03	-0.05	**-0.53**	0.46	**-0.35**	-0.06	**-0.63**	-0.37
SPC	26	-0.02	0.11	-0.13	0.06	0.15	0.07	-0.28	-0.26	-0.16	-0.01	0.16	0.04	-0.11

*Statistically significant r values ($p < 0.05$) are given in boldface.

§Sub-subgroups RC-1, RC-9, and RC-13 correspond to division of the remitting course subgroup into sub-subgroups in accordance with the similarity of parameters 1, 9, and 13, respectively.

**EDSS, a standard evaluation according to expanded scale of disablement.

†FS indexes, an evaluation of damage to functional systems: fs1, pyramidal functions; fs2, cerebellar functions; fs3, functions of brain stem; fs4, sensitive functions; fs5, functions of intestines and urinary bladder; fs6, visual functions; fs7, cerebral (psychical) functions. Sum of indexes includes all characteristics from fs1 to fs7. More detailed statistical analysis is given in [109-110].

Table 5. Coefficients of correlation (*r*) between the standard Poser clinical parameters and titers of Abs to MBP in the blood of 49 MS patients and in subgroups with remitting (RC), primary progressive (PPC), and secondary progressive course (SPC) of the pathology, as well as some correlation coefficients corresponding to subgroups or sub-subgroups after cluster fragmentation of the initial group and subgroups [112]

Number of groups and subgroups	Number of MS patients	Age, years	Age at the onset of MS, years	Duration of disease, years	EDSS**	Rate of progression	FS† fs 1	fs 2	fs 3	fs 4	fs 5	fs 6	fs 7	Sum of indexes
						Number of analyzed parameter								
	1	2	3	4	5	6	7	8	9	10	11	12	13	
Whole group	49	-0.23	-0.30	-0.04	0.05	0.20	0.19	0.08	-0.45	-0.11	-0.18	0.01	-0.28	-0.23
RC	16	0.41	0.55	0.21	-0.25	-0.17	-0.41	-0.06	0.24	-0.47	-0.21	-0.28	0.44	-0.21
PPC	7	0.03	-0.07	0.11	-0.09	-0.11	0.04	0.16	0.27	0.27	0.10	-0.10	0.05	0.21
SPC	26	-0.03	-0.06	0.03	-0.04	0.00	0.01	0.13	0.05	0.09	-0.02	-0.07	0.03	0.03
RC-1§	11	**-0.63***	**-0.63**	-0,14	-0.12	0.20	-0.30	0.08	-0.29	0.23	0.03	0	-0.31	-0.18
RC-9	9	-0.44	-0.58	0.06	0.00	-0.12	0.58	-0.03	-0.09	**-0.90**	0.00	0.08	**-0.74**	-0.26
RC-13	10	**-0.69**	**-0.71**	-0.48	-0.46	0.20	-0.14	-0.25	-0.54	-0.30	-0.41	0.02	-0.49	**-0.84**

*Statistically significant *r* values (*p* < 0.05) are given in boldface.
§Sub-subgroups RC-1, RC-9, and RC-13 correspond to division of the remitting course subgroup into sub-subgroups in accordance with the similarity of parameters 1, 9, and 13, respectively. More detailed statistical analysis is given in [112].
**EDSS, a standard evaluation according to expanded scale of disablement.
†FS indexes, an evaluation of damage to functional systems: fs1, pyramidal functions; fs2, cerebellar functions; fs3, functions of brain stem; fs4, sensitive functions; fs5, functions of intestines and urinary bladder; fs6, visual functions; fs7, cerebral (psychical) functions. Sum of indexes includes all characteristics from fs1 to fs7.

Recently, the levels of auto-Abs to myelin basic protein (MBP) were compared in the blood of 49 patients with multiple sclerosis (MS) and healthy donors [112]. All MS patients showed significantly higher anti-MBP Abs levels as compared to healthy subjects. For all 49 MS patients, the absolute values of *r* for positive (0.01 to 0.09), absent (~0), and negative correlations (-0.02 to -0.07) between anti-MBP Abs and 13 standard clinical parameters were relatively low and statistically non-significant. Several correlation coefficients become higher and reached values up to 0.1 to 0.55 and –0.04 to –0.47 after the cohort was divided into subgroups of patients with primary progressing, secondary progressing and remitting course of the disease (some of values are given in Table 5). Interestingly, the coefficients of correlation between the same two analyzed parameters can be either positive or negative in the case of different subgroups. Thus, for the whole group of 49 MS patients the coefficient of correlation between the titers of anti-MBP Abs and patient age at the moment of MS clinical onset was –0.06, while it was +0.55, –0.30 and –0.07 for primary progressing, remitting, and secondary progressing course subgroups, respectively. A similar situation was observed for other pairs of analyzed parameters [112].

The groups of remitting and secondary progressing course of MS patients were not "homogenous" with respect to the patients' characteristics, and their further subdivision using cluster and factorial analysis revealed statistically significant correlation coefficients [112]. For example, for one sub-subgroup of the remitting course subgroup, a direct dependence between titers of anti-MBP and symptoms of damage of the pyramidal tract was observed ($r = 0.92$). In some cases, correlations of the opposite sign were observed for the same pairs of analyzed parameters for the three subgroups with different MS courses and their sub-subgroups obtained by cluster analysis.

Interestingly, in the case of different MS subgroups the level of anti-DNA Abs correlates with various clinical parameters, more often with the disturbance in the function of cerebrum, bladder, and intestines, and, to a less extent, cerebellum [110]. In contrast to anti-DNA Abs, a positive correlation of anti-MBP titers with disturbed brain stem function was revealed in a relatively large fraction of patients (~37%), while a negative correlation was shown with pyramid function and with the rate of disease progression [110, 112]. It should be mentioned that the correlation between Abs to DNA and to MBP in MS patients was also very weak.

The absence of a definite dependence between titers of anti-DNA and anti-MBP Abs and these parameters with the standard clinical indices may be due to several reasons. MS is an extremely multifactor disease, in which similar pathomorphological and clinical indices manifested as MS may result from very different underlying processes and connections [113, 114]. For example, in each MS patient, the "relative stability" of different organs and their functions to the destructive effect of transient immune system errors can be significantly different depending on the genetic background and environmental stress factors, including geographic ones [113-115]. Some proteins of influenza, herpes, polyoma, Epstein–Barr and other viruses and of some bacteria have been reported to mimic human myelin proteins, and therefore these infections leading to the immunization with their proteins can stimulate subsequent formation of Abs to myelin and finally the development of AI reactions [116-119]. In individual MS patients, the development of AI reactions can be stimulated by different viral or bacterial infections as well as various toxic chemicals. Furthermore, it should be taken also into account that MS is an at least two-phase pathology [118]. The cascade of reactions corresponding to the first inflammatory phase is very complicated and involves many proteins, enzymes, cytokines, and chemokines inducing macrophages and other cells producing NO• radicals and osteopathin [114, 118]. The complex coordinated action of T- and B-cells, complement system, inflammation mediators, and auto-Abs results in formation of demyelinization nidi and interruption of axon conductivity. The neurodegenerative phase of MS that ensues later is directly connected with neural tissue destruction in the patients [114, 118]. Therefore, any analysis of biochemical, immunological and clinical indices must take into account the current phase of the disease. Even then, quite different characteristics of pathologic processes can be obtained in individual patients, as the disease progresses against the background of the continually changing immunoregulation including exhaustion of different compensatory and adaptive mechanisms and systemic metabolic changes. This makes the clinical course of MS hardly predictable in individual patients [114, 118]. Therefore, it is not surprising that we could not find statistically significant correlation of titers of Abs to DNA and MBP with the standard clinical characteristics in the whole group of 49 MS patients, since each patient can be characterized by an individual combination of genetic, environmental, chronic, inflammatory, autoimmune, demyelinating, neurodegenerative and other factors.

The mechanism of autoimmune damage of the thyroid has not been adequately studied, and the pathogenesis of the thyroid gland autoimmune disorders remains unclear; different Abs are believed to play a significant role in the pathogenesis of Hashimoto's thyroiditis (HT) [89, 120]. There are several types of Abs in thyroid diseases: to thyroglobulin, to MFT, superficial AG, the second colloidal AG, thyreostimulating Abs, etc. Damage of thyrocytes by Abs has been suggested, and a pathogenic role of Abs to thyroglobulin and MFT has been proven [89, 90, 120, 121]. Autoantibodies to thyroglobulin, a 660-kDa precursor of thyroid hormones, are found in nearly all patients with HT and in a smaller fraction of healthy individuals [121]. A high concentration of anti-thyroglobulin Abs is one of the indicators of a systemic AI process in patients with HT.

In bronchial asthma, vasoactive intestinal peptide (VIP), widely distributed in the central and peripheral nervous systems, acts as an auto-antigen [17].

Among all these pathologies, only SLE is usually considered to be related to patients' autoimmunization with DNA, since the sera of SLE patients usually contain high concentrations of DNA. Therefore, at first glance it is reasonable to suggest that anti-DNA Abs do not play a significant role in the pathogenesis of most AI or viral diseases except SLE. Disease-specific Abs such as Abs to VIP and thyroglobulin in the case of bronchial asthma [17] and HT [89, 120, 122], respectively, are highly likely to be of primary importance for the development of AI processes. However, although anti-DNA Abs may be considered secondary or accompanying, we argue that non-specific Abs against DNA and RNA, which may arise in any AD, also can play a remarkable role in the AI processes.

Some viral infections (for example, AIDS, hepatitis, tick-borne encephalitis (TBE), etc.) can lead to the formation of Abs to different antigens including DNA and RNA. A comparison of the relative levels of auto-Abs to nat- and den-DNA in the blood of 55 patients with TBE was carried out [123]. 31% of the TBE patients were shown to have an increased level of Abs to nat-DNA, and 40% of the patients demonstrated an increased level of Abs to den-DNA. The percentage of TBE patients with the increased concentration of anti-nat-DNA Abs was higher than that of MS patients (18%) and some other AI diseases (6-18%), but comparable with that for patients with SLE (38%) and systemic polymyositis (42%). In contrast to patients with SLE and MS, the level of Abs to nat-DNA in the patients with TBE was higher than the level of Abs to den-DNA. Correlation coefficients of Ab levels to nat- and den-DNA were estimated for the whole group of patients and for separate subgroups with different disease manifestations (temperature reaction, fever, and meningitis). Correlations between titers of anti-DNA Abs and three standard biochemical markers of TBE (activity of aspartate aminotransferase, alanine aminotransferase, and total bilirubin concentration) for 22 TBE patients were analyzed [123]. Statistically significant correlations were found only between the level of Abs to nat-DNA and activities of aspartate and alanine aminotransferases, with the correlation coefficients 0.44 and 0.48, respectively [123].

A similar situation can occur in HIV-infected patients. A pronounced immune response to the viral components is the most important factor slowing the transition of HIV infection to the stage of AIDS characterized by a progressive decrease in the number of T helpers and their functional insufficiency [124]. HIV-dependent activation of B lymphocytes leads to the production of Abs to viral proteins, auto-Abs to human cell components, and various immune complexes. Similarly to AIDS, the blood of hepatitis patients often contains organ-unspecific autoantigens.

Microbial infections expose the human organism to different components from the parasite's cells, including protein, DNA, RNA, lipids, and polysaccharides. The sera of mice infected with *Salmonella typhimurium* [125, 126], malaria [127], *Plasmodium chabaudi* [128], and the sera of humans infected with *Trypanosoma cruzi* [129] or bacterial pathogens [130, 131] contain a variety of Abs to the parasite's antigens and to human lipids, proteins, and nuclear components, including anti-DNA Abs. The origin of anti-DNA Abs in the infections remains speculative; some of them may arise inadvertently in the course of a normal immune response due to the induction by Abs that bear structures (mimotopes) mimicking DNA [131]. The immunoregulatory effect of the infection seems to be related, at least partially, to the increase in a particular population of Abs, the polyreactive antibodies [126]. It has been proposed that infectious agents can act in some cases through the mechanism of molecular mimicry. For instance, the agents responsible for molecular mimicry in multiple sclerosis include measles, hepatitis B, herpes simplex, influenza, papilloma, and Epstein-Bar viruses [118].

A perpetually growing number of observations suggest that ADs originate from malfunctions of hematopoietic stem cells (HSCs) [132] (see below). Thus, it is possible that different viral and bacterial antigens introduced by infections can, in certain cases, affect the proliferation and differentiation of HSCs and trigger the development of AI processes.

3. THE ORIGIN OF ARTIFICIAL AND NATURAL ABZYMES

Artificial catalytic Abs can be obtained by immunization of animals with chemically stable analogs of transition states of chemical reactions (reviewed in [7-10, 16]). On the other hand, artificial antiidiotypic Abs can also possess catalytic activity [42, 133]. Building on earlier observations on the existence of idiotypic determinants related to the antigen, Jerne proposed that the immune system is self-regulated by a network of idiotype–anti-idiotype interactions [134]. The simplified model of this network may be schematically presented as follows:

$$Ag1 \quad Ag2 \quad Ag3 \quad Ag4$$

$$\bullet \rightarrow Y \rightarrow Y \rightarrow Y \rightarrow$$

$$Ab1 \quad Ab2 \quad Ab3$$

Antibody 1 can effectively bind antigen 1, Ag1. At the same time, the former can also be an antigen inducing generation of secondary Ab2. The latter may also be an antigen causing generation of Ab3, and this can be continued (Ab4, Ab5, etc.). The scheme shows a great similarity between the antigen determinant of Ag1 and the antigen-binding site of Ab2 (the same is true for the pair Ab1-Ab3). Antibodies 1 and 2 are termed idiotype and anti-idiotype, respectively, etc. There is convincing evidence that such idiotype–anti-idiotype networks are actually present in the body. The presence of blood serum Ab4 (in the notation shown in the scheme) has been confirmed in experimental animals [134].

If the active site of an enzyme plays the role of antigen triggering this anti-idiotypic chain, it is logical to suggest that the secondary anti-idiotypic Ab2 may possess the structure, a part of which represents an "internal image" or "mould" of the active site of this enzyme, and, consequently, these Abs may possess some properties of this enzyme. This remarkable property of idiotypic mimicry has been exploited to rise monoclonal antiidiotypic Abzs with acetylcholinesterase [135, 136], carboxypeptidase [137, 138], and β-lactamase-like [139] activities. The catalytic antibody capable of degrading the active site of urease of *Helicobacter pylori* and eradicating the bacterial infection in mouse stomach was successfully obtained [140]. This monoclonal Ab was generated by immunization with a designed recombinant protein UreB, which contained the crucial region of the *H. pylori* urease β-subunit active site. The light chain of this antibody by itself showed a proteolytic activity that substantially degraded both UreB and the intact urease [140].

The origin of natural Abzs in different AI diseases is complex. Natural Abzs hydrolyzing DNA, RNA, polysaccharides, oligopeptides, and proteins have been described from the sera of patients with several AI (SLE, HT, polyarthritis, MS, asthma, rheumatoid arthritis, etc.) and viral diseases with a pronounced immune system disturbance (viral hepatitis and AIDS) (reviewed in [23-27]). Healthy humans and patients with many diseases with insignificant autoimmune reactions usually lack Abzs or develop Abzs with very low catalytic activities, which are often on a borderline of the sensitivity of detection methods [23-27].

It is commonly believed that Abzs are associated with autoimmunization and that auto-Abs in SLE and other AI diseases are most probably of anti-idiotypic nature [141, 142]. However, similarly to artificial Abzs against analogs of transition states of catalytic reactions, naturally occurring Abzs may be Abs raised directly against the enzyme substrates acting as haptens, which, bound to different proteins, could resemble transition states of catalytic reactions [16-27]. For example, Abzs hydrolyzing VIP [17], thyroglobulin [28], and myelin basic protein [31-33] in the sera of patients with asthma, Hashimoto's thyroiditis, and multiple sclerosis, respectively, are Abs against these proteins; the same is true for casein-hydrolyzing human milk Abs against casein [143]. pIgGs from AIDS patients hydrolyzing HIV-1 reverse transcriptase [34] and HIV-1 integrase [35] were the first examples of proteolytic Abzs appearing in humans directly against these proteins due to a viral infection and AI reactions. However, in parallel with formation of Abzs against viral proteins, the production of Abzs hydrolyzing specifically human serum albumin and human casein was revealed in HIV-infected patients [34].

It was suggested that some DNase Abzs of SLE patients are antiidiotypic Abzs to topoisomerase I [144]. Immunization of rabbits with DNase I produces Abs with DNase activity of antiidiotypic nature [145]. Idiotypic Ab1 was obtained by immunization of rabbits with DNase I and then used to elicit a polyclonal anti-idiotypic Ab2, which was able to hydrolyze DNA, indicating the existence of internal images mimicking the enzymatic activity of DNase I.

Taking into account our data concerning Abzs in different AI diseases, it was suggested that polyclonal DNase Abs of AI patients may be a cocktail of Abs against complexes of DNA and RNA with proteins and antiidiotypic Abzs to different DNA-hydrolyzing enzymes (reviewed in [23-27]). To find out which antigens can induce Abzs with DNase and RNase activities in AI diseases, we have immunized rabbits with DNA, RNA, DNase I, DNase II, and pancreatic RNase A [146-150]. Immunization of rabbits with pure DNA and RNA generated Abs interacting with DNA and possessing weak DNase and RNase activities, while Abs from non-immunized rabbits did not hydrolyze nucleic acids [146-150]. Many SLE anti-DNA Abs are directed against DNA bound to proteins, including complexes with histones appearing as a result of internucleosomal cleavage during apoptosis [96]. Therefore, we have emulated such natural complexes using complexes of DNA and RNA with methylated bovine serum albumin (BSA). Immunization of rabbits with complex of DNA and RNA with methylated BSA elicited production of 10-50-fold more active DNase and RNase IgGs, while pIgGs from animals immunized with methylated BSA were catalytically inactive [146, 147].

Immunization of healthy rabbits with bovine DNase I, DNase II, and bovine pancreatic RNase A also produced IgGs with intrinsic DNase and RNase activities [148-150]. An antiidiotypic nature of IgGs against DNase I with DNase activity was demonstrated [145]. It was shown that 74-85% of the total pIgGs with DNase and RNase activities belong to antiidiotypic Abs to RNase A (0.6-0.8% of total polyclonal IgGs), while 15-26% of the activities cannot interact with Sepharose bearing Abs against RNase A and may be Abs to nucleic acids bound to RNase [149]. Interestingly, only ~10% of the total pIgGs with DNase and RNase activities from rabbits immunized with DNase II (~0.1% of total polyclonal IgGs) were of antiidiotypic nature, while the remaining 90% did not interact with Sepharose bearing Abs against DNase II and hence may also be Abs to nucleic acids bound to DNase II [150]. The low content of antiidiotypic Abzs to DNase II hydrolyzing DNA and RNA may be a consequence of relatively low immunogenicity of the active site of DNase II as compared with other antigenic determinants of this protein. Anti-DNA–protein and anti-RNA–protein complexes and other antinuclear antibodies are found in the sera of patients with multisystem connective tissue disease [76]. Thus, one cannot exclude that DNase I, DNase II, and RNase A can interact with RNA and DNA and induce formation of anti-RNA and or anti-DNA Abs, which possess no or low affinity for these enzymes, but could be much more catalytically active than antiidiotypic Abzs. In addition, different proteins interacting with DNA and RNA can differ both in their ability to stimulate the formation of Abs against bound nucleic acids and in the relative nuclease activities of these Abzs.

So far we have discussed different ways of nuclease Abzs formation in healthy animals without AI reactions. Since immunization of AI mice results in a dramatically higher incidence of Abzs with a higher activity than in conventionally used normal mouse strains [151, 152], the formation of Abzs in AI diseases may be much more profuse. It is known that, theoretically, the immune system can produce up to 10^6 different Ab variants in response to a single antigen. In AI diseases the possible number of antigens that can elicit production of DNase and/or RNase Abzs is very high. First, an increased level of apoptosis in AI patients may trigger production of Abzs directly to DNA and RNA and their complexes with various proteins. It is known that the immune response to DNA and RNA, especially in their complexes with proteins, partially depends on the nucleic acid sequence and length [76-79]. The number of different DNA and RNA molecules stimulating the formation of Abs and Abzs may be very high since in the sera of humans, DNA and RNA are significantly fragmented, and even relatively small fragments of different sequences can elicit immune response. As mentioned above, antiidiotypic Abs against active centers of different DNases and RNases can also possess catalytic activity [145-150]; even Abs against human topoisomerase I are catalytically active in the hydrolysis of DNA [144]. It means that potentially many enzymes degrading DNA or RNA can also stimulate formation of DNase and/or RNase Abzs, which can be significantly different in their enzymatic properties.

The data discussed in this section suggest the possibility for Abz production through the pathway described for artificial Abs induced by transition-state analogs. Some antigens may change conformation when they associate with other proteins, and their structure in such complexes could mimic that of a transition state of the antigen's reaction. ADs are accompanied by extensive apoptosis. This may result in abnormally high blood concentrations of both native and partially destroyed proteins, nucleic acids, polysaccharides, etc. The literature data and our results (see above) suggest that both pathways of Abz generation (production of anti-idiotypic Abs and Ig to substrate itself) can function in ADs. The central question is why autoimmunization of AI patients and mice results in a dramatically higher incidence of catalytically inactive Abs and Abzs with enzyme properties as compared with healthy humans and animals.

4. ABZYMES OF HUMAN MILK

Although Abzs with very low activity can sometimes be detected in healthy people, the enzymatic relative activities (RAs) of AI patients are usually significantly higher to the extent where specific Abzs can present a convenient diagnostic marker of some AI pathologies ([23-27] and refs therein). We have shown that the appearance of Abzs specific for various substrates is among the earliest and clear signs of AI reactions in a number of AI diseases (SLE, Hashimoto's thyroiditis, polyarthritis, multiple sclerosis) and viral diseases with strong immune system disturbances (AIDS, hepatitis) [23-27]. According to our data, catalytic activity of nuclease Abzs is usually very easily detectable at the onset of AI diseases when the total concentrations of Abs to DNA or other auto-antigens have not yet increased significantly and correspond to their ranges for healthy donors [23-27].

During pregnancy and immediately after delivery, women are very often characterized by immune processes similar to those in AI patients ([23-27, 153] and refs therein). sIgA and/or IgG possessing DNase, RNase, amylase, and ATPase activities were found in blood serum and milk of pregnant and lactating females [153-160]. We have discovered that milk of clinically healthy human mothers contains very unusual sIgA and/or IgG possessing protein [161-163], lipid [164-166] and polysaccharide kinase activities [167-169]. Many AI pathologies can be "activated" or "triggered" in clinically healthy women during pregnancy and soon after childbirth [170, 171]. Independently of the presence or absence of detectable AI reactions in women during pregnancy, sometimes there may develop postnatal AI pathologies such as SLE, Hashimoto's thyroiditis, phospholipids syndrome, polymyositis, autoimmune myocarditis, etc. [171-173]. One of the most frequently found post-natal AI pathologies is Hashimoto's thyroiditis, with the prevalence of 1.9-16.7% [171-173]. Various manifestations of these AI diseases can be detected during the first 3-6 postnatal months but usually do not last for more than one year.

Analysis of published data suggests that pregnant women may be directly immunized through a specific response of their immune system to certain compounds of viral, bacterial or food origin that can efficiently stimulate production of different Abs and Abzs. Immunization of animals by direct injection of antigens (mainly proteins) into the bloodstream or by oral administration no more than 1-3 months before delivery leads to the production of anti-protein Abs, which then may be detected in the milk at high concentrations [174]. Production of milk Abs starting several months after the immunization supports the existence of a specific "immuno-memory" in pregnant females, The autoimmunization of mothers during pregnancy similar to that occurring in AI patients is very probable; an increased level of DNA in the serum of normal women during the first three months of pregnancy has been reported, resembling the situation in AI diseases [175]. In addition, an increased level of apoptosis during the last 3 months of pregnancy has been demonstrated [176] together with the presence of low numbers of embryonic cells in the blood of pregnant women [177, 178]. This means that, in contrast to healthy humans, pregnant women may be efficiently immunized by compounds of various viruses and bacteria, when they are in contact with such compounds. Interestingly, the relative blood Abz activities significantly increase after delivery and at the beginning of lactation [153, 160]. Nevertheless, enzymatic activities of Abs from the milk of lactating women are 5–600-fold higher than those from the sera of the same women [153, 160]. In addition, the DNase activity of Abzs from blood of healthy pregnant women was 4–5-fold lower than that from pregnant women with pronounced autoimmune thyroiditis [153]. Thus, one cannot exclude that molecular mechanisms of immune system activation leading to production of autoreactive Abs and/or autoantibodies with and without catalytic activities are, to some extent, similar or overlapping in both AI patients and human mothers. Overall, pregnancy and especially the beginning of lactation may be considered important periods associated with the production not only of different Abs and auto-Abs, but also of Abzs.

The mother's milk sIgA are active at the mucosal surfaces protecting them from the invasion of pathogenic microorganisms and limiting the access of environmental antigens [179, 180]. Milk IgGs can penetrate into blood through the intestinal epithelium thus protecting newborns. Therefore, one cannot exclude that, in contrast to auto-Abs of AI patients, Abzs of mother milk could contribute to the protective role of Abs through hydrolysis of different nucleic acids, polysaccharides, and proteins [23-27, 153-169]. Possible differences and similarities in the roles of Abzs as well as in mechanisms of their production in AI patients and in lactating mothers are very interesting. Many questions concerning Abzs can be answered only using experimental animals to model certain immune states but they have not yet been widely used for studying the mechanisms of Abzs accumulation.

5. ASSOCIATION OF DIFFERENT AUTO-ABS AND ABZYMES FORMATION WITH CHANGES IN COLONY FORMATION OF HEMATOPOIETIC PROGENITORS

MRL-lpr/lpr mice spontaneously developing a SLE-like disorder are a very promising model to study the mechanisms of natural Abzs generation and their role in the pathogenesis of pronounced AI disturbances. MRL-lpr/lpr mice are characterized by marked hypergammaglobulinemia, production of numerous auto-Abs, circulating immune complexes, glomerulonephritis and severe lymphadenopathy. A mutation in the *lpr* gene of these mice leads to a deficit in functional Fas ligand and dysregulation of apoptosis in homozygotes [181, 182]. As a result, the mice develop SLE-like phenotype, including accumulation of double-negative T cells ($CD4^-$ $CD8^-$ $B220^+$ TCR^+) in the peripheral lymphoid organs.

MRL/MPJ-*lpr* and SJL mice were used to obtain Abzs with amidase/esterase activity in the expanded sequence space of Ab repertoire using haptenic transition-state analogues with a phosphonate and/or phosphoimidate moiety ([151] and refs therein). A surprising result in this study was that the Abzs were obtained with a dramatically higher incidence in these AI mouse strains than in conventionally used normal mouse strains. Testing the ability of several strains of mice to elicit esterolytic Abs after immunization with a *p*-nitrobenzyl phosphonate hapten revealed that the occurrence of catalytic antibodies in SJL and MRL/lpr autoimmune mice is dramatically higher than in normal mouse strains (e.g., wild-type MRL/++ or BALB/c) [152]. Polyclonal auto-Abs purified from the sera of NZB/W, MRL-lpr/lpr and SJL/J mice show DNase activity, as opposed to those harvested from non-AI BALB/c mice [183], although no standard criteria were checked in this study to attribute this activity to IgGs. The levels of the catalytic activity were strongly dependent on the age of the animal, with the highest levels of catalytic activity found in the sera of mice between 8 and 12 months of age [183].

An affinity-linked oligonucleotide cleavage assay was successfully applied to screen a large number of hybridoma clones derived from non-immunized (NZB x NZW)F1 mice with spontaneous SLE [184]. Three clones producing DNase Abzs were found. It was shown that the DNase center of a monoclonal DNase IgG from AI-prone MRL-lpr/lpr mice is located at the interface between the light and heavy chains, and both L- and H- chains are able to hydrolyze DNA when separated [185].

Recently, IgGs were isolated from the sera of MRL-lpr/lpr mice [186-188]. Convincing evidence was provided using different approaches including several strict criteria that DNase, amylase, and ATPase activities are intrinsic to mouse polyclonal IgGs, similarly to Abzs from SLE patients [186-188]. Although many questions concerning SLE Abzs could be answered using experimental animals for modeling certain states of the immune system, they have not yet been widely employed in studies of the mechanisms of Abzs accumulation. Recently we have carried out the first analysis of possible correlations between the relative catalytic activities of mouse IgGs in the hydrolysis of DNA, ATP, and oligosaccharides with several clinical and biochemical markers of AI pathologies (proteinuria, Ab titers to native and denatured DNA) at various stages of mouse SLE, pregnancy and lactation [189]. An ever-growing number of observations suggested that AI diseases may originate from defects in hematopoietic stem cells [132]. Therefore, lymphocyte proliferation and apoptosis at different stages of the AI disorder development in MRL-lpr/lpr mice were also studied. Hematopoietic progenitor colony formation in the course of spontaneous pathology, pregnancy, lactation, and after immunization of mice was characterized.

It was shown that appearance of pronounced visual symptoms (pink spots, cephalic and dorsal alopecia, general health deterioration, etc.) correlated well with proteinuria ($\geq$ 3-mg/ml concentration of protein in urine) [187-189]. The highest levels of anti-DNA Abs, DNase, ATPase, and amylase Abz activity, proteinuria and visible markers of SLE were observed at 7-12 months of age, but we have used spontaneously diseased mice with all visible symptoms no older than 7 months. Although the state of "health" in the case of AI-prone mice may be considered very provisional, the mouse SLE pathology is nevertheless spontaneous and AI reactions leading to deep pathology develop gradually. In order to distinguish different levels of the pathology development, MRL-lpr/lpr mice demonstrating no typical SLE indices and Abz activities (similar to healthy control non-AI mice) were conditionally designated (independently of age) as healthy MRL-lpr/lpr mice, whereas the animals demonstrating no visual or biochemical SLE indices but having detectable Abz activities were conditionally designated as pre-diseased mice [187-189].

As mentioned above, the beginning of the lactation may be regarded as an important period associated with the production of Abzs [23-27]. Taking this into account, we have analyzed twelve groups of non-AI mice and AI-prone MRL-lpr/lpr mice with and without several pronounced SLE indices mentioned above, as well as pregnant and lactating mice and assayed RAs of their IgGs in the hydrolysis of DNA, ATP, and maltoheptaose (MHO) (Tables 6 and 7).

At 3-7 months of age, control non-AI BALB/c and CBA males and females (groups 1 and 2) demonstrated no proteinuria (0.1-0.12 mg/ml << 3 mg/ml), very low and comparable concentrations of Abs to nat- and den-DNA (0.017-0.04 A_{450}), and non-detectable level of DNase or ATPase activities (Table 6) [187-189]. IgGs of some of these control mice did not possess detectable amylase activity, while other were characterised by low but detectable activity; the average values of IgG amylase activity were ~1 % (Table 6).

The majority of 2-3-months-old MRL-lpr/lpr males and females demonstrated no visible signs of pathology and average biochemical markers similar to those for control healthy BALB/c and CBA mice; the absence of proteinuria (0.37-0.38 mg/ml), higher, but still relatively low concentrations of anti-DNA Abs (0.09 – 0.12 A_{450}), undetectable levels of DNase or ATPase and low amylase Abzs activities (Table 6).

As we have shown previously, detection of Ab DNase and RNase activities in human serum may be considered a good indicator of the onset or a significant progression of AI reactions associated with several AI pathologies [23-27]. Interestingly, detectable levels of nuclease activities of IgGs and/or IgMs in humans sometimes can be revealed up to 2-3 months earlier than a statistically reliable increase in anti-DNA Ab concentrations. Some 7-months-old MRL-lpr/lpr males and females demonstrating no visual symptoms can be conditionally considered as animals soon to succumb to the disease (pre-diseased), since 80-95% of mice at 7-8 months usually develop very deep SLE. Interestingly, all conditionally healthy MRL-lpr/lpr males and females at 7 months of age (groups 5 and 6) demonstrated characteristic values of urine protein concentration (range 0.4-1.2 mg/ml); on average, these values (~0.8-0.9 mg/ml) were statistically significantly higher than in healthy mice (groups 1-4) but lower than ≤ 3 mg/ml (Table 6). These groups were characterized by increased concentrations of Abs against denatured (0.08-0.16 A_{450}) and native (0.11-0.2 A_{450}) DNA as compared with mice of 2-3-months of age (Table 6). A significant difference was observed between male groups 3 and 5 and female groups 4 and 6, respectively, in the case of Abs to native DNA (Table 6). Interestingly, all 7-months-old MRL-lpr/lpr males and females with no visible indices of SLE demonstrated detectable DNase (range 1-9 %, average 3.0-6.1 %) and ATPase (range 0.1-6%, average 0.4-2.4 %) activities (Table 6). Thus, like in the case of human AI patients, only mouse IgG DNase and ATPase activities can be considered statistically significant indicators of pre-disease conditions of spontaneous SLE [187-189].

The MRL-lpr/lpr males and females, also at 7 months of age but with visual symptoms of spontaneous SLE, demonstrated very high proteinuria (5-8 mg/ml) and a moderate and statistically insignificant increase in the concentrations of anti-DNA Abs (0.16-0.23 A_{450}; groups 7 and 8) in comparison with 7-months-old pre-diseased mice (groups 5 and 6; Table 6). Spontaneous pathology in 7-months-old MRL-lpr/lpr mice (groups 7 and 8) is characterized by significant variations in Abz RAs. DNase and ATPase RAs of Abzs from males (group 7) fell in the ranges 2-64% and 4-314%, respectively. Similar ranges of DNase and ATPase RAs were observed for group of diseased 7-months-old females (group 8). The average values of DNase (20-22%) and ATPase (65-68.3%) activities for Abzs from different males and females (groups 7 and 8) were increased 3–7- and 27–171-fold, respectively, as compared with pre-diseased mice (groups 5 and 6; Table 6). The increase in the amylase RAs after the development of SLE by 7-months-old males and females (3.9 and 9.2%, respectively; groups 7 and 8) as compared with young mice (groups 3 and 4) was 1.9–5.0-fold. Since IgGs from healthy control and young AI-prone mice possess amylase activity, this factor cannot be considered a very good marker of severe AI pathology. Thus, the most important markers of mouse severe SLE are very high proteinuria (5-8 mg/ml) and high activity of IgGs in the hydrolysis of DNA and ATP (Table 6) [187-189].

We have immunized conditionally healthy MRL-lpr/lpr males (3 months of age) with complex of DNA and methylated BSA [189]. This led to a minor development of visible markers of SLE 1.5 months after the first immunization, but to drastic effect on proteinuria (~9.5 mg/ml, group 9), which was increased ~25-fold as compared with young males (groups 3 and 4) but was comparable with those for males and females with spontaneous SLE (~5-8 mg/ml, groups 7 and 8) (Table 6). Immunization of the males (group 9) led to the highest and statistically significant increase in the level of Abs against native (on average ~0.6 A_{450}) and denatured DNA (on average ~1.0 A_{450}) in comparison with healthy or diseased mice (groups 1-8; Table 6). For the immunized males, the highest increase in the relative DNase (range 50-510%) and especially ATPase (range 500-1887%) activities was observed, the average activities was estimated as ~360% and ~1333%, respectively (Table 6). As compared with the 7-month-old pre-diseased males (group 5) DNase activity of the immunized mice (group 9) was increased ~120-fold, and ATPase, ~3330-fold (Table 6). The amylase RA was increased in immunized males as compared with healthy males (group 3) by a factor of ~8.8 (Table 6). Interestingly, development of SLE pathology stimulated by immunization is characterized mainly by a significant increase in anti-DNA Abs concentrations (12-19-fold) and Abz RAs (8.8-3330-fold), while indices of proteinuria for the spontaneous and stimulated pathology are comparable (Table 6) [187-189].

5.1. Ab Catalytic Activities in Pregnant and Lactating Mice

In contrast to spontaneous or induced mouse SLE (5–9.5 mg/ml), no pronounced proteinuria (≥3 mg/ml) was detected in the females during pregnancy (0.31 mg/ml), 4 days (0.32 mg/ml), or 2 weeks (0.7 mg/ml) after delivery and at the beginning of lactation (Table 6) [187-189]. The concentrations of anti-DNA Abs (0.24–0.25 A_{450}, group 10) in the pregnant females were ~2.5–3.0-fold higher than in the non-pregnant healthy females (0.08–0.12 A_{450}, group 4) and comparable with these values in the diseased females and males (0.21–0.23 A_{450}, groups 7 and 8; Table 6).

Interestingly, 4 days and 2 weeks after the beginning of lactation the average values of the relative concentrations of Abs to nat-DNA were ~1.8–2.4-fold (0.54–0.57 A_{450}, groups 11 and 12) higher than in the pregnant mice (group 10) and became comparable with those for the males immunized with DNA (0.6 A_{450}; Table 6). The average values of concentrations of Abs to denatured DNA for the lactating females (0.35–0.39 A_{450}) were ~1.4–1.6-fold higher than for the pregnant females, but were remarkably lower than for the immunized mice (1.1 A_{450}; Table 6). Thus, similar to the diseased mice (groups 7 and 8), or the immunized males (group 9), the pregnant and especially lactating females (groups 10-11) were characterized by increased overall concentrations of anti-DNA Abs. However, in contrast to the diseased and immunized mice, the high levels of anti-DNA Abs in the pregnant and lactating mice did not correlate with proteinuria (Table 6).

On average, the 7-months-old pre-diseased females (group 4) demonstrated DNase (6.1%) and ATPase (24%) RAs comparable with those for the pregnant animals (group 10; 6.3 and 39.3%, respectively; Table 6). The average amylase RA of the pregnant females (3.9%) is also comparable with those for the diseased males and females (3.7-9.2%). After the beginning of lactation, the average DNase activity increased sharply to ~44% (range 3-100%) and then after 2 weeks of lactation decreased to ~19% (range 0.3–79%). A similar situation was observed for the IgG amylase activity, which increased between pregnancy and the start of lactation from 3.9 to 31.7%, and then decreased to 13.7% after two weeks of lactation. The most significant increase in the activity was observed for ATPase Abzs in the females. The average relative ATPase activity reached 367% (range 20–1737%) in the mice 4 days after delivery and then decreased to 191% (range 1–567%) two weeks after the delivery (Table 6). Thus, 4 days after delivery, the lactating mice demonstrated 6–9-fold increases in average DNase, ATPase, and amylase RAs, and all these activities decreased ~2-fold after two weeks of lactation (Table 6) [187-189].

5.2. Hematopoietic Progenitor's Colony Formation

Possible relationships between the Abz RAs and the colony formation ability of hematopoietic progenitors were studied [187-189]. In the bone marrow of young MRL-lpr/lpr males and females (groups 3 and 4) demonstrating no detectable Abz DNase and ATPase activities we have found a normal distribution of committed progenitors similar to that for non-AI CBA mice (group 1; Table 7). The number of BFU-E and CFU-GEMM colonies increased ~2 and 16.4–28.4-fold, respectively, in the 7-months-old MRL-lpr/lpr males and females (groups 5 and 6) without SLE clinical manifestations and proteinuria but with low detectable Abzs activities. In the spontaneously diseased males and females (groups 7 and 8) with high Abz RAs, the hematopoietic stem cells (HSC) profile was changed remarkably in comparison with the pre-diseased mice (groups 5 and 6, respectively): the number of BFU-E colonies increased ~2-fold, while the number of CFU-GM and CFU-GEMM colonies decreased 2.6–4-fold and 2.4–3.4-fold.

After the development of SLE induced by immunization, the mice (group 9) were characterized by the highest increase in proteinuria, anti-DNA Abs, Abz activities, and a very specific HSC differentiation profile was observed (Table 7). The numbers of BFU-E and CFU-GEMM colonies were 3.6- and 4.3-fold lower than for the spontaneously diseased males (group 7) while these parameters for CFU-GM colonies were comparable.

Table 6. Autoimmune characteristics of autoimmune-prone MRL-lpr/lpr and control non-autoimmune mice [187-189]

Group description[†]	Group number	Number of mice	Urine protein, mg/ml[*]	Abs to native DNA, A_{450}[*]	Abs to denatured DNA, A_{450}[*]	DNase activity, %[*]	ATPase activity, %[*]	Amylase activity[*]
Control males and females								
(CBA × C57BL) F1 (3-7 mo.)	1	8 (4 females + 4 males)	0.12±0.07	0.04±0.01	0.02±0.01	0[***]	0[***]	1.0±0.5[***]
BALB/c (3-7 mo.)	2	8 (4 females + 4 males)	0.1±0.08	0.03±0.01	0.017±0.004	0	0	1.1±0.5
MRL-lpr/lpr males								
Healthy (2-3 mo.)	3	5	0.38±0.1	0.032±0.01	0.09±0.07	0	0	1.9±1.2
Healthy, pre-diseased (7 mo.)	5	5	0.8±0.3	0.1±0.05[+]	0.16±0.05	3.0±1.0[‡]	0.4±0.25	n.d.[§]
Diseased (7 mo)	7	8	**8.0±3.1**[**]	**0.2±0.05**[+]	**0.23±0.11**	**22.0±24.0**	**68.3±98.0**	**3.7±1.0**
Immunized	9	6	**9.5±1.7**[**]	**0.6±0.17**	**1.1±0.16**	**360.0±230.0**	**1333±530**	**17.6±7.5**
MRL-lpr/lpr females								
Healthy (2-3 mo)	4	5	0.31±0.03	0.08±0.03	0.12±0.06	0	0	1.8±1.1
Healthy, pre-diseased (7 mo)	6	5	**0.9±0.2**	0.18±0.1[+]	0.08±0.04	6.1±2.8	2.4±1.7	n.d.
Diseased (7 mo)	8	5	**5.0±3.8**[**]	**0.23±0.1**[+]	0.21±0.12	**20.0±21.0**	**65.0±93.0**	**9.2±5.4**
Pregnant (2-3 mo)	10	5	0.31±0.2	0.24±0.05	0.25±0.07	7.3±6.0	**39.3±42.8**	3.9±3.6
Lactating (3 mo), 4 days after delivery	11	5	0.32±0.1	**0.54±0.3**	**0.35±0.21**	**44.4±40.6**	**367±548**	**31.7±27.3**
Lactating (3 mo), 14 days after delivery	12	5	0.70±0.3	**0.57±0.28**	**0.39±0.18**	**19.0±24.0**	**191±173**	**13.7±11.0**

[*] For each mouse, the mean and standard deviation of three experiments is shown.
[**] Proteinuria corresponds to ≥3 mg of total protein/ml of urine.
[***] 100% relative activity corresponds to a complete transition of the substrate to its products of hydrolysis in the presence of 0.1 mg/ml IgGs.
[§] Not determined
[†] MRL-lpr/lpr mice demonstrating no typical SLE indices or Abz activities (similar to healthy control non-AI mice) were conditionally control non-A1 mice) were conditionally designated healthy independently of age; the animals showing detectable levels of abzymes were conditionally designated pre-diseased.
[‡] Cohorts with statistically significant ($p \leq 0.05$) differences in the parameters in comparison with conditionally healthy MRL-lpr/lpr males and females are given in boldface.
[+] Values obtained using 10–12 mice.

Table 7. Formation of bone marrow progenitor colonies in AI-prone MRL-lpr/lpr and control non-autoimmune mice [187-189]

Group description[†]	Visual symptoms	Group number	Number of mice	Number of colonies[*]		
				BFU-E	CFU-GM	CFU-GEMM
CBA (3-7 mo)	no	1	8	3.0 ± 0.5	7.3 ± 1.0	0.25 ± 0.05
Males						
Healthy (2-3 mo.)	no	3	5	6.5 ± 1.5	7.0 ± 1.0	0.5 ± 0.1
Healthy pre-diseased (7 mo)	no	5	5	**12.7 ± 1.4**[‡]	**30.0 ± 1.3**	**9.2 ± 1.9**
Diseased (7 mo)	yes	7	5	**25.3 ± 9.8**	7.4 ± 0.4	**3.9 ± 2.0**
Immunized (3 mo)	yes, weak	9	5	7.0 ± 2.1	6.0 ± 2.6	0.9 ± 0.7
Females						
Healthy (2-3 mo)	no	4	5	5.5 ± 0.5	11 ± 2.5	0.5 ± 0.2
Healthy, pre-diseased (7 mo)[ç]	no	6	5	**11.5 ± 2.0**	**23.0 ± 3.0**	**8.2 ± 3.0**
Diseased (7 mo)	yes	8	5	**22.1 ± 8.0**	9.0 ± 3.9	2.4 ± 1.8
Pregnant (3 mo)	no	10	5	6.8 ± 2.0	**7.8 ± 1.5**	**0.1 ± 0.08**
Lactating (3 mo), 4 days after delivery	no	11	5	8.8 ± 2.0	**19.1 ± 1.8**	0.25 ± 0.2
Lactating (3 mo), 14 days after delivery	no	12	5	**21.0 ± 8.0**	9.7 ± 0.5	**2.1 ± 0.7**

[*]For each mouse, the mean and confidence interval of four experiments is shown.

[†]MRL-lpr/lpr mice demonstrating no typical SLE indices or Abz activities (similar to healthy control non-AI mice) were conditionally designated healthy independently of age; the animals showing detectable levels of abzymes were conditionally designated pre-diseased.

[‡]Cohorts with statistically significant ($p \leq 0.05$) differences in the parameters in comparison with conditionally healthy MRL-lpr/lpr males and females are given in boldface.

Pregnancy (group 10) led to a remarkable decrease in the level of HSC proliferation and to a change in the differentiation profile: a 5–82-fold decrease in CFU-GEMM colonies was observed as compared with the female groups 4, 6, and 8, while the number of BFU-E and CFU-GM cell colonies for the pregnant and control healthy mice was comparable (Table 7). During pregnancy (group 10) the relative concentrations of anti-DNA Abs and Abz RAs were higher or, for some indices, comparable with those for the pre-diseased and diseased mice (groups 6 and 8; Table 6), while the levels of all HSC colonies formation, especially BFU-E and CFU-GEMM, were significantly lower for the pregnant females than for the pre-diseased and spontaneously diseased males and females (Table 7). Thus, the profile of HSC differentiation in the pregnant females (group 10) differs from those in the healthy non-pregnant, pre-diseased and diseased mice (groups 4, 6, and 8).

Four days after the beginning of lactation, a statistically significant 2.4-fold increase in the average number of CFU-GM colonies, the progenitors of neutrophils and macrophages, was observed, while the average increase in the formation of BFU-E and CFU-GEMM colonies was not statistically significant (Table 7). The HSC differentiation profile became formally comparable with that for young healthy males and females (groups 3 and 4, Table 7). Two weeks after the beginning of lactation, the indices of the differentiation profile again changed remarkably, the average number of CFU-GM colonies decreasing ~2-fold, with a 2.4- and 8.4-fold increase observed in BFU-E and CFU-GEMM colonies, respectively

Table 7). Interestingly, the changes in HSC differentiation profiles occur in parallel with a significant increase in the IgG RAs with the end of pregnancy and the beginning of lactation (4 days after delivery) and then a remarkable decrease in the Abz activities 14 days after the delivery (Table 6) [187-189].

5.3. Lymphocyte Proliferation in Different Mouse Organs

The relative levels of lymphocyte proliferation from different organs of MRL-lpr/lpr mice in the absence and in the presence of mitogen have been analyzed (Table 8) [187-189]. Spontaneous development of SLE with high proteinuria leads to a remarkable increase in lymphocyte proliferation in all analyzed organs of males and females (groups 8 and 7) as compared with the control young mice (groups 3 and 4). In spite of a significant difference in the RAs of Abzs from the immunized males (group 9) and the males or females spontaneously developing SLE (groups 7 and 8), all these groups were characterized by comparable levels of lymphocyte proliferation, which on average were significantly higher than in the control (groups 3 and 4; Table 8). Interestingly, the pre-diseased males (group 5) demonstrated proliferation indices intermediate between the control (group 3) and the spontaneously diseased males (group 7). In the presence of mitogen, the level of proliferation of lymphocytes from all organs of these mouse groups increased 2–20-fold depending on the organ analyzed, with the highest increase observed for thymus and spleen cells (Table 8).

Transition from the control (group 4) to pregnant females (group 10) associated with an appearance of detectable Abz activities (Table 6) led to a 6.7-fold statistically significant increase in the lymphocyte proliferation only in the thymus (group 10); for other organs, this index was also higher but the differences were not statistically significant (Table 8). The beginning of lactation (4 days after delivery, group 11) associated with the highest increase in different Abz RAs (Table 6) led to statistically significant 3.3- and 6.3-fold increases in proliferation of cells from thymus and spleen, respectively, in comparison with the control females (group 4), while a 1.5–1.8-fold increase in this index for bone marrow and lymph nodes was statistically insignificant (Table 8). From a comparison of the pregnant (group 10) and lactating females (group 11), it can be seen that a statistically significant 6.3-fold increase in lymphocyte proliferation was observed only for cells from the spleen, while proliferation of the cells from thymus and lymph nodes decreased 1.6–2.0-fold in the lactating mice. Interestingly, a 1.9–2.3-fold decrease in RAs of Abzs (Table 6) in the mice lactating for 14 days in comparison with the females 4 days after delivery occurs in parallel with a 2.9- and 1.6-fold decrease in the lymphocyte proliferation in bone marrow and spleen, respectively, while this indices for thymus and spleen cells were comparable (Table 8). Activation of the cells from pregnant and lactating females with mitogen led to a minimal ~2-fold increase in bone marrow cell proliferation, while this factor was significantly higher for cells from other organs (10–44-fold, Table 8) [187-189].

Table 8. Lymphocyte proliferation in mouse organs [187-189]

Group description[†]	Group number	Number of mice	Proliferation level × 10^{-2}, cpm[*]							
			Bone marrow		Lymph nodes		Thymus		Spleen	
			-	+Con A	-	+Con A	-	+Con A	-	+Con A
CBA (3-7 mo)	1	8	28.1±5.4	n.d.**	11±3.2	n.d.	11±2.8	n.d	40±8.7	n.d
Males										
Healthy (2-3 mo)	3	5	nd	nd	12 ± 7.3	24.7±16.3	5.6 ± 0.95	105±22	13.7 ± 5.4	256±59
Healthy pre-diseased (7 mo)	5	5	nd	nd	17.5 ± 3.4	**157 ± 63**[‡]	10.1 ± 3.7	179 ± 53	**38.6 ± 2.2**	405 ± 109
Diseased (7 mo)	7	5	41±15.6	66.6 ± 45.7	14.6±9.1	**249 ± 154**	15.6± 9.3	160 ± 81	29.3± 10.6	300 ± 82.5
Immunized (3 mo)	9	5	37.6±24.7	49.6 ± 35.7	20.4±19.0	**189 ± 144**	7.0± 6.0	84 ± 61	33.0± 23.0	245 ± 163
Females										
Healthy pre-diseased (2-3 mo)	4	5	25.4±12.2	24.8 ± 10.8	4.4±1.8	254 ± 169	2.7± 1.0	106 ± 33	7.1± 4.4	215 ± 83
Diseased (7 mo)	8	5	23±9.1	35 ± 10	7.7±6.0	196 ± 58	7.7± 4.5	186 ± 118	22± 11.8	246 ± 115
Pregnant (2-3 mo)	10	5	36.8±8.4	55.4 ± 23.7	10.3±6.3	279± 85	**18.2± 9.3**	153 ± 57	5.1± 2.4	nd
Lactating (3 mo) 4 days after delivery	11	5	44.9 ± 11.4	**93.1 ± 29.4**	6.6±3.9	340 ± 162	**8.8± 0.9**	108 ± 35	**44.4± 18.4**	**525 ± 115**
Lactating (3 mo) 14 days after delivery	12	5	15.8±5.4	29.6 ± 10.6	7.1±4.4	137 ± 57	6.7± 5.1	69 ± 66	27.1± 18.4	310 ± 159

[*]For each mouse, the mean and confidence interval of three experiments is shown.
**Not determined.
[†]MRL-lpr/lpr mice demonstrating no typical SLE indices or Abz activities (similar to healthy control non-AI mice) were conditionally designated healthy independently of age; the animals showing detectable levels of abzymes were conditionally designated pre-diseased.
[‡]Cohorts with statistically significant ($p \leq 0.05$) differences in the parameters in comparison with conditionally healthy MRL-lpr/lpr males and females are given in boldface.

5.4. Apoptosis Assay

The relative levels of apoptosis in different organs of various groups of MRL-lpr/lpr mice have been analyzed (Table 9) [187-189]. In the control young mice (groups 3 and 4) characterized by the absence of DNase and ATPase Abzs (Table 6), the level of apoptosis was comparable with that in the pre-diseased males (group 5) but was remarkably higher than in the diseased males and females demonstrating Abz activities (groups 7 and 8). The highest and statistically significant 2–3-fold decrease in apoptosis was observed for bone marrow, thymus and spleen of the immunized males (group 9), while the pregnant females (group 10) demonstrated a ~1.8-fold decrease in apoptosis in the bone marrow, lymph nodes, and thymus, and a 13-fold decrease in spleen lymphocyte apoptosis (Table 9). For the other groups of mice with spontaneously developed SLE (groups 8 and 9) or for the lactating females (groups 11 and 12), the average apoptosis indices were remarkably lower but there was no statistically significant difference between them. In the presence of mitogen, the level of apoptosis was increased 1.2–3-fold depending on the group of mice and the organs analyzed (Table 9) [187-189].

Table 9. Apoptosis in MRL-lpr/lpr mouse organs in the presence and in the absence of concanavalin A [187-189]

Group description[†]	Group number	Number of mice	Apoptosis level, fluorescence (relative units)*							
			Bone marrow		Lymph nodes		Thymus		Spleen	
			-	+Con A	-	+Con A	-	+Con A	-	+Con A
CBA (3-7 mo)	1	8	19.8±6.9	nd**	11.8±6.5	nd	12.7±6.4	nd	11.2±7.5	nd
Males										
Healthy (2-3 mo)	3	5	19.0±5.2	nd	11.5±0.5	18.5±1.0	12.2±2.0	23.0±3.0	10.0±1.0	13.2±3.0
Healthy pre-diseased (7 mo.)	5	5	15.0±4.2	nd	12.7±2.0	18.5±2.5	8.7±1.2	24.3±3.2	**17.0±2.1**[‡]	21.3±3.0
Diseased (7 mo)	7	5	9.8±2.3	14.6±6.0	7.6±2.6	9.1±1.9	7.9±4.2	14.6±7.8	11.2±1.9	15.6±5.5
Immunized (3 mo)	9	5	**6.1±2.3**	8.7±3.2	5.7±2.6	9.8±3.7	**6.1±4.2**	11.2±6.4	**4.8±1.9**	10.8±1.7
Females										
Healthy (2-3 mo)	4	5	17.8±5.1	24.6±6.1	15.2±4.3	26.1±8.7	14.4±5.2	22.2±7.3	19.5±5.6	26.6±8.4
Diseased (7 mo)	8	5	15.8±3.4	22.8±5.2	12.2±5.1	18.2±4.5	11.2±4.3	20.8±4.9	13.2±2.6	15.8±4.6
Pregnant (3 mo)	10	5	**9.2±2.7**	16.2±6.8	**7.0±2.3**	9.5±7.5	8.2±1.9	**13.2±2.7**	**1.5±0.5**	nd
Lactating (3 mo), 4 days after delivery	11	5	14.8±4.4	17.3±3.5	10.8±4.5	**9.2±2.7**	10.8±4.6	14.0±3.1	15.3±2.8	20.0±4.2
Lactating (3 mo), 14 days after delivery	12	5	12.2±6.5	13.3±7.2	**7.0±2.5**	9.2±5.0	10.5±4.0	**11.7±4.3**	9.4±4.3	11.8±4.4

*For each mouse, the mean and confidence interval of three experiments is shown.
**Not determined.
[†]MRL-lpr/lpr mice demonstrating no typical SLE indices or Abz activities (similar to healthy control non-AI mice) were conditionally designated healthy independently of age; the animals showing detectable levels of abzymes were conditionally designated pre-diseased.
[‡]Cohorts with statistically significant ($p \leq 0.05$) differences in the parameters in comparison with conditionally healthy MRL-lpr/lpr males and females are given in boldface.

5.5. Conclusion

The data in Table 6 and the analysis of time-dependent changes in mouse proteinuria, anti-DNA Abs, and Abz RAs before and after the development of visible pathological markers allow us to conclude that MRL-lpr/lpr mice of any age undergo a moderate increase in the concentration of urine protein, anti-DNA Abs, and enzymatic RAs 0.5-2.0 months before spontaneously developing pronounced pathology. Interestingly, only the increase in DNase and ATPase activities at a pre-disease stage (groups 5 and 6) was a decisive and unambiguously significant indicator of the beginning of specific AI-reactions (Table 6) [187-189].

Pregnancy and especially lactation, associated with a remarkable increase in anti-DNA Abs and with an appearance of Abz catalytic activities, should be considered special female conditions leading to specific AI reactions without a development of proteinuria and visible SLE markers (Table 6). These findings are in agreement with the literature data that clinically healthy pregnant women may be efficiently immunized by components of various viruses and bacteria, and autoimmunization of mothers may occur during pregnancy, similarly to the situation in AI patients ([23-27] and refs therein). This leads to appearance of anti-DNA Abs and different Abzs in the serum of pregnant women and then to a significant elevation of these markers in the serum and especially in the milk after the beginning of lactation. Interestingly, the level of DNase and ATPase activities of IgGs in the milk of lactating women did not change significantly in the first month after delivery and then slowly decreased by 40-80% during 2-6 months of the postnatal period [153, 160]. In mice, the Abz RAs after 14 days of lactation was ~2-fold lower than in mice lactating for 4 days, but the lactation period is ~7-10 times shorter in mice than in humans.

Although the mice were immunized with DNA, the ATPase and amylase activities of their Abs also increased greatly (Table 6). This was not surprising and was in agreement with the published data that immunization of AI mice produces an unexpectedly high increase in the number of clones secreting various auto-Abs, including Abzs, in comparison with normal mice [23-27, 151-152]. Lower levels of anti-DNA Abs and different Abzs in the diseased and pre-diseased mice as compared with the immunized mice (Table 6) may be due to a wider repertoire of different auto-Abs including DNase, ATPase, and amylase Abzs in the latter.

Table 7 shows significant differences in HSC differentiation profiles for all mouse groups analyzed. Our findings support the existence of specific and diverse relationships between the profile of HSC differentiation, lymphocyte proliferation, apoptosis and the Abz RAs in various mouse groups (Tables 6-9). Interestingly, the largest difference in lymphocyte proliferation in all mouse groups with high Abz activities (groups 7-10, 12) in comparison with the control mice (groups 3 and 4) is observed in the thymus and especially in the spleen, where B-lymphocyte progenitors differentiate into Ab-producing plasmocytes (Table 8).

Since immunized males demonstrate the highest levels of anti-DNA Abs and very high DNase and ATPase activities (Table 6), one can suppose that apoptosis suppression in these males can lead to an increased production of B-lymphocytes secreting anti-DNA Abs and Abzs. The Abzs production in all other mouse groups most probably results from specific balance of HSC proliferation and differentiation, lymphocyte proliferation, and apoptosis in different mouse organs. Taking into account these three factors, one can see two specific groups, the immunized and pregnant mice, significantly deviating from the controls and other mouse groups analyzed (Tables 7-9). Immunization of males leads to the highest increase in Abz activities, occurring in parallel with a significant decrease in apoptosis, especially in bone marrow, thymus and spleen (Table 9). A similar situation is observed in pregnant females (group 10), which demonstrate the largest decrease in apoptosis in all organs and especially in the spleen (Table 9). All other mouse groups show a general tendency towards a decrease in apoptosis in comparison with control groups, but usually it does not reach statistical significance. Thus, a significant decrease in apoptosis in the immunized and pregnant mice may be an important factor providing the increased number of specific lymphocytes producing auto-Abs and Abzs, which are normally eliminated. As a consequence, in contrast to control conditionally healthy young mice (groups 1-4) the serum of pregnant females is characterized by detectable levels of DNase and ATPase RAs, while immunized mice demonstrate the highest levels of these activities.

The pregnant and immunized mice (groups 9 and 10) differ from other groups in the HSC differentiation (Table 8) [187-189]. Interestingly, upon transition from young males or females (groups 3 and 4) to conditionally pre-diseased 7-months-old mice without proteinuria but with high Abz RAs (groups 5 and 6; Table 6), a significant change in HSC differentiation profile occurred: a 2.1–4.3-fold and a 16.4–18.4-fold increase in the number of GFU-GM and CFU-GEMM colonies was observed (Table 7). The higher number of CFU-GEMM was accompanied by a striking increase in their size. Interestingly, after the males and females spontaneously developed SLE associated with proteinuria and an increase in Abz RAs (groups 7 and 8), a significant increase in BFU-E and a decrease in GFU-GM and CFU-GEMM colonies was observed (Table 7). In contrast to the pre-diseased mice, the CFU-GEMM colonies of the diseased animals were of normal size. Thus, all mice demonstrating detectable level of Abzs activities without a significant increase in proteinuria and anti-DNA Abs can be considered pre-diseased; in comparison with conditionally healthy young mice they are characterized by a specific profile of HSC differentiation, increased lymphocyte proliferation in thymus and spleen, and increased apoptosis in spleen (Tables 7-9). The pre-diseased mice differ from the diseased mice (groups 7 and 8) in the profile of HSC differentiation, the size of CFU-GEMM colonies, the level of proteinuria, and Abz RAs, but there is no significant difference in apoptosis and lymphocyte proliferation [187-189].

Interestingly, the profile of HSC differentiation in immunized mice (group 9) is quite different from the pre-diseased (group 5) and spontaneously diseased mice (group 7), but comparable with that for young males and females (groups 3 and 4). In addition, bone marrow cell of the immunized males are characterized by low mitogen responsiveness (a 1.3-fold increase), while cells from the lymph nodes, thymus, and spleen are very sensitive to concanavalin A (a 7.4–12-fold increase, Table 8). These data and the similarity of the HSC differentiation profiles for the immunized and young control mice suggest that immunization with DNA does not remarkably affect bone marrow stem cells and that the significant increase in anti-DNA Abs and DNase or ATPase RAs is provided mostly by changes in proliferation and differentiation of lymphocyte progenitors in other mouse organs. The largest increase in lymphocyte proliferation in immunized males occurs in spleen (Table 8). Thus, the increased levels of anti-DNA Abs and Abzs in immunized mice may be mainly provided by an activation of lymphocyte differentiation and proliferation in different organs, first of all in the spleen, with a concomitant decrease in apoptosis. Very high urine protein concentration and visible markers of SLE demonstrated by the immunized males (Table 6) may be a result of kidney and spleen dysfunction [187-189].

As mentioned above, pre-disease is accompanied with a significant change in the profile of HSC differentiation in the spleen [187-189]. These changes in the mouse immune system are most likely only temporary, since a transition from the pre-diseased (groups 5 and 6) to diseased mice (groups 7 and 8) is associated not only with an increase in the level of anti-DNA Abs and different Abzs, but also with a significant change in the profile of HSC differentiation (Table 7). This change seems to be the most important factor in the irreversible switching of the mouse immune system to an autoimmune mode, since the changes in cell proliferation and apoptosis in different organs occur mainly on transition from healthy to pre-diseased mice and the observed differences in these indices between pre-diseased and diseased mice are insignificant (Tables 7-9).

Pregnant and lactating females are very interesting groups. A transition from control (group 4) to pregnant females (group 10) leads to: a) appearance of Abs catalytic activities (Table 6), b) a remarkable suppression of HSC proliferation (in particular, a 5-fold decrease in CFU-GEMM colonies) accompanied with small changes in the number of BFU-E and CFU-GM colonies (Table 7), c) a significant decrease in apoptosis in all organs and especially in the spleen (Table 9), and d) a change in lymphocyte proliferation in all organs analyzed and especially an increase in thymus cell proliferation (Table 8). These findings are in agreement with the literature data on specific "immuno-memory", a pregnancy-specific mode in which the mammalian immune system collects the information about possible environmental antigens harmful for newborns ([23-27, 153, 160, 174, 175] and refs therein). As a result, parenteral or oral administration of various antigens to animals late in pregnancy leads to the production of the corresponding Abs, which are accumulated at high levels in the serum and even more in milk [174, 175]. Autoimmunization may also occur to some degree during pregnancy. Specific stimulation of production of various Abs, including DNase Abzs, by the immune system of mothers after viral and bacterial infection, and an increase in milk Abzs RAs after allergic diseases during pregnancy were observed [157]. The beginning of lactation represents an important period when the pregnancy "immuno-memory" state switches into a new mode associated with production of different Abs and Abzs, which are found mostly in milk [23-26]. This switch is sometimes very dangerous for females since it may trigger pronounced immune reactions and autoimmune shock, a phenomenon well known in obstetrics. Many postnatal AI pathologies including SLE, Hashimoto's thyroiditis, phospholipids syndrome, polymyositis, AI myocarditis, etc. can be stimulated by pregnancy in initially healthy women [170, 173]. These AI diseases may develop without a strong increase in immune reactions at the beginning of lactation, but more often autoimmune shock is a specific predictive marker of a future development of typical progressive or chronic AI diseases. AI reactions during pregnancy and after delivery are observed much more often than postnatal AI pathologies since AI reactions usually cease with the end of lactation. In contrast to pregnant and lactating women, AI reactions in AI patients are usually permanent and the pathologies have chronic character with temporary remissions and exacerbations. Taking these observations together, one can suppose that there may be a significant difference in the mechanisms of AI reactions in lactating females and in patients with AI pathologies. At the same time, one cannot exclude that the molecular mechanisms of immune system activation leading to the production of autoreactive Abs and/or auto-Abs are, to some extent, similar or overlapping in both AI patients and human mothers. Therefore a comparison of pre-diseased, diseased, pregnant or lactating mice is of a special interest.

During the pregnancy (group 10), a very specific reorganization of the profile of HSC differentiation as compared with other mouse groups occurred (Table 7). While the reorganization of HSC differentiation of the pre-diseased males in comparison with the healthy ones led to a 2–18-fold increase in the number of all colonies (CFU-GEMM, BFU-E, and CFU-GM), the group of pregnant females demonstrated a 1.4-fold decrease in CFU-GM and a statistically significant 5-fold decrease in CFU-GEMM colonies. This indicates not only a significant change in the bone marrow HSC differentiation profile, but also suppression of HSC proliferation in pregnant females. Bone marrow HSC proliferation in the pregnant mice was more significantly suppressed in comparison with the spontaneously pre-diseased and diseased mice; for example, the number of CFU-GEMM colonies in the pregnant females was 24–92-fold lower than in these two groups (Table 7).

Interestingly, in the pregnant females (group 10) as compared with the pre-diseased mice (group 5), a significant decrease in the values characterizing lymphocyte proliferation in the lymph nodes and especially in the spleen was observed, whereas the situation was the opposite in thymus (Table 8). In comparison with the pre-diseased and spontaneously diseased mice, the pregnant females were characterized by a very low level of apoptosis in different organs, which was comparable with that in the immunized males (Table 9). Thus, the immune system characteristics of pregnant females differ not only from those of healthy but also from the pre-diseased and diseased males. The most significant differences were observed in the formation of CFU-GEMM colonies and in the suppression of lymphocyte proliferation in different organs (Tables 7-9).

After the beginning of lactation (4 days after delivery), the profile of HSC differentiation and the level of proliferation of different bone marrow cells were sharply changed: the number of CFU-GEMM and especially CFU-GM colonies increased significantly, while the number of BFU-E colonies barely changed (Table 7). In parallel, we have found a decrease in the proliferation of lymphocytes from lymph nodes and thymus but an increase in the bone marrow cell proliferation (Table 8). A highest and statistically significant 6.3-fold increase in the spleen cell proliferation was observed. In addition, the beginning of lactation was associated with a tendency to increased apoptosis, and the largest and statistically significant 10-fold increase in spleen cell apoptosis was observed at transition from the pregnancy (group 10) to the beginning of lactation (group 11) (Table 9).

Later, 14 days after delivery, when all Abz RAs decreased 2–2.3-fold, a specific and strong change in HSC differentiation was observed again: a statistically significant 2.4- and 8.4-fold increase in the number of BFU-E and CFU-GEMM colonies, respectively, and a 2-fold decrease in the number of CFU-GM colonies was found (Table 7). Interestingly, late in the lactation (14 days after delivery, group 12) as compared with the beginning of lactation (group 11) there was a statistically significant 2.8-fold decrease only in the proliferation of bone marrow lymphocytes and a tendency to decreasing cell proliferation in spleen (1.6-fold decrease), while the proliferation indices for lymph nodes and thymus cells were comparable (Table 8). There was no difference in the apoptosis of lymphocytes from various organs of lactating females at 4 and 14 days after delivery (Table 9). Thus, the profile of HSC differentiation underwent several sequential changes: at the beginning of pregnancy, after delivery and in the late period of lactation. All these female-specific conditions were associated with the appearance of Abzs in the pregnant females, a very significant 6.1–9.3-fold increase in Abs RAs after the delivery, and a ~2-fold decrease in Abz RAs 14 days after the delivery. As was shown previously, different Abzs with very low activity can sometimes be detected in the sera of healthy donors [23-27]. However, we have found neither DNase nor ATPase Abzs in healthy mice, while the amylase activity was detectable in young mice, including the control non-AI mice (Table 6). Thus, Abzs may be ubiquitous even in healthy individuals. At the same time, the production of different Abzs in healthy mammals is most probably suppressed due to apoptosis of specific AI lymphocytes. During pregnancy, the apoptosis significantly decreased (Table 9), which may be the main reason of the increase in the number of clones producing anti-DNA Abs and different Abzs (Table 6). Taken together, our data suggest that during both transition states, pre-disease and pregnancy, significant but different changes in the differentiation and proliferation of bone marrow cell progenitors and in the apoptosis are observed (Table 7). A number of additional changes in the HSC differentiation, cell proliferation or apoptosis following the two transition states (pre-disease and pregnancy) lead to comparable increases in auto-Abs and Abzs production for diseased or lactating mice, but it seems that there may be significant differences in the specific characteristics of an immune system (e.g., clonal differentiation) in these cases in spite of the apparent similarity in the HSC differentiation profiles of the lactating (group 12) and spontaneously diseased females (group 8, Table 7).

It should be emphasized that our data on pregnant and lactating mice do not reveal all processes in their immune systems. Human and animal milk contains IgG, IgM, IgA, and sIgA, of which sIgA is the major component (>85-90%) [190]. After the beginning of lactation, the bulk of Abz activities in milk is due to sIgAs and to less extent to IgGs, while the specific activities of the serum Abzs are significantly lower ([153] and refs therein). sIgA is selectively produced by plasma cells residing in the interstitial tissue underlying the epithelial surfaces of the lactating breast [191]. These lymphoid cells migrate to the breast from the maternal intestinal lymphoid tissues (Peyer's patches) and from the lymphoid centers in the bronchial tree [191, 192]. The germinal-center B cells of Peyer's patches express mainly surface IgA along with some IgM or IgG [192]. Such isotype skewing is the result of B-cell heavy-chain gene switching in the course of clonal differentiation to the precursors of IgA-producing immunocytes, whose preferential induction is the hallmark of gut-associated lymphoid tissue [193]. Milk IgGs may be synthesized locally by such lymphoid tissue and also originate, at least partially, from the mother's circulation [194]. The serum Abs of AI patients are produced mainly by B lymphocytes of different organs.

The literature data (see above) and our findings suggest that AI diseases originate from specific changes in differentiation and proliferation of hematopoietic stem cells. From our point of view, the mechanisms of Abzs production and the biological roles of Abzs in lactating females and in patients with AI pathologies may be significantly different. After the beginning of lactation, female "immuno-memory" may be specifically switched to activate immunocytes in the Peyer's patches and lymphoid tissue producing milk Abs. The increase in Abzs activities in the serum associated with activated lymphocyte proliferation in the thymus and the spleen (Table 8) may be to some extent a side effect, since the change in HSC differentiation in pregnant and lactating females could mainly be aimed to modify the activity of Peyer's patches. As mentioned above, in contrast to AI diseases, all auto-Abs and Abzs usually disappear after the end of lactation. It means that the changes in differentiation and proliferation of bone marrow HSC and cells in other tissues and organs occurring in AI patients cannot be easy normalized, while the easy silencing of the "immuno-memory" in lactating women is a programmed phenomenon. Therefore, we infer that the formally similar profiles of HSC differentiation in lactating females 14 days after delivery and in spontaneously diseased females obscure a real existing difference in their immune status. In spite of the formal similarity of the immune system indices for the diseased and lactating mice, AI reactions in lactating females are not associated with kidney dysfunction and proteinuria, and these groups can differ significantly in a specific cell composition of BFU-E, CFU-GEMM, and CFU-GM colonies and in clonal differentiation of the specific lymphocyte precursors in different mouse organs. Nevertheless, our data also support the hypothesis that the mechanisms of auto-Abs and Abzs production in ill and in pregnant or lactating females overlap to some extent [187-189]. The suppression of AI processes in lactating females after the end of lactation implies an existence of special mechanisms, absent in AI patients, that switch the immune system back to normal.

6. EXTREME DIVERSITY OF ABZYMES IN AUTOIMMUNE DISEASES

As was mentioned in the Introduction, healthy humans cannot develop Abzs with detectable DNase and RNase activities, while IgGs and/or IgMs and IgAs hydrolyzing RNA, DNA, polysaccharides, peptides, and proteins have been described in the sera of patients with several AI and viral diseases. Intact IgGs from patients with asthma are mostly inactive in the hydrolysis of nucleic acids expect rare individuals, but separated light chains of IgGs appear to be more active in the hydrolysis of DNA [195].

During many infections, the human organism is exposed to different bacterial components including protein, DNA, RNA, and polysaccharides [125-131]. Because of their ability to bind a variety of exogenous antigens, including bacterial and viral ones, natural Abs play a major role in the primary line of defense against infections. Some results suggest that the synthesis of auto-Abs and Abs directed against bacterial antigens at least partially follow distinct pathways, but with the existing experimental data it is impossible to determine unambiguously whether these two Ab populations are produced by the same or distinct B-cell subpopulations [125]. Recently, DNase activity in the patients with diseases caused by several bacterial infections has been analyzed [196]. The catalytic activities were significantly lower than in patients with different AI pathologies and increased in the following order: streptococcal infection (erysipelas) < urogenital chlamydiosis associated with arthritis (Reiter's disease) < meningococcal meningitis < shigellosis < suppurative surgical infections caused by *Staphylococcus aureus* < suppurative surgical infections caused by epidermal staphylococci < urogenital ureaplasmosis associated with reactive arthritis. The RAs of IgGs in the hydrolysis of DNA increased in the following order: diabetes ≤ bacterial infections ≤ viral hepatitis < polyarthritis < Hashimoto's thyroiditis < AIDS ≤ MS < SLE ([23-27, 196] and refs therein).

6.1. Structural Diversity of Abzymes

Extreme structural diversity of Abzs with various activities including DNase and RNase was revealed using a number of different methods.

In functional studies, chromatographically separated light chains of IgGs from the sera of asthma patients were found to be active in the hydrolysis of VIP [197, 198]. The light chains hydrolyzed VIP with the specific activity 32-fold greater than that of Fab, and the hydrolytic activity was saturable [199]. The light chain of the VIP Abz was expressed in bacteria, purified, and found to possess an intrinsic catalytic activity [200]. Subsequently, single chain Fv constructs containing the VL domain of the anti-VIP light chain linked via a 14-residue peptide to its natural VH domain partner possessed an increased affinity for the substrate ground state. From these and other data, a model of catalysis by the anti-VIP Abs was proposed. According to the model, the essential catalytic residues are located in the VL domain and additional residues from the VH domain are involved in high-affinity binding of the substrate [198].

DNase, RNase, ATPase, and amylase Abzs may show very different contributions of variable domains of H and L-chains to their active centers. The Abz-dependent hydrolysis of DNA and RNA by isolated light chains of IgGs from SLE, MS, asthma, and other AI patients, as well as from MRL-lpr/lpr mice, is more efficient than by intact Abs [24-27, 186, 195, 201-203]. A similar situation was observed for human milk IgGs and sIgAs with DNase and RNase activities [155, 156]. In addition, both H and L-chains of sIgAs had affinity to DNA-cellulose but only L-subunits hydrolyzed DNA and RNA [156]. It was demonstrated that the catalytic center of recombinant variable fragment (scFv) of DNase IgGs from AI-prone MRL-lpr/lpr mice may be located at the interface between the light and heavy chains and that after separation both of these chains are able to hydrolyze DNA [185].

After mild treatment of IgG from the sera of MRL-lpr/lpr mice with 5% 2-mercaptoethanol followed by reducing SDS-PAGE, the amylase activity was revealed in the bands corresponding to the intact IgG (H_2L_2) and its partially reduced forms (H_2L, HL_2, and HL) as well as in the separated H and L chains [187].

Chemically active derivatives of ATP modify only the L-chain of H_2L_2 human milk pIgGs [160]. However, the separated L and H subunits of ATP-hydrolyzing milk IgG are not capable of hydrolyzing ATP. This activity can be detected only for the original milk IgGs (H_2L_2) and for its partially reduced forms, H_2L and HL. These data strongly suggest that the nucleotide-hydrolyzing activity is an intrinsic property of different oligomeric forms of L- and H-subunits of human milk IgGs and that the active center is localized on the interface between these subunits [160]. In contrast to human milk IgGs, pIgGs from the sera of diseased MRL-lpr/lpr mice and their isolated heavy and light chains efficiently hydrolyze different NTPs, NDPs, AMP, and dAMP, whereas Abs from the sera of control healthy mice are catalytically inactive [188].

The first example of Abzs present in all healthy humans and mammals was Ab with superoxide dismutase activity [133, 204, 205]. Recently we have reported that IgGs from the sera of healthy Wistar rats demonstrate horseradish peroxidase-like activity [206-209]. We have used different approaches to provide convincing evidence that this peroxidase activity and, in addition, a H_2O_2-independent oxidoreductase activity are intrinsic to rat IgGs. It was shown that intact pIgGs and their separated H- and L-chains possess both peroxidase and oxidoreductase catalytic activity [209].

From the crystal structure of a catalytic Ab with esterase-like activity, it was concluded that the ligand *p*-nitrophenyl acetate interacts with amino acid residues of both light and heavy chains of Abzs and that both types of subunits are required for catalysis [210]. Taken together, it is obvious that light and heavy chains of different Abzs can contribute to the active sites of Abzs in different ways. Thus, it is possible that polyclonal IgGs, IgAs, sIgA, and IgMs with different catalytic activities either can contain mixtures of Abzs with catalytic activity residing exclusively in light or heavy chains, or, similarly to mouse monoclonal DNase IgGs [185] and mouse polyclonal ATPase IgGs [188], the active centers may be located at the interface between the light and heavy chains, when only L-chains or a mixture of separated H- and L- chains can catalyze the hydrolysis of substrates.

The next question concerning the structural diversity of Abzs relates to the type of light chains of Abzs. SLE IgGs and IgMs purified on DNA-cellulose were fractionated on Sepharose bearing immobilized monoclonal antibodies against λ or κ L-chains of human Igs;

60-70 % of SLE IgGs and IgMs were adsorbed by Abs against κ L-chains and 30-40%, by Abs against λ L-chains [201, 202]. The fraction containing κ L-chains was 10–50-fold more active in the hydrolysis of both RNA and DNA. Analysis of subfractions of IgG F(ab) fragments by the same method led to identical conclusion.

IgGs from the sera of MS patients [203] and from milk of healthy human mothers with both λ ands κ L-chains also efficiently hydrolyze DNA and RNA [156, 157]. IgGs from MS patients containing light chains of the λ type are several fold more active in the hydrolysis of DNA than Abs with light chains of the κ type. At the same time, MS IgGs containing λ and κ light chains demonstrated comparable relative activities in the hydrolysis of human myelin basic protein (hMBP) [211].

Interestingly, different fractions of polyclonal IgGs from AI patients with DNase and RNase activities demonstrated different net charges when separated by chromatography on DEAE cellulose [212] and varied in their stability to heating and "acidic shock" [201, 202].

We have recently analyzed DNase activity of electrophoretically homogeneous preparations of IgGs from the sera of SLE patients after their separation by isoelectric focusing (Kuznetsova, personal communication). DNase activity was associated with many fractions of IgGs with the isoelectric points in the range 3–8. The same situation was observed for DNase IgGs from the sera of MRL-lpr/lpr mice that had spontaneously developed pronounced AI symptoms. Thus, in contrast to canonical enzymes, such as DNases I and II from human blood, subfractions of catalytic Abs can differ in their isoelectric points. This approach can also be used for additional characterization of structural diversity of polyclonal Abzs.

The next question concerning structural diversity of Abzs is related to a possibility of existence of catalytic Abs of different subclasses. IgGs of IgG1–IgG4 subclasses were analyzed for catalytic activity in the hydrolysis of hMBP [211]. IgGs of all four subclasses were catalytically active, with their contribution to the total MBP-hydrolyzing activity of Abzs and its 19-mer peptide increasing in the order: IgG1 (1.5–2.1 %) < IgG2 (4.9–12.8 %) < IgG3 (14.7–25.0 %) < IgG4 (71–78 %). Our findings suggest that the immune systems of individual MS patients generate a variety of anti-hMBP abzymes with different catalytic properties, which can attack hMBP of the myelin-proteolipid axon sheath, playing an important role in MS pathogenesis.

It was demonstrated that small fractions of MS IgGs of all four subclasses (IgG1–IgG4) are catalytically active in the hydrolysis of DNA and their relative activity (nM supercoiled DNA/1mg IgG/1 h) increases in the order: IgG1 (0.58) < IgG2 (0.94) < IgG3 (1.4) < IgG4 (4.1), while their approximate relative contribution to the total activity of Abzs increases in the following order: IgG1 (6.9 %) < IgG3 (9.3 %) < IgG2 (18.2 %) < IgG4 (65.6%) (Parkhomenko T., personal communication).

According to the catalytic center structure, canonical proteases belong to one of the following types: serine, thiol, acidic, and metal-dependent. Proteolytic IgGs from the sera of 95-100% of patients with AI diseases, including VIP-hydrolyzing IgGs from asthma [17], casein-hydrolyzing Abzs from human milk [143] and from HIV-infected patients [34], are serine protease-like, and their activity is greatly reduced after Abs incubation with the specific serine protease inhibitors PMSF or AEBSF.

Table 10. Inhibition of proteolytic activity of individual IgGs from ten AIDS patients by specific inhibitors of proteases of different types [35].

No. of prepration	Inhibition, %*				
	AEBSF	Leupeptin	Pepstatin A	Iodoacetamide	EDTA
IgG9	42±5	74±8	51±5	85±9	0
IgG10	0	70±7	0	83±9	96±9
IgG11	0	0	0	66±7	0
IgG12	0	0	0	66±5	44±5
IgG13	0	0	59±6	98±8	98±8
IgG14	0	0	0	87±7	3±1
IgG15	0	11±3	0	33±4	45±4
IgG16	0	0	0	78±8	40±3
IgG17	49±5	0	0	12±1.5	0
IgG19	0	0	0	49±5	2±1

*The decrease in the intensity of the initial IN band estimated from SDS-PAGE electrophoresis data, the initial IN intensity in the absence of inhibitor was taken for 100%. For each preparation, a mean and standard deviation of three experiments are shown.

Recently, we have analyzed possible catalytic diversity of the proteolytic activity of polyclonal IgGs and IgMs from MS patients [32, 33]. Specific inhibitors of thiol and acidic proteases did not significantly affect the Ab-dependent hydrolysis of hMBP. The strongest inhibition of the proteolytic activity of IgGs and IgMs was observed after incubation of these Abzs with specific inhibitors of serine proteases (PMSF, AEBSF or benzamidine) or with EDTA. The effects of specific inhibitors of serine and metal-dependent proteases on the IgG-dependent hydrolysis of hMBP varied significantly from patient to patient: observed inhibition effects were 30-70% and 10-80%, respectively. Abs hydrolyzing MBP was the first example of Abzs with metalloprotease activity [32-33]. These data support the view of catalytic diversity of polyclonal hMBP-hydrolyzing Abz from MS patients.

The most surprising results were obtained for Abzs from HIV-infected patients specifically hydrolyzing viral integrase [35]. Inhibition of serine protease-like activity was observed only in two of ten preparations (Table 10). Five of ten AIDS IgGs were significantly (≥40%) inhibited by EDTA (Table 10), which was comparable with the picture for IgGs from MS patients [33-34]. A significant effect of pepstatin A (inhibition >5-10%) on the proteolytic activity of two Abz preparations, IgG9 and IgG13, was revealed. Iodoacetamide, a specific inhibitor of thiol proteases, usually does not significantly affect the activity of proteolytic Abzs (≤3-7% inhibition) [30-34, 143]. Therefore, it was surprising that the integrase-hydrolyzing activity of AIDS IgGs could be suppressed in all 10 preparations for 12–98% (mean ± S.D., 65.7±20.6 %; Table 10), which is quite different from other known proteolytic Abzs.

Our findings support the idea that anti-integrase pIgGs of AIDS patients can contain Abzs of four types resembling thiol, serine, acidic, and metal-dependent proteases, the ratio of which may be individual for every patient [35]. Since the proteolytic activity of IgG9 was suppressed significantly (42-85%) by specific inhibitors of serine, acidic, and thiol proteases, it is possible that the immune system of HIV-infected patients produces anti-integrase Abzs with a combined structure of the active center, which may carry amino acid residues typical of different proteases. We also suggest that IgG10 may be Abzs with the combined structure of the active center containing structural elements of thiol and metal-dependent proteases, while IgG13 in addition can contain a carboxylic side chain.

Taking these data together, it is obvious that catalytic Abs may be very different in their structural properties, which may change significantly depending on the Ab enzymatic activity, specific AI disease, and even patient analyzed.

6.2. Diversity of Enzymatic Functions of Abzymes

Canonical enzymes usually catalyze only one chemical reaction [213, 214]. For example, DNases hydrolyze only DNA and are inactive in the hydrolysis of RNA, while RNases cannot hydrolyze DNA. However, there are some examples of enzymes possessing several enzymatic functions, for example phosphomonoesterases and phosphodiesterases can hydrolyze non-specifically RNA and DNA with comparable efficiency [213, 214]. Interestingly, the same polyclonal IgGs, IgAs and IgMs from the sera of patients with several studied AI and viral diseases or from human milk possess both DNase and RNase activities and their relative activity in the hydrolysis of RNA is often significantly higher than in the hydrolysis of DNA [23-27, 156, 157, 201, 202, 215-219]. Several monoclonal mouse SLE IgGs against B-DNA of different sequences efficiently hydrolyze single- and double-stranded DNA and RNA in a sequence-independent manner, with the hydrolysis of RNA being 30–100-fold faster than of DNA [220].

The properties of the ATP-hydrolyzing milk IgG distinguish it from other nucleotide-hydrolyzing enzymes. In contrast to known ATPases [221, 222], milk IgGs utilize not only ATP, but also other NTPs and dNTPs as substrates with comparable efficiencies [160]. In addition, catalytic IgGs from the serum and milk of human mothers were shown to hydrolyze not only NTPs, but also NDPs and NMPs. It is known that some phosphatases are also capable of hydrolyzing not only NMPs, but also NDPs and NTPs at a significantly lower rate [221, 222]. Nevertheless, in contrast to known phosphatases, milk catalytic IgGs hydrolyze NTPs faster than NMPs and are activated by Mg^{2+} ions.

Similarly to human milk Abs, pIgGs from the sera of diseased MRL-lpr/lpr mice utilize ATP and other NTPs, NDPs, and AMPs as substrates with comparable efficiencies [188]. The affinity of human milk IgGs for ATP is 1–2 orders of magnitude higher than that of other ATPases and phosphatases [221, 222]. Interestingly, the relative affinity of nucleotide-hydrolyzing mouse IgGs for nucleotides [188] is 500–1000-fold lower than that of human milk IgGs [160]. At the same time, mouse IgGs hydrolyze ATP and AMP 80–2600-fold faster than human milk IgGs. Some other catalytic properties of human milk and mouse IgGs are similar. Orthophosphate (P_i) is the main product of hydrolysis of all nucleotides and formation of di- (PP_i) or triphosphate (PPP_i) was not observed. Moreover, both catalytic IgGs did not hydrolyze p-nitrophenylphosphate or α-naphtylphosphate, two typical substrates of known phosphatases [221, 222]. Overall, the substrate specificity of human milk and mouse serum catalytic IgG is completely different from those of known ATPases and phosphatases.

Since the NTP-, NDP, and NMP-hydrolyzing activities of human and mouse IgGs were studied using the same preparation of catalytic Abs, it was interesting to consider why the same IgGs can demonstrate different or similar properties in hydrolysis of nucleoside-5'-

mono, di-, and triphosphates. On one hand, it is plausible that these two catalytic activities reside within the same protein, since monoclonal lupus IgGs which recognize different specific DNA sequences show both DNase and RNase activities [185]. On the other hand, a mixture of different catalytic Abs that hydrolyze ATP, ADP, or AMP may be present in the polyclonal pool of milk IgGs. At the same time, it seems possible that the fraction of polyclonal IgG may contain a mixture of a limited number of ATP/AMP-hydrolyzing Abs and a greater number of catalytic IgGs hydrolyzing only AMP [160].

It should be noted that the same pIgG preparations from the sera of diseased MRL-lpr/lpr mice possess DNase and nucleotide-hydrolyzing activity [188]. We therefore addressed the question whether the same monoclonal fractions of pIgGs can hydrolyze both DNA and mononucleotides. Using mouse pIgGs it was shown that mononucleotides and DNA are hydrolyzed by different subfractions of pIgG, and only AMP effectively competes with ATP (and vice versa) for the nucleotide-binding site of the specific subfractions of mouse pIgGs [188]. In addition, four preparations of monoclonal mouse IgGs efficiently hydrolyzed both ATP and AMP, but did not hydrolyze plasmid scDNA or short oligonucleotides. Only one of four monoclonal IgGs possessed a very low 5'-phosphatase activity removing the phosphate group from the 5'-end of $d(pN)_{10}$ oligonucleotides Thus, the same monoclonal Abzs cannot hydrolyze DNA and mononucleotides. However, some Abzs combine to some extent the enzymatic properties of canonical ATPases and phosphatases. It was interesting how monoclonal Abs possessing two or more activities may be produced by individual immune systems. We tried to understand this phenomenon of Abzs using model experiments; healthy rabbits were immunized with DNA, RNA, DNase I, DNase II, and pancreatic RNase A [146-150].

Table 11. Relative content (RC) and relative total activity (RA) of IgGs from rabbits immunized with different immunogens in the hydrolysis of scDNA and poly(C) in five subfractions (protein peaks) separated by chromatography on DNA-cellulose [146-150]

Peak no.[#]	Elution conditions*	Non-immunized		DNA		RNA	
		RC, %	RA, DNase (RNase), %	RC, %	RA, DNase (RNase), %	RC, %	RA, DNase (RNase), %
0	Non-fractionated	100*	0 (0)	100	100 (100)*	100	100 (100)
1	0.0 M NaCl	68.8	0 (0)	22.5	87.4 (38.3)	56.0	0 (0)
2	0.1 M NaCl	9.3	0 (0)	5.7	12.6 (26.2)	11.0	30.0 (0)
3	0.5 M NaCl	17.1	0 (0)	66.6	0 (35.5)	29.0	68.7 (100)
4	3 M NaCl	4.8	0 (0)	5.2	0 (0)	4.0	1.3 (0)
5	pH 2.6	0	0 (0)	0	0 (0)	0	0 (0)
		DNAse I		DNase II		Ribonuclease A	
0	Non-fractionated	100	100 (100)	100	100 (100)	100	100 (100)
1	0.0 M NaCl	37.3	9.3 (0)	55.6	5.5 (19.7)	45.0	6.0 (0)
2	0.1 M NaCl	18.2	29.5 (0)	11.1	25.7 (52.9)	22.6	67.5 (44.7)
3	0.5 M NaCl	34.2	54.6 (100)	28.3	27.8 (27.4)	15.8	6.4 (55.3)
4	3 M NaCl	0	0.0 (0)	2.0	22.3 (0.0)	7.8	11.3 (0)
5	pH 2.6	10.3	6.6 (0)	3.0	18.6 (0.0)	8.8	8.8 (0)

*Salt concentration of the buffer used for elution of the IgG fraction from DNA-cellulose are shown (see Figure 1).
[#]Peak numbers are the same for all five chromatographies as in Figure 1

It is known that different auto-Abs, including Abs to DNA and to different enzymes interacting with DNA, are contained in the sera not only from AI patients but also from healthy human and mammals [223, 224]. DNase and RNase pIgGs from the sera of AI patients are usually very heterogeneous in their affinity for DNA and can be separated into several fractions by chromatography on DNA-cellulose ([23-27] and refs therein). In addition, DNA and DNA-cellulose can interact not only with anti-DNA Abs but also with Abs against phospholipids, polysaccharides, cell surface proteins, etc., demonstrating cross-reactivity with DNA [27, 223-225].

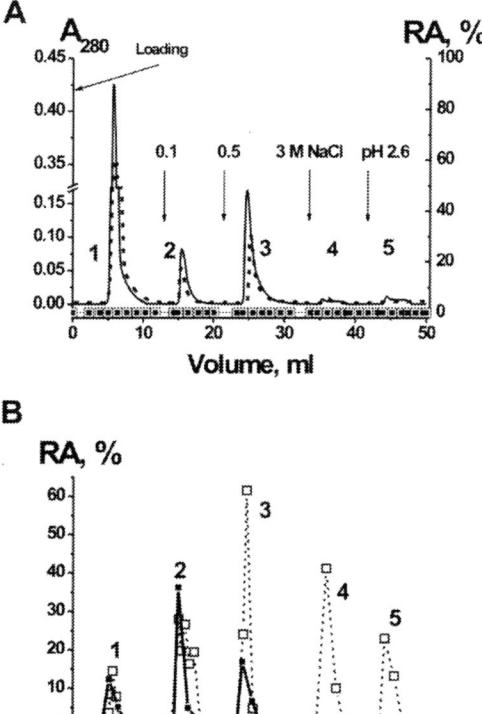

Figure 1. Affinity chromatography of pIgG preparations from the sera of two rabbits on DNA cellulose: (—) and (- - -), absorbance at 280 nm for non-immunized and immunized rabbit IgGs respectively (A). The relative (RA) DNase (□) and RNase (■) activities of IgG fractions eluted from the sorbent by different concentrations of NaCl are shown for the non-immunized (A) and immunized rabbit (B). The complete conversion of 4.43 nM scDNA to its hydrolyzed forms after 18 h and the complete hydrolysis of 140 μM poly(C) after 2.5 h were taken for 100% RA in the hydrolysis of DNA and RNA, respectively. Errors in the initial rate determination from two experiments for each fraction did not exceed 7–12% [150]

We have compared the affinity of pIgGs from the sera of non-immunized rabbits and the animals immunized with DNA, RNA, DNase I, DNase II, and RNase A for DNA by chromatography on DNA-cellulose using the same conditions of chromatography [146-150]. The proteins were eluted with the same buffer containing different concentrations of NaCl (0.1–3 M) and then with 50 mM glycine-HCl, pH 2.6; finally, five peaks of Abs possessing different affinity for DNA were obtained for every immunogen. For example, Figure 1 demonstrates representative data for IgGs from the rabbit immunized with DNase II and non-immunized animals [150]. Similar to IgGs from healthy humans [23-27], a fraction of pIgGs from non-immunized rabbits (26–31% depending on the rabbit) interacted with DNA cellulose, but all fractions eluted from the resin were catalytically inactive (Figure 1A). Immunization of rabbits with DNA, RNA, DNase I, DNase II, and RNase A led to an increase in the fraction of pIgGs interacting with DNA cellulose, depending on the immunogen, to 44–77.5% under the condition used.

The data for all immunogens are summarized in Table 11. The pIgG fractions of the first peak with very low affinity for DNA, eluted in the flow-trough, possessed detectable DNase activity in the case of all immunogens except RNA, while RNase activity was not observed for RNA, DNase I, and RNase A as immunogens (Table 11). Interestingly, an immunization by each of five antigens induced a specific repertoire of Abzs. For example, anti-DNA and anti-RNA Abs did not contain Abz subfractions with high affinity for DNA-cellulose (eluted with 3 M NaCl and acidic buffer), while immunization of rabbits with DNase I, RNase and DNase II results in an appearance of such subfractions [146-150]. Only pIgGs of the peak eluted with 0.5 M NaCl possessed both DNase and RNase activity in the case of anti-DNase I [148], and anti-RNA [147] abzymes, while several peaks with both activities were observed for anti-DNA (peaks 1 and 2), anti-RNase (peaks 2 and 3), and anti-DNase II Abzs (peaks 1-3, Figure 1). Only in the case of anti-DNA Abzs the fractions of the third peak eluted with 0.5 M NaCl hydrolyzed only RNA and were inactive with DNA (Table 11). Abs against all five antigens corresponding to five possible peaks resolved by chromatography on DNA-cellulose demonstrated very different k_{cat} values and ratios of these values in the hydrolysis of DNA and RNA (Tables 12 and 13). The k_{cat} values characterizing the hydrolysis of DNA and RNA by non-fractionated IgGs from rabbits immunized with DNA, RNA, DNase I, RNase, and DNase II varied in a wide range: $1.7 \times 10^{-6} - 2.5 \times 10^{-4}$ min^{-1} (DNA) and 0.025–0.22 min^{-1} (RNA) Thus, DNA- and RNA-hydrolyzing Abzs may be of very different nature and with very different properties, hydrolyzing only DNA, only RNA or both these substrates, like monoclonal mouse anti-DNA Abs [220]. In addition, each immunogen stimulating the formation of DNase and RNase Abzs induces a specific repertoire of Abzs with very different enzymatic properties.

A very interesting question is why all immunogens (DNA, RNA, DNase I, DNase II, and RNase A, and most probably other enzymes hydrolyzing nucleic acids) can stimulate the formation of Abzs with RNase and DNase activities, while canonical enzymes usually possess only one of these activities. The immune system can theoretically produce up to 10^6 different Ab variants in response to a single antigen. At the same time, chemical and structural patterns of DNA and RNA, as well as different nucleases hydrolyzing DNA and RNA, have a number of similarities. One can propose that 10^6 possible Ab variants against one immunogen may vary in their closeness of fit to the structure of antigen, some of them possess better complementarity to other cognate antigens than to immunogen itself. In addition, spontaneous mutagenesis of lymphocyte DNA coding for Abzs could also produce Abs somewhat mismatched to the immunogen used.

As mentioned above, immunization of healthy animals leads mainly to the changes in differentiation and proliferation of lymphocytes of different organs, while the Abzs production in diseased AI mice is associated with combinations of changes in proliferation and differentiation of bone marrow hematopoietic stem cells and lymphocytes in different mouse organs [187-189]. Therefore, immunization of AI mice produces an unexpectedly high increase in the number of clones secreting various auto-Abs, including Abzs, as compared with normal mice [27, 151, 152]. Thus, catalytic reaction diversity of different abzymes in AI patients can be much more significant.

6.3. Affinity and Relative Catalytic Activity Diversity of Abzymes

In principle, some Abzs can be produced not only in AI patients, but also in healthy humans (see above). However, even plasmid scDNA nicking, the most sensitive DNase assay, did not detect DNase activity of Abs from healthy humans [23-27]. Similar results were obtained for healthy mice, in which detectable activity of IgGs was revealed only after immunization with DNA or spontaneous development of SLE [186, 189].

Interestingly, separated light chains of IgGs interacting with DNA are usually more active that intact IgGs and sometimes, using scDNA, it is possible to reveal a very low activity of a small fraction of healthy human IgGs after their reduction with 2-mercapthoethanol [23-27]. On one hand, it may be hypothesized that the activity of light chains arises from their ability to recognize the transition state of the reaction of substrate hydrolysis and therefore they are more active than oligomeric forms of intact Abzs. However, it may be a consequence of a higher affinity of intact Abs, as compared with separated light chains, for different substrates due to interaction of the substrates with both light and heavy chains of Abzs. In such cases, separation of the light chains can lead to a decrease in the lifetime of the existence of the complex and, as a consequence, to an increase in the turnover number and V_{max} of the reaction catalyzed by L-chains.

Several examples of Abzs with amylase and protease activities from AI patients were described above. The generation of all discussed Abzs with different catalytic activities is associated with AI processes in autoimmune or healthy humans and animals; however all healthy humans and other mammals possess Abzs with oxidoreductase activities [204-209].

As we have shown previously, the fraction of polyclonal Abzs with different catalytic activities including nuclease Abzs in the serum of AI patients usually does not exceed 1–7% of total Igs [22-26]. At the same time, no current method can efficiently separate Abzs from catalytically inactive Abs, or separate catalytic Abs with, for example, only RNase and only DNase activities. Chromatography of pAbs on different affinity sorbents leads usually only to a partial enrichment of individual fractions of Abzs with specific activity; the specific activities of the individual monoclonal subfractions in a pAb pool may be significantly higher than those of the non-fractionated or partially purified pAbs. Therefore, the specific activities of polyclonal Abs were usually characterised using the total concentration of non-fractionated or partially purified Abs [23-27]. To provide a quantitative estimate of the Abzs activities, the reactions are usually performed under pseudo first order conditions within the linear regions of the time courses. In this case, catalytically inactive Ab subfractions, either interacting with specific substrate or not, do not affect the apparent K_M values. The measured k_{cat} values usually characterize the relative content of catalytically active Abzs subfractions in the total pool of physically homogeneous pAbs. Since polyclonal Abzs usually contain a major subfraction characteristic of each pathology and the individual patient, the relative activities of non-fractionated Abs typically characterize the activity of the major subfraction with the highest activity [23-27].

The catalysis mediated by artificial Abzs is usually characterized by relatively low reaction rates: k_{cat} values are 10^2-10^6-fold lower than for canonical enzymes [16]. The known k_{cat} values for natural Abzs from AI patients catalyzing many different chemical reactions vary in the range of 0.001–40 min^{-1} ([23-27] and refs therein).

Polyclonal DNase Abzs from AI patients and from human milk usually demonstrate relatively low specific activities, 0.001–5% of those of known human DNases and RNases, Abzs from human milk usually being more active [27]. However, the RAs of Abs from the sera of AI patients vary markedly from patient to patient. Figure 2 illustrates cleavage of plasmid DNA by Abs from various patients with different ADs after 2 h of incubation. During this time, some Abs cause only single breaks in one strand of supercoiled DNA converting it to the relaxed form (lanes 1-3), whereas others cause multiple breaks causing DNA linearization (lanes 4-6). The most active Abs hydrolyze DNA into short and medium-length oligonucleotides (lanes 7-10). It should be reiterated that Figure 2 illustrates a range of possible changes in the relative DNase activities in patients with different AI and viral diseases. The percentage of patients with low (only DNA relaxation), intermediate (partial DNA degradation) and high DNase activity (cleavage into short oligonucleotides) usually significantly changes from one pathology to another ([23-27] and refs therein). Interestingly, the specific DNase and RNase activities of IgM from the sera of SLE patients usually exceed those of IgG 5–20-fold [201, 202], and we have recently observed a similar situation for IgMs and IgAs with MBP-hydrolyzing activity from MS patients [32]. The switch from production of IgM to IgG antibodies may be accompanied by selection of Abzs possessing lower catalytic efficiency [32].

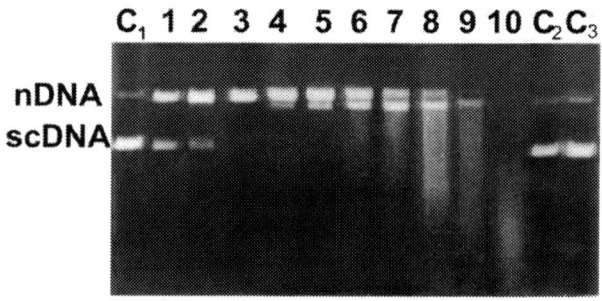

Figure 2. DNase activities of catalytic IgGs from patients with different ADs in the cleavage of supercoiled (sc) and nicked (n) plasmid DNA. Lanes 1–10, IgGs from the sera of 10 different patients; C_1, scDNA incubated alone; C_2 and C_3, scDNA incubated with Ab from the sera of two healthy donors [195, 196, 202, 203, 212, 216, 227, 249, 262, 263]

The RAs of IgGs from the sera of patients with different infectious diseases significantly varied from patient to patient but most of the Abs had detectable DNase activity [48, 196]. Interestingly, no IgGs from the patients with infectious diseases were found to fragment scDNA under conditions described above, and only relaxed plasmid DNA was formed. In these experiments the relative DNase activity corresponding to the complete transition of 10 µg/ml of scDNA to the relaxed form (3.35 nM, 100%) in the presence of 0.1 mg/ml Abs is equal to 16.7 nM nicked DNA / 1 h / 1 mg of Abs. The relative activities of IgGs corresponding to these patients increased in the following order: streptococcal infection (17.2 ± 7.0 %) ≤ urogenital chlamydiosis associated with arthritis (17.8 ± 10.1) ≤ meningococcal meningitis (19.0 ±13.7 %) ≤ shigellosis (21.3 ± 13.7 %) ≤ suppurative surgical infections caused by *S. aureus* (32.1 ± 7.4 %) ≤ suppurative surgical infections caused by epidermal staphylococci (34.5 ± 9.6 %) < urogenital ureaplasmosis associated with reactive arthritis (96.3 ± 1.1 %).

In contrast to canonical DNase I and Abzs from AI patients [23-27] and similarly to patients with diseases caused by bacterial infections [48, 196], IgGs from healthy rabbits immunized with DNA, RNA, DNase I, DNase II, and RNase A formed only relaxed DNA and were not able to produce linear DNA, and the type of scDNA hydrolysis did not depend on the Ab concentration and the time of incubation [146-150]. The k_{cat} values (0.5–8.7×10^{-4} min^{-1}) characterizing scDNA hydrolysis by rabbit IgG subfractions (Tables 12 and 13) are significantly lower than for the hydrolysis of scDNA by IgGs from SLE patients (k_{cat} = 14–40 min^{-1}) [226] or k_{cat} values (2.7×10^{-2}–11.3 min^{-1}) estimated for d(pN)$_{10-13}$ oligonucleotide hydrolysis by polyclonal Abzs from SLE patients and from human milk [156, 157, 201, 202]. These k_{cat} values are also lower than those for Abzs from patients with bacterial infections (0.1–7.0×10^{-2} min^{-1}) [146-150] and comparable with those for artificial Abzs obtained by immunization of healthy non-AI animals. Overall, all kinetic and thermodynamic characteristics of DNase Abzs from patients with bacterial infections are closer to those for healthy animals immunized with DNA, RNA, and nucleases than to the parameters of Abzs from patients with different AI pathologies. The relative DNase activity of Abs was strongly dependent on individual patients or immunized animals, but in general increased in the following order: immunized rabbits ≤ diabetes < bacterial infections < hepatitis < polyarthritis <AID ≤ HT< MS ≤ SLE.

Interestingly, the specific activities of RNase IgGs and IgMs from the sera of patients with different AI diseases may be 10–1000-fold higher than those of DNase Abzs from the same patients. RNase activities of AI Abzs were 0.1–20% of that of RNase A and of six known human sera RNases, while poly(A) was hydrolyzed by AI Abzs 2–10 times faster than by RNase A, one of the most active RNases known [19, 212, 216, 217, 227]. The specific activity of homogeneous Abs of several SLE and MS patients was 40–400% of that of RNase A [227]. The pH dependences and salt effects also varied in different patients but the activity was specifically stimulated by Mg^{2+} ions, which nearly completely inhibit all known human RNases.

Among the most active were Abzs from MRL-lpr/lpr mice hydrolyzing different nucleotides; the k_{cat} values for ATP and AMP as substrates varied in the range 82–370 min^{-1} [188]. Interestingly, the highest k_{cat} values were observed for IgGs from healthy Wistar rats with H_2O_2-independent peroxidase and H_2O_2-independent oxidoreductase activities [206-209]. In the absence of external metal ions, the specific peroxidase activity of IgGs from the sera of different rats varied in the range 1.6–26% (as compared with horseradish peroxidise, HRP; k_{cat} = 1.1×10^4 min^{-1} taken for 100%) and increased up to 13–198% after addition of Fe^{2+} or Cu^{2+} ions. The oxidoreductase activity of HRP is 24-fold lower than its peroxidase activity, while oxidoreductase and peroxidase activities of IgGs are comparable. Oxidoreductase activities of different rat IgGs in the absence of external metal ions varied from 22 to 800%, and in the presence of Fe^{2+} or Cu^{2+} ions, from 37 to 1100% in comparison with the HRP oxidoreductase activity [207]. It should be mentioned that peroxidase and oxidoreductase activities of IgGs from the sera of healthy humans are about 1-2 order of magnitude lower than those for rats (Tolmacheva A., personal communication).

Table 12. K_m and k_{cat} values characterizing five pIgG fractions (Figure 1) from the sera of rabbits immunized with DNA, RNA, DNase I, DNase II, and RNase A in the hydrolysis of plasmid scDNA [146-150]*

No. of the fraction[#]	Conditions of IgG elution from DNA-cellulose**	Immunogen used; apparent K_m and k_{cat} values in the hydrolysis of plasmid scDNA			
		K_m, nM*	$k_{cat} \times 10^4$, min^{-1}*	K_m, nM*	$k_{cat} \times 10^4$, min^{-1}*
		DNA		RNA	
0	Non-fractionated	58.9±13.9	2.5±0.3	20.0±5.0	0.017 ± 0.002
1	0.0 M NaCl	68.1±11.4	6.9±0.7	0	0
2	0.1 M NaCl	21.5 ± 4.0	4.7 ± 0.4	21.0 ± 5.0	0.07 ± 0.02.
3	0.5 M NaCl	0.0	0.0	12. 0 ±3.0	0.12.0± 0.2
		DNase I		DNase II	
0	Non-fractionated	8.8±1.0	1.28 ± 0.02. 0.28 ± 0.02	15.8±2.0	1.0±0.1
1	0.0 M NaCl	68.7 ± 8.8	0.1 ± 0.015	60.8 ± 10.5	0.53 ± 0.08
2	0.1 M NaCl	9.5 ± 1.5	0.28 ± 0.035	18.3 ± 3.5	2.2 ± 0.4
3	0.5 M NaCl	7.0 ±0.8	0.46 ± 0.07	13.5 ±2.5	8.7 ± 1.7
4	3 M NaCl	0.0	0.0	0.8 ± 0.1	3.9± 0.5
5	pH 2.6	0.36 ± 0.05	0.16 ± 0.02	0.5 ± 0.09	1.1 ± 0.2
		RNase A			
0	Non-fractionated	1.0 ± 0.4 15.4 ± 3.7	0.16 ± 0.05 0.61 ± 0.22		
1	0.0 M NaCl	18.3 ± 3.3	0.32 ± 0.04		
2	0.1 M NaCl	15.6 ± 1.6	4.7 ± 1.0		
3	0.5 M NaCl	11.3 ± 3.0	0.18 ± 0.03		
4	3 M NaCl	0.8 ± 0.1	0.3 ± 0.05		
5	pH 2.6	0.5 ± 0.1	0.45 ± 0.06		

*Five fractions for every immunogen were obtained by affinity chromatography of total pIgGs on DNA-cellulose as in Figure 1.

**Salt concentration of the buffer used for elution of the IgG fraction from DNA-cellulose are shown (see Figure 1).

[#]Peak numbers are the same for all five chromatographies as in Figure 1

The affinity of Abzs with DNase activity for DNA is usually high and corresponds to the typical affinity of Abs for nucleic acids [23-27]. The affinity of scDNA for DNase IgGs from rabbits immunized with DNA, RNA, DNase I, DNase II, and RNase A in terms of K_m (0.5–60.8 nM, Table 12) is comparable with the affinity of plasmid scDNA for IgGs from SLE (K_m = 43-92 nM) [226] and multiple sclerosis patients (0.36 nM) [203]. The DNA affinity characterizing different subfractions of rabbit pIgGs [146-150] and Abzs from AI patients [27, 201-203] is 3–4 orders of magnitude higher than that of bovine DNase I (K_m = 46–58 µM) [226].

Table 13. K_m and k_{cat} values characterizing five pIgG fractions (Figure 1) from the sera of rabbits immunized with DNA, RNA, DNase I, DNase II, and RNase A in the hydrolysis of poly(C) [146-150]*

No. of the fraction[#]	Conditions of IgG elution from DNA-cellulose**	Immunogen used; apparent K_m and k_{cat} in the hydrolysis of poly(C)			
		K_m, μM*	k_{cat}, min^{-1}*	K_m, μM*	k_{cat}, min^{-1}*
		DNA		RNA	
0	Non-fractionated	33.9 ± 7.8	0.22 ± 0.02	13.0 ± 2.0	0.025 ± 0.005
1	0.0 M NaCl	73.2 ± 14.8	0.32 ± 0.03	0	0
2	0.1 M NaCl	28.5 ± 3.0	3.5 ± 0.4	0	0
3	0.5 M NaCl	25.2 ± 5.6	1.1 ± 0.1	14.0 ± 2.0	0.1 ± 0.02
-	-	DNase I		DNase II	
0	Non-fractionated	13.4 ± 2.0	0.028 ± 0.003	32.9 ± 3.7	0.18 ± 0.02
1	0.0 M NaCl	0	0	83.7 ± 9.8	0.07 ± 0.01
2	0.1 M NaCl	0	0	34.2 ± 4.9	0.88 ± 0.09
3	0.5 M NaCl	12.2 ± 1.8	0.11 ± 0.015	15.4 ± 2.0	0.17 ± 0.025
-	-	RNase A			
0	Non-fractionated	18.4 ± 2.7	0.12 ± 0.2		
1	0.0 M NaCl	0.0	0.0		
2	0.1 M NaCl	18.4 ± 2.2	0.39 ± 0.04		
3	0.5 M NaCl	18.7 ± 2.6	0.69 ± 0.08		

*Five fractions for every immunogen were obtained by affinity chromatography of total pIgGs on DNA-cellulose as in Figure 1.
**Salt concentration of the buffer used for elution of the IgG fraction from DNA-cellulose are shown (see Figure 1).
[#]Peak numbers are the same for all five chromatographies as in Figure 1

Table 14 summarizes the RAs of human RNases and Abzs isolated from blood of patients with various ADs in various hydrolytic reactions. Interestingly, all IgG and IgM abzymes efficiently hydrolyzed poly(A), whereas RNase A and related human blood RNases were barely active with this substrate [19, 215-218, 227]. It is possible to discriminate the studied ADs on the basis of substrate specificity of the hydrolytic reaction catalyzed by the respective Abzs [217, 218]. The ratio of the rates of poly(A) to poly(C) hydrolysis catalyzed by RNases and Abzs is especially telling (Table 14).

The data concerning Abzs from the sera of patients with different AI diseases were indicative of catalytic and affinity heterogeneity of non-fractionated polyclonal Abs. The differences in the catalytic properties of Ab subfractions making up the total polyclonal Ab pool and their variations between patients may be demonstrated most clearly by comparison of the kinetics of hydrolysis of different substrates. Were polyclonal Abs to contain only one type of Abzs, the dependence of the initial rate on the substrate concentration for non-fractionated Abs should be consistent with Michaelis–Menten kinetics and give only one pair of K_m and V_{max} values. If polyclonal Abs contain more that one type of monoclonal Abzs, these dependences may be inconsistent with Michaelis–Menten kinetics and represent a sum of several hyperbolic curves corresponding to different Ab subfractions, but the contribution of some of them to the total curve may be small or indistinguishable from comparable K_m and k_{cat} values.

Table 14. Relative specific activities of pIgGs from the sera of patients with different autoimmune diseases in comparison with those for pancreatic RNase A and RNases from human blood in the hydrolysis of various ribopolynucleotides and cycloCMP [202, 212, 215, 216, 227]

Preparation	Relative specific activities, %*				
	cCMP	poly(U)	poly(A)	poly(C)	total RNA
RNases					
RNase A	100	2 *(200)***	0.01	100 *(10000)*	15 *(1500)*
Human blood RNases	not determined	3-16	0	100	5-10
IgGs					
Healthy donors	0	0	0	0	0
Hepatitis B	4-5	0.02 *(0.3)*	0.06	0	Not determined
Polyarthritis	4	0.2 *(10)*	0.02	14 *(700)*	3 (150)
Hashimoto's thyroiditis	10	0.2 *(13)*	0.016	10 *(625)*	2 (125)
SLE	35	0.5-0.8 *(4)*	0.2	4 *(20)*	5.0 (25)
MS	4-8	0.6-4.0 *(8)*	0.1-0.2	5-7 *(43)*	10-15 (83)

*All specific activities were estimated per mole of protein. The specific activities of pancreatic RNase A in the hydrolysis of poly(C) and cCMP were taken for 100%; the specific activities of all catalysts in the hydrolysis of poly(U), poly(A), and total yeast RNA was calculated relatively to that for poly(C) hydrolysis by RNase A.

**The ratios of the rates of hydrolysis of the analyzed substrate and poly(A) by the same enzyme or abzyme are given in the parentheses.

In several papers, we have used different kinetic data plotting techniques. However, determination of the K_m and V_{max} values using the Cornish-Bowden representation was the most appropriate for illustration of the different ranges of these values in different Ab preparations; the common intersection point of the lines usually gives K_m and V_{max} values as shown in Figure 3A [201]. A situation where the initial rate data obtained at increasing concentrations of RNA substrate was consistent with Michaelis-Menten kinetics was observed with all human RNases (Table 15) but only with one IgG of 10 preparations and one IgM of 10 preparations. Two IgM preparations demonstrated two apparent pairs of K_m and V_{max} values (Figure 3B). Five of the 10 analyzed preparations of catalytic IgM showed fan-like Cornish-Bowden dependences showing smooth changes of the apparent K_m and V_{max} values with an increase in the substrate concentration, in which cases there were no evident intersection points. An example of one of these IgM preparations is given in Figure 3D. The remaining three IgM preparations were intermediate between the first and the third cases above: they gave many points of intersection showing a change in the apparent K_m in the range from 40 to 500 nM (Figure 3C).

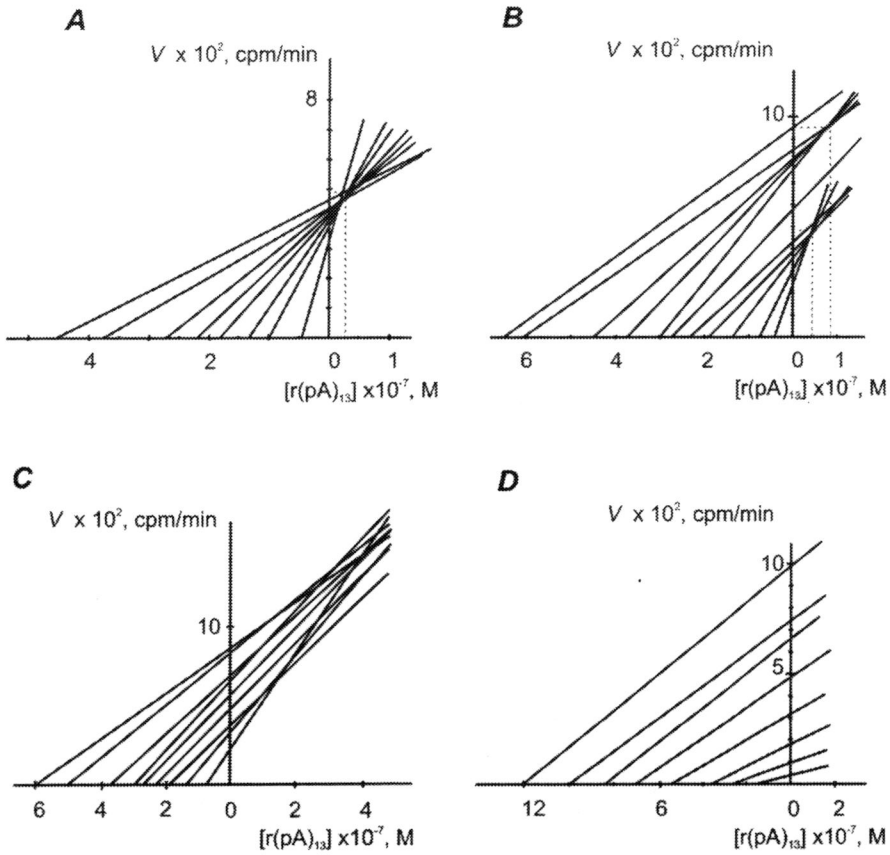

Figure 3. Initial rates of IgM-dependent hydrolysis of $[5'-^{32}P](pA)_{13}$ oligonucleotide as a function of its concentration for Ab preparations from sera of four different SLE patients [201]. The K_m and V_{max} values were determined from Cornish-Bowden plots (A-D). The common intersection point gives the values of K_m and V_{max} in the case of IgM-1 (A) and two values of both K_m and V_{max} values for IgM-2 (B); a set of intersection points for $(pA)_{13}$ shows a range of K_m and V_{max} values of IgM-3 (C); no obvious intersection points are evident in the IgM-4 preparation (D)

A similar situation was observed for SLE IgGs [202]. Three IgGs (IgG-2 – IgG-4) demonstrated several apparent values of both K_M and V_{max} (Figure 4B). The apparent K_M and k_{cat} values for hydrolysis of $(pA)_{13}$ for these 3 IgGs gave many points of intersection covered the ranges 10–2000 nM and 0.01–2.5 min^{-1}, respectively. Two IgGs (IgG-5 - IgG-6) demonstrated fan-like Cornish-Bowden dependences showing smooth changes in the apparent K_M and V_{max} values with increasing substrate concentration, and no evident intersection points (Figure 4C). At saturating concentration of $(pA)_{10}$ (50 µM) these two IgGs gave k_{cat} values of 2.2 and 5.1 min^{-1}. The data for IgGs IgG1 - IgG-4 are summarized in Table 16. RNase A and two alkaline RNases from the sera of SLE patients demonstrated classical Cornish-Bowden dependences and only one K_M value (Table 16). Taking into account very similar enzymatic properties of all five human blood nucleases, it was reasonable to believe that even the use of a mixture of all these nucleases could not lead to the observed very unusual Cornish-Bowden dependences.

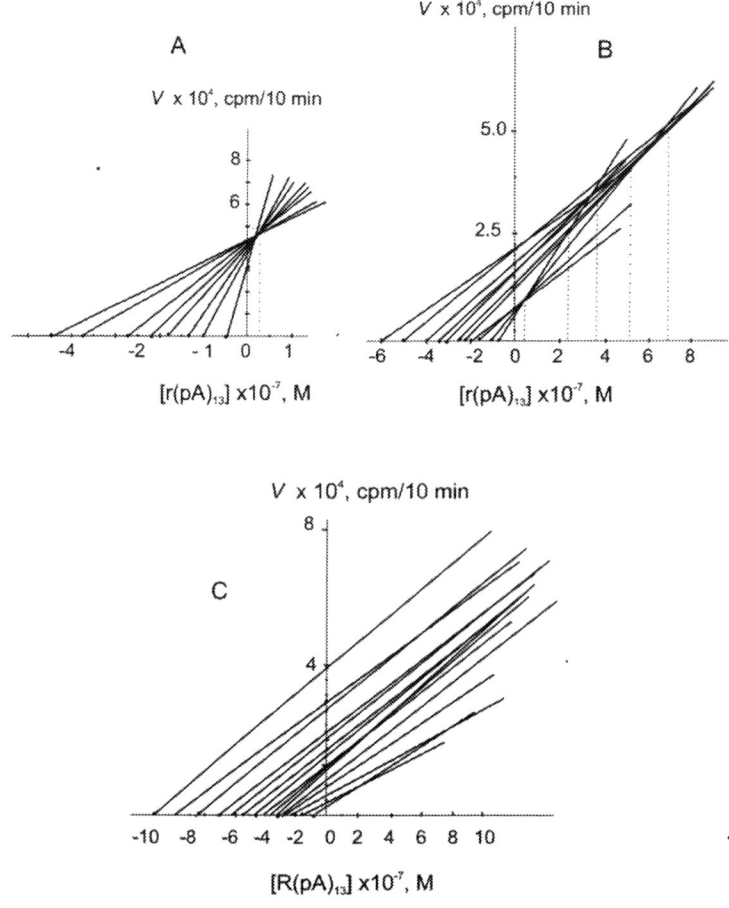

Figure 4. Initial rates of hydrolysis of $[5'-^{32}P](pA)_{13}$ oligonucleotide as a function of its concentration for IgGs from three different SLE patients [202]. The K_m and V_{max} values were determined from Cornish-Bowden plots (A - C). The common intersection point gives the values of K_M and V_{max} for IgG-1 (A) and several values of K_M and V_{max} for IgG-2 (B); no obvious intersection points are evident for IgG-5 (C)

Since the pIgMs were mostly extremely heterogeneous in their composition of monoclonal IgM subfractions, we have examined the hydrolysis of $p(A)_{13}$ in detail using only two single preparations of catalytic IgM demonstrating one and two K_m values, respectively (Table 15). Catalytic IgM-1 possessed comparable affinities for $(pA)_{13}$ and $d(pA)_{13}$, while the rate of oligoriboadenylate cleavage was about 150-fold greater that that for the oligodeoxyriboadenilate. A similar situation was observed for all IgM preparations analyzed, independently of their "catalytic heterogeneity". At fixed concentrations of both substrates and catalytic IgM, all preparations hydrolyzed different oligo- and polyribonucleotides 100-200 times faster than deoxyribo-substrates. It is interesting that the IgGs from the sera of SLE patients also hydrolyze homooligoribonucleotides 50-100 times faster than oligodeoxyribonucleotides [19, 202, 228]. Nevertheless, in contrast to SLE IgG, for which $d(pA)_n$ and $(pA)_n$ are the best substrates and the hydrolysis of $d(pT)_n$ and $(pU)_n$ is 10-15 times slower [19], catalytic IgM preferentially hydrolyzes $(pU)_n$, for which its affinity is about one order of magnitude lower than for $(pA)_n$ (Table 15). Interestingly, mouse monoclonal lupus

IgGs, which recognize different specific DNA sequences, show both DNase and RNase activities, the RNase activity being 50–100-fold greater than the DNase activity [220].

Table 15. Kinetic parameters of hydrolysis of different oligonucleotides by catalytic IgMs from the sera of SLE patients, human sera RNases, and pancreatic ribonuclease A [201]

Substrate	Preparation	K_m^*, M	k_{cat}, min^{-1}	k_{cat}/K_m, $M^{-1} min^{-1}$
IgM antibodies				
$d(pA)_{13}$	IgM-1	5.4×10^{-8}	2.7×10^{-2}	5.0×10^5
$(pA)_{13}$		4.3×10^{-8}	1.5	3.4×10^7
$p(U)_{10}$		1.3×10^{-7}	5.8	4.5×10^7
$p(A)_{13}$	IgM-2	8.7×10^{-8} (K_{m1})	1.8	2.1×10^7
		10.2×10^{-8} (K_{m2})	3.2	3.1×10^7
RNases				
$p(A)_{13}$	Pancreatic RNase A	3.4×10^{-6}	2.2×10^{-2}	6.4×10^3
$p(A)_{13}$	Human blood RNase 3	4.9×10^{-6}	1.7×10^{-2}	3.5×10^3
$p(U)_{10}$		2.1×10^{-6}	37	1.8×10^7
$p(A)_{13}$	Human blood RNase 4	7.2×10^{-6}	5.2×10^{-2}	7.2×10^3
$p(U)_{10}$		5.6×10^{-6}	26	4.6×10^6

*The errors of the values were within ± 10-20%.

Table 16. Kinetic parameters for hydrolysis of different oligonucleotides by catalytic IgGs from the sera of SLE patients, human serum RNases, and pancreatic ribonuclease A [202]

Substrate	Preparation	K_m, M^*	k_{cat}, min^{-1}
Human blood IgGs			
$d(pA)_{13}$	IgG-1	7×10^{-8}	2.0×10^{-2}
$(pA)_{13}$		4×10^{-8}	1.4
$d(pA)_{13}$	IgG-2	$4.7 \times 10^{-8} - 3.0 \times 10^{-7**}$	$2.0 \times 10^{-3} - 7.1 \times 10^{-2**}$
$(pA)_{13}$		$5.1 \times 10^{-8} - 4.4 \times 10^{-7**}$	$0.12 - 0.84^{**}$
$p(U)_{10}$		$9.0 \times 10^{-8} - 4.1 \times 10^{-7**}$	$3.2 \times 10^{-3} - 1.3 \times 10^{-2**}$
$(pA)_{13}$	IgG-3 – IgG4	$1 \times 10^{-8} - 2 \times 10^{-6**}$	$1.0 \times 10^{-2} - 2.5^{**}$
Different RNases			
$p(A)_{13}$	RNase A	3.4×10^{-6}	2.2×10^{-2}
$p(A)_{13}$	Human RNase 3	4.9×10^{-6}	1.7×10^{-2}
$p(U)_{10}$		2.1×10^{-6}	37
$p(A)_{13}$	Human RNase 4	7.2×10^{-6}	5.2×10^{-2}
$p(U)_{10}$		5.6×10^{-6}	26

*The errors of the values were within 10–20%.
**These range corresponds to several K_m and k_{cat} values, which fall within the range (see text).

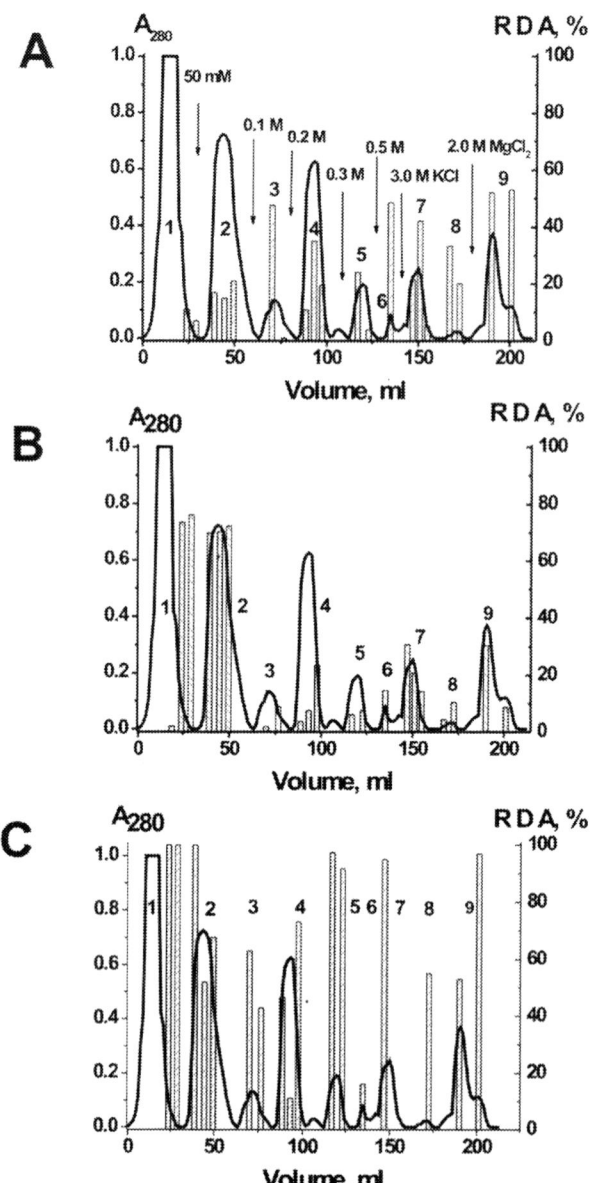

Figure 5. Affinity chromatography of polyclonal IgG preparation from the serum of a diseased mouse with high proteinuria on DNA-cellulose: (—), absorbance at 280 nm (A, B, C) [230]. The relative DNase activity (RDA) of the IgG fractions eluted from the resin by different concentrations of KCl and 2 M MgCl$_2$ in the presence of Ca^{2+} (A), Mg^{2+} (B), and Mn^{2+} ions (C) is shown by the bars. The relative activity was normalized to standard conditions corresponding to 5 µl of the eluate and 10-min incubation; the highest RDA among the fractions determined in the presence of Mn^{2+} ions (C) was taken for 100%. Errors in the initial rate determination from three experiments for any Me^{2+} did not exceed 7–12%

We have obtained homogeneous preparations of two previously described RNases (RNases 3 and 4 [229]) from human serum and compared these enzymes and pancreatic RNase A with catalytic IgM of SLE patients. Table 15 demonstrates that the affinity of the catalytic IgMs for $(pA)_{13}$ and $(pU)_{10}$ is 16–170-fold higher than that of all RNases analyzed. The reaction rate constants (apparent k_{cat}) for $(pA)_{13}$ hydrolysis by the IgMs are 29–190-fold greater than those for all RNases analyzed (Table 15). Even with oligo(U), one of the best substrates for most known mammalian RNases, the reaction rate constants for the IgMs are only 4.5–6.4-fold lower than for human sera RNases (Table 15). The specific activities of ten samples of catalytic IgM with a poly(U) substrate varied in the range 10–60% of those of human RNases 3 and 4. A similar situation was observed for pIgGs from SLE patients (Table 16).

Similarly to Abs from AI patients, one to several pairs of K_m and k_{cat} values were observed for polyclonal Abzs with ATPase [160], lipid [165-166], and polysaccharide kinase activities [167, 168] from human milk.

We have analyzed possible diversity of Abzs in their affinity for different substrates by chromatography on sorbents bearing the immobilized substrates. Interestingly, when IgGs from SLE and MS patients [201-203], diseased MRL-lpr/lpr mice [230], and milk of healthy human mothers [156, 157] were eluted from DNA-cellulose by a KCl gradient (0–3 M), the protein, DNase, and RNase activities were distributed all over the chromatography profiles. In all cases we have found specific Ab subfractions with very high affinity for DNA, which were eluted from DNA-cellulose only with 2–3 M $MgCl_2$ or with acidic buffer (pH 2.6). Figure 5 shows the chromatography of pIgG from the serum of one diseased MRL-lpr/lpr mouse on DNA-cellulose [230].

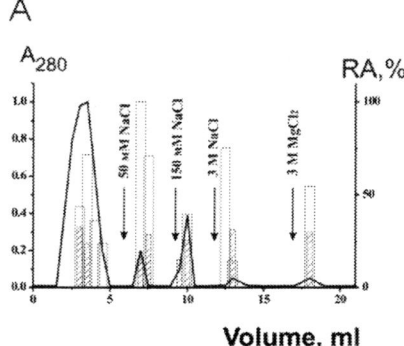

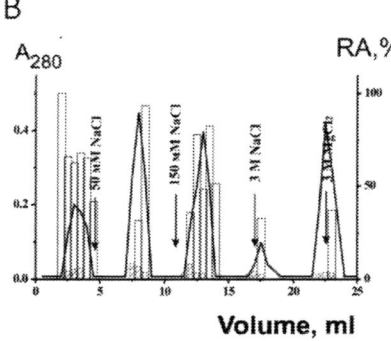

Figure 6. Affinity chromatography of polyclonal human milk IgGs (A) and sIgAs (B) on ATP-Sepharose: (—), absorbance at 280 nm (A and B) [165]. The relative lipid kinase activity (RA) of the Ab fractions eluted from the resin by different concentrations of NaCl and 3 M $MgCl_2$ was estimated in the presence of $[\gamma\text{-}^{32}P]$ATP and $[^{32}P]$orthophosphate (white and grey bars, respectively). The highest RA among the fractions was taken for 100%

In addition, we have observed similar distribution of human milk Abzs with protein kinase [162-163], lipid kinase [165, 166], polysaccharide kinase [167, 168], and nucleotide-hydrolyzing [160] activities upon their affinity chromatography on ATP-Sepharose. Abzs with casein- (from human milk [143] and the sera of HIV-infected patients [33]), MBP- (from MS patients) [30], reverse transcriptase and integrase-hydrolyzing (from HIV infected patients) [143] activities produced chromatography profiles of the same type on affinity resins with immobilized cognate proteins. Figure 6 illustrates the extreme diversity in the affinity and catalytic activity of human milk polyclonal sIgAs (A) and IgGs (B) with lipid kinase activity; the profiles of affinity chromatography of these Abzs on Sepharose bearing immobilized ATP are provided.

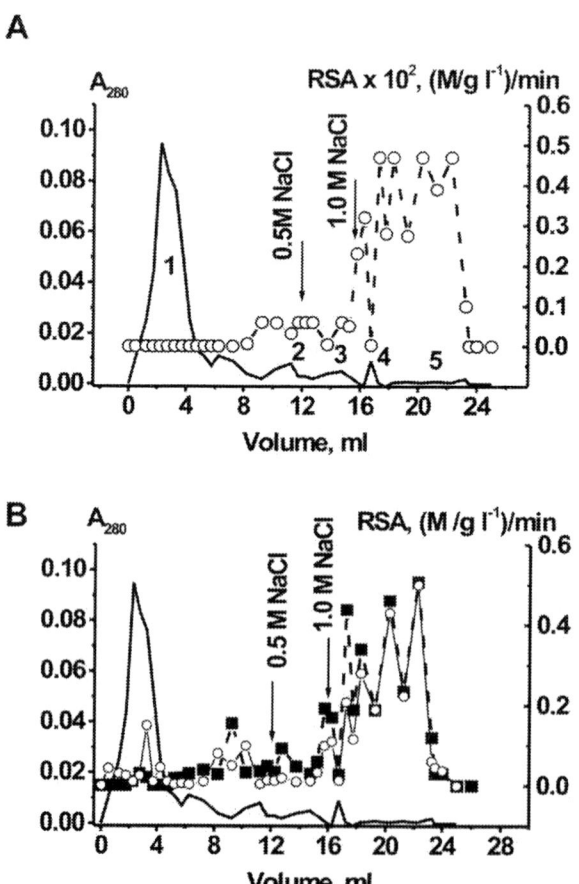

Figure 7. Chromatography of rat IgGs on Chelex-100 and the analysis of peroxidase activity in the presence and in the absence of metal ions [207]. A mixture of IgGs from four rats was chromatographed on Chelex-100; (−), absorption at 280 nm. The relative specific peroxidase activity (RSA, M/g l^{-1}/min) was measured in the eluted fractions in the absence (A) of external metal ions (O) and in the presence (B) of 1.4 mM FeSO$_4$ (■) or 5 mM CuCl$_2$ (O)

A similar situation was observed in the chromatography of Abs obtained by immunization of healthy rabbits with DNA, RNA, DNase I, DNase II, and RNase A [146-150]. As shown in Figure 1, the nuclease activity of IgG from DNase II-immunized rabbits was distributed all over the profile. The K_M and k_{cat} values for RNA and DNA were measured for different fractions of rabbit IgGs after their chromatography on affinity resins (Tables 12 and 13). The affinity of Abz fractions for these substrates (in terms of K_m values) increased gradually with the increase in eluting NaCl concentration (Tables 12 and 13). All these data are indicative of the extreme diversity of Abzs with different activities in their affinity for specific substrates and in their relative specific activities (V_{max} or k_{cat}).

Chromatography of IgGs from Wistar rats on Chelex-100 resin that chelates metal ions led to adsorption of a small fraction of IgG that contained bound metal ions and to its separation to many subfractions demonstrating various affinities for the chelating resin and different increased oxidoreductase and peroxidase specific activities, as compared with the non-chromatographed preparation and IgG fractions having no affinity for this resin (Figure 7) [207].

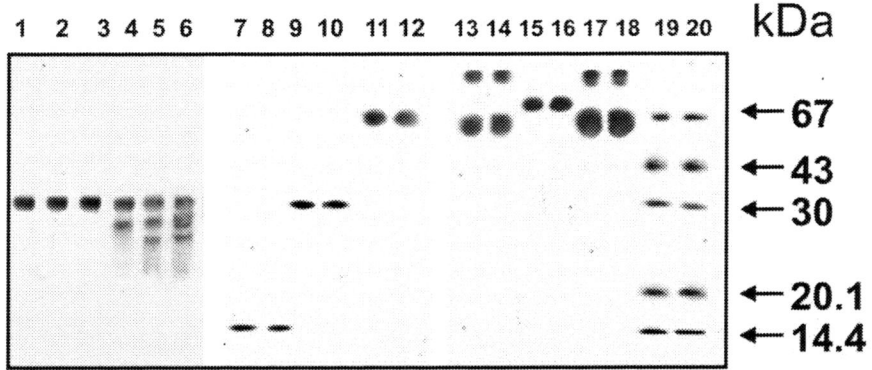

Figure 8. SDS-PAGE analysis of protein hydrolysis by pIgGs [35]. HIV-1 IN (0.2 mg/ml) was incubated for 16 h in the absence (lane 1) or in the presence of 0.1 mg/ml pIgGs from two healthy donors (lanes 2 and 3) and pIgGs from two AIDS patients (lanes 4 and 5, IgG7 and IgG18), or with 0.01 mg/ml AIDS IgGs purified on IN-Sepharose (6). Preparations of other proteins (0.2-0.4 mg/ml) were incubated for 16 h without (odd numbers) or with 0.05 mg/ml AIDS IgGs purified on IN-Sepharose (even numbers): lysozyme (7 and 8); human milk casein (9 and 10), p66 HIV-1 reverse transcriptase (11 and 12); human serum albumin (13 and 14); human milk lactoferrin (15 and 16); bovine serum albumin (17 and 18); a mixture of protein molecular mass markers (19 and 20).

Thus, Abzs with different activities and from various sources demonstrate extreme diversity in their k_{cat} values and affinity for the cognate substrates. More often, at the onset of ADs one can reveal only one or two pairs of K_m and V_{max} values for the substrate analyzed. Then, after a prolonged period of pathology, pAbs usually demonstrate several well-distinguishable K_m and V_{max} values. During exacerbation or after very long-duration AI diseases, the number of monoclones, producing different Abzs, and, as a consequence, the number of K_m and V_{max} values may be very large; usually it is impossible to establish how many values of these parameters in total characterize the full repertoire of Abzs making up the polyclonal Abs pool of these patients.

6.4. Diversity of Abzymes in Their Substrate Specificity

Many canonical proteases can hydrolyze all proteins. In contrast, a number of reports show that anti-protein auto-Abzs from the sera of healthy donors and patients with AI and viral diseases usually specifically hydrolyze only the antigen but not other tested proteins: VIP (asthma and healthy donors [16]), thyroglobulin (Hashimoto's thyroiditis, rheumatoid arthritis, and healthy donors [27]), casein (milk of healthy mothers and HIV infected patients [34, 143]), MBP (multiple sclerosis [31-33]), HIV reverse transcriptase and integrase (AIDS [34, 35]), and human serum albumin and casein (HIV-infected patients [34]). Figure 8 illustrates the specific hydrolysis of HIV-1 integrase only by IgGs from HIV-infected patients [35].

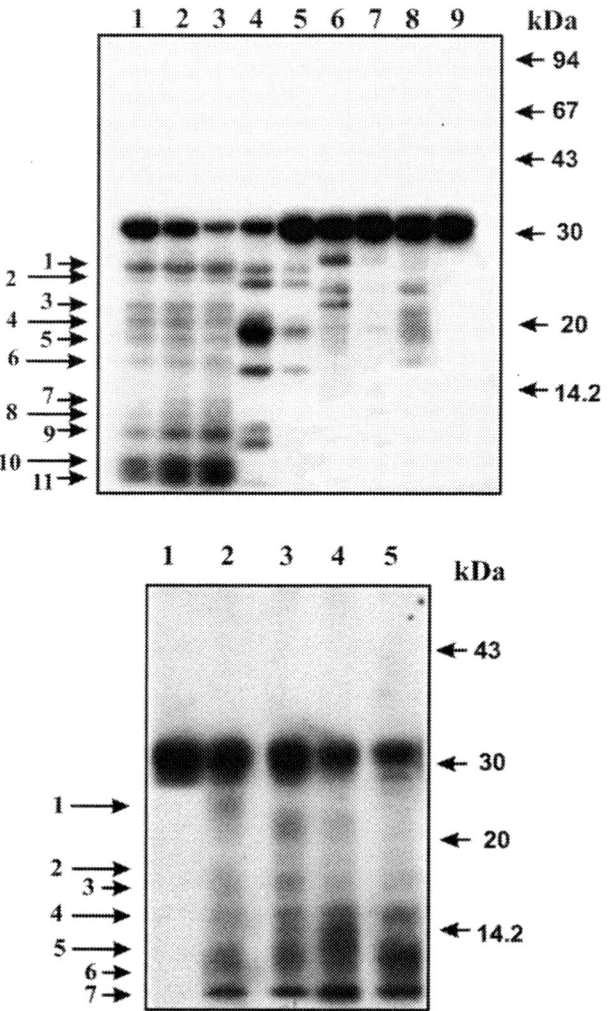

Figure 9. SDS-PAGE analysis of the products of [^{32}P]casein hydrolysis by different proteases, human milk sIgA (A), and IgGs from HIV-1 infected patients (B) [143]. A, Lanes 1, 2, and 3, [^{32}P]β-casein incubated with sIgAs for 20, 40, and 60 min, respectively; lanes 4 and 5, incubation with trypsin for 10 and 15 min; lanes 6 and 7, incubation with proteinase K for 10 and 15 min; lane 8, incubation with chymotrypsin for 10 min; 9, casein incubated alone for 60 min. B, Lane 1, β-casein incubated alone; lane 2, 3, and 4, incubation for 14 h, 7 h, and 14 h, respectively in the presence of pIgGs from three different HIV-1 infected patients. The reaction mixture (10 μl) contained 6.2 μg/ml casein and sIgAs or enzymes at the following concentrations: 0.32 μg/ml trypsin, 0.064 μg/ml chymotrypsin, 0.1 μg/ml proteinase K, and 20-50 μg/ml sIgAs or IgGs

It was shown that IgGs from HIV-infected patients hydrolyze viral integrase in the central and C-terminal domains and that three cleavage sites correspond to the immunodominant regions of integrase (Baranova S. and Odintsova L., personal communication).

The patterns of the same protein hydrolysis by Abs specific to only one protein and canonical proteases are usually quite different. For example, Figure 9A demonstrates an SDS-PAGE analysis of products of [^{32}P]casein hydrolysis by human milk sIgA and several canonical proteases. In the case of sIgA, formation of ~11 detectable ^{32}P-labeled polypeptides (apparent molecular mass: 27.4, 25.4, 22.5, 21.5, 20.1, 18.8, 13.9, 12.9, 12.0, 10.7, 9.8 kDa) was observed (lanes 1–3). The products of hydrolysis in this molecular mass range in the case of trypsin (27.1, 24.8, 19.2, 15.9, 12.4, and 11.7 kDa), chymotrypsin (24.0, 26.7, 16.8, and 15.1 kDa) and proteinase K (24.0, 26.7, 16.8, and 15.1 kDa) were not the same as for sIgA. In addition, hydrolysis of β-casein with sIgA but not with other proteases produced ^{32}P-labeled products with low molecular masses (9.8 and 10.7 kDa; lanes 1–3). This can be indicative of a limited number of sites in a β-casein molecule that can be digested with proteolytic polyclonal sIgA. Similar differences in the cleavage patterns were observed for canonical proteases and Abzs specific to other proteins [31-35, 143].

All studied sIgAs from human milk demonstrated comparable patterns of β-casein hydrolysis [143]. However, IgGs from the sera of HIV-infected patients produced three different patterns of β-casein cleavage, which were different from the patterns generated by human milk sIgAs (Figure 9B) [34]. These data suggest that casein-hydrolyzing Abzs in organisms of healthy women and HIV-infected patients may be produced in significantly different ways.

pIgGs from the sera of two asthma patients hydrolyzed six peptide bonds localized between amino acid residues 14–22 in VIP, while IgGs from the second patient cleaved an additional peptide bond between the residues 7 and 8 [199, 231]. IgMs of HIV-infected patients hydrolyzed virus envelope gp120 protein within several peptides [232].

The sites of MBP cleavage determined by mass spectrometry were localized within four different immunodominant MBP regions [233]. The Abzs also cleaved recombinant substrates containing encephalytogenic MBP peptides. Interestingly, although these Abzs efficiently cleaved only MBP but not other protein substrates tested [31-33], they effectively hydrolyzed several peptide bonds of oligopeptides corresponding to four known IgG-dependent specific cleavage sites of hMBP, as well as many non-specific oligopeptides (Legostaeva G., personal communication). Hence, proteolytic Abzs may be more specific for intact target proteins than at the level of short oligopeptides. As mentioned above, the catalytic center of proteolytic Abzs is usually located on the light chain, while the heavy chain is more often responsible for the specific antigen recognition and the increased antigen affinity for Abs. Intact proteins often can interact with both light and heavy chains of Abzs, thus ensuring the specificity of the target protein recognition and its cleavage. At the same time, short oligopeptides may interact only with the light chain, which possesses lower affinity for substrates, and therefore their hydrolysis may be less specific or completely non-specific.

IgGs and IgMs from the sera of patients with MS and SLE were found to possess amylolytic activity hydrolyzing α-(1→4)-glucosyl linkages of maltooligosaccharides, glycogen, and several synthetic substrates [234-236]. The specific amylolytic activity of individual IgMs from the analyzed patients was about three orders of magnitude higher than that for healthy donors, whereas IgG from only a few patients had high amylolytic activity [236, 237]. Fractions of auto-Abs from human milk [154] and from the sera of patients with different AI pathologies [154, 234-237] revealed different modes of action in the hydrolysis of maltooligosaccharides, p-nitrophenyl maltooligosaccharides and p-nitrophenyl α-D-glucopyranoside; several samples of Abzs demonstrated β-xylosidase activity, which is not observed in known mammalian polysaccharide-hydrolyzing enzymes.

In contrast to canonical ATPases, Abs from the milk of healthy mothers [160] and SLE mice [188] hydrolyze not only ATP but all NTPs, NDPs, and AMP. At the same time, they cannot hydrolyze p-nitrophenylphosphate and α-naphtylphosphate, which are typical substrates of known phosphatases.

Interestingly, polyclonal Abzs from the sera of patients with different ADs usually hydrolyze both single- and double-stranded DNA with comparable efficiency, or hydrolysis of double-stranded (ds) plasmid DNA is much faster [23-25]. Later it was shown that Abzs from patients with atherosclerosis, which is not generally regarded as a pathology with immune status disbalance, also possess DNase activity, but this Abzs efficiently hydrolyze only single-stranded (ss) DNA. In addition, IgGs from the sera of patients with AI diabetes demonstrate very low activities in the hydrolysis of ss deoxyoligonucleotides, while hydrolysis of plasmid DNA by these Igs is detected very rarely [195].

The mouse monoclonal anti-DNA IgG BV 04-01 and its F(ab) fragment hydrolyzed the both ss- and ds DNA in the presence of Mg^{2+} ions, with efficient hydrolysis of the C-rich region of the $A_7C_7ATATAGCGCGT_7$ oligonucleotide and a preference for cleavage within CG-rich regions of double-stranded DNA [238].

The oligonucleotide cleavage patterns were distinct for different MS patients [203]; some Abzs were sequence-dependent whereas others produced both 5'-phosphate-terminated products like those of DNase I and 3'-phosphate terminated products typical for DNase II, or hydrolyzed hetero-ODN in a sequence-independent manner (Figure 10). Hydrolysis of oligonucleotides was also strongly dependent on the reaction conditions and on the presence of EGTA, $MgCl_2$, or NaCl. MS IgGs demonstrated different combinations of endo- and exonuclease activities, but the properties of the DNase Abzs distinguished them from other known DNases [203].

We have shown that the specificity of IgG abzymes from patients with HT and polyarthritis [216], SLE [19], MS [227], and different types of hepatitis [212] for classic homopolynucleotide poly(N) substrates, cCMP, and $tRNA^{Phe}$ with a compact stable structure [216-219] was different, correlated with the disease, and was distinguishable from the specificity of the known pro- and eukaryotic RNases. Table 14 demonstrates a difference in average RNase RAs of IgGs from the sera of patients with different AI and viral diseases in the case of different polynucleotide substrates. Although the RNase RAs were strongly dependent on the patient, in general they increased in the following order: hepatitis < polyarthritis < HT < SLE ≤ MS.

Table 17 demonstrates the difference in the substrate specificity of canonical mammalian ribonucleases and IgMs from the sera of several SLE patients, which is comparable with that for SLE IgGs (see the discussion regarding the nuclease specificity of SLE IgM in section 6.3).

Overall, the diversity of RNase activity of polyclonal Abzs is much greater than that of their DNase activity [23-27]. An *in vitro* transcript of human mitochondrial tRNA^{Lys} was used to assay RNA hydrolysis by IgGs from the sera of 50 patients with different autoimmune or viral diseases [216-219]. Homopolynucleotide substrates and tRNA^{Phe}, which have relatively stable three-dimensional structures in solution, showed a correlation between the disease, the patients' IgG cleavage specificity, and the specific pattern of substrate cleavage. Such specific patterns allow one distinguish different autoimmune or viral diseases [216-219]. The level of activity with the *in vitro* tRNA^{Lys} transcript, which is less structurally stable than tRNA^{Phe} or homopolynucleotides, was strongly dependent on the patient, but in general increased in the following order: hepatitis B ≤ Hashimoto's thyroiditis < SLE [218]. The pH dependences and effects of various salts also varied for Abzs from different diseases. Nevertheless, the RNase activity of all IgGs was specifically stimulated by Mg^{2+} ions, which nearly completely suppress the activity of all known human RNases. In contrast to the classical substrates, no correlation between the IgG cleavage specificity and a specific disease was revealed; each patient demonstrated an individual repertoire of polyclonal RNase IgGs independently of the disease and an individual pattern of tRNA^{Lys} hydrolysis [218].

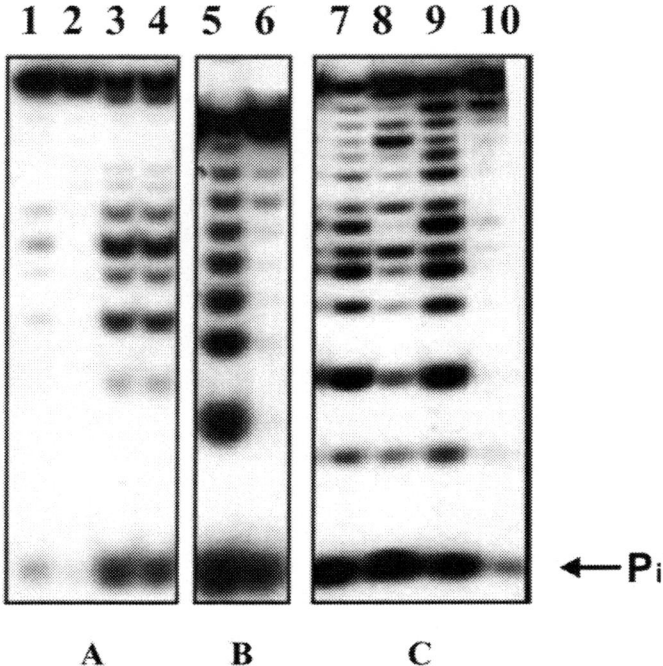

Figure 10. Influence of some reaction components on the hydrolysis pattern of various 5 nM [5'-^{32}P]ODNs [203] (A, dAGCAGTGGCGCCCGA; B, d(pT)$_{10}$; C, dCCAGTCACGACGTT) by IgGs from sera of different MS patients (lanes 1-4 - Abz3; lanes 5-8 - Abz1; lanes 9-10 - Abz2) in 20 mM Tris-Hepes, pH 7.4, containing (with the exception of lane 10) 5 mM MgCl$_2$ and: lane 1 – 7 nM plasmid DNA; lane 2 – 0.2 μM none-labeled ODN of the same sequence; lane 3, 5, 7, 9 – no additions; lane 4 - 100 mM NaCl; lane 6 – 2 mM potassium phosphate; lane 8 – 0.3 mM EGTA; lane 10 – 1 mM EDTA

Table 17. Substrate specificity of catalytic IgMs from the sera of a health donor, three SLE patients, pancreatic ribonuclease A, and two human blood RNases [201]

Preparations	Specific activity, unit/mg*			
	IgM			
	poly(A)	poly(C)	poly(U)*	total yeast RNA
Healthy donor	~0	~0	~0	~0
SLE patient 1	420 ± 20	100 ± 7	500 ± 40	620 ± 30
SLE patient 2	200 ± 20	100 ± 12	700 ± 70	800 ± 60
SLE patient 3	140 ± 12	40 ± 5	500 ± 30	440 ± 25
	Ribonucleases			
RNase A	~0	5800 ± 480	300 ± 15	1300 ± 100
Human RNase 3	~0	4000 ± 300	200 ± 15	1200 ± 100
Human RNase 4	~0	4300 ± 200	200 ± 10	970 ± 50

*1 unit is equal to the amount of the protein producing 0.1 A_{260} unit of acid-soluble fraction from the polymer substrate after incubation of the reaction mixture for 10 min at 37°C.

In contrast to canonical human RNases, some RNase IgGs isolated from blood of AI patients were activated by high concentrations of mono- and divalent metal ions; they hydrolyzed the substrates under the conditions totally inhibiting all known human RNases [216-219]. Under certain conditions, some RNase Abzs exhibited a substrate specificity similar to that of RNases from bacteria, viruses, and also from cobra and viper venom, which is highly toxic for humans [216-219]. The change in pH revealed minor Abzs subfractions with very different patterns of cleavage of various tRNA; there were Abs effectively hydrolyzing RNA at a comparable rate within the pH range 4.5–9.5.

Substrate specificity of Abzs from human milk is of special interest. On one hand, DNase and RNase IgGs and sIgAs are less diverse in their substrate specificity as compared with Abzs from AI diseases [23-27]. At the same time, human milk contains extremely unusual Abzs, which have not been found so far in the sera of AD patients, and their substrate specificities are completely different in comparison with canonical enzymes. Human milk protein-, lipid-, and polysaccharide kinase sIgAs and IgGs were the first examples of natural Abzs with synthetic activities and of natural bisubstrate Abzs.

All known protein, lipid, and polysaccharide kinases including the only milk protein kinase can use only ATP as the phosphate group donor. Milk sIgA and IgG abzymes phosphorylating about 15 milk proteins as well as unusual minor lipids, oligo- and polysaccharides tightly bound with Abzs can use almost any deoxy- or ribonucleoside-5'-triphosphate as the phosphate donor [161-162, 165-168]. Figure 11 demonstrates the ability of small fractions of polyclonal sIgAs (A) and pIgGs (B) from human milk to phosphorylate selectively β-casein (A) and two minor lipids tightly bound with Abs in the presence of different [^{32}P] substrates.

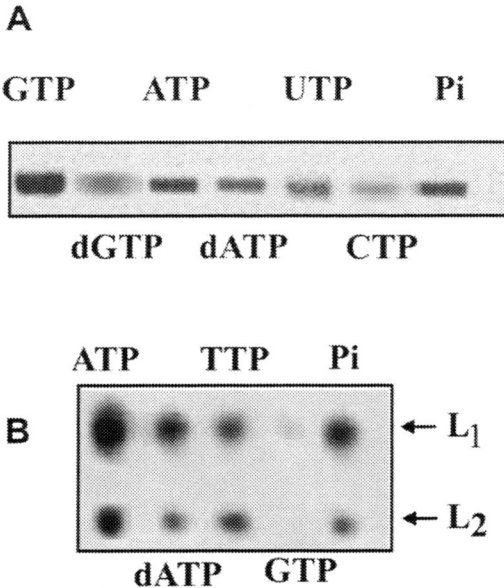

Figure 11. B, Comparison of the incorporation of ^{32}P label into human β-casein by SDS-PAGE (A) and into minor L1 and L2 lipids tightly bound to sIgA by TLC on Kieselgel plates using a system chloroform–methanol–7 M NH$_4$OH 60:35:5 (B) [163, 166]. Before the analysis, sIgA were incubated with 50 μM ^{32}P-labeled substrates of the same specific radioactivity in the presence (A) or in the absence of 2 mg/ml casein (B). The lipids were then extracted with a chloroform–methanol mixture

To our knowledge there are no examples of kinases that can use inorganic *ortho*phosphate directly as a phosphate group donor. Interactions of proteins with *ortho*phosphate leading to formation of covalent bonds are extremely rare. For example, it was shown that incubation of alkaline pyrophosphatase with *ortho*phosphate leads to the protein phosphorylation [239-241]. However, we could find no reported example of enzymes catalyzing transfer of *ortho*phosphate from solution to any substrate (protein, lipid, polysaccharide, etc.). At the same time, milk catalytic IgG and sIgA possess such a unique capability. Incubation of IgG or sIgA in the presence of [^{32}P]*ortho*phosphate leads to the efficient phosphorylation of proteins, lipids, and oligo- or polysaccharides (Figure 11) [163, 165-168].

The levels of phosphorylation of human milk proteins and minor lipids in the case of ATP (100%) and *ortho*phosphate (10–90%) were comparable for both IgG and sIgA abzymes and we did not find milk enzymes (except milk Abs) capable of using [^{32}P]*ortho*phosphate as a substrate [163]. It was shown that the products of sIgA-dependent oligosaccharide phosphorylation with [^{32}P]*ortho*phosphate and [γ-^{32}P]ATP are also comparable [167]. But in contrast to protein and lipid kinase activities of sIgAs, their oligosaccharide kinase activity preferred [^{32}P]*ortho*phosphate over [γ-^{32}P]ATP as a substrate. Thus, the phosphate donor specificity of milk catalytic sIgAs is completely different from those of known canonical kinases.

As mentioned above, milk Abs with kinase activities are bisubstrate abzymes. The canonical human milk protein kinase specifically phosphorylates casein, whereas milk IgGs and sIgAs with protein kinase activity accept not only casein, but approximately 15 other human milk proteins as substrates [23-27, 163].

Lipids tightly bound to milk sIgAs and IgGs represent a very minor fraction of human milk lipids belonging to gangliosides, in which one ore more sialic (or N-acetylneuraminic) acid residues are usually attached to the sugars of glycosylceramide ([164] and refs therein). Known gangliosides contain one (GM1, GM3) or two (GD3) sialic acid moieties as part of carbohydrate group and are acidic. In contrast to these gangliosides, both L1 and L2 minor lipids contain only one residue of sialic acid. The results of alkaline methanolysis of L1 and L2 demonstrate that each of these lipids contain five alkaline-labile bonds [165, 166], whereas GM1 and GM3 are mono-esters and GD3 contains two fatty acid moieties. In contrast to GM1, GM3 and GD3 glycosylceramides, L1 and L2 lipids cannot be oxidized with sodium periodate. Since among known lipids only GM1, GM3 and GD3 contain residues of sialic acid, it is obvious that the minor lipids L1 and L2 tightly bound to milk IgGs and IgMs may be viewed as new milk lipids [165-166].

As mentioned above, several oligo- and polysaccharides bound to human milk sIgAs and IgGs can be phosphorylated when Abs are incubated with [γ-^{32}P]ATP or [^{32}P]*ortho*phosphate. Since the oligosaccharides are very tightly bound to sIgAs and IgGs, their exhaustive phosphorylation allows estimating the relative amount of Abs containing oligosaccharides. By complete phosphorylation of oligosaccharides at saturating concentrations of [^{32}P]*ortho*phosphate (or ATP) with relatively long reaction time (3-10 h) we have calculated that, depending on the donor, different purified milk Ab preparations contain 1–3% of Abzs tightly bound to oligosaccharides [167, 168].

[^{32}P]oligo- and polysaccharides were efficiently cleaved by some polysaccharide-hydrolyzing enzymes (for example, Figure 12). As can be seen from PAGE (Figure 12A) and TLC data (Figure 12B), some of the twelve enzymes used efficiently hydrolyzed the [^{32}P]compounds, while others did not remarkably decrease the amount of radioactivity corresponding to the starting labeled material. The data obtained are summarized in Table 18. Four enzymes (β-glucosidase, cellobiohydrolase, galactosidase and β-1,3-glucanase) had either no or a weak effect on the polymeric (Figure 12A) or oligomeric (Figure 12B) [^{32}P]saccharides. The highest level of hydrolysis (oligosaccharides number I-IV, lane 7, Fig 12B) was observed in the case of α-mannosidase releasing mannose from α-mannosides. At the same time, an incubation of polysaccharides with this enzyme led to a significant decrease in ^{32}P-label corresponding only to the third band and there was no significant decrease in the first and second product of phosphorylation (lane 7, Figure 12A). Lichenase (hydrolysis of α-(1,4)-glucan linkages, lane 6), and glucoamylase (hydrolysis of 1,4-α-D-glucan linkages, lane 3) hydrolyzed the oligosaccharides only partially, being virtually inactive on the polymeric compound 3 but significantly degrading polysaccharide 1. Interestingly, several hydrolases (β-glucanase, α-amylase, endo-β-*N*-acetylglucosaminidase F, chitinase, α-L-fucosidase) that cleave different linkages between various saccharide moieties (see Table 18) effectively hydrolyzed polysaccharide 1, but had no significant effect on the polymeric product 2 (Figure 12A).

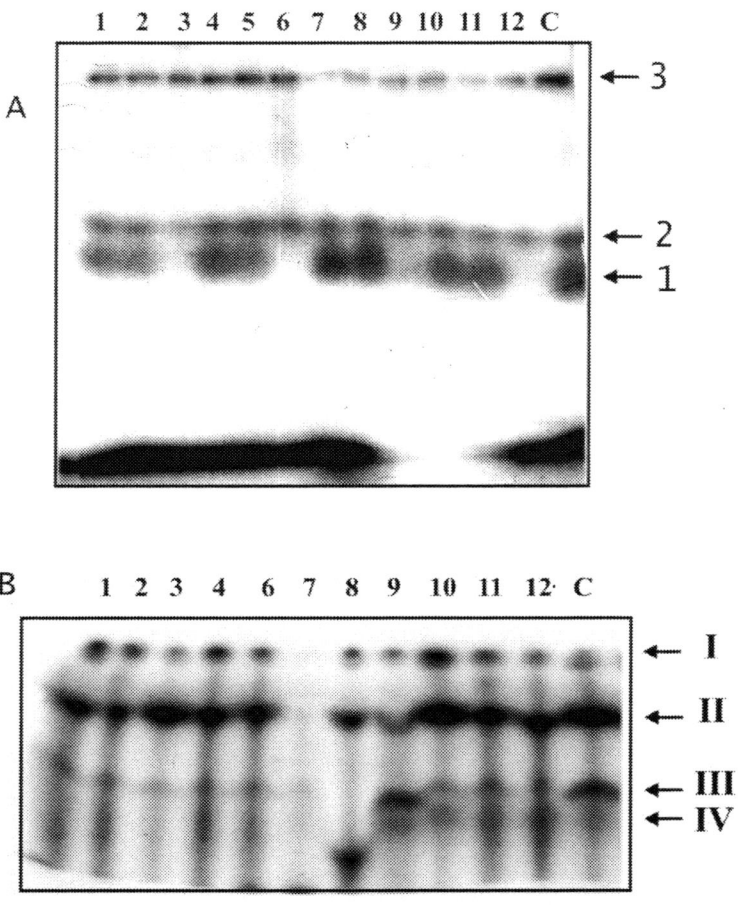

Figure 12. Hydrolysis of [^{32}P]poly- and oligosaccharides by 12 different polysaccharide-hydrolyzing enzymes analyzed by 30% SDS-PAGE (A) and TLC (B) [167]. The following enzymes were used: β-glucosidase (lane 1), cellobiohydrolase (lane 2), glucoamylase (lane 3), galactosidase (lane 4), β-1,3-glucanase (lane 5), lichenase (lane 6), α-mannosidase (lane 7), β-glucanase (lane 8), α-amylase (lane 9), Endo F (lane 10), chitinase (lane 11), α-L-fucosidase (lane 12). C, a mixture of [^{32}P]oligo- and polysaccharides incubated alone. The mixture of [^{32}P]poly- and oligosaccharides was obtained using human milk sIgA and [^{32}P]*ortho*phosphate as a phosphate donor [174]

Only two of these enzymes, α-amylase and α-L-fucosidase, effectively hydrolyzed polysaccharide 1 (Figure 12A). None of these enzymes, except β-glucanase and α-amylase, hydrolyzed (or hydrolyzed only partially) some of the oligosaccharides I–IV (Figure 12B). Taken together, our results clearly show that labeled polysaccharides 1–3 are not homopolymeric and contain different monomers including even acetamido-2-deoxy-D-glucosides (hydrolysis by chitinase, Table 18). The data are indicative of an unusual and most probably highly branched structure of these polysaccharides, where different monomeric units can be connected through different linkages. It is easy to imagine that some of the oligosaccharides I–IV can represent fragments of larger milk polysaccharides. At the same time, it cannot be excluded that some of them are unrelated to polysaccharides or represent internal parts of polysaccharides, since these oligosaccharides are hydrolyzed efficiently by α-mannosidase and exo-1,3-β-glucanase, which release terminal carbohydrate moieties and do not hydrolyze polysaccharides to any extent (Table 18). A significant difference in the hydrolysis of oligo- and polysaccharides by the same enzymes can indicate a very complicated structure of branched polysaccharides. Our data suggest that human milk sIgAs are tightly bound to several different oligo- and polysaccharides, which can be phosphorylated during their incubation with [γ-^{32}P]ATP or [^{32}P]*ortho*phosphate.

Table 18. Hydrolysis of different [^{32}P]oligo- and polysaccharides (phosphorylated by sIgA) by different polysaccharide-hydrolyzing enzymes [167]

Enzyme/source	Enzymes and type of hydrolyzed linkages	No. of enzyme	Electrophoretic band number*			TLC spot number **			
			1	2	3	I	II	III	IV
Cellobiohydrolase from *Geotrichum candidum*	1,4-β-D-Glucan cellobiohydrolase; EC 3.2.1.91	2					+	+	+
Glucoamylase from *Asprgillus awamori*	1,4-α-D-glucan glucanohydrolase, EC 3.2.1.3	3	++	+	-	+		++	++
α-Galactosidase from *Trichoderma reesei*	α-D-galactoside galactohydrolase, mellibiase, EC 3.2.1.22	4					+	+	+
Lichenase from *Bacillus licheniformis*	1,3-1,4-β-D-glucan 4-glucanohydro-lase, EC 3.2.1.73	6	++				+	+	+
α-Mannosidase from *Oerskovia sp.*	α-D-Mannoside mannohydrolase; EC 3.2.1.24	7		++		+++	+++	+++	+++
Exo-1,3-β-Glucanase from *Trichoderma viride*	1,3-β-D-glucan glucanohydrolase; EC 3.2.1.58	8		++			+	+++	+++
α-Amylase from pancreas	1,4-α-D-glucan glucanohydrolase EC 3.2.1.1.	9	+	+	+	+	++		
Endo F from *Chryseobacterium meningsepticum*	Endo-β-N-acetylglu-cosami-dase F; EC 3.2.1.96	10		+			+		
Chitinase from *Serratia marcescens*	α-(1,4-β-[2-acetamido-2-deoxy-D-glucoside)] glycanohydrolase EC 3.2.1.14	11		+			+	+	
α-L-Fucosidase from *Thermus sp.*	α-L-fucoside fucohydrolase; EC 3.2.1.51	12	++	+	+	+	+	++	

** The relative efficiency of poly- and oligosaccharide hydrolysis analyzed by PAGE and TLC, respectively (Figure 12).

A similar analysis of the structure of [^{32}P]oligo- and polysaccharides bound to human milk IgGs was carried out [168]. Overall, we have obtained similar results indicating the complicated and highly branched structure of polysaccharides bound with milk sIgA and IgGs [167, 168]. However, glucoamylase and α-L-fucosidase caused virtually no hydrolysis of polysaccharides isolated from IgGs while efficiently hydrolyzing polysaccharides from sIgAs [167]. α-Mannosidase was the only enzyme that efficiently cleaved polysaccharides bound to both sIgAs [167] and IgG [168]. 1,3-Glucanase and endo-β-*N*-acetylglucosaminidase F relatively weakly cleaved polysaccharides obtained both from sIgAs and IgGs [167, 168].

Thus, our data show that minor oligo- and polysaccharides, which are phosphorylated and tightly bound to IgGs and sIgAs, may be similar in their mobility on TLC and electrophoresis but nevertheless differ in their structure.

An extreme diversity in the substrate specificity was observed for IgGs from the sera of healthy Wistar rats with H_2O_2-dependent peroxidase and H_2O_2-independent oxidoreductase activities [208]. These IgGs can efficiently oxidize not only 3,3'-diaminobenzidine but also *o*-phenylendiamine, phenol, *p*-dihydroquinone, α-naphthol, and NADH, but, unlike HRP, cannot oxidize adrenalin. In contrast to IgGs, HRP cannot oxidize phenol, *p*-dihydroquinone, or α-naphthol in the absence of H_2O_2. IgGs were also more universal in their metal dependence than known plant and mammalian peroxidases [207, 209, 242].

Taking these observations together, it is evident that the substrate specificity of Abzs of different classes and sub-classes from the sera of AI patients and human milk distinguishes them from canonical enzymes. In principle, the repertoire of Abzs with different activities in each AI patient or diseased animal may be very individual.

6.5. pH Optima Diversity of Abzymes

The pH optima for Abzs with different activities were studied in several works. It was shown that, in contrast to all canonical enzymes including human RNases which have one pronounced pH optimum (6.8–7.5) for hydrolysis of poly(A) [229, 243, 244], catalytic SLE IgGs usually have high activity over a wide pH range (6.0–9.5, Figure 13A) [202]. For $(pA)_{13}$ hydrolysis (Figure 13A) IgG-1 had a pronounced optimum at pH 8.8; IgG-2 demonstrated three marked pH optima at pH 8.5, 7.7, and 7.2, while IgG-5 had no optimum and the hydrolysis proceeds with comparable rates at pH from 6.0 to 9.5. Two other preparations (IgG-3 and IgG-4), like IgG-2, also showed several pronounced pH optima between 6.0 and 9.5, while IgG-6 had no pH optimum, like IgG-5.

Very significant differences in the number of pH optima distributed between pH 5.0 and 10 or comparable rates at all pH values were also observed for SLE IgMs and MS IgGs with DNase and RNase activities [201, 202]. Figure 13B demonstrates the influence of pH on the relative RNase activity of IgMs from the sera of three different SLE patients [201].

In contrast to all human DNases (for example, Figure 14), all IgGs from the sera of MRL-lpr/lpr mice demonstrated high or detectable activity over a wide pH range (5.5–9.5) with a pronounced or at least visible tendency for an increase in RA at pH 5.8, 6.6, 7.4, 8.6, and 9.4 [230]. The heights of the peaks corresponding to various optima were different and the ratios of RAs at these pH values were individual for each IgG preparation. Only IgG preparation demonstrated a significant increase in the activity at pH >9.0 as compared with its activity at other pH values. IgG-2 and IgG-3 demonstrated comparable RAs at acidic (5.0–6.2), neutral and alkaline pH (7.5–9.5), while IgG-4 showed a lower activity at acidic pH (4.0–5.0) than at neutral and alkaline pH (6.0–9.0). IgGs from the sera of Wistar rats efficiently catalyzed oxidation of 3,3'-diaminebenzidine over the wide pH range (5.0–9.0) demonstrating several pronounced bell-shaped pH optima [209].

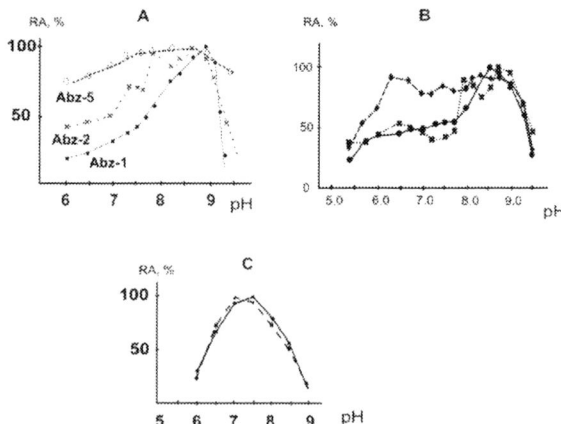

Figure 13. pH dependence of the relative RNase activity of human blood RNases and IgGs and IgMs from the sera of six SLE patients in the hydrolysis of [5'-^{32}P](pA)$_{13}$ oligonucleotide [202, 202]. Results for three electrophoretically and immunologically homogeneous IgGs (A) [202]; and IgMs (B) [201] and human sera RNase 3 (●) and RNase 4 (◆) (C) [201, 202] are shown

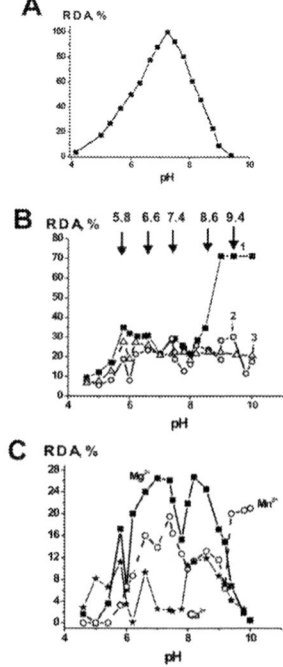

Figure 14. pH dependence of the relative DNase activities (RDAs) of human urine DNase I (A) and three polyclonal IgG preparations (1–3) from three different mice (B) in the presence of 2 mM (or 10 mM for DNase I) MgCl$_2$ [230]. (C), pH dependences of the RDAs of a polyclonal IgG preparation from another mouse in the presence of 2 mM Mg^{2+}, Mn^{2+}, or Ca^{2+}. The arrows in Panel B indicate common optimal pH values in the presence of Mg^{2+} for all four preparations (Figure B and C) expressed as the peaks or at least prominent shoulders in the pH dependencies. The relative activity of IgG-1 (B) or DNase I (A) was taken for 100 %, all other Ab RDAs were normalized to the standard condition corresponding to IgG-1. Errors in the initial rate determination from three experiments for any Me^{2+} and pH did not exceed 7–10%

As mentioned above, DNA and RNA Abzs from AI patients are much more heterogeneous in their substrate specificity than proteolytic Abzs. At the same time, proteolytic Abzs can also demonstrate very different pH optima. It is well known that canonical mammalian, bacterial, and plant proteases, depending on their biological function, can have optimal pH values ranging from acidic (2.0) to neutral and alkaline (8–10) [245, 246]. Since the range of optimal pH of MBP-hydrolyzing MS Abzs was not known, we have measured the relative activity of IgGs at pH from 2.6 to 10.5 and compared the results with the pH optima of canonical mammalian proteases [211]. First, we have analyzed the pH dependences of the initial rates of hMBP hydrolysis by five individual MS IgGs. The pH profile of each IgG was unique (Figure 15). In contrast to all human proteases, which have one pronounced pH optimum, catalytic IgGs demonstrated high hMBP-hydrolyzing activity within a wide pH range (2.6–10). Interestingly, one of the pIgG preparations (IgG-1) had a single pronounced optimum of hMBP hydrolysis at pH 2.6; four preparations (IgG-2–IgG-5) demonstrated a notable pH optimum at pH 4.2–5.4, while only three of them (IgG-2–IgG-4) have visible optima at pH 8.2–9.8. The hydrolysis of the substrate proceeded with very different rates at pH 5.3–8.2 (Figure 15). These results demonstrate that IgGs from individual MS patients likely consist of different sets of catalytic IgG subfractions demonstrating quite distinct enzymatic properties. At pH 2.6, IgGs are usually partially denatured, but the duration of the reaction still allows them to hydrolyze hMBP with detectable or high efficiency (Figure 15). Taking this into account, one cannot exclude that human immune system could in principle produce Abzs with a proteolytic activity similar to that of gastric acidic proteases (Odintsova E. and Baranova S., personal communications).

A similar situation of several optima over a very wide pH range was recently observed for human milk sIgA hydrolyzing casein and for integrase-cleaving IgGs and IgMs from HIV-infected patients.

IgGs obtained from the sera of healthy Wistar rats efficiently catalyzed oxidation of substrates due to H_2O_2-dependent peroxidase and H_2O_2-independent oxidoreductase activities in the wide range of pH (5.0–9.0) and H_2O_2 concentrations (0.1–50 mM, demonstrating several pronounced pH optima and discrete bell-shaped dependences of the reaction rates on the substrate concentration [209].

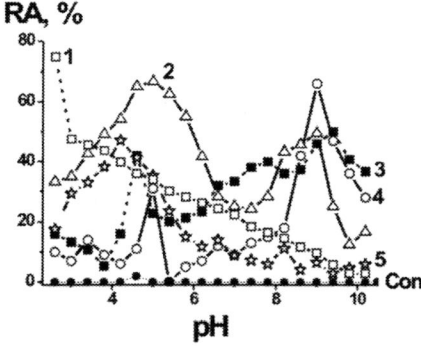

Figure 15. pH dependence of the relative hMBP-hydrolyzing activity (RA) of IgGs from the sera of five different MS patients (1–5) [211]. Hydrolysis of hMBP incubated alone was used as control ("Con.") The RA completely converting 0.19 mg/ml hMBP to shorter fragments after 1.5 h in the presence of 0.1 mg/ml pIgGs was taken for 100%. Errors in the initial rate determination from two experiments did not exceed 7-10 %

Table 19. Relative content of metal ions in the lyophilized IgGs samples from the plasma of nine rats [242].

Metal	Metal x 10^4, %*									Average value x 10^4, %
	Number of the rat (IgG preparations)									
	1	2	3	4	5	6	7	8	9	
Fe	12	11	5.0	7.0	4.0	10	8.0	2.0**	23	9.1 ± 6.2***
Pb	7.7	8.7	8.7	5.7	1.7	20	6.7	1.7	17	8.7 ± 6.2
Zn	6.0	2.5	1.5	0.5	0.1	0.3	4.5	0.1	16	3.5 ± 5.1
Cu	2.6	2.6	2.6	1.6	2.6	1.6	1.6	0.3	8.6	2.7 ± 2.4
Al	3.0	3.0	2.0	3.0	2.0	2.0	1.0	1.0	4.0	2.3 ± 1.0
Ca	0.1	0.15	3.0	3.0	3.0	0.2	0.3	0.1	10	2.2 ± 3.2
Ni	0.3	0.3	0.3	0.3	0.4	0.4	0.4	0.3	3.3	0.7 ± 1.0
Mn	0.05	0.2	0.1	0.1	0.1	0.1	0.7	0.1	0.3	0.2 ± 0.2
Co	≤0.1	≤0.1	≤0.1	≤0.1	≤0.1	≤0.1	≤0.1	≤0.1	≤0.1	≤0.1
Mg	≤0.1	≤0.1	≤0.1	≤0.1	≤0.1	≤0.1	≤0.1	≤0.1	≤0.1	≤0.1

*The content was determined by two-jet arc plasmatron atomic emission method; the errors in the values from two experiments were within 5–7%.
**The maximal and minimal values for each metal are marked in bold.
***Mean ± S.D.

Again, the discussed data continue the same diversity theme: a pool of many auto-Abs may contain very different monoclonal Abzs with various pH optima. In this connection it should be mentioned that the RAs of Abzs from different AI patients are usually compared at one fixed pH, in which all samples are active. However, Abzs from different donors can remarkably vary in their pH optima in any chemical reaction. Changing the reaction pH, one can reveal not only the major fraction of Abzs in different individuals analyzed, but also other subfractions of Abs, the activity of which may be comparable with or less than that of the major subfraction. In addition, the number of K_M and V_{max} values, characterizing interaction of different monoclonal of polyclonal Abzs with their specific substrates, can significantly increase when they measured at several pH values.

6.6. Metal Dependence Diversity of Abzymes

Human and mammalian Abs and auto-Abs are known to interact with different metal ions. The relative content of different metals was analysed in the rat blood plasma, decreasing in the following order: Ca > Mg > Fe > Cu > Zn > Al ≥ Sr > Ti ≥ Mo ≥ Mn ≥ Pb ≥ Co ≥ Ni > Ag [242]. We have recently shown that rat IgGs lose most bound metal ions during the standard procedure of purification to electrophoretic homogeneity [207]. Approximately 9–12% of purified rat IgGs was adsorbed by Chelex free from metal ions, while a fraction of the rest of IgGs (16-27%) could bind to this resin charged with Cu^{2+} or Fe^{2+}. In contrast to blood plasma, purified rat IgGs did not contain detectable amount of Sr, Ti, Mo, Cr, or Ag. Although the plasma samples were characterized by high Mg content, the relative amount of this metal bound to purified IgGs was very low. The contents of different metals in each rat were distinctive, but on average, the relative amount of different metals bound to IgGs decreased in the order: Fe ≥ Pb ≥ Zn ≥ Cu ≥ Al ≥ Ca ≥ Ni ≥ Mn > Co ≥ Mg (Table 19) [242]. All IgGs contained comparable amounts of Ni, the ratio between its maximal and minimal values was 1.3-fold. The highest-to-lowest ratio of other metal ions bound to IgGs from the sera of nine rats differed from ~4 for Al to ~160 for Zn (Table 19). The relative amount of Fe in different IgGs was 33–460-fold higher than that of Ni, Mn, Co, or Mg. A similar situation was observed after a standard purification of electrophoretically homogeneous IgGs from the sera of MS patients, but the relative amounts of MS IgG-bound metals decreased in a different order: Fe ≥ Ca > Cu ≥ Zn ≥ Mg ≥ Mn ≥ Pb ≥ Co ≥ Ni [33]. sIgAs from human milk showed yet another order of bound metal content: Ca > Mg ≥ Al > Fe ≈ Zn ≥ Ni ≥ Cu ≥ Mn (Odintsova, personal communication). These data demonstrate that Abs from individual humans and animals can interact with various metal ions demonstrating significant differences in the bound metal ions in spite of the comparable content of the main types of metals in the milk and blood plasma.

It is known that DNase II is a metal-independent nuclease [247, 248], while DNase I hydrolyzes DNA only in the presence of Mg^{2+} or some other metal ions [248]. As shown above, many characteristics of DNase Abzs from human milk and the sera of patients with different AI diseases are quite different from those of canonical DNases. At the same time, IgGs and/or IgMs with DNase activity from the sera of patients with SLE, MS, polyarthritis, Hashimoto's thyroiditis, asthma hepatitis, HIV and bacterial infections were similar to DNase I in their Me^{2+} dependence; they were activated mainly by Mg^{2+} and Mn^{2+}, although some Ab preparations from some individuals were better activated by other metal ions [23-27, 201-203, 212, 228, 249].

In contrast to DNase activity of Abzs from AI patients, human milk sIgA was only slightly activated by Mg^{2+}, Mn^{2+}, or Zn^{2+}, and the cleavage of DNA substrates was inhibited by Ca^{2+} and Cu^{2+} [156] Importantly, the minimal products of hydrolysis of oligodeoxyribonucleotides by known DNases are dinucleotides [250], while degradation of $d(pN)_n$ oligonucleotides by milk sIgAs generated mononucleotides as the main final products of the reaction.

Rabbit IgGs against DNase I, RNase A, RNase A, DNA, and RNA, similarly to AI Abzs, were inactive in the presence of EDTA, while an addition of Mg^{2+} ions to the dialyzed preparations of IgGs increased their DNase activity [146-150]. In the presence of externally added 5 mM Mg^{2+} the rabbit IgGs were 17–25-fold more active than the same IgG preparations containing intrinsic metal ions before their dialysis.

The most detailed study of Me-dependent diversity of DNase Abs was carried out for IgGs from diseased MRL-lpr/lpr mice [230]. Polyclonal DNase IgGs were not active after dialysis against EDTA, but could be activated by several externally added Me^{2+} ions, with the level of activity decreasing in the following order: $Mn^{2+} ≥ Mg^{2+} > Ca^{2+} ≥ Cu^{2+} > Co^{2+} ≥ Ni^{2+} ≥ Zn^{2+}$, whereas Fe^{2+} did not stimulate hydrolysis of scDNA by the Abs. The data for some metals ions are given in Figure 16 [230].

The dependences of the initial rate on the concentration of different Me^{2+} ions were generally bell-shaped, demonstrating one to four maxima at different concentrations of Me^{2+} ions in the 0.1–12 mM range, depending on the ion. In the presence of all Me^{2+} ions, IgGs pre-dialyzed against EDTA produced only the relaxed form of scDNA, followed by sequence-independent hydrolysis of the relaxed DNA. An addition of Cu^{2+}, Zn^{2+}, or Ca^{2+} inhibited Mg^{2+}-dependent hydrolysis of scDNA, while Ni^{2+}, Co^{2+}, and Mn^{2+} activated this reaction (Figure 17). Mn^{2+}-dependent hydrolysis of scDNA was activated by Ca^{2+}, Ni^{2+}, Co^{2+}, and Mg^{2+} ions but was inhibited by Cu^{2+} and Zn^{2+}. After addition of the second metal ion, accumulation of linear DNA (single strand breaks closely spaced in the opposite strands of DNA) was observed only in the case of Mg^{2+} and Ca^{2+} or Mn^{2+} ions. Chromatography on DNA-cellulose separated DNase IgGs into many subfractions with various affinities for DNA and very different levels of the relative activity (0–100%) in the presence of Mn^{2+}, Ca^{2+}, and Mg^{2+} ions (Figure 5) [230]. In contrast to all human DNases having a single pH optimum, mouse DNase IgGs demonstrated several pronounced pH optima between 4.5 and 9.5, and these dependences were different in the presence of Mn^{2+}, Ca^{2+}, and Mg^{2+} ions (Figure 14). These findings underscore the diversity of the ability of mouse IgGs to function at different pH and to be activated by different optimal metal cofactors.

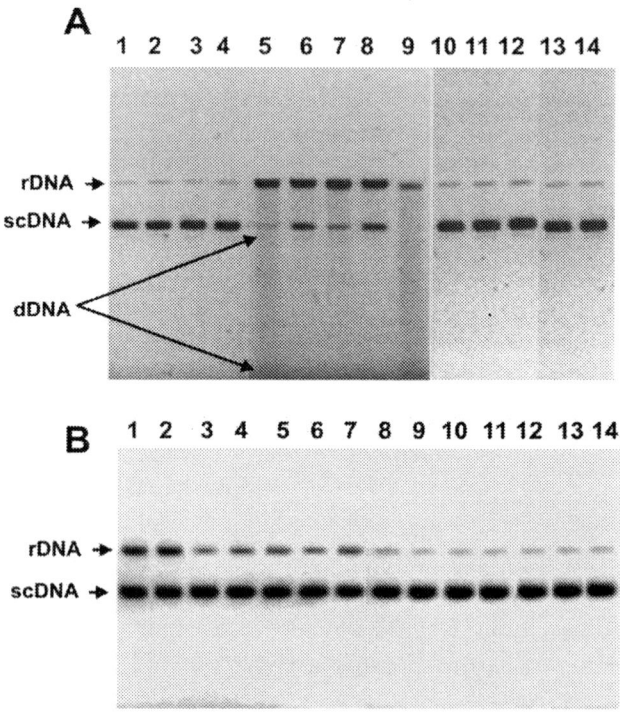

Figure 16. A, Cleavage of sc pBluescript DNA after a 30-min incubation in the presence of 0.03 mg/ml IgGs from five different mice (previously dialyzed against EDTA) and 2 mM $NiCl_2$ (lanes 5–9) or $FeCl_2$ (lanes 10–14) [230]. Lanes 1 and 2 correspond to scDNA incubated with $NiCl_2$ or $FeCl_2$, respectively, in the absence of Abs; lanes 3 and 4, incubation of scDNA with $NiCl_2$ and $FeCl_2$ in the presence of IgGs from a healthy mouse. B, IgG-dependent cleavage of scDNA under special conditions leading to a formation of only relaxed DNA (rDNA) in the presence of IgGs from different mice and different Me^{2+} ions (2 mM): 1, Mg^{2+}; 2 and 3, Mn^{2+}; 4, Cu^{2+}; 5, Ca^{2+}; 6, Co^{2+}; 7, Ni^{2+}; 8, Zn^{2+}. Lanes 9-14 correspond to the incubation of scDNA without Abs in the presence of different ions (2 mM): 9, Mg^{2+}; 10, Mn^{2+}; 11, Cu^{2+}; 12, Ca^{2+}; 13, Co^{2+}; 14, Ni^{2+}. In order to limit scDNA cleavage only to the plasmid relaxation, the time of incubation was varied from 8 to 30 min and the Abs were used in the concentrations 2×10^{-5}–1×10^{-3} mg/ml

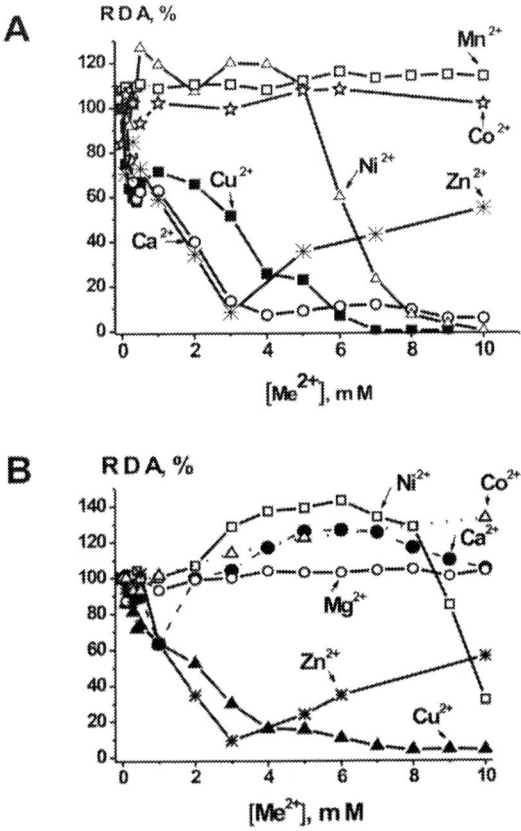

Figure 17. The influence of the second Me^{2+} ion on the relative DNase activity (RDA) of Mg^{2+}-dependent (A) and Mn^{2+}-dependent (B) cleavage of sc pBluescript DNA catalyzed by an equimolar mixture of four dialyzed IgG preparations [230]. The RDAs measured in the presence of different metal ions were normalized to the same concentration of Abs and time of incubation, the specific activities of the IgG mixture in the presence of Mg^{2+} or Mn^{2+} ions but in the absence of other Me^{2+} ions were taken for 100%. Errors in the initial rate determination from three experiments for any concentration of Me^{2+} ions did not exceed 7–12 %

The data discussed through the paper clearly demonstrate that RNase IgMs and IgGs purified from the sera of various SLE patients consist of different sets of catalytic Ab subfractions demonstrating quite distinct enzymatic properties. Nevertheless, all these subfractions share common properties that distinguish them from other known human RNases [201, 202]. All five human sera RNases are activated 1.7–2.7-fold by 50–100 mM NaCl [229, 243, 251-253]. In contrast, all analyzed catalytic IgGs and IgMs were strongly inhibited by low NaCl concentrations (5–10 mM) and were almost completely inactive in 50 mM NaCl. The catalytic Abs of all SLE patients were activated by $MgCl_2$ and $MnCl_2$ similarly to the five human alkaline RNases, but the effect of $MgCl_2$ and $MnCl_2$ on the rates of Abz-dependent hydrolysis of oligoribonucleotides was significantly greater (5.5–6.5-times) than in the case of the canonical RNases (1.5–2.0 times) [252]. The RNase activity of all IgGs and IgMs was specifically stimulated by 50–150 mM $MgCl_2$, the concentrations that nearly completely inhibit all known human RNases. In addition, affinity chromatography of SLE Abs on DNA-cellulose separated IgGs into many subfractions with various affinities for RNA and very different relative RNase activities in the presence of different metal ions [201-202].

Most Mg^{2+}-dependent Abzs from AI and viral patients display no sequence specificity but are rather sensitive to the structural features of tRNAs specific for Phe, Lys, Asp, and Gln [216-219]. Abzs from some patients demonstrate a major RNase A-type specificity with minor differences (preference for CpA and UpA sequences), while others contain a major subfraction possessing an RNase T1-type specificity. The Mg^{2+}-stimulated IgG-associated RNase in most cases demonstrates a cobra venom RNase V1-like action on $tRNA^{Phe}$ with a unique Mg^{2+}-activated specificity for double-stranded regions [217, 218]. In spite of some similarities, SLE Abzs show specificities quite different from those of RNase V1, and the observed specificity differs remarkably from patient to patient. Thus Abzs can discriminate, especially in the presence of Mg^{2+}, between sequences and structural changes, including stability and folding. They may become tools for investigating RNA structure in solution but, since their specificities are multiple, any further application will require the development of monoclonal Abzs.

IgGs from the sera of patients with MS contained several chelated metals, the relative amount of which decreased in the following order: Fe ≥ Ca > Cu ≥ Zn ≥ Mg ≥ Mn ≥ Pb ≥ Co ≥ Ni [33]. In contrast to IgGs, IgA, and IgM of healthy individuals, Abs of MS patients effectively hydrolyze MBP [33]. A specific metal-dependent fraction was obtained by chromatography of highly purified IgGs from MS patient on Chelex-100. This IgG fraction did not hydrolyze human MBP in the absence of Me^{2+} ions but was activated after addition of Me^{2+} ions as follows: $Mg^{2+} > Mn^{2+} > Cu^{2+} > Ca^{2+}$ [33]. Proteolytic activities of IgGs from some MS patients were also activated by other metal ions (Ni^{2+}, and, to a less extent, Fe^{2+}, Co^{2+}, Zn^{2+}, Pb^{2+}, and Co^{2+}). The observed properties of MS Abzs distinguish them from other known mammalian metalloproteases and demonstrate their pronounced catalytic diversity.

Metal-dependent IgGs from MS patients were the first example of Abzs with metal-dependent proteolytic activity. Later we presented the evidence that sIgAs from the milk of healthy human mothers contain intrinsically bound metal ions after the standard purification (Ca > Mg ≥ Al > Fe ≈ Zn ≥ Ni ≥ Cu ≥ Mn), the removal of which by dialysis against EDTA lead to a significant decrease of β-casein-hydrolyzing activity of these Abs [143]. Affinity chromatography of sIgAs on benzamidine-Sepharose interacting with canonical serine proteases separates a small metalloprotease sIgA fraction (6.8 ± 1.8%) from the main part of these Abs and sIgAs with serine protease-like β-casein-hydrolyzing activity (Odintsova et al., personal communication). The relative activity of this metalloprotease sIgA fraction containing internal metal ions increases 1.2–1.9-fold after an addition of metal ions ($Mg^{2+} > Fe^{2+} > Cu^{2+} \geq Ca^{2+} \geq Mn^{2+}$) but decreased by 85 ± 7% after removal of intrinsically bound metals. The metalloprotease sIgA fraction free of intrinsic metal ions demonstrated high β-casein-hydrolyzing activity in the presence of individual externally added metal ions ($Fe^{2+} > Ca^{2+} > Co^{2+} \geq Ni^{2+}$) and especially several combinations of metals: $Co^{2+}+Ca^{2+} < Mg^{2+}+Ca^{2+} < Ca^{2+}+Zn^{2+} < Fe^{2+}+Zn^{2+} < Fe^{2+}+Co^{2+} < Fe^{2+}+Ca^{2+}$. The patterns of hydrolysis of a 22-mer peptide corresponding to one of sIgA-dependent specific cleavage site in β-casein depended significantly on the metal used. Metal-dependent sIgAs were extremely variable in their ability to bind casein-Sepharose, metal-charged iminodiacetate-Sepharose, and different metal ions.

We have analyzed the IN-hydrolyzing activity of ten AIDS pIgGs [35]. The proteolytic activity of five preparations was inhibited by 40-96 % after an incubation of the IgGs with EDTA (Table 10).

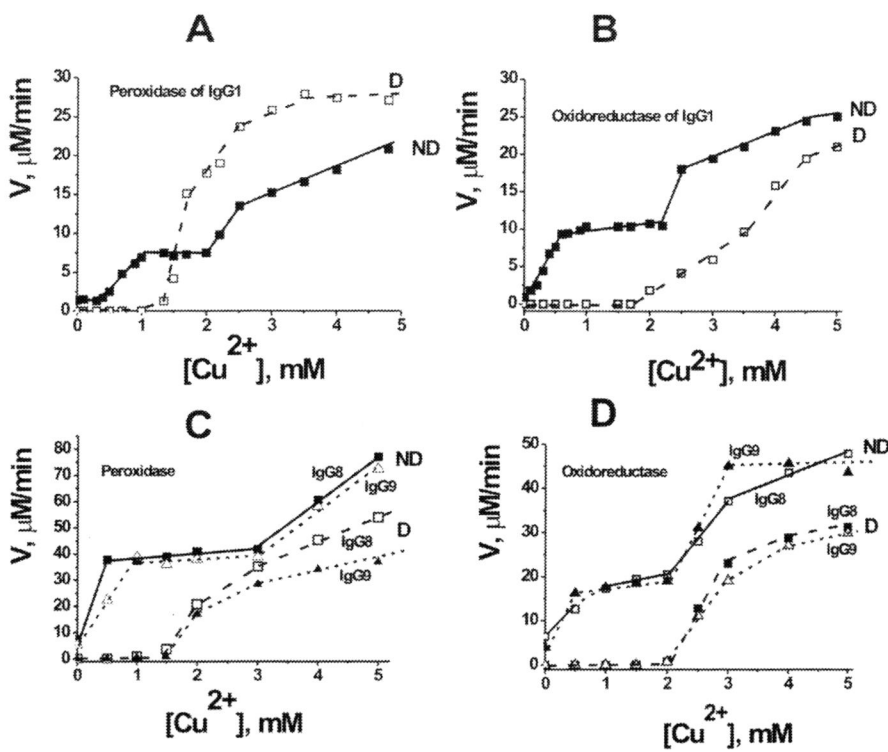

Figure 18. Dependences of the peroxidase and oxidoreductase activities in the IgG-catalyzed oxidation of 3,3'-diaminobenzidine (0.2 mg/ml) on the concentration of $CuCl_2$ [242]. Plots corresponding to dialyzed (D) and non-dialyzed (ND) IgGs (5 µg/ml) and numbers of IgG preparations are indicated in Panels A-D. Errors in the initial rate determination from two experiments for any Cu^{2+} concentration did not exceed 5–10%

As mentioned above, proteolytic Abzs are less diverse in their substrate specificity than Abs with other activities. However, monoclonal fractions of these polyclonal Abzs are also extremely different toward optimal metal cofactor (Bezuglova A., Legostaeva G., personal communications).

We have shown recently that polyclonal IgGs from the blood of Wistar rats possess HRP-like H_2O_2-dependent peroxidase and H_2O_2-independent oxidoreductase activities [206-209]. IgGs lose these activities after removing the bound metal ions by dialysis against EDTA [207, 242]. Externally added Cu^{2+} or Fe^{2+} significantly stimulated both activities of non-dialyzed IgGs containing different internal metals (Fe ≥ Pb ≥ Zn ≥ Cu ≥ Al ≥ Ca ≥ Ni ≥ Mn > Co ≥ Mg) showing pronounced biphasic dependences corresponding to ~0.1–2 and ~2–5 mM Me^{2+}, while the curves for Mn^{2+} were nearly linear (Figures 18 and 19) [242]. Cu^{2+} alone significantly stimulated both the peroxidase and oxidoreductase activities of dialyzed IgGs only at high concentration (≥2 mM), while Mn^{2+} weakly stimulated the peroxidase activity at >3 mM but was active in the oxidoreductase stimulation at a low concentration (<1 mM) (Figure 20). Fe^{2+}-dependent peroxidase activity of dialyzed IgGs was observed at 0.1–5 mM, but Fe^{2+} was completely unable to support the oxidoreductase reaction. Mg^{2+}, Ca^{2+}, Zn^{2+}, Al^{2+}, and especially Co^{2+} and Ni^{2+} were not able to activate dialyzed IgGs, but slightly activated non-dialyzed IgGs. The combinations $Cu^{2+}+Mn^{2+}$, $Cu^{2+}+Zn^{2+}$, $Fe^{2+}+Mn^{2+}$, and $Fe^{2+}+Zn^{2+}$ converted the biphasic curves into hyperbolic ones and significantly increased the activity as compared with Cu^{2+}, Fe^{2+} or Mn^{2+} ions taken separately; the rates of the oxidation catalyzed by non-dialyzed and dialyzed IgGs became comparable (Figures 19 and 20). Mg^{2+}, Co^{2+}, and Ni^{2+} markedly activated the Cu^{2+}-dependent oxidation catalyzed by dialyzed IgGs, while Ca^{2+} inhibited these reactions [242].

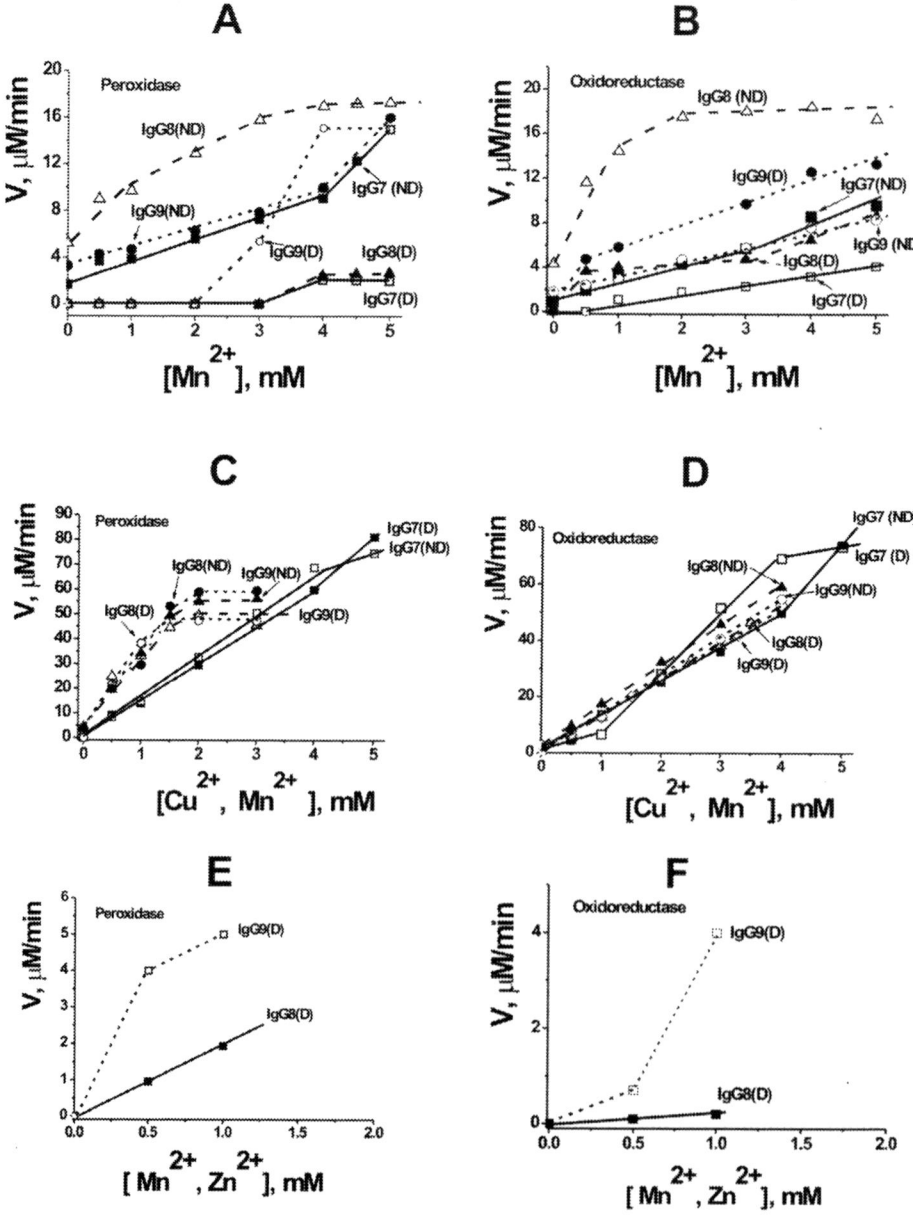

Figure 19. Dependences of the peroxidase and oxidoreductase activities in the IgG-catalyzed oxidation of 3,3'-diaminobenzidine (0.2 mg/ml) on the concentration of $MnCl_2$ and its equimolar mixture with $CuCl_2$ or $ZnCl_2$ [242] Plots corresponding to dialyzed (D) and non-dialyzed (ND) IgGs (5 µg/ml) and numbers of IgG preparations are indicated in Panels A-F. Errors in the initial rate determination from two experiments for any Me^{2+} concentration point did not exceed 5–10%. At the concentrations of Cu^{2+} + Zn^{2+} exceeding 1 mM, precipitation of the reaction mixtures components was observed

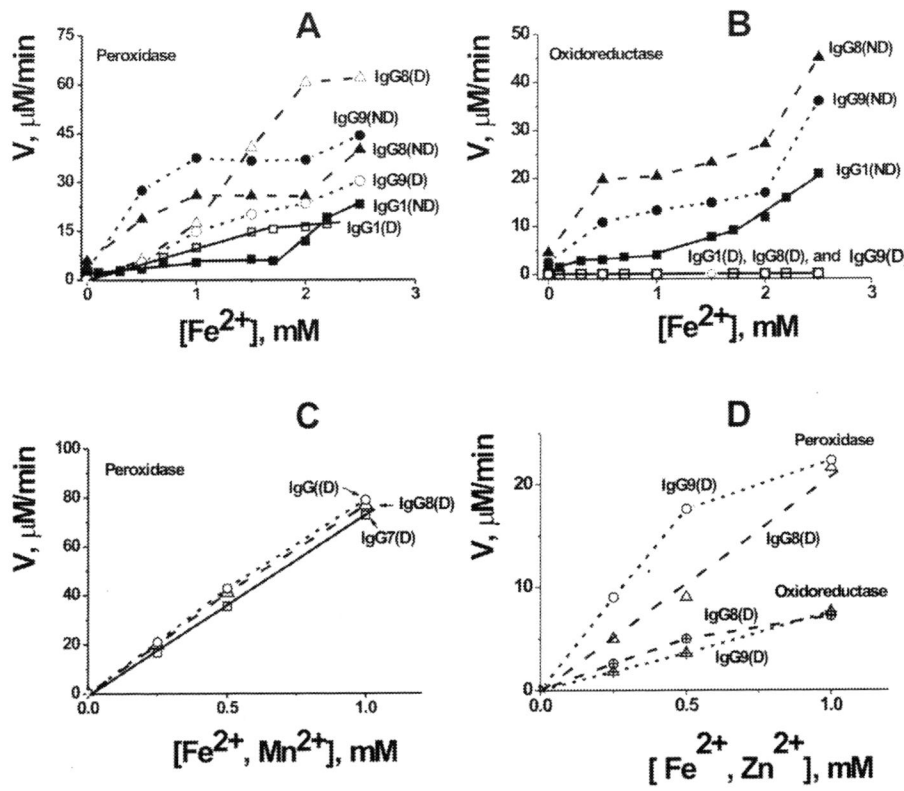

Figure 20. Dependences of the peroxidase and oxidoreductase activities in the IgG-catalyzed oxidation of DAB (0.2 mg/ml) on the concentration of FeCl$_2$ and an equimolar mixture of FeCl$_2$ with MnCl$_2$ or ZnCl$_2$ [242]. Plots corresponding to dialyzed (D) and non-dialyzed (ND) IgGs (5 μg/ml) and numbers of IgG preparations are indicated in Panels A-D. Errors in the initial rate determination from two experiments for any Fe^{2+} concentration with or without other metals did not exceed 5–10%

Taken together, our data indicate that only three types of metal ions, Cu^{2+}, Fe^{2+} and Mn^{2+}, are able to stimulate peroxidase and/or oxidoreductase activity of dialyzed IgGs when used alone [242]. It was concluded that such metal ions as Ca^{2+}, Mg^{2+}, Al^{3+}, and Zn^{2+} cannot directly participate in oxidation reactions but can affect the catalytic activity of Abs indirectly due to an interaction with the variable or constant domain of Abs and induction of conformation changes in Abz molecules. On the other hand, each of these metal ions can serve as a second electrophilic metal cofactors in Ab catalytic centers supplementing the main variable oxidation state cofactors Fe^{2+}, Cu^{2+}, and Mn^{2+}, similar to the Zn^{2+} cofactor in Cu,Zn-dependent superoxide dismutase [242].

Activation of IgGs by two metal ions with variable oxidation state seems more likely to rely on the second metal as electrophilic cofactor, or on both metal ions directly participating in the oxidation reaction, than on conformational changes due to metal interactions with the variable or constant domain of Abs. Since dialyzed and non-dialyzed IgGs did not demonstrate biphasic dependences and had a significantly higher activity in the presence of Cu^{2+} together with Mn^{2+} and Zn^{2+} ions, some fractions of IgG molecules most probably can function as Cu/Cu, Cu/Mn, and Cu/Zn peroxidases or oxidoreductases [242]. Similar conclusions can be drawn for other pairs of metal ions. The second metal ion may be of variable ($Cu^{2+}+Cu^{2+}$, $Cu^{2+}+Mn^{2+}$, $Cu^{2+}+Co^{2+}$, $Cu^{2+}+Ni^{2+}$, $Fe^{2+}+Fe^{2+}$, $Fe^{2+}+Mn^{2+}$, $Mn^{2+}+Mn^{2+}$) or constant oxidation state nature ($Fe^{2+}+Zn^{2+}$, $Cu^{2+}+Zn^{2+}$, $Cu^{2+}+Mg^{2+}$), and both types of the second metal ion, in principle, can activate IgGs directly or indirectly, but a direct participation of two metal ions with variable oxidation state in the oxidation reaction seems more probable [242].

6.7. Conclusion

Polyclonal Abzs with many catalytic activities from patients with different AI diseases and from the milk and blood of healthy humans described above can be Abs of different classes and sub-classes (IgG1-IgG4, sIgA1, sIgA2, etc.) containing light chain of λ- or κ-type. All these Abzs are catalytically very heterogeneous; they can contain subfractions of monoclonal Abzs differing in the structure of catalytic centers (e.g., similar to serine, thiol, acidic, and metalloproteases, Me-dependent and independent nucleases and proteases, H_2O_2-dependent and independent oxidoreductases), net charge, thermal stability, pH optimum, dependence on different metal ions, substrate specificity, the affinity for substrates, etc. The data strongly suggest that some Abzs may have chimeric active centers, combining parts of the active centers of several canonical enzyme types. For example, in contrast to canonical DNases and RNases, monoclonal Abzs hydrolyze DNA and RNA [220], but they do not possess properties of phosphonomoesterases and phosphodiesterases cleaving DNA and RNA with comparable rates. In contrast to typical ATPases, Abzs hydrolyze not only ATP, but also all ribo- and deoxyribo-5'-mono-, di-, and triphosphates, and can thus be compared to phosphatases, which remove a phosphate from all mononucleotides. However, unlike phosphatases, Abzs cannot hydrolyze trinitrophenolphosphate; these Abzs share properties of canonical ATPases and phosphatases only to some extent [157, 160].

The observed heterogeneity of DNase polyclonal Abzs is not unexpected since a mammalian immune system can theoretically produce up to 10^6 variants of Abs against one antigen. In the case of ADs, including the MRL mouse model, a possible number of antigens that can stimulate production of DNase Abzs is significantly greater than those for healthy mammals. First, due to an increased level of apoptosis, Abzs directly to DNA and its complexes with various proteins may be produced. It is known that an immune response to DNA, especially in its complexes with proteins, depends to a certain extent on the DNA sequence and the length of DNA fragments [77-79]. The number of different DNA molecules stimulating the formation of Abs may be very high since the sera of autoimmune mammals contain highly fragmented nuclear DNA from apoptotic cells, and even relatively small DNA fragments of different sequences can trigger immune response. As mentioned above, antiidiotypic Abs against active centers of DNases can also possess catalytic activity. For example, it was shown that Abs against DNase I, DNase II, RNase A [145, 148-150] and even against human topoisomerase I are catalytically active in the hydrolysis of DNA [144]. It means that potentially any enzyme degrading DNA or RNA can also stimulate formation of DNase Abzs, which can be significantly different in their enzymic properties.

Different anti-DNA Abs in AI diseases and bacterial infections may form in different ways. It was shown that bacterial DNA is more immunogenic for healthy mammals than mammalian DNA and that it can induce formation of anti-DNA Abs, since it is rich in GC dinucleotides and methylated adenosine and possesses unique immunogenic epitopes [254]. Some data [126, 255] demonstrate that bacterial DNA can induce AI response against DNA mostly in organisms lacking correct mechanisms of tolerance to autoantigens, while healthy mammals mainly respond with specific Abs against bacterial DNAs.

During the spontaneous development of a profound SLE-like pathology in MRL-lpr/lpr mice, the specific reorganization of immune system is associated with changes in the differentiation profile and the level of proliferation of bone marrow hematopoietic stem cells and with production of DNase, ATPase, and amylase Abzs [187-189]. Immunization of healthy mice with DNA also leads to production of these Abzs but it is associated only with an increased lymphocyte proliferation and suppression of lymphocyte apoptosis in different organs (especially in spleen), but not with altered differentiation of bone marrow cells [187-189]. Immune processes after the exposure of mammals to bacterial DNA during many infectious diseases may be considered similar to those after immunization of healthy mice with DNA. In addition, the RAs of DNase Abs increased with the progress of the AI pathology [23-27], while the time course of immunization associated with infections is usually not so long as compared with chronic AI diseases. At the onset of AI diseases, Abs are usually contain catalytic Abzs produced by a single clone, or at least a relatively narrow repertoire of Abzs with relatively low RAs. In the course of chronic pathology development, the repertoire of Abzs constantly widens and Abs with significantly higher RAs can be found. In addition, the number of Abzs with high RAs usually increases during exacerbation of AI pathologies [23-27].

Metal ions usually catalyze hydrolysis of peptide and phosphodiester bonds by activating water molecules and increasing their nucleophilicity or forming OH⁻ anions [219-220]. However, metal-independent nucleases and proteases are known (for example, RNase A, DNase II), which activate H_2O through its binding to nucleophilic groups of amino acids in the active centers [213-214]. Our data indicate that a small fraction of proteolytic Abzs can hydrolyze peptide bonds in similar ways by activation of H_2O in a Me-dependent or Me-independent fashion.

Some Abzs can catalyze hydrolytic or oxidative reactions in the presence of only one type of metal ions, but the best activation was often observed in the presence of a combination of several metal ions ([242] and refs therein). A better Abz activation in presence of two different Me^{2+} could be explained as follows. It is known that active centers of some hydrolases contain two sites for binding identical or different metal ions, since two metal ions convert water molecules to more nucleophilic OH⁻ anions more efficient and therefore increase the rate of nucleophilic substitution to a higher degree [213-214]. Therefore, we can suppose that small subfractions of metalloprotease Abzs and other Me^{2+}-dependent Abzs may be simultaneously activated by two metal ions. Additionally, in some Abzs both separated light and heavy chains are active in the hydrolysis of substrates; the examples include monoclonal DNA-hydrolyzing IgGs [185], polyclonal nucleotide-hydrolyzing Abs from MRL-lpr/lpr mice [188], and polyclonal rat IgGs with oxidoreductase activity [209]. Therefore, one cannot exclude that the effect of two different metals may reflect dependence of the active centers in light and heavy chains on different metal ions.

Interestingly, several metal ions can activate metalloprotease Ab fractions containing internally bound metal ions but inhibit the same fractions after removal of the internal metal ions by dialysis against EDTA, or vice versa (Odintsova et al., personal communication). For example, Ni^{2+} and Co^{2+} activate the casein-hydrolyzing metalloprotease sIgA fraction free of metal ions but inhibit the reaction catalyzed by the same fraction containing internal metal ions and demonstrate very complicated dependences of the RAs on the metal concentration. A similar situation with some metal ions was observed for DNase IgGs from MRL-lpr/lpr mice [230], and oxidoreductase IgGs from Wistar rats [242]. However, it is not surprising since all metal ions and their combinations demonstrate different properties as electrophilic cofactors of Ab metalloproteases, nucleases and oxidoreductases. Competition between external and internal metal ions for the Abzs should form their new combinations, which may either increase or decrease the reaction rate as compared with the initial combination of metals intrinsically bound to the Abzs.

In the case of DNase Abzs from MRL-lpr/lpr mice, the relationship between different Me^{2+} ions taken separately or in various combinations is very specific and has no correlation with that of known pro- or eukaryotic DNases [230]. Like for DNase I, the second metal probably stabilizes the Ab conformation optimal for producing linear DNA. However, one cannot exclude that some of the second metal ions are not involved directly in the catalysis and can interact, for example, with the constant part of IgGs and influence the reaction through an allosteric mechanism.

It is reasonable to suggest that, similar to other Abzs specifically hydrolyzing different proteins (VIP, thyroglobulin, MBP, etc; reviewed in [23-27]), casein- [143], MBP- [33], and HIV integrase-hydrolyzing Abzs [35] are most probably Abs directly to these proteins. The amino acid sequences of these proteins serving as antigenic determinates in principle can be bound to different metal ions. In this case one could expect formation of very specific subfractions of Abs and Abzs having affinity for the proteins complexed with different Me^{2+} ions. However, Abs could preferentially form complexes with the proteins charged with a specific metal ion, and protein hydrolysis by such Abzs may be faster in the presence of these specific Me^{2+} ions. This mechanism of Abz formation in principle can generate Abzs highly diverse with respect to their catalytic properties, affinity for different proteins and metal ions, and protein sequence specificity. In this case, various subfractions of metalloprotease Abzs may be optimally activated by specific metal ions, and a better activation of Abzs by the combinations of different metals may be a sum of activation of different subfractions by their respective optimal metal ions. From our point of view, protein-hydrolyzing Abzs many be formed in very different ways, which can be reflected in an extreme diversity of their properties.

Abzs formed after immunization of rabbits with DNA, RNA, DNase I, DNase II, or RNase can hydrolyze either DNA or RNA, or, similarly to the mouse monoclonal IgGs against DNA [220], possess a combined specificity capable of hydrolysis of both DNA and RNA by the same Ab molecule. In the active site of RNase A, RNA cleavage and the following hydrolysis of the terminal 2',3'-cyclophosphate intermediate are effected by the imidazole rings of two histidine residues [213, 214]. Interestingly, Abzs from patients with different AI diseases efficiently hydrolyse both RNA of any sequence and cCMP [23-26]. Since IgGs from rabbits immunized with DNA, RNA, DNase I, DNase II, or RNase did not hydrolyze cCMP, the active sites of RNase pIgG may contain only one histidine residue, only sufficient for the catalysis of the first step of RNA hydrolysis. This hypothesis is in agreement with the observation that the introduction of one histidine residue into the variable part of the light chain of Jel-103 monoclonal antibody specifically interacting with poly(rI) converts it into an Abz that hydrolyze poly(rI) [256]. In addition, formation of Abzs catalyzing two steps of RNA hydrolysis, observed in the case AI patients, may be associated with changes in the differentiation profile and the level of proliferation of patient bone marrow hematopoietic stem cells similar to that in diseased MRL-lpr/lpr mice [189].

The data concerning extreme diversity of Abzs from AI patients were obtained using different methods of polyclonal Abs analysis. As a consequence, the apparent number of monoclonal Abzs with different catalytic properties within the polyclonal Abs pool may be significantly underestimated since it is impossible to separate Abzs with comparable affinities for a specific substrate or to distinguish monoclonal Abzs with similar kinetic parameters. Some minor monoclonal Abzs with a relatively high activity and even major Abzs with low activity may be masked by major Abzs with high activity. Therefore, we have tried recently to analyze a possible number of monoclonal Abzs in the sera of SLE patients using phage display. Phage particles displaying light chains of SLE IgGs were separated by affinity chromatography on DNA-cellulose (Kuznetsova et al., personal communication). The adsorbed particles were eluted with buffers containing different concentrations of NaCl (0.1–3 M) and then with 50 mM glycine-HCl (pH 2.6); nine peaks of particles containing light chains with different affinity for DNA were obtained. Light chains corresponding to all peaks were active in the hydrolysis of DNA and RNA. From the peak eluted in 0.5 M NaCl, fifteen monoclonal preparations of light chains with high DNase and/or RNase activities were obtained and characterized. These preparations were different in their pH optimum, dependence on different metal ions, substrate specificity, and relative activity. In fact, our preliminary data show that the peak of phage particles eluted in 0.5 M NaCl may contain at least 25–30 monoclonal light chains with different characteristics. A similar situation was observed when the same was used to select MBP-hydrolyzing monoclonal light chains (Bezuglova et al., personal communication). Assuming that every of the nine peaks contains 15–30 monoclones, the total number of different nucleolytic Abzs in the analyzed DNA library may be more than 135–270. Thus, a possible number of monoclonal Abzs with different catalytic activities in the pool of polyclonal Abs in patients with SLE and other AI diseases may be very large. This speculation agrees with our analysis of the catalytic diversity of preparations of polyclonal Abzs by different physicochemical methods described above.

Thus, AI mammals can be considered as a promising reservoir of new type of biocatalysts with new and very diverse enzymatic properties.

7. BIOLOGICAL FUNCTION OF ABZYMES

Abzs have been studied primarily in the context of AI diseases where their biological role remains unknown: do they have a function or represent a dysfunction? It is quite possible that some Abzs play positive roles while others are harmful. In bronchial asthma, it has been suggested that the respiratory tract dysfunction may stem from the protease activity of auto-Abzs resulting in a deficit of VIP, which plays a major role in the pathophysiology [257, 258].

Recently, it was shown that hMBP-hydrolyzing activity is an intrinsic property of IgGs, IgMs, and IgAs from the sera of MS patients [31-33, 211]. Later the hMBP-hydrolyzing activity of IgG from MS patients was confirmed and the specific sites of the neural antigen cleaved by Abs were established [233]. Recognition and degradation of MBP peptides by serum auto-Abs was confirmed as a novel biomarker for MS [259]. In MS, the protease activity of anti-hMBP Abzs can attack hMBP of the myelin-proteolipid sheath of axons. An established MS drug Copaxone appears to be a specific hMBP-hydrolyzing Abzs inhibitor [233]. Consequently, the Abzs may play an important negative role in MS pathogenesis.

Abzs hydrolyzing DNA or RNA could a priori be viewed as non-specific side-products of the AI process since they occur in the sera of patients with many AI and viral diseases. However, at least in SLE, DNase Abzs are cytotoxic with the efficacy approaching that of tumour necrosis factor, a well-known inducer of apoptosis [70, 92, 260]. Complement-independent cytotoxicity of DNase Abzs is suggested by further evidence. DNase Abzs from lymphoproliferative patients are cytotoxic [92] and DNA-hydrolyzing Bence-Jones proteins from multiple myeloma patients enter the nucleus and cause DNA fragmentation; catalytically active Abs preparations were significantly cytotoxic and their activity was related to the progressive clinical status deterioration [261].

It should be mentioned that Abzs obtained by immunization of healthy rabbits with DNA, RNA, DNase I, DNase II, or RNase were not cytotoxic toward different tumour cells. In addition, only 30–40% of DNase IgGs from MS patients are cytotoxic, while nearly 90–100% of Abzs of SLE patients show cytotoxicity [26]. Therefore, it is possible that formation of cytotoxic nuclease Abzs is a consequence of specific immune processes in AI patients associated with changes in the differentiation profile and the levels of proliferation of bone marrow hematopoietic stem cells [189] and widening of the repertoire of Abzs in AI mammals.

A decrease in Abzs hydrolyzing nucleic acids is most probably a positive sign in many AI diseases. For example, it was shown for 120 patients with Hashimoto's thyroiditis that the relative activities of DNase Abzs correlate with the concentration of thyroid hormones and other biochemical and immunological indices of this pathology, and are related to the progressive deterioration of the clinical status, including exacerbation of thyroid gland damage [262, 263]. The very widely used therapy of patients by thyroxine led only to a temporary change in the hormone concentration in the blood but did not affect the level of DNA-hydrolyzing antibodies. However, treatment with the immunosuppressive drug plaquenil (7-chloro-4(β-diethylamino-α-methylbutylamino)quinoline), significantly decreased the DNA-hydrolyzing activity of Abs, which correlated with rising thyroid hormone concentrations, enhanced thyroid gland function, and an improvement of the clinical state of the patients [262, 263].

High-affinity anti-DNA Abs have been recently identified as a major component of the intrathecal IgG in brain and CSF of MS patients [108]. In addition, it was shown that DNase Abzs from MS patients are cytotoxic and induce apoptosis [26]. Moreover, MS IgGs and IgMs possess a high polysaccharide-hydrolyzing activity [237]. Taking these data into account, it is reasonable to suggest that polysaccharide-hydrolyzing, DNase, and especially hMBP-hydrolyzing Abzs may cooperatively promote neuropathologic mechanisms in this chronic inflammatory disorder [31-33].

In Hashimoto's thyroiditis, Abzs hydrolyzing thyroglobulin have been considered a positive factor, since they could minimize AI responses to thyroglobulin and prevent formation of immunocomplexes [264]. Proteolytic IgGs from patients with sepsis may participate in control of disseminated microvascular thrombosis and play a role in recovery from the disease [49].

In contrast to DNase Abzs, polysaccharide-hydrolyzing Abs are usually present even in the sera of healthy humans and their activity remarkably increases in the sera of human patients and animals with autoimmune diseases [187, 189, 236, 237, 265, 270] and especially with pathologies caused by infections. Formation of specific Abs against bacterial DNA during bacterial infections in healthy mammals suggests that the specific catalytic Abs can mostly hydrolyze bacterial DNA [48]. One cannot exclude that combined action of Abzs with proteolytic and polysaccharide-hydrolyzing activities can at least partially degrade bacterial cell wall and facilitate the entry of DNase Abs into bacterial cells to hydrolyze bacterial DNA. This cooperative action of abzymes with different catalytic activities may have a protective effect against infectious diseases [48].

In HIV-infected patients, the proteolytic anti-integrase Abzs can hydrolyze integrase and therefore may play an important role in AIDS pathogenesis and protection of patients from the disease development [35]. Abzs hydrolyzing integrase significantly suppress 3'-processing and integration reactions catalysed by this enzyme. Recently it was shown that the serum of HIV-infected patients also contains Abzs hydrolyzing HIV reverse transcriptase [34] and DNA [255, 266]. The immune response to virus components is the most important factor slowing down transition of HIV infection to the stage of AIDS [124]. Therefore, reverse transcriptase-, integrase-, and DNA-hydrolyzing Abzs may cooperatively protect HIV-infected patients from AIDS development.

In healthy humans, some Abzs may also play important protective roles. As was shown recently, mono- and polyclonal Abs from different sources have an intrinsic ability to intercept singlet oxygen $^1O_2$ and catalytically reduce it to H_2O_2 [204, 205]. From isotope incorporation experiments and kinetic data, Abs were shown to use H_2O as an electron source, facilitating its addition to $^1O_2$ to form H_2O_3 as the first intermediate in a reaction cascade that eventually leads to H_2O_2. These findings suggest a protective function of Abs against $^1O_2$ and raise the question of whether the need to detoxify $^1O_2$ has played a decisive role in the evolution of the immunoglobulin fold [204, 205]. Thus, Abzs offer a mechanism by which oxygen can be reduced and recycled during the oxidative burst in macrophages, thereby potentiating the microbicidal action of the immune system.

We have recently shown that intact IgGs from the sera of healthy Wistar rats oxidize 3,3'-diaminobenzidine in the presence and in the absence of H_2O_2 similarly to HRP [206-209, 242]. It was demonstrated that the peroxidase and oxidoreductase activities of IgGs can efficiently oxidize not only 3,3'-diaminobenzidine but also *o*-phenylendiamine, phenol, *p*-dihydroquinone, α-naphthol, and NADH but, in contrast to HRP, cannot oxidize adrenalin [208]. In contrast to IgGs, HRP cannot oxidize phenol, *p*-dihydroquinone, or α-naphthol in the absence of H_2O_2. In contrast to plant and mammalian peroxidases, IgGs were more universal in their metal dependence. As mentioned above, human serum contains Abzs with superoxide dismutase activity [204, 205]. Therefore, it seems likely that some Abzs can reduce oxygen from $^•O_2^-$ to H_2O_2, while other Abzs neutralize the latter. Our data indicate that substrate specificity of peroxidase and oxidoreductase IgGs can be extremely wide. Taking these observations together, we suggest that the specific repertoire of polyclonal mammalian Abs can serve as an additional natural system of detoxification of reactive oxygen species, and can destroy toxic, carcinogenic, and mutagenic compounds.

All mammalian neonates are essentially agammaglobulinemic at their mucosal surfaces at birth [267]. Milk contains a wide array of Abs to bacterial, viral, and protozoal antigens [179, 180, 267, 268] with antimicrobial activities, which reach mucosal surfaces of the intestinal and respiratory tracts and protect infants from infection and disease. Passive immunity may also be acquired by the child due to mother's milk IgG after their transfer across the intestinal epithelium to the newborn's circulation [269]. It seems likely that catalytic Abzs of mother's milk may also provide protection to breast-fed newborns. For example, it is known that increased amounts of DNases and RNases in human blood or therapy of patients with nucleases protects them from different viral and bacterial diseases ([23] and refs. therein). An inverse correlation between mammary tumour incidence and the amount of RNase activity in human milk was revealed [270]. One could suppose that DNA- and RNA-hydrolyzing Abs from milk are can neutralize viral and bacterial nucleic acids not only by binding these antigens, but also through their hydrolysis; the DNA-hydrolyzing activity of Abs raises the possibility that these Abzs may protect newborns through the hydrolysis of viral and bacterial nucleic acids.

Phosphorylation of proteins, lipids, and polysaccharides is very important for signal transduction and regulation. Lipids containing sialic acid are involved in mediating cell surface phenomena, function as membrane receptors, and may control many other processes of living cells [271-274]. Various oligo- and polysaccharides and their complexes with milk proteins posses a number of different protective function [275, 276]. Considering the crucial role of breast milk sIgAs and IgGs in the passive immunity in newborns, protein, lipid, and polysaccharide kinase activities of Abzs can be very important for protecting infants from different bacterial and viral diseases. Specific stimulation of production of various Abs including catalytic ones by the mother's immune system as a result of autoimmunization and infections may be a way of strengthening the protective function of breast milk and may play a very important role in the passive immunity of neonates and contribute to mucosal immunity by policing the function of some cells.

8. ABZYMES AS DIAGNOSTIC TOOLS

Auto-Abs are found not only in AI patients but also in healthy humans; different auto-Abs including anti-DNA IgGs can be detected in the sera of healthy donors [80, 81, 86, 112]. However, healthy humans do not develop Abzs with detectable DNase, RNase, ATPase, MBP, HIV reverse transcriptase and integrase activities, which are either totally absent or present at the levels on the borderline of sensitivity of the detection methods [23-27].

We have shown that the appearance of Abzs specific for various substrates is among the earliest and clear signs of AI reactions in a number of AI diseases (SLE, HT, polyarthritis, MS) and viral diseases with strong immune system disturbances (AIDS, hepatitis) [23-27]. According to our data, catalytic activity of nuclease [23-27, 188, 189], ATPase [23-27, 188, 189], MBP-hydrolyzing Abzs [31-33] usually can be very easily detected at the onset of AI diseases when the concentrations of Abs to DNA or other auto-antigens are still low and correspond to their ranges in healthy donors. For example, the serum of ~95% of SLE [201, 202, 228], ~90% of MS [203, 227], and 65% of Hashimoto's thyroiditis [262, 263] patients contains DNase Abzs, while only 35, 17, and 23% of these patients, respectively, reveal increased levels of anti-DNA Abs [80]. In all cases (SLE, MS, HT, polyarthritis, and viral hepatitis) the relative levels of these activities increase during exacerbation and decrease during remissions of the disease [23-27]. The statistically significant ($p < 0.05$) coefficients of correlation between the anti-DNA Abs titers and RAs of Abzs for patients with different AI, viral and bacterial infections are usually in the range from 0.6 to 0.8 [23-27, 47].

Since Abzs possess catalytic activity, in contrast to ELISA, it is possible to reveal even small amounts of Abzs with low activity in the polyclonal Abs pool due to catalyst turnover and increase in the detection signal with time. Therefore, assays for some types of Abzs could in principle be used as diagnostic tools for AI diseases. This conclusion was confirmed by the analysis of the ratios of anti-DNA Abs and RAs of DNase, ATPase, and amylase activities in the course of spontaneous development of SLE in autoimmune-prone MRL-lpr/lpr mice [187-189]. Detectable ATPase and DNase activities were revealed in conditionally pre-diseased mice and it was the earliest statistically significant marker of spontaneous SLE, whereas the further significant increase in their activities correlated with the appearance of visible SLE markers and with an increase in the concentrations of anti-DNA Abs and urine protein.

Admittedly, the analysis of Abz activities for diagnostic purposes needs further refinement. Abzs hydrolyzing certain proteins (VIP or thyroglobulin [17, 28]) were found not only in AI patients, but also in norm and in patients with diseases like sepsis [49], which causes many deaths in intensive care units and results from a deleterious systemic host response to infection. The level of Abs with amylase activity in healthy donors was ~40–100-fold lower than in AI patients [235-237, 265, 266]. Although Abzs with low activity can sometimes be detected in healthy people, the RAs of Abzs from AI patients are usually 1–3 orders of magnitude higher [23-27]. Therefore, an appearance of some Abzs or a 10–100-fold increase in the activity of others over the average Abz indices for healthy donors may be used as the earliest markers of AI reactions in mammals.

Although DNase, RNase, and ATPase Abzs are absent from healthy humans and these Abzs can be easily detected at the onset of SLE, MS, polyarthritis, and HT [23-27], diagnostic use of these activities has its own problems. This is because DNase and RNase Abzs with low but easy detectable activity exist in patients with some bacterial and viral infections [48, 196, 212, 249]. In contrast to AI pathologies, the nuclease Abzs are usually present in the sera of infected patients only temporary and disappear soon after clearance of the infectious agent. Thus, diagnostics cannot rely solely on nuclease Abzs analysis. Yet, diseases caused by bacterial and viral infection are diagnosed as a rule by independent specific methods, which should be used to exclude infections if AI diseases were to be diagnosed by Abz assays. Even in the absence of specific indications of viral and bacterial infections, the AI diseases diagnostics using detection of nuclease, ATPase and amylase Abzs should be performed in conjunction with all standard clinical, immunological, biochemical and other indices of AI pathologies. The detection of high levels of nuclease, ATPase, and amylase Abzs can help to make more exact diagnosis or justify more detailed clinical tests for the patient. In addition, as discussed in sections 6.4 and 6.6, the major fractions of RNase Abzs from the sera of patients with different AI-diseases demonstrate different and quite specific patterns of cleavage of tRNA^{Phe} and some other tRNA [215-219]. This criterion can add to more precise diagnostics of AI pathology (SLE, MS, polyarthritis, HT, and viral hepatitis). In addition, a comparison of the substrate specificity of RNase Abzs toward poly(A), poly(U), poly(C), and poly(G) can also distinguish different types of AI pathologies [216, 217].

For diagnostics of MS, thirteen Poser's medical indices are often used [111], but a clinically definite MS diagnosis is usually based on tomographic detection of specific plaques in the brain, which appear on late stages of this disease. Anti-DNA Abs in MS patients, for their lack of a clear pathogenetic meaning, were generally regarded only as an additional evidence of a systemic immunoregulation disbalance. However, cloning of the IgG repertoire directly from active plaques and periplaque regions and from B-cells recovered from the cerebrospinal fluid of MS patients revealed only anti-DNA Abs [108]. These data were interpreted as an evidence of a leading role of anti-DNA Abs in MS pathogenesis [108]. We have described three patients producing Abzs with high DNase activity but not fulfilling the Poser's criteria at that moment. Approximately 1.5–2 years later these patients met the Poser's criteria, and after 2–3 years, specific brain plaques were revealed.

Assays for Abzs (IgG, IgA and IgM) hydrolyzing MBP can provide a more reliable test for MS development [31-33]. Recognition and degradation of MBP peptides by serum auto-Abs was proposed as a novel biomarker for MS [259]. We argue that determination of RAs of both DNA and MBP-hydrolyzing Abzs is more appropriate for MS diagnostics since according to our preliminary data the RAs of these Abzs and their ratio can significantly depend on the stage and phase (remission or exacerbation) of this disease.

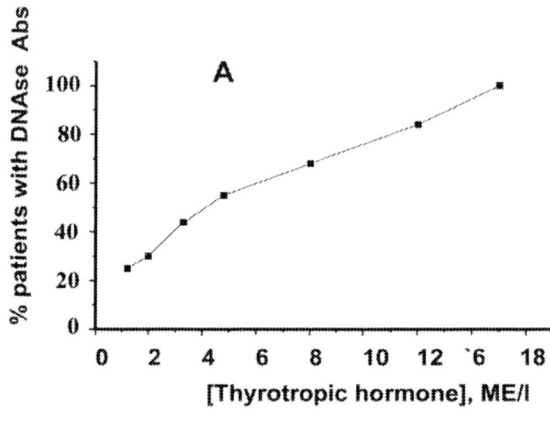

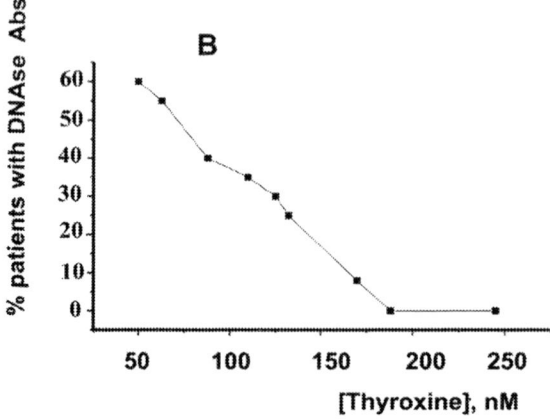

Figure 21. Dependence of the percentage of HT patients containing DNA-hydrolyzing activity on the patient's serum concentration of thyrotropic hormone (A) or thyroxine (B). Most HT patients (83 of 120) can be binned in groups demonstrating comparable concentration (within 20%, see Figure) of thyrotropic or thyroxine hormone, each group containing 6–16 patients. Percentage of patients with Abzs out of all patients in each bin is then calculated. The details of the analysis are given in [262]

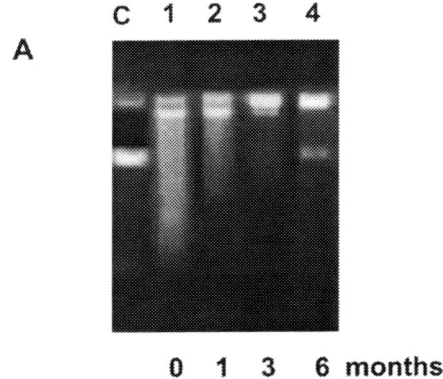
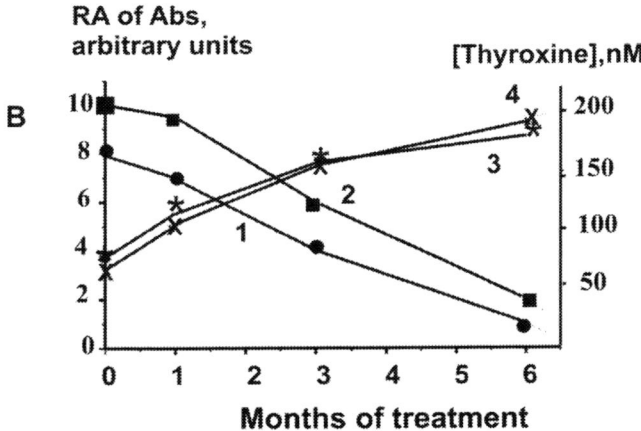

Figure 22. (A), Agarose gel analysis of DNase activity of IgG from the sera of one HT patient (corresponding to curve 1 of Fig 22B) before (lane 1) and after treatment with plaquenil during 1 (lane 2), 3 (lane 3) and 6 months (lane 4) using pBR322 DNA (15 µg) and Ab (5 µg/ml), lane 1 - DNA incubated alone [262]. (B), Time dependencies of the decrease of relative DNase activity of IgG (lanes 1 and 2) and of increase of thyroxine concentration (lanes 3 and 4) of two patients treated with plaquenil. The relative activity of Abs is expressed in arbitrary units (see Figure 4A); curves 1 and 3 correspond to Abs of patients demonstrating an initial activity of about 8 arbitrary units, curves 2 and 4 to other patient with an initial activity of about 10 arbitrary units

Whereas the diagnostic use of Abz assays is entailed with some difficulties, they can be more successfully applied to evaluate the efficiency of therapeutic intervention in AI patients with a known diagnosis. IgGs from 78 out of 120 patients with Hashimoto's thyroiditis possessed DNase activity, the relative level of which correlated with biochemical and immunological indices and the thyroid hormone status [262, 263]. We found nearly linear relationships between the fraction of patients with detectable Abzs and the increase in thyrotropic hormone and the decrease in thyroid hormone concentrations (Figure 21). All patients with increased thyrotropic hormone (13 ME/l) and/or very low thyroxin (50 nmole/ml), typical of hypothyrosis, contained DNase Abzs and showed a correlation of Abz activity with exacerbation of thyroid gland damage, while patients at the initial stage or during a remission of the pathology had no or reduced Abz activity. The specific activity of DNase IgGs increases with the relative amount of anti-thyroglobulin Abs and therefore provides a good indicator of the progress of this AI pathology. The very widely used therapy with thyroxin led to a temporary change in blood hormone concentration but not of Abz levels or AI status, but the immunosuppressive drug plaquenil significantly decreased the DNase activity of Abs, which correlated with rising thyroid hormone concentrations, enhanced thyroid gland function, and an improvement of the clinical state of the patients (Figure 22).

We consequently believe that Abzs offer good indicators of alteration of AI processes in different AI diseases.

9. ABZYMES AS THERAPEUTIC AGENTS

Abzs represent an absolutely new group of physiologically active substances with dual characteristics: they come from a pool of canonical auto-Abs and possess catalytic activity. Monoclonal Abs are suitable for therapeutic applications due to their excellent target binding characteristics (specificity, affinity) and long half-life *in vivo*. Abzs can be developed into a new generation of therapeutics with enhanced antigen inactivation capability. The field of monoclonal Abzs with immunotherapeutic potential has recently been reviewed [53-59]. Some general possibilities of present and future therapeutic Abs and Abzs application were discussed in [56]. Abs and Abzs can be used to neutralize pathogens, toxins and endogenous mediators of pathology. As cell-targeting reagents, Abs can be used to modulate cytoplasmic cascades or to tag specific cells for complement- or effector-mediated lysis. Abs can also be modified to deliver toxic or modulatory payloads (small molecules, radionuclides and enzymes) and engineered to bind multiple epitopes or even to have novel catalytic activity. The modular structure of Igs and the availability of Ab fragment libraries also make it possible to produce variable-domain therapeutics (Fab, single-chain and domain Abs). Although exhibiting less favorable kinetics in vivo, these fragments are straightforward to express and easily penetrate tissues, making them especially useful as neutralizing or delivery agents. The number of approved Abs is expected to increase in the near term, as the platform is adopted as a viable alternative to small molecule discovery [56]. The Abzs strategy can be employed for new methods of drug synthesis, as well as for in vivo therapies. Catalytic antibodies seem to be a promising tool for therapeutic purposes, because of their specificity and stereoselectivity. For instance, cocaine-hydrolyzing Abzs have been developed, and may provide a novel approach to the problems of drug addiction [57, 277].

Possible application of Abzs for prodrug activation and their potential utility in clinical oncology was also discussed [55]. Abzs have two distinct advantages over canonical enzymes: first, they can be selected to perform reactions not catalyzed by endogenous enzymes, and second, they can be humanized to minimize their immunogenicity [56].

Among monoclonal Abzs, proteolytic Abs with different substrate specificities are of special value. Abzs that cleave HIV envelope gp120 protein may find their use in the treatment of AIDS [53, 56]. The strategy exploits the natural tendency of the immune system to synthesize serine protease-like Abzs. Igs in uninfected humans recognize residues 421-433 located in the B-cell superantigenic site of gp120 and cleave this peptide. The catalytic activity resides in the variable region, and is robustly present in IgMs and IgAs but poor in IgGs. Mucosal IgAs are highly catalytic and neutralize HIV, suggesting that they constitute a first line of defense against HIV. SLE patients produce the Igs at higher levels. Homology of the 421-433 region to an endogenous retroviral sequence and a bacterial protein may provide clues about the antigen driving anti-superantigenic site synthesis in SLE patients and uninfected subjects. The potency and breadth of HIV neutralization brings hopes of clinical application of catalytic anti-421-433 Igs as immunotherapeutic and topical microbicide reagents. The properties of the Abz can provide valuable guidance in designing a prophylactic vaccine that amplifies protective catalytic immunity to HIV [53, 56, 59].

pIgG degrading gp120 was obtained taking advantage of the susceptibility of SJL mice to a peptide-induced AI disorder, experimental AI encephalomyelitis [278]. Immunization of specific pathogen-free SJL mice with structural fragments of gp120 fused in-frame with the encephalitogenic MBP(85-101) peptide resulted in a pronounced disease-associated immune response against these antigens. This strategy can be generalized to create catalytic vaccines against viral pathogens [278].

Affinity chromatography-purified Abs from the sera of HIV-infected patients hydrolyze viral reverse transcriptase and integrase and strongly inhibit the reactions catalyzed by these enzymes [34, 35]. These polyclonal and corresponding monoclonal Abzs with these proteolytic activities are potentially interesting for designing new anti-HIV agents.

The appearance of factor VIII (FVIII)-neutralizing Abs in haemophilic patients following therapeutic administration of exogenous FVIII is one of the major factors complicating the treatment of this disease [64-66]. Most anti-FVIII Abs described to date are directed towards epitopes involved in the procoagulant activity of FVIII. However, recent data suggest that some FVIII inhibitors may be catalytic antibodies hydrolyzing FVIII. The characterization of these Abs as site-specific proteases may provide new approaches to the treatment of haemophilia [64-66].

Immunoglobulins that bind amyloid β peptide (Aβ) are under clinical trials for immunotherapy of Alzheimer's disease [53, 62]. IgMs and recombinant Ig fragments that hydrolyze Aβ have been identified. Hydrolysis of peripheral Aβ by the IgMs may induce increased Aβ release from the brain. The catalytic IgMs are increased in patients with Alzheimer's disease, presumably reflecting a protective AI response. Reduced Aβ aggregation and neurotoxicity attributable to the catalytic function were evident. These findings provide a foundation for development of catalytic Igs for Alzheimer disease immunotherapy [62].

Monoclonal Abzs catalyzing specific degradation against the β subunit of *H. pylori* urease have been developed [68]. The heavy chain of Abzs also exhibits the specific degradation of urease. These Abzs were reported to be prepared for medicinal use.

As mentioned above, mammalian Abzs with superoxide dismutase activity can reduce $^{\bullet}O_2^-$ to H_2O_2 [204, 205] while other Abzs with peroxidase activity can convert toxic H_2O_2 to O_2 and H_2O [206-209]. In addition, Abzs with H_2O_2-dependent peroxidase and H_2O_2-independent oxidoreductase activity efficiently oxidize different toxic, mutagenic, and carcinogenic compounds [206-209]. Thus, these Abzs can be used for detoxification of reactive oxygen species and oxidation of different mutagenic and carcinogenic compounds in human blood.

In conclusion, a number of studies of Abzs show the extremely wide potential of the immune system in producing Abzs possessing very different enzymatic activities, which very often are not comparable with those of known enzymes, and natural Abs with specified and novel functions may have wide potential for biotechnology and medicine.

ACKNOWLEDGMENTS

This research was made possible in part by grants from the Presidium of the Russian Academy of Sciences (Molecular and Cellular Biology Program) and Russian Foundation for Basic Research.

ABBREVIATIONS

Abs	antibodies
Abzs	abzymes, or catalytically active antibodies
AG	antigen
AI	autoimmune
AD	autoimmune disease
AIDS	human autoimmune deficit syndrome
BSA	bovine serum albumin
CC	correlation coefficient
HSCs	hematopoietic stem cells
sc	supercoiled
ss and ds	single- and double-stranded, respectively
CBA	(CBAxC57BL)F1 mice
HT	Hashimoto's thyroiditis
hMBP	human myelin basic protein
MFT	microsomal fraction of thyrocytes
MBP	myelin basic protein
MS	multiple sclerosis
nat-DNA and den-DNA	native and denatured DNA, respectively
MHO	maltoheptaose
pAbs and pIgGs	polyclonal Abs and IgGs, respectively
RF	rheumatoid factor
SLE	systemic lupus erythematosus
SDS-PAGE	SDS-polyacrylamide gel electrophoresis
TBE	tick-borne encephalitis
VIP	vasoactive intestinal peptide
RA	relative activity
CFU-GM	granulocytic-macrophagic colony-forming unit
BFU-E	erythroid burst-forming unit
CFU-GEMM	granulocytic-erythroid-megakaryocytic- macrophagic colony-forming unit.

REFERENCES

[1] Pauling, L. (1946). Molecular basis of biological specificity. *Chem. Eng. News*, *24*, 13751-377.

[2] Jencks, W. (1969). *Catalysis in chemistry and enzymology*. New York: McGraw-Hill.

[3] Schochetman, G. & Massey, R. (1985). International Patent no. W085/02414.

[4] Pollack, S. J., Jacobs, J. W. & Schultz, P. G. (1986). Selective chemical catalysis by an antibody. *Science*, *234*, 1570-1573.

[5] Tramontano, A., Janda, K. D. & Lerner, R. A. (1986). Catalytic antibodies. *Science*, *234*, 1566-1570.

[6] Tramontano, A., Janda, K. D. & Lerner, R. A. (1986). Chemical reactivity at an antibody binding site elicited by mechanistic design of a synthetic antigen. *Proc. Natl. Acad. Sci. USA*, *83*, 6736-6740.

[7] Lerner, R. A. & Tramontano, A. (1987). Antibodies as enzymes. *Trends in Bioch. Sci.*, *12*, 427-438.

[8] Benkovic, S. J. (1992) Catalytic antibodies. *Annu. Rev. Biochem.*, *61*, 29-54.

[9] Stewart, J. D. & Benkovic, S. J. (1993). Recent developments in catalytic antibodies. *Int. Rev. Immunol.*, *10*, 229-240.

[10] Martin, A. B. & Schultz, P. G. (1999). Opportunities at the interface of chemistry and biology. *Trends Cell Biol.*, *9*, 24-28.

[11] Nevinsky, G. A., Semenov, D. V. & Buneva, V. N. (2000). Catalytic antibodies (abzymes) induced by stable transition-state analogs. *Biochemistry (Moscow)*, *65*, 1233-1244.

[12] Tanaka, F. (2002). Catalytic antibodies as designer proteases and esterases. *Chem Rev.*, *102*, 4885-4906.

[13] Deng. S. X., de Prada, P. & Landry, D. W. (2002). Anticocaine catalytic antibodies. *J. Immunol. Methods*, 269, 299-310.

[14] Dias, S., Jovic, F., Renard, P. Y., Taran, F., Créminon, C., Mioskowski, C. & Grassi, J. (2002). Immunologically driven chemical engineering of antibodies for catalytic activity. *J. Immunol. Methods*, *269*, 81-98.

[15] Tanaka, F. & Barbas, C. F. 3rd. (2002). Reactive immunization: a unique approach to catalytic antibodies. *J. Immunol. Methods*, *269*, 67-79.

[16] Keinan, E. E. (Eds.) (2005). *Catalytic antibodies*, pp. 1-586. Weinheim: Wiley-VCH Verlag GmbH and Co. KgaA.

[17] Paul, S., Volle, D. J., Beach, C. M., Johnson, D. R., Powell, M. J. & Massey, R. J. (1989). Catalytic hydrolysis of vasoactive intestinal peptide by human autoantibody. *Science*, *244*, 1158-1162.

[18] Shuster, A. M., Gololobov, G. V. Kvashuk, O. A. Bogomolova, A. E. . Smirnov, I. V & . Gabibov, A. G. (1992). DNA hydrolyzing autoantibodies. *Science*, *256*, 665-667.

[19] Buneva, V. N., Andrievskaia, O. A., Romannikova, I. V., Gololobov, G. V., Iadav, R. P., Iamkovoi, V. I. & Nevinskii, G. A. (1994). Interaction of catalytically active antibodies with oligoribonucleotides. *Mol. Biol. (Moscow) 28*, 738-743.

[20] Suzuki, H. (1994). Recent advances in abzyme studies. *J. Biochem.*, *115*, 623-633.

[21] Tramontano, A., Gololobov, G. & Paul, S. (2000). Proteolytic antibodies: origins, selection and induction. *Chem. Immunol.*, *77*, 1-17.

[22] Gololobov, G., Tramontano, A. & Paul, S. (2000). Nucleophilic proteolytic antibodies. *Appl. Biochem. Biotechnol.*, *83*, 221-231.

[23] Nevinsky, G. A., Kanyshkova, T. G. & Buneva, V. N. (2000). Natural catalytic antibodies (abzymes) in normalcy and pathology. *Biochemistry (Moscow)*, *65*, 1245 - 1255.

[24] Nevinsky, G. A. & Buneva, V. N. (2002). Human catalytic RNA- and DNA-hydrolyzing antibodies. *J. Immunol. Methods*, *269*, 235-245.

[25] Nevinsky, G. A., Favorova, O. O. & Buneva, V. N. (2002). Natural Catalytic Antibodies - New Characters in the Protein Repertoire. In E. Golemis (Eds.), *Protein-protein interactions; a molecular cloning manual*, pp. 532-534. New York, Cold Spring Harbor: Cold Spring Harbor Lab. Press.

[26] Nevinsky, G. A. & Buneva, V. N. (2003). Catalytic antibodies in healthy humans and patients with autoimmune and viral pathologies. *J. Cell. Mol. Med.*, *7*, 265-276.

[27] Nevinsky, G. A. & Buneva, V. N. Natural catalytic antibodies-abzymes. In E. Keinan, (Eds.), *Catalytic antibodies*, pp. 503-567. Weinheim: Wiley-VCH Verlag GmbH and Co. KgaA.

[28] Kalaga, R., Li, L., O'Dell, J. R. & Paul, S. (1995). Unexpected presence of polyreactive catalytic antibodies in IgG from unimmunized donors and decreased levels in rheumatoid arthritis. *J. Immunol.*, *155*, 2695-2702.

[29] Thiagarajan, P., Dannenbring, R., Matsuura, K., Tramontano, A., Gololobov, G. & Paul, S. (2000). Monoclonal antibody light chain with prothrombinase activity. *Biochemistry*, *39*, 6459-6465.

[30] Lacroix-Desmazes, S., Moreau, A., Sooryanarayana, Bonnemain, C., Stieltjes, N., Pashov, A., Sultan, Y., Hoebeke, J., Kazatchkine, M. D. & Kaveri, S. V. (1999). Catalytic activity of antibodies against factor VIII in patients with hemophilia A. *Nat. Med.*, *5*, 1044-1047.

[31] Polosukhina, D. I., Kanyshkova, T., Doronin, B. M., Tyshkevich, O. B., Buneva, V. N., Boiko, A. N., Gusev, E. I., Favorova, O. O. & Nevinsky, G. A. (2004). Hydrolysis of myelin basic protein by polyclonal catalytic IgGs from the sera of patients with multiple sclerosis. *J. Cell. Mol. Med.*, *8*, 359 - 368.

[32] Polosukhina D. I., Buneva, V. N., Doronin, B. M., Tyshkevich, O. B., Boiko, A. N., Gusev, E. I., Favorova, O. O. & Nevinsky, G. A. (2005). Hydrolysis of myelin basic protein by IgM and IgA antibodies from the sera of patients with multiple sclerosis. *Med. Sci. Monit.*, *11*, BR266- BR 272.

[33] Polosukhina D. I., Kanyshkova, T. G., Doronin, B. M., Tyshkevich, O. B., Buneva, V. N., Boiko, A. N., Gusev, E. I., Favorova, O. O. & Nevinsky, G. A. (2006). Metal-dependent hydrolysis of myelin basic protein by IgGs from the sera of patients with multiple sclerosis. *Immunol. Lett.*, *103*, 75-81.

[34] Odintsova, E. S., Kharitonova, M. A., Baranovskii, A. G., Siziakina, L. P., Buneva, V. N. & Nevinsky, G. A. (2006). Proteolytic activity of IgG antibodies from blood of acquired immunodeficiency syndrome patients, *Biochemistry (Moscow)*, *71*, 251-261.

[35] Baranova, S. V., Buneva, V. N., Kharitonova, M. A., Sizyakina, L. P., Calmels, C., Andreola, M. L., Parissi, V. & Nevinsky, G. A. (2009). HIV-1 integrase-hydrolyzing antibodies from sera of HIV-infected patients. *Biochimie*, *91*, 1081-1086.

[36] Iverson, B. L. & Lerner, R. A. (1989). Sequence-specific peptide cleavage catalyzed by an antibody. *Science*, *243*, 1184-1188.

[37] Ersoy, O., Fleck, R., Blanco, M. J. & Masamune, S. (1999). Design and syntheses of three haptens to generate catalytic antibodies that cleave amide bonds with nucleophilic catalysis. *Bioorg. Med. Chem.*, 7, 279-86.

[38] Gao, Q. S. & Paul, S. (1995). Site-directed mutagenesis of antibody-variable regions. *Methods Mol. Biol.*, 51, 319-327.

[39] Miller, G. P., Posner, B. A. & Benkovic, S. J. (1997). Expanding the 43C9 class of catalytic antibodies using a chain-shuffling approach. *Bioorg. Med. Chem.*, 5, 581-590.

[40] Roberts, V. A., Stewart, J., Benkovic, S. J. & Getzoff, E. D. (1994). Catalytic antibody model and mutagenesis implicate arginine in transition-state stabilization. *J. Mol. Biol.*, 235, 1098-1116.

[41] Stewart, J. D., Krebs, J. F., Siuzdak, G., Berdis, A. J., Smithrud, D. B. & Benkovic, S. J. (1994). Dissection of an antibody-catalyzed reaction. *Proc. Natl. Acad. Sci. USA*, 91, 7404-7409.

[42] Barbas, C. F., 3rd, Heine, A., Zhong, G., Hoffmann, T., Gramatikova, S., Bjornestedt, R., List, B., Anderson, J., Stura, E. A., Wilson, I. A. & Lerner, R. A. (1997). Immune versus natural selection: antibody aldolases with enzymic rates but broader scope. *Science*, 278, 2085-2092.

[43] Gouverneur, V. E., Houk, K. N., de Pascual-Teresa, B., Beno, B., Janda, K. D. & Lerner, R. A. (1993). Control of the exo and endo pathways of the Diels-Alder reaction by antibody catalysis. *Science*, 262, 204-208.

[44] Janda, K. D., Lo, L. C., Lo, C. H., Sim, M. M., Wang, R., Wong, C. H. & Lerner, R. A. (1997). Chemical selection for catalysis in combinatorial antibody libraries. *Science*, 275, 945-948.

[45] Thayer, M. M., Olender, E. H., Arvai, A. S., Koike, C. K., Canestrelli, I. L., Stewart, J. D., Benkovic, S. J., Getzoff, E. D. & Roberts, V. A. (1999). Structural basis for amide hydrolysis catalyzed by the 43C9 antibody. *J. Mol. Biol.*, 291, 329-345.

[46] Slobin, L. I. (1966). Preparation and some properties of antibodies with specificity toward rho-nitrophenyl esters. *Biochemistry*, 5, 2836-2841.

[47] Kul'berg, A. I, Docheva, I. V., Tarkhanova, I. A. & Spivak, V. A. (1969). Proteolytic activity in preparations of purified immunoglobulin G and rabbit antibodies. *Biokhimiia (Moscow)*, 34, 1178-1183.

[48] Parkhomenko, T. A., Odintsova, E. S., Buneva, V. N., Kunder, E. V., Zhyltsov, I. V., Senkovich, S. A., Generalov, I. I., Nevinsky, G. A. (2009). DNA-hydrolyzing activity of IgG antibodies from the sera of patients with diseases caused by different bacterial infections. *J. Cell. Mol. Med.*, 13, 2875-2887.

[49] Lacroix-Desmazes, S., Bayry, J., Kaveri, S. V., Hayon-Sonsino, D., Thorenoor, N., Charpentier, J., Luyt, C. E., Mira, J. P., Nagaraja, V., Kazatchkine, M. D., Dhainaut, J. F., Mallet, V. O. (2005). High levels of catalytic antibodies correlate with favorable outcome in sepsis. *Proc. Natl. Acad. Sci. USA*, 102, 4109-4113.

[50] Paul, S. (1996). Natural catalytic antibodies. *Mol. Biotechnol.*, 5, 197-207.

[51] Paul, S. (1998). Mechanism and functional role of antibody catalysis. *Appl. Biochem. Biotechnol.*, 75, 13-24.

[52] Paul, S., Nishiyama, Y., Planque, S., Taguchi, H. (2006). Theory of proteolytic antibody occurrence. *Immunol. Lett.*, 103, 8-16.

[53] Tellier, C. (2002). Exploiting antibodies as catalysts: potential therapeutic applications. *Transfus. Clin. Biol.*, 9, 1-8.

[54] Zhou, Y. X., Karle, S., Taguchi, H., Planque, S., Nishiyama, & Y., Paul, S. (2002). Prospects for immunotherapeutic proteolytic antibodies. *J. Immunol. Methods, 269,* 257-268.

[55] Nishi, Y. (2003). Enzyme/abzyme prodrug activation systems: potential use in clinical oncology. *Curr. Pharm. Des., 9,* 2113-2130

[56] Stockwin, L.H. & Holmes, S. (2003). Antibodies as therapeutic agents: vive la renaissance! *Expert Opin. Biol. Ther. 3,* 1133-1152.

[57] Hanson, C. V., Nishiyama, Y, & Paul, S. (2005). Catalytic antibodies and their applications. *Curr. Opin. Biotechnol., 16,* 631-636.

[58] Planque, S., Nishiyama, Y., Taguchi, H., Salas, M., Hanson, C. & Paul, S. (2008). Catalytic antibodies to HIV: physiological role and potential clinical utility. *Autoimmun. Rev. 7,* 473-479.

[59] Wójcik, T. & Kieć-Kononowicz, K. (2008). Catalytic activity of certain antibodies as a potential tool for drug synthesis and for directed prodrug therapies. *Curr. Med. Chem., 15,* 1606-1615.

[60] Thiagarajan, P. & Paul, S. (2000). Prothrombin cleaving antibody light chains. *Chem. Immunol., 77,* 115-129.

[61] Taguchi, H., Planque, S., Nishiyama, Y., Symersky, J., Boivin, S., Szabo, P., Friedland, R., P., Ramsland, P. A., Edmundson, A. B., Weksler, M. E. & Paul, S. (2008). Autoantibody-catalyzed hydrolysis of amyloid beta peptide. *J. Biol. Chem., 283,* 4714-4722.

[62] Tguchi, H., Planque, S., Nishiyama, Y., Szabo, P. & Weksler, (2008). Catalytic antibodies to amyloid beta peptide in defense against Alzheimer disease. *Autoimmun Rev., 7,* 391-397.

[63] Lacroix -Desmazes, S., Misra, N., Bayry, J., Villard, S., Kazatchkine, M. D. & Kaveri, S. V. (2002). Antibodies with hydrolytic activity towards factor VIII in patients with hemophilia A. *J. Immunol. Methods, 269,* 251-256.

[64] Wootla, B., Dasgupta, S., Mallet, V., Kazatchkine, M. D., Nagaraja, V., Friboulet, A., Kaveri, S. V. & Lacroix-Desmazes, S. (2006). Physiopathology of catalytic antibodies: the case for factor VIII-hydrolyzing immunoglobulin G. *Blood Coagul. Fibrinolysis, 17,* 229-234.

[65] Lacroix -Desmazes, S., Kazatchkine, M. D. & Kaveri, S. V. (2003). Catalytic antibodies to factor VIII in haemophilia A. *Blood Coagul. Fibrinolysis, 14*; Suppl. 1, S31-S34.

[66] Bayry, J., Lacroix-Desmazes, S., Pashov, A., Stahl, D., Hoebeke, J., Kazatchkine, M. D. & Kaveri, S. V. (2003). Autoantibodies to factor VIII with catalytic activity. *Autoimmun. Rev., 2,* 30-35.

[67] Lacroix-Desmazes, S., Wootla, B., Delignat, S., Dasgupta, S., Nagaraja, V., Kazatchkine, M. D. & Kaveri, S. V. (2006). Pathophysiology of catalytic antibodies. *Immunol. Lett., 103,* 3-7.

[68] Taizo, U., Hifumi, E. & Okamura, Y. (2006). Super catalytic antibodies (antigenase) capable of destroying *H. pylori* urease. *Nippon Rinsho., 64,* 286-292.

[69] Parren, P. W., Leusen, J. H. & van de Winkel, J. G. (2003). Antibody-catalyzed water oxidation: state-of-the-art immunity or ancient history? *Trends Immunol., 24,* 467-469.

[70] Gabibov, A. G., Kozyr, A. V. & Kolesnikov, A. V. (2000). Disease association and cytotoxic effects of DNA-hydrolyzing autoantibodies. *Chem. Immunol., 77,* 130-156.

[71] Zouali, M. (2001). B cell tolerance to self in systemic autoimmunity. *Arch. Immunol. Ther. Exp. (Warsz)*, *49*, 361-365.

[72] Pisetsky, D. (2001). Immune response to DNA in systemic lupus erythematosus. *Isr. Med. Ass. J. 3*, 850-853.

[73] Earnshaw, W. C. & Rothfield, N. (1985). Identification of a family of human centromere proteins using autoimmune sera from patients with scleroderma. *Chromosoma*, *91*, 313-321.

[74] Raptis, L. & Menard, H. A. (1980). Quantitation and characterization of plasma DNA in normals and patients with systemic lupus erythematosus. *J. Clin. Invest.*, *66*, 1391-1399.

[75] Reimer, C., Raska, I., Tan, E. M. & Sheer, U. (1987). Human autoantibodies: probes for nucleolus structure and function. *Virchows. Arch. B Cell Pathol. Incl. Mol. Pathol.*, *54*, 131-36.

[76] Gottieb, A. A. & Shwartz, R. H. (1972). Antigen-RNA interactions. *Cell Immunol.*, *5*, 341-362.

[77] Kubota, T. (1977). Lessons from a monoclonal antibody to double-stranded DNA. *J. Med. Dent. Sci.*, *44*, 37-44.

[78] Mitsuhashi, S., Saito, R., Kurashige, S. & Yamashugi, N. (1978). Ribonucleic acid in the immune response. *Moll. Cell. Biochem.*, *20*, 131-147.

[79] Marion, T. N., Krishan, M. R., Desai, D. D., Jou, N. T. & Tillman, D. M. (1997). Monoclonal anti-DNA antibodies: structure, specificity, and biology. *Methods*, *11*, 3-113.

[80] Shoenfeld, Y., Ben-Yehuda, O., Messinger, Y., Bentwitch, Z., Rauch, J., Isenberg, D. I., Gadoth, N. (1988). Autoimmune diseases other than lupus share common anti-DNA idiotypes. *Immunol. Lett.*, *17*, 285-291.

[81] Nevinsky, G. A., Polosukhina, D. I. Doronon, B. M., Tyshkevich, O. B., Favorova, O. O. & Buneva V. N. (2004). Possible role of Abs hydrolyzing basic myelin protein in pathogenesis and diagnostics of multiple sclerosis. *Konsilium (Russ.) 4*, 30-34.

[82] Hhachn B. Ch. (1996). Systemic lipus erythematosus. In E. E. Braunvald, K.D. Isselbakher, R.G. Petersdorf, D. D., Wilson, D.B. Martin & A.S. Fauchi (Eds.), *Internal diseases*, pp. 407-419. Moscow: Medicine.

[83] Jager, L. (1988). *Klinishe immunologie and allergologie*, vol. 3, pp. 270-279. VEB Gustav Fischer Verlag.

[84] Yee, C. S., Hussein, H., Skan, J., Bowman, S., Situnayake, D. & Gordon C. (2003). Association of damage with autoantibody profile, age, race, sex and disease duration in systemic lupus erythematosus. *Rheumatology*, *42*, 276-279.

[85] Liu, G., Wang, Z., Wang, L., Xie Q., Zhang, R., Zuo, C. & Lin, M. (2002). The correlation between anticardiolipin antibodies and diseases activity in patients with systemic lupus erythematosus *Hua Xi Yi Ke Da Xue Xue Bao.*, *31*, 223-225.

[86] Korovkina, E. S., Zonova, E. V., Buneva, V. N., Konenkova, L. P. & Nevinsky G. A. (2006). Interdependency analysis between antibody level to different antigenes and clinical data of systemic lupus erythematosus. *Allergology and Immunology (Russ.)*, *7*, 498-507.

[87] Nasonov, E. L. (1994). *Klinics and immunopathology of rheumatic diseases*. Moscow: Binom.

[88] Dobrovolskii, A. B. & Panchenko E. P. (2002). In V. A. Tkachuk (Eds.), *Klinical biochemistry*. Moscow: Geotar-medicine.

[89] Boger, U., Hegedus, L., Hansen, J. M., Finke, R. & Shleusener, H. (1995). Thyroid cytotoxic antibodies in atrophic and goiters autoimmune thyroiditis. *Eur. J. Endocrinol., 132*, 69-74.

[90] Engler, H., Riesen, W. F. & Keller, B. (1994). Anti-thyroid peroxidase (anti-TPO) antibodies in thyroid diseases, non-thyroidal illness and controls. Clinical validity of a new commercial method for detection of anti-TPO (thyroid microsomal) autoantibodies. *Clin. Chem. Acta., 225*, 123-136.

[91] Shoenfeld, Y., Teplizki, H. A., Mendlovic, S., Blank, M. & Mozes, E. & Isenberg, D. A. (1989). The role of the human anti-DNA idiotype 16/6 in autoimmunity. *Clin. Immunol. Immunopathol., 51*, 313-325.

[92] Kozyr, A. V., Kolesnikov, A. V., Aleksandrova, E. S., Sashchenko, L. P., Gnuchev, N. V., Favorov, P. V., Kotelnikov, M. A., Iakhnina, E. I., Astsaturov, I. A., Prokaeva, T. B., Alekberova, Z. S., Suchkov, S. V. & Gabibov, A. G. (1998). Novel functional activities of anti-DNA autoantibodies from sera of patients with lymphoproliferative and autoimmune diseases. *Appl. Biochem. Biotechnol., 75*, 45-61.

[93] Gololobov, G. V., Mikhalap, S. V., Starov, A. V., Kolesnikov, A. F. & Gabibov, A. G. (1994). DNA-protein complexes. Natural targets for DNA-hydrolyzing antibodies. *Appl. Biochem. Biotechnol., 47*, 305-314.

[94] Sugiama, Y. & Yamamota, T. (1996). Characterization of serum anti-phospholipid antibodies in patients with multiple sclerosis. *Tohoku J. Exp. med., 178*, 203-215.

[95] Bigazzi, P. E. (1983). In: S. Cohen, P. E Wozd, & R. T. McKlaskie (Eds), *Mechanisms of Immunology*, pp. 181-206. Moscow: Meditsina.

[96] Founel, S. & Muller, S. (2002). Antinucleosome antibodies and T-cell response in systemic lupus erythematosus. *Ann. Med. Interne (Paris), 153*, 513-519.

[97] Blanco, F., Kalsi, J. & Isenberg, D. A. (1991). Analysis of antibodies to RNA in patients with systemic lupus erythematosus and other autoimmune rheumatic diseases. *Clin. Exp. Immunol., 86*, 66-70.

[98] Sato, T., Uvhiumi, T., Arakawa, M. & Kominami, R. (1994). Serological association of lupus autoantibodies to a limited functional domain of 28S ribosomal RNA and to the ribosomal proteins bound to the domain. *Clin. Exp. Immunol., 98*, 35-39.

[99] Hirokawa, K., Takasaki, Y., Takeuchi, K., Kaneda, K., Ikeda, K., Hashimoto, H. & Ikeda, R. (2002). Anti-TS1-RNA: characterization of novel antibodies against sequence-specific RNA by random RNA selection in patients with Sjogren's syndrome. *J. Rheumatol., 29*, 931-937.

[100] Ikeda, R., Takasaki, Y., Hirokawa, K., Takeuchi, K. & Hashimoto, H. (2003). Clinical significance of antibodies to TS1-RNA in patients with mixed connective tissue disease. *J. Rheumatol., 30*, 998-1005.

[101] Dabelic, N. & Cices, N. (1997). Clinical importance of antinuclear antibodies. *Lijec Vjesn., 119*, 236-242.

[102] O'Connor, K. C., Bar-Or, A. & Hafler, D. A. (2001). Neuroimmunology of multiple sclerosis. *J. Clin. Immunol., 21*, 81-92.

[103] Archelos, J. J., Storch, M. K. & Hartung, H. P. (2000). The role of B cells and autoantibodies in multiple sclerosis. *Ann. Neurol., 47*, 694-706.

[104] Hemmer, B., Archelos, J. J. & Hartung, H. P. (2002). New concepts in the immunopathogenesis of multiple sclerosis. *Nat. Rev. Neurosci.*, *3*, 291-301.

[105] Niehaus, A., Shi, J., Grzenkowski, M., Diers-Fenger, M., Archelos, J., Hartung, H. P., Toyka, K., Bruck, W. & Trotter, J. (2000). Patients with active relapsing-remitting multiple sclerosis synthesize antibodies recognizing oligodendrocyte progenitor cell surface protein: implications for remyelination. *Ann. Neurol.*, *48*, 362-371.

[106] Iglesias, A., Bauer, J., Litzenburger, T., Schubart, A. & Linington, C. (2001). T- and B-cell responses to myelin oligodendrocyte glycoprotein in experimental autoimmune encephalomyelitis and multiple sclerosis. *Glia*, *36*, 220-234.

[107] Cross, A. H., Trotter, J. L. & Lyons, J. (2001). B cells and antibodies in CNS demyelinating disease. *J. Neuroimmunol.*, *112*, 1-14.

[108] Williamson, R. A., Burgoon, M. P., Owens, G. P., Ghausi, O., Leclerc, E., Firme, L., Carlson, S., Corboy, J., Parren, P. W., Sanna, P. P., Gilden, D. H. & Burton, D. R. (2001). Anti-DNA antibodies are a major component of the intrathecal B cell response in multiple sclerosis. *Proc. Natl. Acad. Sci. USA*, *98*, 1793-1798.

[109] Ershova, N. A., Garmashova, N.V., Buneva, V. N., Mogel'nitskii, A. S., Tyshkevich, O. B., Doronin, B. M., Konenkova, L. P., Boiko, A. N., Slanova, A.V., Nesterova, V. A., Gusev, E. I., Favorova, O. O. & Nevinskii, G. A. (2003). Association between DNA antibodies levels in the blood of patients with multiple sclerosis and clinical presentation of the disease. *Zh. Nevrol. Psikhiatr. Im. S. S. Korsakova*, *2*, 25-33.

[110] Ershova, N. A., Garmashova, N. V., Mogel'nitskii, A. S., Tyshkevich, O. B., Doronin, B. M., Konenkova, L. P., Buneva, V. N. & Nevinskii, G. A. (2007). Antibodies to DNA in the blood of patients with multiple sclerosis. *Russ. J. Immunol.*, *1*, 229-245.

[111] Poser, C. M. (1984). *The diagnosis of multiple sclerosis*, pp. 3-13. NY: Thieme-Stratton.

[112] Polosukhina, D. I., Garmashova, N. V., Tyshkevich, O. B., Doronin, B. M., Buneva, V. N. & Nevinskii, G. A. (2009). Autoantibodies to myelin basic protein in patients with multiple sclerosis. *International Journal of Immunorehabilitation* (Russ), *11*, 10-18.

[113] Boiko, A. N. & Favorova O. O. (1995). Multiple sclerosis: molecular and cellular mechanisms. *Mol. Biol. (Moscow)*, *29*, 727-749.

[114] Gusev, E. I., Demina, T. L. & Boiko, A. N. (1997). *Multiple Sclerosis.* Moscow: Oil and Gas.

[115] Pihlaja, H. & Rantamaki, T. (2003). Linkage disequilibrium between the MBP tetranucleotide repeat and multiple sclerosis is restricted to a geographically defined subpopulation in Finland. *Genes and Immunity*, *4*, 138-146.

[116] Andersen, O., Lygner, P. E. & Bergstrom, T. (1993). Viral infections trigger multiple sclerosis relapses: a prospective seroepidemiological study. *J. Neurol.*, *240*, 417-422.

[117] Meinl, E. (1999). Concepts of viral pathogenesis of multiple sclerosis. *Curr. Opin. in Neurol.*, *12*, 303-307.

[118] Steinman, L. (2001). Multiple sclerosis: a two-stage disease. *Nat. Immunol.*, *2*, 2762-2764.

[119] Talbot, P. J., Paquette, J. S. & Ciurli C. (1996). Myelin basic protein and human coronavirus 229E cross-reactive T cells in multiple sclerosis. *Ann. Neurol.*, *39*, 233-240.

[120] Klinishe immunologie and allergologie (1988). , Jager L. (Ed.,). Jena, 3, 270-279.

[121] Senda, Y., Nishibu, M., Kawai, K., Mizukami, Y. & Hashimoto, T. (1995). Estimation of anti-thyroid peroxidase autoantibody and anti-thyroglobulin autoantibody in patients with various thyroid disease-comparison between histopathological findings and serological results in patients with Hashimoto's thyroiditis. *Rinsho-Byori*, *43*, 1243-1250.

[122] Paul, S., Li, L., Kalaga, R., O'Dell, J., Dannenbring, R. E., Jr., Swindells, S., Hinrichs, S., Caturegli, P. & Rose, N. R. (1997). Characterization of thyroglobulin-directed and polyreactive catalytic antibodies in autoimmune disease. *J. Immunol.*, *159*, 1530-1536.

[123] Garmashova, N. V., Kazanskiĭ, V. E., Tyshkevich, O. B., Doronin, B. M., Buneva, V. N. & Nevinskiĭ, G. A. (2004). Antibodies to DNA in the blood of patients with tick-borne encephalitis. *Mol. Biol. (Moscow)*, *38*, 723-730.

[124] Fauci, A.S., Braunwald, E, Kasper, D.L. et al. (2008). *Harrison's Principles of Internal Medicine, 17th Edition*. McGraw-Hill Professional.

[125] Matsiota-Bernard, P., Mahana, W., Avrameas, S. & Nauciel, C. (1993). Specific and natural antibody production during *Salmonella typhimurium* infection in genetically susceptible and resistant mice. *Immunology*, *79*, 375-380.

[126] Matsiota-Bernard, P., Hentati, B., Pie, S., Legakis, N., Nauciel, C., Avrameas, S. (1996). Beneficial effect of *Salmonella typhimurium* infection and of immunoglobulins from *S. typhimurium*-infected mice on the autoimmune disease of (NZB x NZW) F1 mice. *Clin. Exp. Immunol.*, *104*, 228-235.

[127] Hentati, B., Sato, M. N., Payelle, B., Avrameas, S. & Ternynck, T. (1994). Beneficial effect of polyclonal immunoglobulins from malaria-infected BALB/c mice on the lupus-like syndrome of (NZB x NZW)F1 mice. *Eur. J. Immunol.*, *24*, 8-15.

[128] Ternynck, P., Falanga, B., Unterkircher, C., Gregoire, J., Da Silva, L.P. & Avrameas, S. (1991). Induction of high levels of IgG autoantibodies in mice infected with Plasmodium chabaudi. *Int. Immunol.*, *3*, 29-37.

[129] Unterkircher, C., Avrameas, S. & Ternynck, T. (1993). Autoantibodies in the sera of Trypanosoma cruzi-infected individuals with or without clinical Chagas disease. *J. Clin. Lab. Anal.*, *7*, 60-69.

[130] Boekel, E. T., Siegert, C. E., Vrielink, G .J., Ceelen, A. & De Kievet, W. (2007). Analyses of CD27(++) plasma cells in peripheral blood from patients with bacterial infections and patients with serum antinuclear nntibodies. *J. Clin. Immunol.*, *27*, 467-76.

[131] Wun, H. L., Leung, D. T., Wong, K. C., Chui, Y. L. & Lim, P. L. (2001). Molecular mimicry: anti-DNA antibodies may arise inadvertently as a response to antibodies generated to microorganisms. *Int. Immunol.*, *13*, 1099-1107.

[132] Ikehara, S., Kawamura, M. & Takao, F. (1990). Organ-specific and systemic autoimmune diseases originate from defects in hematopoietic stem cells. *Proc. Natl. Acad. Sci.* USA, *87*, 8341-8344.

[133] Wentworth, P., Jr., Liu, Y., Wentworth, A. D., Fan, P., Foley, M. J. & Janda, K. D. (1998). A bait and switch hapten strategy generates catalytic antibodies for phosphodiester hydrolysis. *Proc. Natl. Acad. Sci.* USA, *95*, 5971-5975.

[134] Jerne, N. K. (1974). Towards a network theory of the immune system. *Ann. Immunol. (Paris)*, *125C*, 373-389.

[135] Izadyar, L., Friboulet, A., Remy, M. H., Roseto, A. & Thomas, D. (1993). Monoclonal anti-idiotypic antibodies as functional internal images of enzyme active sites: production of a catalytic antibody with a cholinesterase activity. *Proc. Natl. Acad. Sci. USA, 90*, 8876-8880.

[136] Kolesnikov, A. V., Kozyr, A. V., Alexandrova, E. S., Koralewski, F., Demin, A. V., Titov, M. I., Avalle, B., Tramontano, A., Paul, S., Thomas, D., Gabibov, A. G. & Friboulet, A. (2000). Enzyme mimicry by the antiidiotypic antibody approach. *Proc. Natl. Acad. Sci. USA, 97*, 13526-13531.

[137] Hu, R., Xie, G.Y., Zhang, X., Guo, Z.Q. & Jin, S. (1998). Production and characterization of monoclonal anti-idiotypic antibody exhibiting a catalytic activity similar to carboxypeptidase A. *J. Biotechnol., 61.* 109-115.

[138] Friboulet, A., Izadyar, L., Avalle, B., Roseto, A. & Thomas, D. (1994). Abzyme generation using an anti-idiotypic antibody as the "internal image" of an enzyme active site. *Appl. Biochem. Biotechnol., 47*, 229-237.

[139] Debat, H., Avalle, B., Chose, O., Sarde, C.-O., Friboulet, A., Thomas, D. (2001). Overpassing an aberrant V(kappa) gene to sequence an anti-idiotypic abzyme with (beta)-lactamase-like activity that could have a linkage with autoimmune diseases. *FASEB J., 15*, 815-822.

[140] Hifumi, E., Morihara, F., Hatiuchi, K., Okuda, T., Nishizono, A. & Uda, T. (2008). Catalytic features and eradication ability of antibody light-chain UA15-L against Helicobacter pylori. *J. Biol. Chem., 283*, 899-907.

[141] Shuster, A. M., Gololobov, G. V., Kvashuk, O. A. & Gabibov, A. G. (1991). DNA-specific catalytic antibodies in human blood sera. *Dokl. Akad. Nauk SSSR, 318*, 1262-1264.

[142] Gabibov, A. G., Gololobov, G. V., Makarevich, O. I., Schourov, D. V., Chernova, E. A. & Yadav, R. P. (1994). LND hydrolyzing autoantibodies. *Appl. Biochem. Biotechnol., 47*, 293-302.

[143] Odintsova, E. S., Buneva, V. N. & Nevinsky, G. A. (2005). Casein-hydrolyzing activity of sIgA antibodies from human milk. *J. Mol. Recognit., 18*, 413-421.

[144] Bronshtein, I. B., Shuster, A. M., Gololobov, G. V., Gromova, I. I., Kvashuk, O. A., Belostotskaya, K. M., Alekberova, Z. S., Prokaeva, T. B. & Gabibov, A. G. (1992). DNA-specific antiidiotypic antibodies in the sera of patients with autoimmune diseases. *FEBS Lett., 314*, 259-263.

[145] Crespeau, H., Laouar, A. & Rochu, D. (1994). Polyclonal DNase abzyme produced by anti-idiotypic internal image method. *CR Acad. Sci III., 317*, 819-823.

[146] Krasnorutskii, M. A., Buneva, V. N,, & Nevinsky, G. A.. (2008). Antibodies against DNA hydrolyze DNA and RNA. *Biochemistry (Moscow), 73*, 1547-1560.

[147] Krasnorutskii, M. A., Buneva, V. N. & Nevinsky, G. A. (2008). Antibodies against RNA hydrolyze RNA and DNA. *J. Mol. Recognit., 21*, 337–346.

[148] Krasnorutskii, M. A., Buneva, V. N. & Nevinsky, G. A. (2008). Immunization of rabbits with DNase I produces polyclonal antibodies with DNase and RNase activities. *J. Mol. Recognit., 21*, 233–242.

[149] Krasnorutskii, M. A., Buneva, V. N. & Nevinsky G. A. (2008). Anti-RNase Antibodies against pancreatic ribonuclease A hydrolyze RNA and DNA. *Int. Immunol., 20*, 1031-1040.

[150] Krasnorutskii, M. A., Buneva, V. N. & Nevinsky, G. A. (2009). Immunization of rabbits with DNase II leads to formation of polyclonal antibodies with DNase and RNase activities. *Int. Immunol., 21*, 349-360.

[151] Nishi, Y. (2002). Evolution of catalytic antibody repertoire in autoimmune mice. *J. Immunol. Methods, 269*, 213-233.

[152] Tawfik, D. S., Chap, R., Green, B. S., Sela, M. & Eshhar, Z. (2002). Unexpectedly high occurrence of catalytic antibodies in MRL/lpr and SJL mice immunized with a transition-state analog: is there a linkage to autoimmunity? *Proc. Natl. Acad. Sci. USA, 92*, 2145-2149.

[153] Buneva, V. N., Kudryavtseva, A. N., Gal'vita, A. V., Dubrovskaya, V. V., Khokhlova, O. V., Kalinina, I. A., Galenok, V. A. & Nevinsky, G. A. (2003). Dynamics of antibody nuclease activity in blood of women during pregnancy and lactation. *Biochemistry (Moscow), 68*, 890-900.

[154] Savel'ev, A. N., Kanyshkova, T. G., Kulminskaya, A. A., Buneva, V. N., Eneyskaya, E. V., Filatov, M. V., Nevinsky, G. A. & Neustroev, K. N.(2001). Amylolytic activity of IgG and sIgA immunoglobulins from human milk. *Clin. Chim. Acta, 314*, 141-152.

[155] Kanyshkova, T. G., Semenov, D. V., Khlimankov, D., Buneva, V. N. & Nevinsky, G. A. (1997). DNA-hydrolyzing activity of the light chain of IgG antibodies from milk of healthy human mothers. *FEBS Lett., 416*, 23-26.

[156] Nevinsky, G. A., Kanyshkova, T. G., Semenov, D. V., Vlassov, A. V., Gal'vita, A. V. & Buneva, V. N. (2000). Secretory immunoglobulin A from healthy human mothers' milk catalyzes nucleic acid hydrolysis. *Appl. Biochem. Biotechnol., 83*, 115-129.

[157] Buneva, V. N., Kanyshkova, T. G., Vlassov, A. V., Semenov, D. V., Khlimankov, D., Breusova, L. R. & Nevinsky, G. A. (1998). Catalytic DNA- and RNA-hydrolyzing antibodies from milk of healthy human mothers. *Appl. Biochem. Biotechnol., 75*, 63-76.

[158] Semenov, D. V., Kanyshkova, T. G., Kit, Y. Y., Khlimankov, D. Y., Akimzhanov, A. M., Gorbunov, D. A., Buneva, V. N. & Nevinsky, G. A. (1998). Human breast milk immunoglobulins G hydrolyze nucleotides. *Biochemistry (Moscow), 63*, 944-951.

[159] Nevinskii, G. A., Kanyshkova, T. G., Semenov, D. V. & Buneva, V. N. (2001). Catalytically active antibodies and their expected biological function. *Vestn. Ross. Akad. Med. Nauk, 2*, 38-45.

[160] Semenov, D. V., Kanyshkova, T. G., Karotaeva, N. A., Krasnorutskii, M. A., Kuznetsova, I. A., Buneva, V. N. & Nevinsky, G. A. (2004). Catalytic nucleotide-hydrolyzing antibodies in milk and serum of clinically healthy human mothers. *Med. Sci. Monit., 10*, BR23-BR33.

[161] Kit, Yu., Semenov, D. & Nevinskii, G. A. (1995). Do catalytically active antibodies exist in healthy people? *Mol. Biol. (Moscow), 29*, 893-906.

[162] Kit, Yu.Ya., Semenov, D. V. & Nevinsky, G. A. (1996). Phosphorylation of different human milk proteins by human catalytic secretory immunoglobulin A. *Biochem. Mol. Biol. Int., 39*, 521-527.

[163] Nevinsky, G. A., Kit, Y., Semenov, D. V., Khlimankov, D. & Buneva, V. N. (1998). Secretory immunoglobulin A from human milk catalyses milk protein phosphorylation. *Appl. Biochem. Biotechnol., 75*, 77-91.

[164] Gorbunov, D. A., Semenov, D. V., Shipitsin, M.V. & Nevinsky, G. A. (2001). Unusual phospholipids of human breast milk. *Dokl. Biochem. Biophys., 377*, 62-64.

[165] Gorbunov, D. V., Semenov, D. V., Shipitsin, M. V., Kit, Yu. Yu., Kanyshkova, T. G., Buneva, V. N. & Nevinsky, G. A. (2000). Phosphorylation of minor lipids of human milk tightly bound to secretory immunoglobulin A. *Rus. J. Immunol.*, *5*, 267-278.

[166] Gorbunov, D. V., Karataeva, N. A., Buneva, V. N. & Nevinsky, G. A. (2005). Lipid kinase activity of antibodies from milk of clinically healthy human mothers. *Biochim. Biophys. Acta*, *1735*, 153-166.

[167] Karataeva, N. A., Gorbunov, D., Prokudin, I. V., Buneva, V. N., Kulminskaya, A. A., Neustroev, K. N. & Nevinsky, G. A. (2006). Human milk antibodies with polysaccharide kinase activity. *Immunol. Lett.*, *103*, 58-67.

[168] Karataeva, N. A., Buneva, V. N. & Nevinsky, G. A. (2006). Polysaccharide kinase activity of human milk IgG antibodies. *Biochemistry (Moscow)*, *71*, 1488-1504.

[169] Karataeva, N. A. & Nevinsky, G. A. (2007). Enzymes phosphorylating lipids and polysaccharides. *Biochemistry (Mosc)*, *72*, 367-379.

[170] Amino, N., Mori, H., Iwatani, Y., Tanizawa, O., Kawashima, M., Tsuge, I., Ibaragi, K., Kumahara, Y. & Miyai, K. (1982). High prevalence of transient post-partum thyrotoxicosis and hypothyroidism. *N. Engl. J. Med.*, *306*, 849-852.

[171] Tanaka, A., Lindor, K., Ansari, A. & Gershwin, M. E. (2000). Fetal microchimerisms in the mother: immunologic implications. *Liver Transpl.*, *6*, 138-143.

[172] Dayan, C. M. & Daniels, G. H. (1996). Chronic autoimmune thyroiditis. *New Engl. J. Med.*, *335*, 99-107.

[173] Freeman, R., Rosen, H. & Thysen, B. (1986). Incidence of thyroid dysfunction in an unselected post-partum population. *Arch. Intern. Med.*, *146*, 1361-1364.

[174] Fey, H. R., Burtler, R. & Marti, F. (1973). The production in the pregnant cow of anti-human immunoglobulin to be used for the antiglobulin test. *Vox Sang*, *25*, 245-253.

[175] Mestecky, J. & McGhee, J. R. (1987). Immunoglobulin A (IgA): molecular and cellular interactions involved in IgA biosynthesis and immune response. *Adv. Immunol.*, *40*, 153-245.

[176] Kazakov, V. I., Bozhkov, V. M., Linde V. A., Repina, M. A., Mikhailov, V. M. (1995). Extracellular DNA of pregnant women blood. *Tsitologiia (Moscow)*, *37*, 232-235.

[177] Newman, J. (1995). How breast milk protects newborns. *Sci. Am.*, *273*, 76-79.

[178] Mikhailov, V. M., Linde, V. A., Rozanov, I. M., Kottsova, N. A., Susloparov, L. A. & Konycheva, E. A. (1992). DNA synthesis and content in human decidual cells at different stages of differentiation based on flow cytometry data. *Tsitologiia (Moscow)*, *34*, 67-71.

[179] Redhead, K., Hill, T. & Mulloy, B. (1990). Antimicrobial effect of human milk on Bordetella pertussis. *FEMS Microbiol Let.*, *58*, 269-273.

[180] Gillin, F. D., Reiner, D. S. & Wang, C. S. (1983). Human milk kills parasitic intestinal protozoa. *Science*, *221*, 1290-1292.

[181] Nagata, S. & Suda, T. (1995). Fas and Fas ligand: *lpr* and *gld* mutations. *Immunol. Today*, *16*, 39-43.

[182] Watanabe-Fukunada, R., Brannan, C. I. & Copeland, N. G. (1992). Lymphoproliferation disorder in mice explained by defects in Fas antigen that mediates apoptosis. *Nature*, *356*, 314-317.

[183] Ponomarenko, N. A., Durova, O. M., Vorobiev, I. I., Telegin, G. V., Chamborant, O. G., Sidorik, L. L., Suchkov, S. V., Alekbarova, Z. S., Gnuchev, N. V. & Gabibov, A. G.

(2002). Catalytic antibodies in clinical and experimental pathology: human and mouse models. *J. Immunol. Methods*, *269*, 197-221.

[184] Mouratou, B., Rouyre, S. & Guedson, J. L. (2002). A method for the detection and screening of catalytic anti-DNA antibodies. *J. Immunol. Methods*, *269*, 147-155.

[185] Kim, J. S., Lee, S. Y., Lee, W. R., Sohn, J. N., Chung, Y. C., Shim, H. K., Lee, S. C., Kwon, M. H. & Kim, Y. S. (2006). Heavy and light chain variable single domains of an anti-DNA binding antibody hydrolyze both double- and single-stranded DNAs without sequence specificity. *J. Biol. Chem.*, *281*, 15287-15295.

[186] Dubrovskaya, V. V., Andryushkova, A. S., Kuznetsova, I. A., Toporkova, L. B., Buneva, V. N., Orlovskaya, I. A. & Nevinsky, G. A. (2003). DNA-hydrolyzing antibodies from sera of autoimmune-prone MRL/MpJ-lpr mice. *Biochemistry (Moscow)*, *68*, 1081-1088.

[187] Andryushkova, A. A., Kuznetsova, I. A., Orlovskaya, I. A., Buneva, V. N. & Nevinsky, G. A. (2006). Antibodies with amylase activity from the sera of autoimmune-prone MRL/MpJ-lpr mice. *FEBS Lett.*, *580*, 5089-5095.

[188] Andryushkova, A. S., Kuznetsova, I. A., Orlovskaya, I. A., Buneva, V. N. & Nevinsky, G. A. (2009). Nucleitide-hydrolyzing antibodies from the sera of autoimmune-prone MRL-lpr/lpr mice. *Int. immunol.*, *21*, 935-945.

[189] Andryushkova, A. S., Kuznetsova, I. A., Buneva, V. N., Toporkova, L. B., Sakhno, L. V., Tichonova, M. A., Chernykh, E. R., Orlovskaya, I. A. & Nevinsky, G. A. (2007). Formation of different abzymes in autoimmune-prone MRL-lpr/lpr mice is associated with changes in colony formation of haematopoetic progenitors. *J. Cell. Mol. Med.*, *11*, 531-551.

[190] Hanson, L. A., Carlsson, B. & Cruz, J. R. (1979). Colostrum-derived immunity and maternal–neonatal interaction, pp. 145-157. In: P. L Ogra and D. H. Dayton (Eds.), *Immunology of Breast milk*. New York: Raven Press.

[191] Roux, M. E., McWilliams, M., Phillips-Quagliata, J. M., Weisz-Carrington, P. & Lamm, M. E. (1977). Origin of IgA-secreting plasma cells in the mammary gland. *J. Exp. Med.*, *146*, 1311-1322.

[192] Butcher, E. C., Rouse, R. V., Coffman, R. L., Nottenburg, C. N., Hardy, R. R. & Weissman, I. L. (1982). Surface phenotype of Peyer's patch germinal center cells: implications for the role of germinal centers in B cell differentiation. *J. Immunol.*, *129*, 2698-2707.

[193] Brandtzaeg, P., Farstad, I.N., Johansen, F. E., Morton, H. C., Norderhaug, I. N. & Yamanaka, T. (1999). The B-cell system of human mucosae and exocrine glands. *Immunol. Rev.*, *171*, 45-87.

[194] Kim, K., Keller, M. A. & Heiner, D. C. (1992). Immunoglobulin G subclasses in human colostrum, milk, and saliva. *Acta Paediatr.*, *81*, 113-118.

[195] Galvita, A. V., Baranovskii, A. G. Kuznetsova, I. A., Vinshu, N. V., Galenok, V. A., Buneva, V. N. & Nevinsky G. A. (2007). A peculiarity of DNA hydrolysis by antibodies from patients with diabetes. *Russ. J. Immunol.*, *1*, 116-131.

[196] Odintsova, E. S., Parkhomanko, T. A., Buneva, V. N., Generalov, I. I. & Nevinsky, G. A. (2006). IgG antibodies from the sera of patients with some infectional diseases. *Immunopathology. Allergology and Infectology (Russian)*, *2*, 23-31.

[197] Sun, M., Li, L., Gao, Q. S., Paul, S. (1994). Antigen recognition by an antibody light chain. *J. Biol. Chem.*, *269*, 734-738.

[198] Sun, M., Gao, Q. S., Kirnarskiy, L., Rees, A., Paul, S. (1997). Cleavage specificity of a proteolytic antibody light chain and effects of the heavy chain variable domain. *J. Mol. Biol.*, *271*, 374-385.

[199] Mei, S., Mody, B., Eklund, S. H., Paul, S. (1991). Vasoactive intestinal peptide hydrolysis by antibody light chains. *J. Biol. Chem.*, *266*, 15571-15574.

[200] Tyutyulkova, S., Gao, Q. S., Thompson, A., Rennard, S., Paul, S. (1996). Efficient vasoactive intestinal polypeptide hydrolyzing autoantibody light chains selected by phage display. *Biochim. Biophys. Acta*, *1316*, 217-223.

[201] Andrievskaya, O. A., Buneva, V. N., Naumov, V. A. & Nevinsky, G. A. (2000). Catalytic heterogeneity of polyclonal RNA-hydrolyzing IgM from sera of patients with lupus erythematosus. *Med. Sci. Monit.*, *6*, 460 –470.

[202] Andrievskaya, O. A., Buneva, V. N., Baranovskii, A. G., Gal'vita, A. V., Benzo, E. S., Naumov, V. A. & Nevinsky, G. A. (2002). Catalytic diversity of polyclonal RNA-hydrolyzing IgG antibodies from the sera of patients with systemic lupus erythematosus. *Immunol. Lett.*, *81*, 191-198.

[203] Baranovskii, A. G., Ershova, N. A., Buneva, V. N., Kanyshkova, T. G., Mogelnitskii, A. S., Doronin, B. M., Boiko, A. N., Gusev, E. I., Favorova, O. O. & Nevinsky, G. A. (2001). Catalytic heterogeneity of polyclonal DNA-hydrolyzing antibodies from the sera of patients with multiple sclerosis. *Immunol Lett.*, *76*, 163-167.

[204] Wentworth, P. Jr., Jones, L. H., Wentworth, A. D., Zhu, X., Larsen, N. A., Wilson, I. A., Xu, X., Goddard, W. A. 3rd, Janda, K. D., Eschenmoser, A. & Lerner, R. A. (2001). Antibody catalysis of the oxidation of water. *Science*, *293*, 1806-1811.

[205] Wentworth, A. D., Jones, L. H., Wentworth, P. Jr., Janda, K. D., Lerner, R. A. (2000). Antibodies have the intrinsic capacity to destroy antigens. *Proc. Natl. Acad. Sci. USA*, *97*, 10930-10935.

[206] Ikhmyangan, E. N., Vasilenko, N. L., Buneva, V. N. & Nevinsky, G. A. (2005). IgG antibodies with peroxidase-like activity from the sera of healthy Wistar rats. *FEBS Lett.*, *579*, 3960-3964.

[207] Ikhmyangan, E. N., Vasilenko, N. L., Buneva, V. N. & Nevinsky, G. A. (2006). Metal ions-dependent peroxidase and oxidoreductase activities of polyclonal IgGs from the sera of Wistar rats. *J. Mol. Recognit.*, *19*, 91-105.

[208] Ikhmyangan, E. N., Vasilenko, N. L., Sinitsina, O. I., Buneva, V. N. & Nevinsky, G. A. (2006). Substrate specificity of rat sera IgG antibodies with peroxidase and oxidoreductase activities. *J. Mol. Recognit.*, *19*, 432-440.

[209] Ikhmyangan, E. N., Vasilenko, N. L., Sinitsina, O. I., Buneva, V. N. & Nevinsky, G. A. (2006). Catalytic heterogeneity of immunoglobulins G with peroxidase activity derived from blood of healthy Wistar rats. *Immunopathology, Allergology, Infectology (Russian)*, *2*, 32-48.

[210] Golinelli-Pimpaneau, B., Gigant, B., Bizebard, T., Nazava, J., Saludjian, P., Zemel, R., Tawfik, D. S., Eshhar, Z., Green, B. S. & Knossow, M. (1994). Crystal structure of catalytic antibody Fab with esterase-like activity. *Current Biology, Structure*, *2*, 175-183.

[211] Legostaeva, G. A., Polosukhina, D. I., , Bezuglova, A. M., Doronin, B. M. Buneva, V. N. & Nevinsky, G. A. (2010) Affinity and catalytic heterogeneity of polyclonal myelin basic protein-hydrolyzing IgGs from sera of patients with multiple sclerosis. *J. Cell Mol. Med.*, *14*, 699-709.

[212] Baranovskii, A. G., Matushin, V. G., Vlassov, A. V., Zabara, V. G., Naumov, V. A., Buneva, V. N., Nevinskii, G. A. (1997). DNA- and RNA-hydrolyzing antibodies from the blood of patients with various forms of viral hepatitis. *Biochemistry (Moscow)*, *62*, 1358-1366.

[213] Fersht, A. (1985). *Enzyme Structure and Mechanism*, 2nd ed. N.Y.: W. H. Freeman, Co.

[214] Dixon, M. & Webb, E. C. (1979). Enzymes, Third addition, Longman Group Ltd.

[215] Vlassov, A. V., Andrievskaya, O. A., Kanyshkova, T. G., Baranovsky, A. G., Naumov, V. A., Breusov, A. A., Giege, R., Buneva, V. N. & Nevinsky, G. A. (1997). RNA-hydrolyzing antibodies from peripheral blood of patients with lupus erythematosus, *Biochemistry (Moscow). 62*, 474-479.

[216] Vlasov, A. V., Baranovskii, A. G., Kanyshkova, T. G., Prints, A. V., Zabara, V. G., Naumov, V. A., Breusov, A. A., Giege R., Buneva, V. N. & Nevinskii, G. A. (1998). Substrate specificity of serum DNA- and RNA-hydrolyzing antibodies of patients with polyarthritis and autoimmune thyroiditis. *Mol. Biol. (Mosk)*, *32*, 559-569.

[217] Vlassov, A, Florentz, C., Helm, M., Naumov, V, Buneva, V, Nevinsky, G. & Giege, R. (1998). Characterization and selectivity of catalytic antibodies from human serum with RNAse activity. *Nucleic Acid Research*, *26*, 5243-5250.

[218] Vlassov, A. V., Helm, M., Florentz, C., Naumov, V., Breusov, A. A. Buneva V. N, Giege, R. & Nevinsky, G. A. (1999). Variability of substrate specificity of serum antibodies obtained from patients with different autoimmune and viral deseases in reaction of tRNA hydrolysis. *Russ. J. Immunol.*, *4*, 25-32.

[219] Vlasov, A. V., Helm, M., Naumov, V. A., Breusov, A. A., Buneva, V. N., Florentz, C., Giege, R. & Nevinskii, G. A. (1999). Features of tRNA hydrolysis by autoantibodies from blood serum of patients with certain autoimmune and virus diseases. *Mol. Biol. (Moscow)*, *33*, 866-872.

[220] Andrievskaia, O. A., Kanyshkova, T. G., Iamkovoi, V. I., Buneva, V. N. & Nevinskii, G. A. (1997). Monoclonal antibodies to DNA hydrolyze RNA better than DNA. *Dokl. Akad. Nauk*, *355*, 401-403.

[221] Komoda, T., Koyama, I., Hasegawa, M. & Sakagishi, Y. (1983). Alkaline phosphatase - with special reference to alkaline phosphatases of the blood cells. *Rinsho Byori*, *31*, 682-691.

[222] Hardonk, M. J. & Koudstaal, J. (1976). Enzyme histochemistry as a link between biochemistry and morphology. *Prog. Histochem. Cytochem.*, *8*, 1-68.

[223] Berneman, A., Cuilbert, B., Enschrich, S. & Avrames, S. (1993). IgG auto- and polyreactivities of normal human sera. *Mol. Immunol.*, *30*, 1499-1510.

[224] Coutinho, A., Kazatchkine, M. D. & Avrameas, S. (1995). Natural autoantibodies. *Curr. Opin. Immunol.*, *7*, 812-818.

[225] Raz, E., Ben-Bassat, H., Davidi, T., Shlomoz, Z. & Eilat, D. (1993). Cross-reactions of anti-DNA autoantibodies with cell surface proteins. *Eur. J. Immunol.*, *23*, 383-390.

[226] Gololobov, G. V., Chernova, E. A., Schourov, D. V., Smirnov, I. V., Kudelina, I. A. & Gabibov, A. G. (1995). Cleavage of supercoiled plasmid DNA by autoantibody Fab fragment: application of the flow linear dichroism technique. *Proc. Natl. Acad. Sci. USA*, *92*, 254-257.

[227] Baranovskii, A. G., Kanyshkova, T. G., Mogelnitskii, A. S., Naumov, V. A., Buneva, V. N., Gusev, E. I., Boiko, A. N., Zargarova, T. A., Favorova, O. O. & Nevinsky, G. A.

(1998). Polyclonal antibodies from blood and cerebrospinal fluid of patients with multiple sclerosis effectively hydrolyze DNA and RNA. *Biochemistry (Moscow). 63*, 1239-1248.

[228] Andrievskaia, O. A., Buneva, V. N., Zabara, V. G., Naumov, V. A., Iamkovoi, V. I. & Nevinskii, G. A. (1998). Class M immunoglobulins from blood serum of patients with systemic lupus erythematosus effectively cleave RNA. *Mol. Biol. (Moscow), 32*, 908-915.

[229] Akagi, K., Murai, K., Hirao, N. & Yamanaka, M. (1976). Purification and properties of alkaline ribonucleases from human serum. *Biochim. Biophys. Acta, 442*, 368-378.

[230] Kuznetsova, I. A., Orlovskaya, I. A., Buneva, V. N. & Nevinsky, G. A. (2007). Activation of DNA-hydrolyzing antibodies from the sera of autoimmune-prone MRL-lpr/lpr mice by different metal ions. *Biochim. Biophys. Acta, 1774*, 884-896.

[231] Paul, S., Mei, S., Mody, B., Eklund, S. H., Beach, C. M., Massey, R. J. & Hamel, F. (1991). Cleavage of vasoactive intestinal peptide at multiple sites by autoantibodies. *J. Biol. Chem., 266*, 16128-16134.

[232] Paul, S., Karle, S., Planque, S., Taguchi, H., Salas, M., Nishiyama, Y., Handy, B., Hunter, R., Edmundson, A, & Hanson, C. (2004). Naturally occurring proteolytic antibodies: selective immunoglobulin M-catalyzed hydrolysis of HIV gp120. *J. Biol. Chem., 279*, 39611-30619.

[233] Ponomarenko, N. A., Durova, O. M., Vorobiev, I. I., Belogurov, A. A., Kurkova, I. N., Petrenko, A. G., Telegin, G. B., Suchkov, S. V., Kiselev, S. L., Lagarkova, M. A., Govorun, V. M., Serebryakova, M. V., Avalle, B., Tornatore, P., Karavanov, A., Thomas, D., Friboulet, A. & Gabibov, A. G. (2006). Autoantibodies to myelin basic protein catalyze site-specific degradation of their antigen. *Proc. Natl. Acad. Sci. USA, 103*, 281-286.

[234] Savel'ev, A. N., Eneyskaya, E. V., Shabalin, K. A., Filatov, M. V. & Shabalin, K. A., (1999). Autoantibodies with amylolytic activity. *Prot. Pept. Lett., 6*, 179-184.

[235] Ivanen, D. R., Kulminskaya, A. A., Shabalin, K. A., Isaeva-Ivanova, L. V., Ershova N. A., Saveliev, A. N., Nevinsky, G. A. & Neustroev, K. N. (2004). Catalytic properties of IgMs with amylolytic activity isolated from patients with multiple sclerosis. *Med. Sci. Monit., 10*, BR273-BR280.

[236] Neustoev, K. N., Ivanen, D. R., Kulminskaya, A. A., Brumer, I. H., Saveliev, A. N. & Nevinsky, G. A. (2003). Amylolytic activity and catalytic properties of IgM and IgG antibodies from patients with systemic lupus erythematosus. *Human antibodies, 12*, 31-34.

[237] Savel'iev, A. N., Ivanen, D. R., Kulminskaya, A. A., Ershova, N. A., Kanyshkova, T. G., Buneva, V. N., Mogelnitskii, A. S., Doronin, B. M., Favorova, O. O. & Nevinsky, G. A. & Neustroev, K. (2003). Amylolytic activity of IgM and IgG antibodies from patients with multiple sclerosis. *Immunol. Lett., 86*, 291-297.

[238] Gololobov, G. V., Rumbley, C. A., Rumbley, J. N., Schourov, D. V., Makarevich, O. I., Gabibov, A. G., Voss, E. W., Jr. & Rodkey, L. S. (1997). DNA hydrolysis by monoclonal anti-ssDNA autoantibody BV 04-01: origins of catalytic activity. *Mol. Immunol., 34*, 1083-1093.

[239] Kasho, V. N. & Baykov, A. A. (1989). Two pathways for phosphate/water oxygen exchange by yeast inorganic pyrophosphatase. *Biochem. Biophys. Res. Commun., 161*, 475-480.

[240] Shestakov, A. A., Baykov, A. A. & Avaeva, S. M. (1990). Tightly bound pyrophosphate in *Escherichia coli* inorganic pyrophosphatase. *FEBS Lett.*, *262*, 194-196.
[241] Smirnova, I. N., Shestakov, A. S., Dubnova, E. B. & Baykov, A. A. (1989). Spectral and kinetic studies of phosphate and magnesium ion binding to yeast inorganic pyrophosphatase. *Eur. J. Bioche.*, *182*, 451-456.
[242] Tolmacheva, A. S., Zaksas, N. P., Buneva, V. N., Vasilenko, N. L. & Nevinsky, G. A. (2009). Oxidoreductase activities of polyclonal IgGs from the sera of Wistar rats are better activated by combinations of different metal ions. *J. Mol. Recognit.*, *22*, 26-37.
[243] Sorrentino, S. & Libonaty, M. (1994). Human pancreatic-type and nonpancreatic-type ribonucleases: a direct side-by -side comparison of their catalytic properties. *Biochemistry*, *312*, 340-344.
[244] Sorrentino, S. & Libonaty, M. (1997). Structure-function relationships in human ribonucleases: main distinctive features of the major RNase types. *FEBS Lett.*, *404*, 1-5.
[245] Horl, W. H., Wanner, C. & Schollmer, P. (1987). Proteinases in catabolism and malnutrition. *JPEN J. Parenter. Enteral Nutr.*, *11*, 98S-103S.
[246] Rao, M. B., Tanksale, A. M., Ghatge, M. S. & Deshhange, V. V. (1998). Molecular and biotechnological aspects of microbial proteases. *Microbiol. Mol. Biol. Rev.*, *62*, 597-635.
[247] Bernardi, G. (1971). In Boyer, P.D. (Eds.), *The enzymes*. New York: Academic Press.
[248] Suck, D. (1994). DNA recognition by DNase I. *J. Mol. Recognit.*, *7*, 65 -70.
[249] Odintsova, E. S., Kharitonova, M. A., Baranovskii, A. G., Siziakina, L. P., Buneva, V. N. & Nevinskii, G. A. (2006). DNA-hydrolyzing IgG antibodies from the blood of patients with acquired immune deficiency syndrome. *Mol. Biol. (Moscow)*, *40*, 857-864.
[250] Shapot, V. S. (1968). *Nucleases*, pp. 1-162. Moscow; Medicine Press.
[251] Sierakowska, H. & Shugar, D. (1977). Mammalian nucleolytic enzymes. *Progr. Nucleic Acid Res. Mol. Biol.*, *20*, 59-130.
[252] Akagi, K., Yamanaka, M., Murai, K. & Omae, T. (1978). Purification and properties of acid ribonucleases in humam serum and leukocytes. *Cancer Res.*, *38*, 2163-2167.
[253] Sorrentino, S., Libonaty, M. (1994). Human pancreatic-type and nonpancreatic-type ribonucleases: a direct side-by-side comparison of their catalytic properties. *Arch. Biochem. Biophys.*, *312*, 340-348.
[254] Krieg, A. M. ,Yi, A. K., Matson, S., Waldschmidt, T. J., Bishop, G. A., Teasdale, R., Koretzky, G. A. & Klinman, D. M. (1995). CpG motifs in bacterial DNA trigger direct B-cell activation. *Nature*, *374*, 546-549.
[255] Gilkeson, G. S., Grudier, J. P., Karounos, D. G. & Pisetsky, D. S. (1989). Induction of anti-double stranded DNA antibodies in normal mice by immunization with bacterial DNA. *J. Immunol.*, *151*, 1614-1626.
[256] Fletcher, M. C., Kuderova, A., Cygler M. & Lee, J. S. (1998). Creation of a ribonuclease abzyme through site-directed mutagenesis. *Nat. Biotechnol.*, *16*, 1065-1067.
[257] Paul, S. (1994). Catalytic activity of anti-ground state antibodies, antibody subunits, and human autoantibodies. *Appl. Biochem. Biotechnol.*, *47*, 241-253.

[258] Paul, S., Said, S. I., Thompson, A. B., Volle, D. J., Agrawal, D. K., Foda, H. & de la Rocha, S. (1989). Characterization of autoantibodies to vasoactive intestinal peptide in asthma. Characterization of autoantibodies to vasoactive intestinal peptide in asthma. *J. Neuroimmunol.*, *23*, 133-142.

[259] Belogurov, A. A., Kurkova, I. N., Friboulet, A., Thomas, D., Misikov, V. K., Zakharova, M. Y., Suchkov, S. V., Kotov, S. V., Alehin, A. I., Avalle, B., Suslova, E. A., Morse 3rd, H. C., Gabibov, A. G, & Ponomarenko, N. A. (2008). Recognition and degradation of myelin basic protein peptides by serum autoantibodies: novel biomarker for multiple sclerosis. *J. Immunol.*, *180*, 1258-1267.

[260] Kozyr, A. V., Sashchenko, L. P., Kolesnikov, A. V., Zelenova, N. A., Khaidukov, S. V., Ignatova, A. N., Bobik, T. V., Gabibov, A. G., Alekberova, Z. S., Suchkov, S. V. & Gnuchev, N. V. (2002). *Immunol. Lett.*, *80*, 41-47.

[261] Sinohara, H. & Matsuura, K. (2000). Does catalytic activity of Bence-Jones proteins contribute to the pathogenesis of multiple myeloma? *Appl. Biochem. Biotechnol.*, *83*, 85-94.

[262] Nevinsky, G. A., Breusov, A. A., Baranovskii, A. G., Prints, A. V., Kanyshkova, T. G., Galvita, A. V., Naumov, V. A. & Buneva, V. N. (2001). Effect of different drugs on the level of DNA-hydrolyzing polyclonal IgG antibodies in sera of patients with Hashimoto's thyroiditis and nontoxic nodal goiter. *Med. Sci. Monit.*, *7*, 201-211.

[263] Breusov, A. A., Gal'vita, A. V., Benzo, E. S., Baranovskii, A. G., Prints, A. V., Naumov, V. A., Buneva, V. N. & Nevinsky, G. A. (2001). Comparison of the level of DNA-hydrolyzing polyclonal IgG antibodies in sera of patients with Hashimoto's thyroiditis and nontoxic nodal goiter. *Rus. J. Immunol.*, *6*, 17-28.

[264] Li, L., Paul, S., Tyutyulkova, S., Kazatchkine, M. D. & Kaveri, S. (1995) Catalytic activity of anti-thyroglobulin antibodies. *J. Immunol.*, *154*, 3328-3332.

[265] Ivanen, D. R., Kulminskaya, A. A., Eneyskaya, E. V., Ershova N. A., Shabalin, K. A., Savel'ev, A. N., Kanyshkova, T. G., Buneva V. N., Nevinsky G. A. & Neustroev, K. N. (2002). Human autoantibodies with amylolytic activity. *Biologia (Bratislava)*, *57*, suppl. 11, 253-260.

[266] Savel'ev, A. N., Kulminskaya, A. A., Ivanen, D. R., Nevinsky G. A. & Neustroev, K. N. (2004). Human antibodies with amylolytic activity. *Trends in Glycoscience and Glycotechnology*, *16*, 17-31.

[267] Tomasi, T. B. (1979). Introduction In P. L. Ogra, & D. H. Dayton (Eds.), *Immunology of Breast milk*. New York: Raven Press.

[268] Fiat, A. M. & Jolles, P. (1989). Caseins of various origins and biologically active casein peptides and oligosaccharides: structural and physiological aspects. *Mol. Cell. Biochem.*, *87*, 5-30.

[269] Brambell, F. W. (1970). *The transmission of passive immunity from mother to young*. Amsterdam: North-Holland.

[270] Ramaswamy, H., Swamy, C. V. & Das, M. R. (1993). Purification and characterization of a high molecular weight ribonuclease from human milk. *J. Biol. Chem.*, *268*, 4181-4187.

[271] Wiegandt, H. (1985). *Glycolipids*. Amsterdam: Elsevier.

[272] Meyer zu Heringdorf D., van Koppen, C. J. & Jacobs, K. H. (1997). Molecular diversity of sphingolipids signalling. *FEBS Lett.*, *410*, 34-38.

[273] Kates, M. (1972). *Techniques of lipidology*. New York: Elsevier.

[274] Jensen, R.G. (1989). *The lipids of human milk*, pp. 65-92. Boca Raton, Fla: CRC Press.
[275] Coppa, G. V., Bruni, S., Morelli, L., Soldi, S. & Gabrielli, O. (2004). The first prebiotics in humans: human milk oligosaccharides. *J. Clin. Gastroenterol.*, *38*, (6 Suppl), S80-S83.
[276] Newburg, D.S. (1999). Human milk glycoconjugates that inhibit pathogens. *Curr. Med. Chem.*, *6*, 117-127.
[277] De Prada, P., Winger, G. & Landry, D. W. (2000). Application of artificial enzymes to the problem of cocaine. *Ann. N.Y. Acad. Sci.*, *909*, 159-169.
[278] Ponomarenko, N. A., Vorobiev, I. I., Alexandrova, E. S., Reshetnyak, A. V., Telegin, G. B., Khaidukov, S. V., Avalle, B., Karavanov, A., Morse, H. C. (3rd), Thomas, D., Friboulet, A. & Gabibov, A. G. (2006). Induction of a protein-targeted catalytic response in autoimmune prone mice: antibody-mediated cleavage of HIV-1 glycoprotein GP120. *Biochemistry*, *45*, 324-330.

Chapter 2

LUPUS NEPHRITIS: FRONTIERS AND CHALLENGES: A COMPREHENSIVE OVERVIEW

Hussein Sheashaa[1,], Tarek Abbas[1], Fatma Moustafa[2], Khaled Mahmoud[1], Amgad el-Agroudy[1], Anil Chandraker[3], Nidyanandh Vadivel[3], Rashad Hassan[1], Ashraf Bakr[4], Mohamed Zedan[4], Noha Tharwat[4], Wael Elkady[5], and Mohamed Sobh[1]*

[1] Urology and Nephrology Center, Mansoura University, Egypt
[2] Pathology dept, Mansoura University, Egypt
[3] Brigham and women's Hospital, Harvard Medical School, Harvard University, USA
[4] Pediatric hospital, Mansoura University, Egypt,
[5] Surgery, Transplantation, The Methodist Hospital, Houston, TX, USA

ABSTRACT

Lupus nephritis (LN) is a major cause of morbidity and mortality, affecting over half of systemic lupus erythematosis (SLE) patients. It affects adult and pediatric patients. Kidney biopsy remains the cornerstone of LN diagnosis, and there are new International Society of Nephrology/Renal Pathology Society classifications of LN. Although prognosis of LN has improved with the combined use of cytotoxic and steroid therapy, up to 20% of these patients progress to renal failure. Moreover, toxicity of the current regimens remains a major concern. The accelerating advances in molecular and cellular immunology have paved the way for development biologic agents that target specific pathways that contribute to the inflammatory response, but there is no strong evidence of their safety and efficacy. Moreover, the increased risk of renal allograft thrombosis and recurrence of lupus nephritis constitute a substantial risk that should be thoroughly explored. The aim of this chapter is to explore all these aspects in a comprehensive manner. In addition, we will explore the major advances that necessitate the evolution of basic and clinical research to explore the magic management of this syndrome dilemma.

---

[*] Corresponding author: Assistant professor of Nephrology, Urology and Nephrology Center, Mansoura University, Egypt, E-mail: drhattia@yahoo.com

INTRODUCTION

Systemic lupus erythematosus is an autoimmune disease, which involves multiple organs. The disease has a female predominance. It may present as articular and mucocutaneous involvement, renal disease, hematological abnormalities, and central nervous system disease [1]. Despite advances in diagnosis and management, complications still cause substantial morbidity [2]. The survival of SLE patients improved in the past 50 years, with 5-year survival increasing from 50% in 1955 to 94% in 1994 This improvement has been attributed to a number of different factors, including the more judicious use of corticosteroids, refinements in immunosuppressive therapy, more effective treatment of hypertension and cardiovascular disease, and greater availability of dialysis and renal transplantation [3].

Although the prognosis of lupus nephritis has considerably improved over the years, a number of patients may still develop end stage renal disease. For these patients, as well as for most other uremic patients, kidney transplantation is generally considered to be the treatment of choice. Nevertheless, some SLE patients may pose some particular problems which have to be faced, both before and after transplantation [4]. Lupus nephritis occurs in 50% to 80% of SLE patients [4] and has a strong impact on the prognosis; the high morbidity and mortality of patients with SLE are associated with the severity of lupus nephritis [5]. Various clinical and demographic factors have been associated with outcome in lupus nephritis, such as World Health Organization (WHO) class of nephritis, the presence or absence of biological markers, treatment regimens, adherence to treatment, and socio-economic status (SES) and ethnicity of the patient [6].

Immunopathogenesis of Systemic Lupus Erythematosus Nephritis

Introduction

Lupus nephritis results from a complex interplay of autoantibodies in association with nucleosomes and histones, inflammatory cells, stimulated resident cells, complement, cytokines, and reactive nitrogen and oxygen species. Anti double-stranded DNA (Anti-dsDNA) antibodies are believed to participate in the pathogenesis of LN by binding directly or indirectly with renal antigens. Anti-dsDNA antibodies that bind to cell surface targets and/or penetrate into the cell might influence cell activation, proliferation and death, and induce expression of a large number of immunological mediators. While some of these mediators are pathogenic, others are a consequence of disease or are produced to regulate the immune response in SLE [7].

History and origin of anti-DNA antibodies

Antibodies that bind to cell nuclei are present in SLE and many other autoimmune diseases. These antibodies form the basis of the fluorescent antinuclear antibody test used in clinical practice, in which patient serum is incubated on glass slides coated with HEp-2 cells, followed by a fluorescent-labeled anti-immunoglobulin antibody for detection of any bound serum antibody.

Antibodies to DNA, were first described in 1957 [8], constitute a subgroup of antinuclear antibodies that bind single-stranded DNA, double-stranded DNA, or both. Anti-dsDNA antibodies are thought to play a crucial role in the pathogenesis of lupus nephritis [9].

Clinically, anti-dsDNA antibodies can be eluted from the kidneys of patients with active nephritis [10], suggesting that these antibodies might contribute to the induction of tissue damage.

In many patients with SLE, increased renal disease activity is associated with rising titres of anti-DNA antibodies, while prophylactic treatment of serologically active lupus patients with corticosteroids significantly reduces the number of subsequent disease flares [11]. Antibodies to single-stranded and double-stranded DNA are part of the normal repertoire of natural autoantibodies; most of these are low-affinity IgM antibodies that react weakly with several self-antigens. However, these natural antibodies can undergo an isotype switch (from IgM to IgG) that increases their potential to be pathogenic. In addition, somatic mutations in the encoding immunoglobulin genes might result in the production of high-affinity IgG antibodies to DNA [12].

Pathogenicity of Autoantibodies

Although anti-dsDNA was once thought to cause glomerulonephritis by forming complexes with DNA that are passively trapped in the glomeruli [13], some investigators believe that anti-dsDNA antibodies are pathogenic to the kidney via direct (cross-reactivity) or indirect (via a nuclear antigen bridge) binding to glomerular structures [14].

One intracellular effect of anti-DNA antibodies is to enhance cell growth and proliferation, or conversely induce apoptosis. Madaio *et al*. reported that nuclear localizing anti-DNA antibodies bind to DNAse I in living cells and inhibit the activity of this enzyme, making the cells more resistant to apoptosis [15]. This observation might explain the finding of glomerular hypercellularity in mice injected with penetrating antibodies [15]. In contrast, the cytopathic effects of anti-dsDNA antibodies to induce cell death have been demonstrated by others [16]. Up-regulation of apoptosis by anti-DNA antibodies would be consistent with the observation that anti-DNA antibodies can enhance cleavage of DNA [17].

In addition to cell viability, anti-dsDNA antibodies might influence pro-inflammatory pathways upon their binding to cell membrane antigens and/or entry into the cell cytosol. Anti-dsDNA antibody purified from lupus patients was shown to up-regulate the expression and release of von Willebrand factor [18] and adhesion molecules [19] (ICAM-1 and VCAM-1) in human umbilical vein endothelial cells.

Furthermore, there was heightened mRNA expression of IL-1 a, IL-1 receptor-1, IL-8 and TGFb 1, and increased IL-1b and IL-6 proteins in supernatants of anti-dsDNA-treated cells [20, 21]. Sabry et al [22] speculated that Egyptian patients with SLE have altered cytokine profile different from their healthy control subject. TNF-alpha and IL-6 are significantly increased in Egyptian patients with LN compared to the healthy control subjects and these levels are well correlated with SLE disease activity. It was reported that serum levels of intercellular adhesion molecules (ICAM-1) are elevated in SLE patients; these levels are significantly higher in hypertensive patients and those with active LN when compared to normotensive and inactive patients. These findings suggest that sICAM-1 measurement may serve as an additional serologic marker of disease activity in patients with SLE [23].

Nucleosomes

Accumulating evidence suggests that autoantibody interactions occur with nucleosomes (complexes of DNA and histone-containing pairs of histone peptides around which double-stranded DNA is wrapped twice), discounting a central role for DNA as the sole candidate autoantigen in LN. Studies on nephritis have shown that free DNA and DNA/anti-DNA complexes are not present in the circulation, and that intravenous injection of DNA/anti-DNA preparations fail to localize to the glomerulus [24].

On the contrary, accumulating data suggest that nucleosomes are the targets and mediators of autoantibody-related glomerular immune-complex deposition, along with the major autoantigens that elicit the autoimmune response [24-26].

These antibodies are immunoglobulin G in isotype, and bind to the glomerular basement membrane via nucleosomes [27].

The injection of syngeneic apoptotic cells into normal mice has been shown to generate antinuclear antibodies and immune deposition in kidneys [28]. It has been proposed that the IgG autoantibody/nucleosome complex binds heparin sulphate and precipitates glomerular injury, which is supported by the observation of histones and nucleosomes in the glomerular deposits of human lupus nephritis [29].

Apoptosis

Apoptosis is a tightly regulated process of programmed cell death that regulates the late phase of immune responses. Disordered regulation of both apoptosis and the clearance of apoptotic products have been implicated in the pathogenesis of SLE and LN [30].

The fundamental abnormality in SLE is selective loss of tolerance and self/non-self recognition and the development of autoantibodies. In normal immune circumstances, activity against self antigens is prevented by several mechanisms, including the Apo-1/Fas pathway of apoptosis, which has been shown to be involved in the process of immune tolerance by deletion of unwanted autoreactive T cells and B cells [31]. The cascade of caspases (cysteine proteases that are specifically activated in apoptotic cells, and are involved in signalling for initiation of apoptosis) is then set off and this ultimately leads to cell death [32].

Human SLE subjects had increased levels of circulating apoptotic mononuclear cells and dermal keratinocytes. The SLE patients had greater levels of circulating products of apoptosis such as nucleosomes than the controls. Autoantibodies associated with SLE reacted against the granzyme-cleaved nuclear products presented in the surface membrane blebs of apoptotic cells [30].

Reactive nitrogen and oxygen species:

Other putative mediators that might contribute to renal damage in LN are reactive species of nitrogen, such as nitric oxide (NO) and oxygen, such as superoxide or reactive oxygen species (ROS). Elevated levels of NO have been reported to be pathogenic in two murine models of LN, in which specific and non-specific inhibitors of iNOS have been successful in preventing and treating renal disease. As iNOS inhibitors do not alter autoantibody production, the effects of excessive NO production appear to occur after immune complex deposition and complement fixation [33].

Mycophenolate mofetil (MMF) is known to induce remission of LN in human [34], and alleviate murine LN through inhibition of iNOS transcription [35] and NO production [36], which are believed to be one of the major mechanisms by which MMF acts to suppress LN.

Immune complex

The pattern of glomerular injury seen in SLE is primarily related to the site of formation of the immune deposits, which are primarily due to anti-DNA. It is generally accepted that LN is initiated by the glomerular deposition of immune complexes [37].

Immune complexes in the mesangium or subendothelium that contact the extravascular space appear to recruit inflammatory cells, whereas the glomerular basement membrane prevents the recruitment of inflammatory cells to the subepithelial space. The isotype of the deposited antibody also influences pathogenicity [38]. The site of immune complex formation is related to the characteristics of both the antigen and antibody where large intact immune complexes or anionic antigens (which cannot cross the anionic charge barrier in the glomerular capillary wall) are deposited in the mesangium and subendothelial space [39, 40]. The degree of immune deposition then determines whether the patient develops mild disease limited to the mesangium or a more severe focal or diffuse proliferative glomerulonephritis.

Another important determinant of the site of immune complex formation may be related both to the charge of the antibody and to its antigen-binding region, since the antibody may bind to antigens at different sites in the glomerular capillary wall, thereby leading to different histologic and clinical manifestations [41-43].

It has also been suggested that the IgG subclass may be a determinant of the inflammatory response that is induced by immune complex deposition. IgG1 and IgG3 fix complement, while IgG2 and IgG4 do so less avidly [44]. Thus, the latter two subclasses should lead to less inflammation. Consistent with this hypothesis are the observations that anti-DNA antibodies are associated with diffuse proliferative glomerulonephritis and tend to be IgG1 and IgG3 [45], while the immune deposits in membranous nephropathy are more likely to be IgG2 and IgG4 [46]. However, separation of the immune deposits from the circulation by the glomerular basement membrane is probably a more important determinant of the lack of inflammatory change in membranous nephropathy [40].

BK VIRUS AND SYSTEMIC LUPUS ERYTHEMATOSUS

Few clinical studies and several mechanistic studies link BK viral infection as a potentially important trigger in SLE. This sector analyzes the association between BK virus in SLE as a potential causative agent versus a condition resulting from immunosuppressive treatment of this condition.

The BK Virus (BKV) is a polyoma virus and was named after the initials of a patient from whom it was first isolated. It belongs to the papovaviridae family and has high homology to JC Virus (JCV) and SV40. BK virus particles consist of a small circular protein capsid that surrounds a single copy of the approximately 5000 base-pair dsDNA genome. Vast majority of the human population is exposed to BK virus and 60-80% of the adults have serologically positive antibodies confirming prior exposure. Most of the primary infection occurs during childhood [47]. Primary infection is normally followed by a life-long silent persistence or latency. Route of infection or the target organ for persistence has not been clearly proven. However the possibility of gastrointestinal and respiratory route of transmission has been raised. It has been hypothesized that primary BK virus associated viremia results in seeding of the kidney and urothelial tract, where clinical latency occurs. Intermittent reactivation and asymptomatic viruria was primarily noted in immunocompromised hosts such as patients with SLE, AIDS, renal, cardiac and bone marrow transplant recipients and in pregnancy.

Experimental basis for association between BK virus and Lupus

Taguchi et al isolated BK virus in the urine of patients with SLE in 1978 [48]. Subsequently an intense research effort to address the causative role of BK virus in the etiopathogenesis of SLE has been taken. Among viral infections in humans, BK virus has been shown to incorporate their protein to host cell histones. Human DNA is a weak antigen. Autoantibodies against DNA are induced, if the DNA interacts with a foreign protein. Hence it was hypothesized from the below mentioned studies that BK virus infection in human may generate the auto-antibodies through this pathway [49]. Upon infection, BKV releases its genome into the host cell. BK viral DNA is replicated and then transcribed to mRNA in the host cell nucleus. Then mRNA is translated to viral proteins (such as LT-ag) in the host cell cytoplasm. LT-ag then binds to the host cell chromatin and it is released to the circulation on cell death. These complexes are more antigenic and are internalized by the DNA- specific B cells. These B cells process the chromatin fragments into DNA, cellular and LT-ag fragments. T cells specific to these proteins bind to these antigen presenting B cells, resulting in IL-2 production and autoimmune T cell activation [50]. These T cells may then stimulate B cells to proliferate and differentiate into anti-DNA producing plasma cells.

Flaegstad et al [51] inoculated purified infectious BK virus without any adjuvant into five rabbits. Two out of five rabbits produced antibodies to nucleosome, histone and dsDNA epitopes in addition to antibodies to structural viral proteins. These anti-histone antibodies recognized the histones from monkey vera cells and some histone classes from chicken erythrocyte chromatin and calf thymus confirming the auto-immune nature of BK viral infection in vivo. Moens et al [52] then showed that immunizing mice with plasmid DNA containing non-expressible LT-ag or Plasmid DNA that expresses a foreign non-DNA binding luciferase protein does not generate auto-antibodies. This suggests that plasmid DNA on its own is not immunogenic and highlighted the importance of BKV protein binding with DNA in the induction of auto-antibodies. Rekvig et al [53] proceeded to test whether LT-ag expression is sufficient to generate anti-dsDNA antibodies. Injecting LT-ag in immunologically normal mice generated auto-antibodies against dsDNA, histone and other cellular DNA-binding proteins. No antibodies were noted against non-DNA proteins, thus arguing against nonspecific B cell proliferation.

Clinical studies studying the association between BKV and Lupus

Fredriksen et al [54] demonstrated that anti-dsDNA antibodies are also induced in humans after naturally acquired BK virus infection. Fifty-nine children were examined over time for serological signs of primary BK virus infection. Eight children acquired primary BK viral infection and all of them developed anti-BK dsDNA antibodies. In 4 of the 8 patients the antibodies cross-reacted significantly with mammalian dsDNA, and weak cross-reactions were also noted in at least three other patients. They compared these anti-BK DNA antibodies to anti-dsDNA antibodies obtained from 10 SLE patients. In contrast, most anti-dsDNA antibodies from SLE patients cross-reacted extensively with viral and mammalian origin dsDNA. They concluded that patients undergoing a primary BK virus infection develop anti-dsDNA antibodies with a more restricted specificity than the spontaneously produced anti-dsDNA antibodies in SLE.

Sundsfjord et al [55] compared the prevalence and persistence of BK viruria and new infection versus relapse in 44 SLE and 88 age- and sex- matched healthy controls. They noted high prevalence of BK Viruria in SLE patients (66%) compared to healthy controls (0%). They did not observe any significant temporal relationship between immunosuppressive therapy and periodic and persistent polyoma viruria. They questioned the possibility of an unknown inherent immunological defect in patients with SLE contributing to persistent BK viruria. They also noted that BKV have predominantly archetypal regulatory regions with stable specific nucleotide sequences in the same patient at intervals of 1–3 years, indicating viral persistence and not reinfection as a cause of continuous or intermittent urinary shedding. This finding was also noted in the pregnant women. During second and third trimester of pregnancy increasing number of women excrete BK viruria due to reactivation rather than primary infection [56]. Bendiksen et al [57] found no difference in the BK viral strains between SLE and immuno competent individuals, thus arguing against the SLE specific BK Viral strains. Colla et al [58] studied the prevalence of BKV infection in 40 patients with SLE nephritis and 29 healthy controls. Prevalence of BK viremia and viruria among SLE nephritis patients did not significantly differ from the healthy subjects. This study was in stark contrast to the earlier study by Sundsfjord. One of the reasons authors speculated is that, the healthy control group was mostly comprised of nephrology and virology operators. This may not represent the healthy general population since this group had a major susceptibility to acquire BK virus through contact. Most importantly, among SLE nephritis patients, no statistically significant difference between BKV DNA positive and negative groups were noted in-terms of clinical characteristics of renal disease such as renal function, CD4+/CD8+ ratio and index of renal and systemic activity. In this study, SLE nephritis patients with BKV DNA infection tend to have more membranous nephropathy. However due to small number of patients enrolled in this study, no firm conclusion could be drawn.

Diagnosis of SLE

Although renal biopsy is crucial for diagnosing LN, the hallmark of diagnosis of SLE is the presence of antibodies directed against nuclear antigens (ANA) and especially against DNA (anti-DNA) antibodies, and are commonly used to monitor the course of patients with SLE. Autoantibodies ANA's are a highly sensitive screen for SLE, being found in more than 90% of untreated patients, but they are not specific for SLE and occur in many other rheumatologic diseases as well as a variety of infectious diseases The titer of the ANA does not correlate well with the presence of the severity of renal involvement in SLE [59]. Autoantibodies directed against double stranded DNA (anti-dsDNA) are a more specific but less sensitive marker of SLE and are found an almost 75% of untreated patients with active SLE. These antibodies may be detected by different techniques including the radioimmunoassay, an immunofluorescence test directed against the DNA and by ELISA [60]. A variety of other antibodies directed against ribonucleic antigens are commonly present in lupus patients. These include anti-Sm and anti-nRNP against extracted nuclear antigen (ENA). Anti-Sm antibodies, although very specific for SLE are found in only about 25% of lupus patients. In some studies, patients who are anti-Sm-positive have had a greater incidence of renal and CNS disease or more cutaneous vasculitis, cardiopulmonary disease, and a worse prognosis. Levels of total hemolytic complement (CH50) and complement components are usually decreased during active SLE and especially active renal disease. Levels of C4 and C3 often decline before a clinical flare of active lupus [61].

Histological Classification of Lupus Nephritis Lesions

Several classification systems have been proposed and no one is perfect and uniformly accepted. However, the WHO system which incorporates I/F and E/M studies is the most used. It has been recently modified [62].

In order to reasonably exclude a focal lesion, the biopsy should contain a minimum of 10 glomeruli for light microscopic analysis [63]. It is important to realize that the renal biopsy findings, per se, can't be used to establish a diagnosis of SLE. The renal biopsy findings must be interpreted by the referring clinician in the context of the patient's entire clinical presentation, including serologic findings.

Classification of Lupus Glomerulonephritis (LGN)

According to the 2003 International Society of Nephrology(ISN) / Renal pathology society (RPS) ISN/RPS classification of lupus nephritis [62], LGN is classified into the following:

Class I: (Figure 1)
Glomeruli have only mesangial immune deposits, identified by immunofluorescence alone, or both immunofluorescence and electron microscopy, but without light microscopic abnormalities.

Class II (pure mesangial lesions): (Figure 2)
Light microscopy shows mesangial hypercellularity (of any degree) or mesangial matrix expansion but there is no subendothelial deposit by electron microscopy or any global or segmental glomerular scars. There is no significant change in tubular, interstitial and vascular components.

Immunofluorescence microscopy: Glomerular immune deposits almost always contain dominant polyclonal IgG, as well as C3 and in most instances C1q, with variable co-deposits of IgA and IgM. If glomerular immunoglobulin deposits are restricted to IgA or IgM, diagnostic possibilities other than lupus nephritis should be considered in correlation with serologic and clinical findings.

Clinical picture of class II: Minimal clinical evidence of renal involvement with mild to moderate proteinuria and hematuria. Hypertension is uncommon, and the nephrotic syndrome and renal insufficiency are virtually never seen. The renal prognosis is excellent and no specific therapy is indicated unless the patient progresses to more advanced disease.

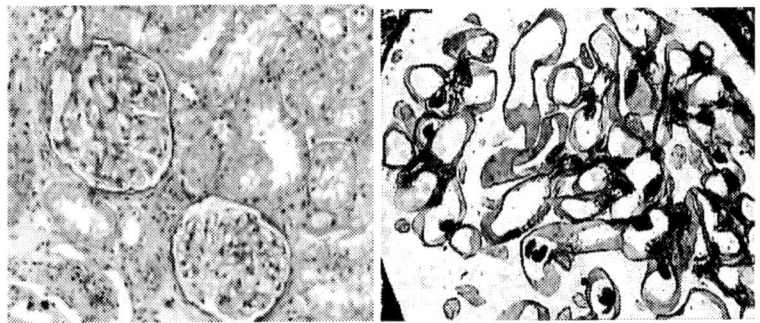

Figure 1. Class I lupus nephritis. No abnormalities detected by light microscopy

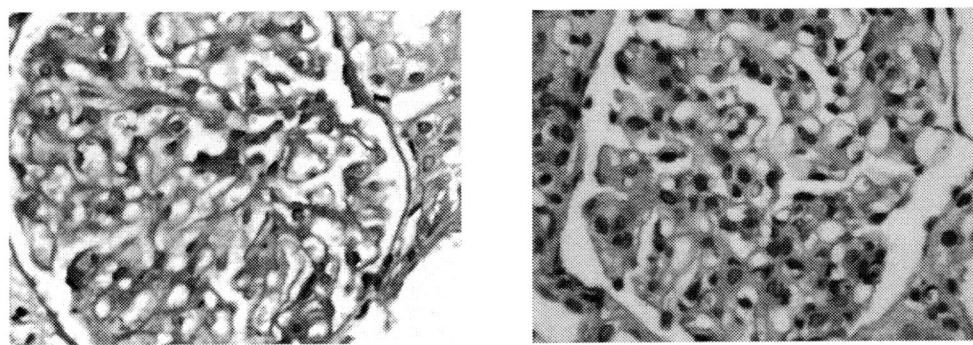

Figure 2. a). Lupus nephritis WHO Class II. Mesangial matrix expantion (PAS x400), (b): Lupus nephritis WHO Class II. Mesangial hypercellularity (HX & E x400)

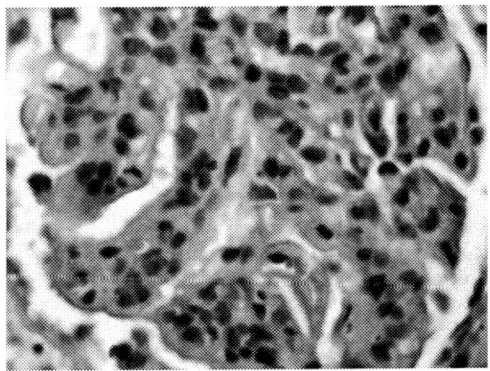

Figure 3. Mesangial hypercellularity (HX & E x 400)

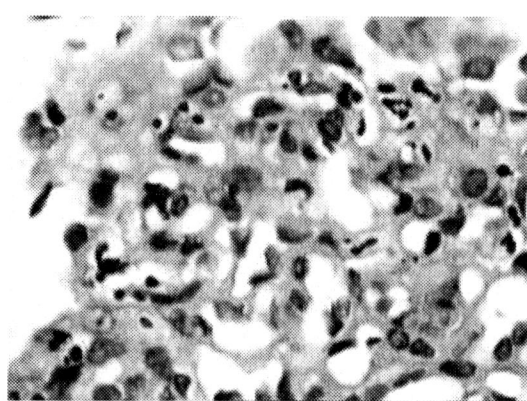

Figure 4. Endocapillary hypercellularity

Definition of active and chronic glomerular lesions [62]

Active lesions: Found with classes III and IV

1. **Mesangial hypercellularity** (Figure 3) may be diffuse or focal and segmental or global in a response to mesangial deposits. The mesangial immune deposits are more diffuse and regular in distribution than the mesangial proliferative response. There is often a poor correlation between the size and extent of the mesangial immune deposits and the severity of the mesangial hypercellularity.

2. **Endocapillary hypercellularity** (Figure 4): It is due to a proliferation of endothelial cells and mesangial cells together with infiltrating mononuclear cells as lymphocytes and monocytes or polymorphnuclear leukocytes that significantly narrows or occludes the glomerular capillary lumen.

3. **Hyaline lesions** (Figures 5-7) include the characteristic wire loop lesions and hyaline thrombi. Glomerular immune deposits can be frequently identifiable by light microscopy because of their large size and widespread distribution. Deposits frequently have a glassy, hyaline, hypereosinophilic appearance with the hematoxylin-eosin stain, special stains help to differentiate the deposits from the eosinophilic mesangial matrix, glomerular basement membrane, and cytoplasm of the glomerular cells. Particularly helpful stains are the trichrome stain, which demarcates the deposits as red (fuchsinophilic) against the blue-staining glomerular mesangium and basement membranes and Jones methenamine silver or combination methenamine silver Masson Ponceau stains which stain the deposits pink or red, against the black-staining mesangial matrix and glomerular basement membrane

    Wire loops (Figure 5, 6) refers to a capillary wall thickening due to the extensive subendothelial deposits. Subendothelial immune deposits are regularly encountered in class III and class IV lupus nephritis. They are relatively focal and segmental in class III and more global and diffuse in class IV. They appear as rigid thick linear brightly eosinophilic refractile thickening of the capillary walls by hematoxylin and eosin. The periodic acid silver methenamine stain gives a double contoured appearance. Silver stain reveals the deposits to be entirely or largely subendothelial, with preservation of an outer peripheral layer of glomerular basement membrane producing a double contoured appearance.

Hyaline intracapillary thrombi (Figure 7). This term is actually a misnomer, because they do not represent true fibrin thrombi but are massive intracapillary immune deposits with the same composition by immunofluorescence as the neighboring subendothelial deposits. Serial sectioning discloses that these intraluminal deposits which are apparently not attached to the capillary basement membranes are actually in continuity with large subendothelial deposits in a deeper plane of section. These hyaline thrombi are most common in class IV lupus nephritis, particularly in specimens with extensive wire loop deposits

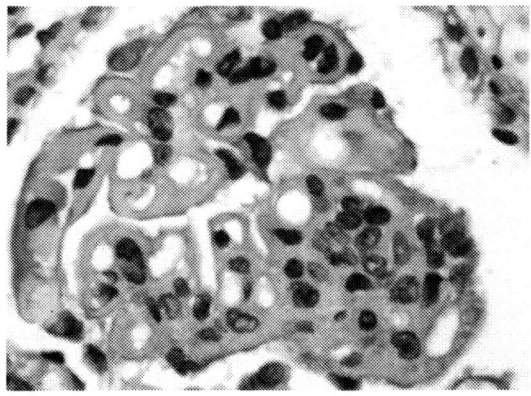

Figure 5. Mesangial hypercellularity and wire loop lesion (HX & E x 400)

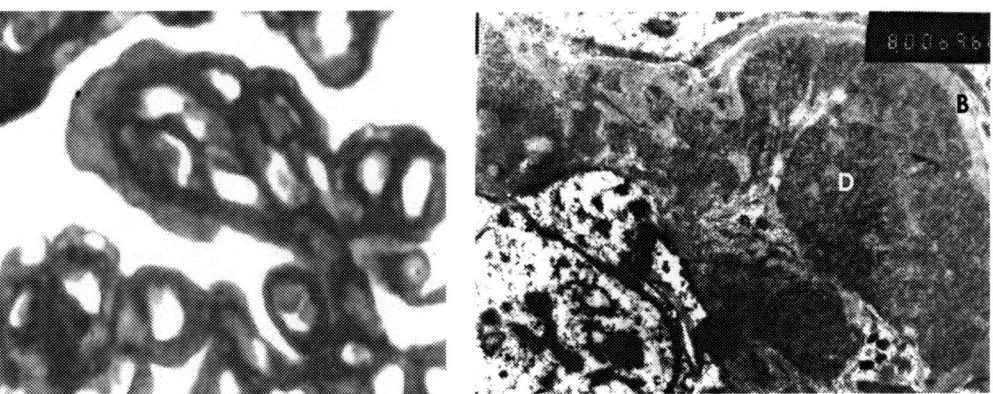

Figure 6. (a). Wire loop lesions. (b): Subendothelial deposits corresponding to wire loop lesions seen by light (Figure ure 6.a) microscopy. (B) basement membrane. .(D) electron dense deposits. . (Uranyl acetate and lead citrate x 8000)

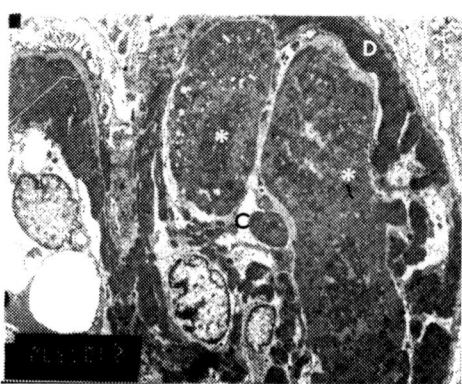

Figure 7. Subendothelial deposits (D), intracapillary thrombi (*), capillary lumen (C). (Uranyl acetate and lead citrate x 2000).

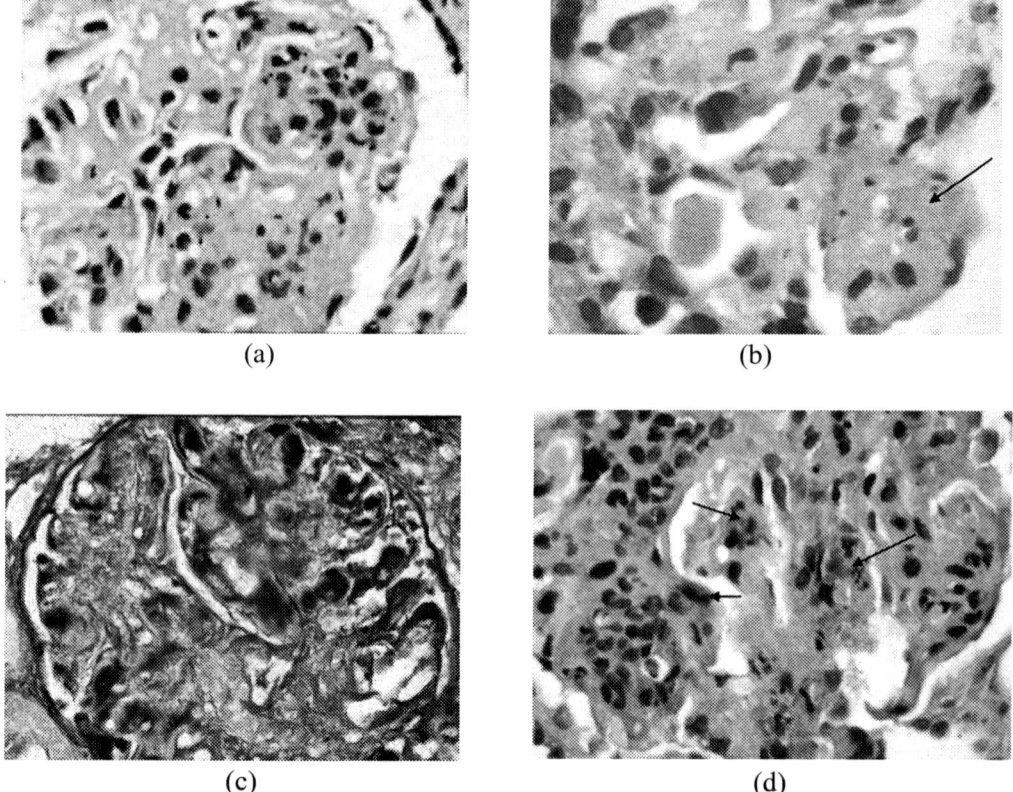

Figure 8. (a) Karyorrhexis necrosis (HX&E x 400). (b) Fibrinoid necrosis (HX & E x 400). (c) Fibrinoid necrosis (Phosphotungestic acid hematoxylin stain x400). (d) hematoxylin bodies (arrows), mesangial hypercellularity & wire loop thickening of basement membranes (x 400).

4. **Necrosis** (Figure 8): Glomerular necrosis is a feature of class III or IV lupus nephritis and is never observed in pure mesangial proliferative (class II) or membranous (class V) lupus nephritis. It is seen in the following forms:

Gaps in the capillary basement membranes.

Karyorrhexis or apoptosis of infiltrating neutrophils and endogenous glomerular cells forming pyknotic or karyorrhectic nuclear debris

Fibrinoid necrosis: It appears as amorphous eosinophilic material staining bright red in trichrome staining and presents most often in the context of an extracapillary proliferative lesion.

Hematoxylin bodies are considered the pathognomonic lesion of lupus nephritis although they are relatively infrequent. They usually occur in glomeruli with very active proliferative and necrotizing features that display other readily identifiable features of full-blown lupus nephritis. Hematoxylin bodies consist of isolated or clustered rounded, smudgy, dark pink-staining structures that are generally smaller than normal nuclei. They usually have indistinct borders and appear to merge into the background tissue with surrounding flecks of hematoxyphilic material. They differ from the dark basophilic, smaller, and distinctly punctuate nuclear fragments observed in foci of karyorrhexis or pyknosis. Hematoxylin bodies are the tissue equivalent of the LE body and consist of naked nuclei, whose chromatin has been altered by binding to ANA.

5. **Frequent neutrophil infiltration** (Figure 9). In computing an activity index, Balow and Austin et al use exudation of more than two neutrophils outside the glomerular capillaries per glomerulus as one of the features of glomerular activity but do not consider lymphocyte or monocyte infiltration. Because neutrophil exudation outside the glomerular capillaries is rare, except in areas of necrosis, this criterion is very important in the formulation of the activity index [64-66].

6. **Crescents** (Figure 10), cellular or fibrocellular, represent a feature of active lupus nephritis that may be encountered frequently in class III or IV lupus nephritis, but never in pure class II or class V disease except in combined lesions. Cellular Crescents can be seen overlie the necrotizing lesions, as well as in glomeruli with nonnecrotizing segmental or global endocapillary proliferation.

7. **Interstitial inflammatory infiltrate.** Most commonly encountered in class III, IV and to less extend in class V. The interstitial infiltrates consist predominantly of mononuclear leucocytes, including lymphocytes, monocytes, and plasma cells. Neutrophils and eosinophils are rarely identified.

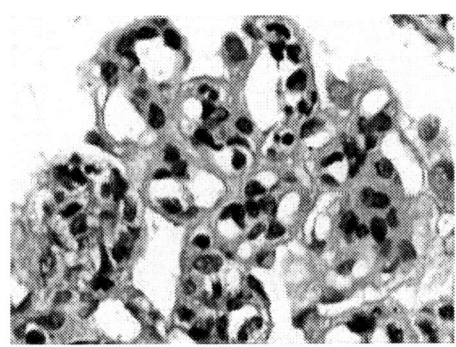 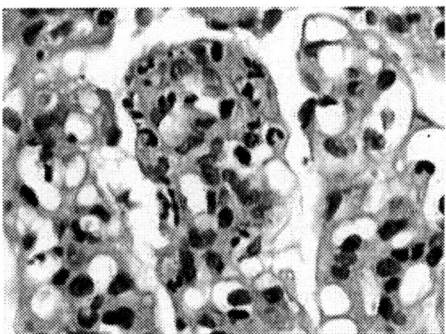

Figure 9. Frequent neutrophil infiltration in mesangial & intracapillary. (Hx & E x400).

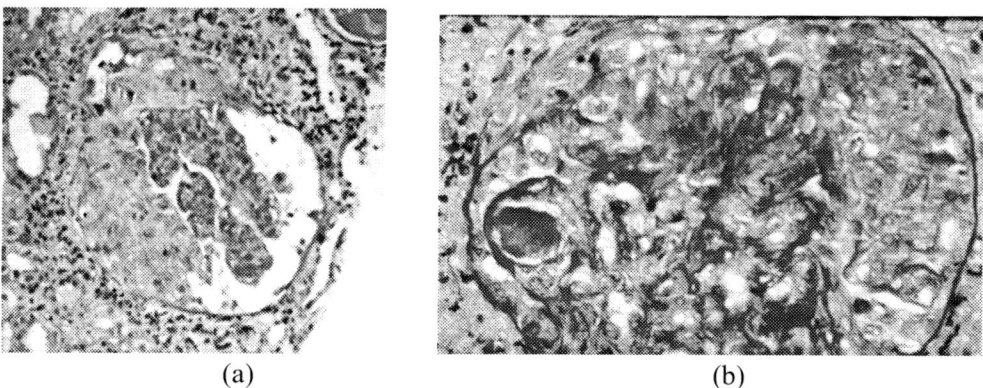

Figure 10. cellular crescent (HX &E x 250). (b) Cellular crescent A thrombus is seen in the efferent arteriole.

Chronic lesions (Figure 11)

Glomerular sclerosis, fibrous adhesions, Fibrous crescents, tubular atrophy, and interstitial fibrosis are chronic lesions encountered in the course of class III, IV, or V lupus nephritis.

Glomerular sclerosis (segmental or global): Occurs In class III lupus nephritis, the glomerular scarring is often initially focal and segmental, mirroring the distribution of the proliferative and necrotizing lesions. In chronic class IV lupus nephritis, the glomerular scarring is typically more global and diffuse, although segmental sclerosis may affect some glomeruli.

Distinguishing "active" and"sclerosing" lesions may help determine prognosis and sensitivity to treatment in both lupus and other glomerulonephritides [67]. Lesions that are potentially sensitive to treatment and reversible are characterized by hypercellularity, leukocyte exudation, necrosis/karyorrhexis, cellular crescents, hyaline deposits, and interstitial inflammatory infiltrate. Renal thrombotic microangiopathy associating SLE may be treatable with plasmapheresis similar to primary hemolytic uremic syndrome or thrombotic thrombocytopenic purpura [68].

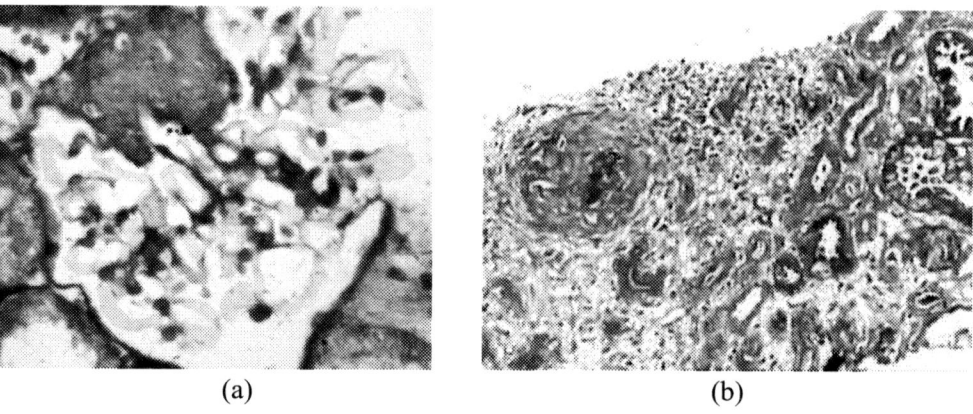

Figure 11 (a). Chronic changes Segmental sclerosis (Masson trichrome x 400). (b). Global sclerosis, fibrous crescents. tubular atrophy and interstitial fibrosis. (Masson trichrome x 400).

Glomerulosclerosis, fibrous crescents, tubular atrophy, and interstitial fibrosis are less sensitive to treatment.

Class III (Figure 12)

Light microscopy: Less than 50 percent of glomeruli are affected with active or inactive segmental or global endocapillary or extracapillary glomerulonephritis. Hypercellularity of the glomerular tuft is frequent. It can be segmental or global, but characteristically is almost never uniform and may vary widely from one glomerulus to another. Hypercellularity may be due to proliferation of mesangial, endothelial, and epithelial cells, and to some extent to monocytes and polymorphonuclear cell exudation. Active necrotizing lesion is sharply delineated areas of segmental proliferation, foci of fibrinoid necrosis with karyorrhexis and or crescent formation.

Subclasses of class III represent the presence of active and/or chronic lesions as following:

> **Class III (A),** which is class III disease with active lesions. This is also called focal proliferative lupus nephritis.
> **Class III (A/C),** which is associated with active and chronic lesions. This is referred to as focal proliferative and sclerosing lupus nephritis.
> **Class III (C),** in which chronic inactive lesions with scarring are observed. This is also called focal sclerosing lupus nephritis.

Immunofluorescence: Capillary wall granular as well as mesangial deposits of full battery of immunoglobulins as well as complement deposits (IgG, C3, and frequently also IgM, IgA, and Clq).

Although less than 50 percent of glomeruli are affected on light microscopy, immunofluorescence microscopy (for IgG and C3) involves all the glomeruli [68].

E/M: Subendothelial and mesangial deposits and more rarely subepithelial deposits, mainly confined to segmental proliferative lesions.

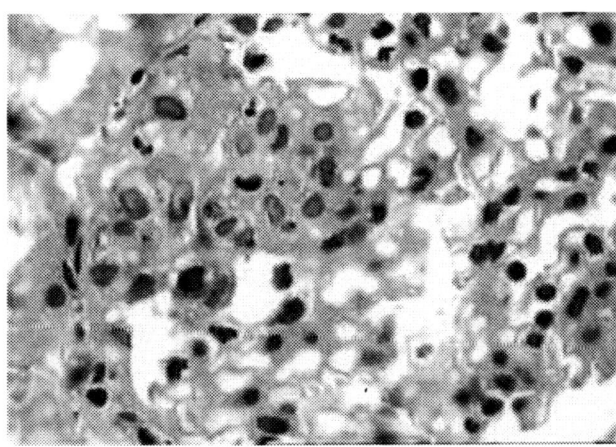

Figure 12. Class III. Segmental area of fibrinoid necrosis (arrow) and mesangial hypercellularity. (Hx & E x 400)

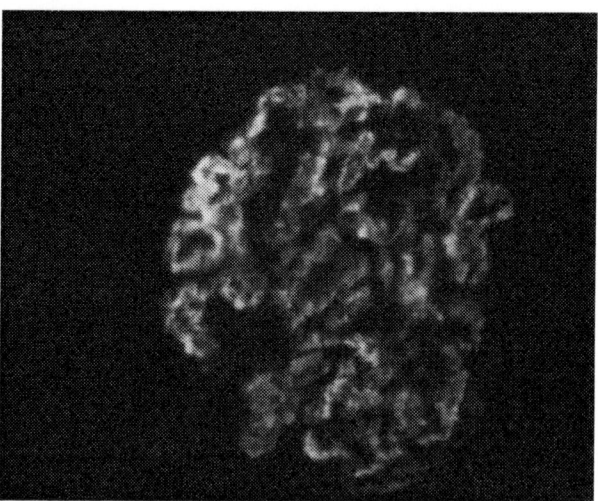

Figure 13. Lupus nephritis class IV: Capillary wall deposits of IgG (x400)

Clinical Correlations of Class III

Hematuria and proteinuria are seen in almost all patients, some of whom also have nephrotic syndrome, hypertension, and an elevated plasma creatinine concentration. Progressive renal dysfunction in focal proliferative lupus nephritis appears to be uncommon [69].

More widespread or severe involvement (40 to 50 percent of glomeruli affected with areas of necrosis or crescent formation, nephrotic range proteinuria, and/or hypertension) is associated with a long-term prognosis that is similar to that of class IV diffuse proliferative lupus nephritis [70]. In 50 percent of the cases serum C3 and C4 are lowered.

Progression of class III lesion: The lesions can progress to diffuse proliferative (class IV) or membranous lupus glomerulonephritis. Progression is possibly predicted by the presence of subendothelial and subepithelial deposits.

Class IV (Figure 13-15)

It appears to be a continuation of class III.

L/M: Diffuse lupus nephritis or class IV disease, more than 50 percent of glomeruli display endocapillary or extracapillary glomerulonephritis.

It is not infrequent to find in some cases diffuse wire loop deposits, but with little or no glomerular proliferation. This is also considered class IV disease.

Additional subclasses of class IV disease are categorized as follows:

- **Class IV-S (A),** which is class IV-S with active lesions. This is also called diffuse segmental proliferative nephritis.
- **Class IV-G (A),** which is class IV-G associated with active lesions. This is also referred to as diffuse global proliferative nephritis.
- **Class IV-S (A/C),** which is associated with active and chronic lesions. This is also called diffuse segmental proliferative and sclerosing nephritis.

- **Class IV-G (A/C),** which is class IV-G with active and chronic lesions. This is also called diffuse global proliferative and sclerosing nephritis.
- **Class IV-S (C),** which is associated with chronic inactive lesions with scars. This is also referred to as diffuse segmental sclerosing lupus nephritis.
- **Class IV-G (C),** which is class IV-G with chronic inactive lesions with scars. This is also called diffuse global sclerosing lupus nephritis

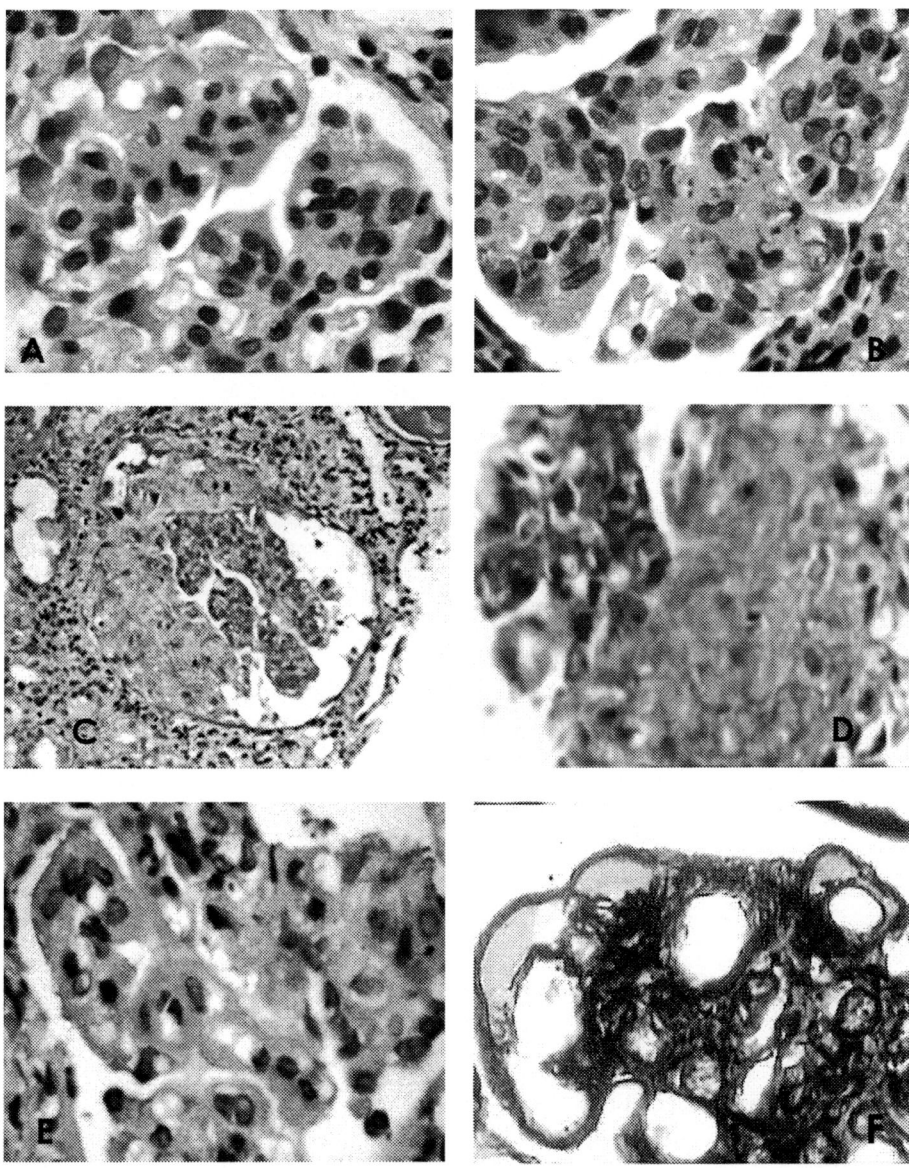

Figure 14. SLE Class IV : Figure ures through A-F are from a biopsy of the same patient. (A) Mesangial hypercellularity. (B) Hypercellularity and karyorrhexis necrosis. (C & D) Cellular crescent. (E) wire loop lesion (F) PAS stain showing the double contoured appearance due to subendothelial deposits.

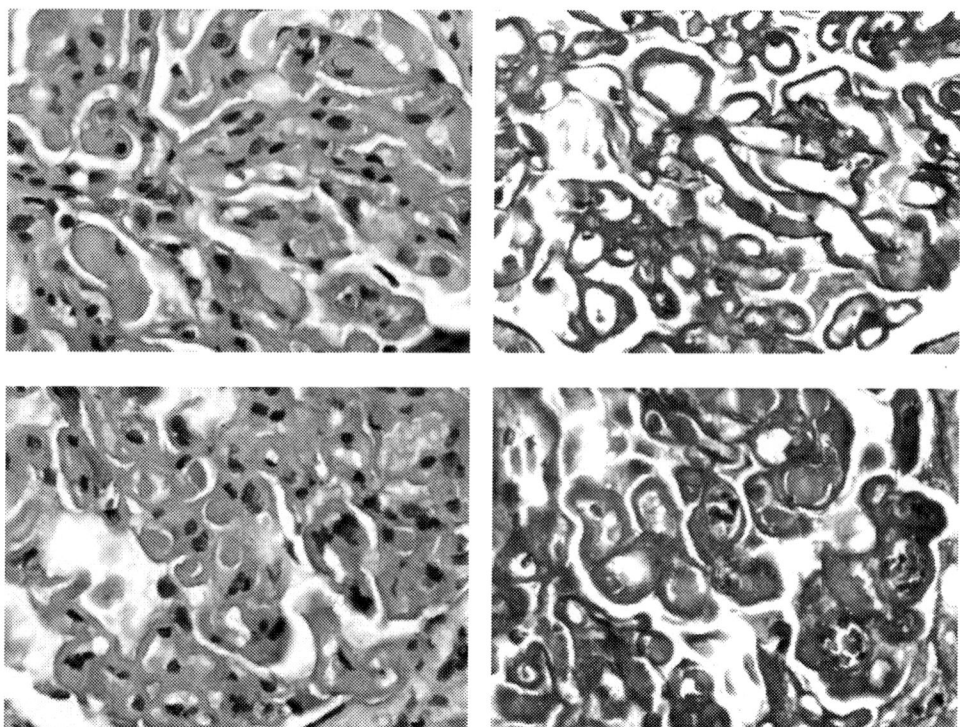

Figure 15. class IV with only diffuse global hyaline lesion (wire loops and hyaline thrombi), but with little or no glomerular proliferation. (Figure ures to the left are stained by HX & E x400. Those to the right are stained by Masson trichrome x 400).

I/F: Coarsely granular deposits of immunoglobulins and complement deposits in the mesangium and capillary walls.

E/M:
Similar to class III: Abundant subendothelial deposits accompanied by large mesangial deposits. Subepithelial and intramembranous deposits are also identified. Mesangial hypercellularity with circumferential mesangial interposition are frequently present. A pattern similar to membranoproliferative glomerulonephritis.

Occasionally, the electron-dense deposits show an organized or crystalline pattern which has been termed a "finger print" pattern. It is suggested that this pattern is accompanied by cryoglobulins because similar structures are seen in patients with idiopathic mixed cryoglobulinemia.

Clinicopathological Correlations of Class IV

Class IV lupus nephritis is the most common and most severe form of lupus nephritis [71].

Hematuria and proteinuria are seen in almost all cases, and the nephrotic syndrome, hypertension, and renal insufficiency are all frequently seen. Affected patients typically have significant hypocomplementemia and elevated anti-DNA levels, especially during active disease [72]. Despite effective immunosuppressive therapy, progressive scarring can occur over a period of years after the inflammation has resolved.

Class V (Figure 16)

L/M: It is a diffuse membranous glomerulopathy. Generalized thickening of the peripheral capillary walls. Spikes are seen by silver methenamine stain.

Abundant, regularly distributed subepithelial deposits are the defining feature of membranous lupus nephritis class V, Glomerular basement membrane spikes and a vacuolated texture where cut obliquely can usually be identified with the silver stain.

Immunofluorescence: Capillary wall granular deposits of immunoglobulins and complement. Occasional mesangial deposits of IgA staining and intense C1q deposits. Mesangial, small subendothelial and tubular basement membrane deposits.

E/M: Typical epimembranous nephropathy with subepithelial and intramembranous deposits. It differs from the typical membranous nephropathy by the presence of mesangial deposits.

The following findings [73], if present, strongly suggest underlying lupus rather than idiopathic membranous nephropathy

(a) Glomerular hypercellularity
(b) Tubuloreticular structures in the endothelial cells on electron microscopy
(c) Concurrent subendothelial or prominent mesangial deposits as in the proliferative forms of lupus nephritis
(d) Immune deposits along the tubular basement membranes and in the small blood vessels.

Clinical picture of class V lupus nephritis

Usually, Patients present with heavy proteinuria. Microscopic hematuria and hypertension also may be seen, and plasma creatinine concentration is usually normal or only slightly elevated. Most patients with membranous lupus maintain a normal or near normal plasma creatinine concentration for five years or more and may not require immunosuppressive therapy.

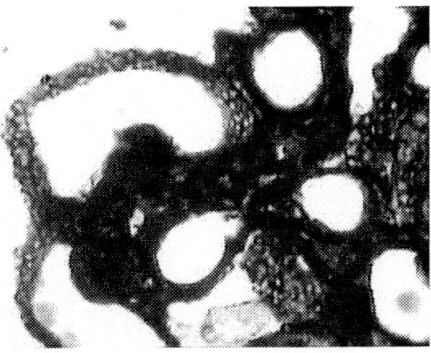
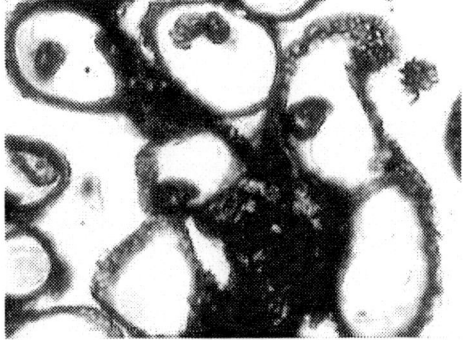

Figure 16. class V membranous lupus

(Class VI) Advanced sclerosing lupus nephritis

Class VI disease is characterized by global sclerosis of more than 90 percent of glomeruli. It represents healing of prior inflammatory injury, as well as the advanced stage of chronic class III, IV, or V lupus nephritis.

Additional Pathological Features Associated with SLE

(i) Tubulointerstitial nephritis: Commonly seen in class III and IV

Tubulointerstitial disease (interstitial infiltrate, tubular injury) with or without immune deposits along the tubular basement membrane is a common finding in lupus nephritis, almost always being seen with concurrent glomerular disease.

Tubulointerstitial immune deposits can be detected by immunofluorescence and electron microscopy in approximately 50% of patients.

Cellular infiltration in the active states is usually formed of lymphocytes, plasma cells and sometimes eosinophils and neutrophils whereas in chronic disease there is interstitial fibrosis and accumulation of monocytes, macrophages and plasma cells.

(ii) Vascular lesions in lupus nephritis

Lupus vasculopathy carries an ominous prognosis prognosis, with frequent, severe renal insufficiency, active urinary sediment, active lupus serologies, hypertension, and rapid progression to renal failure [74].

Lupus vasculitis may present in the following forms:

1. Uncomplicated vascular immune deposits
2. Non inflammatory necrotizing vasculopathy (so-called lupus vasculopathy) (Figure 17)
3. Thrombotic microangiopathy
4. Arteriosclerosis and arteriolosclerosis.
5. Necrotizing vasculitis (PAN type)

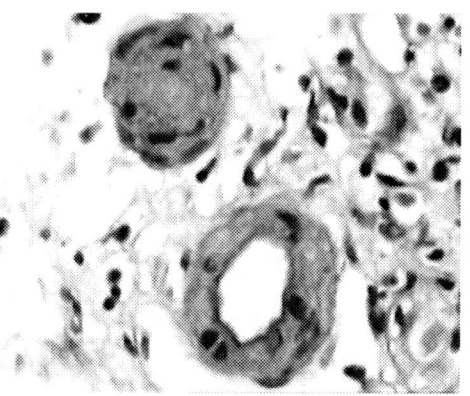 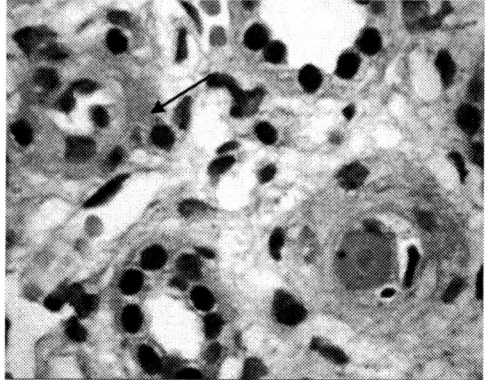

Figure 17. Non inflammatory Necrotizing Vasculopathy. The affected vessels show fibrinoid necrosis in the wall (arrow) that extends into the media. Arterioles are severely narrowed and occluded by luminal deposits of glassy eosinophilic material (HX& E x 400).

Lupus nephritis activity and chronicity indices [64, 75]:

Activity index: It is a total score of 24 counted from the total number of glomerular affection by the following active lesions:

(i) Glomerular cellular proliferation
(ii) Hyaline lesions (wire loops and hyaline thrombi)
(iii) Karyorrhexis and fibrinoid necrosis.
(iv) Cellular crescents.

The scoring depends on the percentage of glomeruli affected. If 25% of glomeruli are affected (given 1), if affect 25-50% of glomeruli (given 2) and if more than 50% of glomeruli are affected (given 3).
However, on scoring necrosis and cellular crescents the net score is multiplied by 2

(v) Leukocyte exudation is scored as the number of neutrophils /glomerulus:
2 cells (given 1), 3 cells (given 2), more than 3cells (given 3)
(vi) Interstitial inflammation.

If less than 20% of the interstitium is affected (given 1), 20-40% of the interstitium (given 2), more than 40% of the interstitium (given 3)

Chronicity index: It is a total score from 12 counted from the total number of the following chronic lesions:

(i) Glomerular sclerosis:
(ii) Fibrous crescents:

The scoring depends on the percentage of glomeruli affected. If 25% of glomeruli are affected (given 1), if affect 25-50% of glomeruli (given 2) and if more than 50% of glomeruli are affected (given 3).

(iii) Tubular atrophy.
(iv) Interstitial fibrosis:

If less than 20% of the interstitium is affected (given 1), 20-40% of the interstitium (given 2), more than 40% of the interstitium (given 3)

What is the value of renal biopsy in a patient with SLE?

In our view, renal biopsy may have a role in the following situations:

(a) Establishing a diagnosis of SLE or lupus nephritis.
(b) It provides information about the class, severity, activity, and chronicity of the renal disease.
(c) It can discriminate between patients who have the most severe lesions from patients who don't.

(d) It helps in guiding therapies; the more the aggressive the pathology the more the energetic therapy and vice versa. So, we avoid unnecessary immunosuppressive medications for patients with advanced chronic changes.

What is the value of re-biopsy and when is it indicated?

Lupus nephritis is one of the few renal diseases for which follow-up renal biopsies are routinely performed in some centers 6 months or more after therapy to gauge the efficacy of treatment and guide further therapeutic management. With increased amount of subendothelial deposits, aggressive steroid and cytotoxic therapy is confirmed.

It is wise to repeat renal biopsies in any patient with a sudden change in clinical findings (e.g., new onset of proteinuria, new activity of the urinary sediment, declining glomerular filtration rate) that may denote a transformation in the class of lupus nephritis or reactivation of disease requiring reinstitution or adjustment of therapy.

Diagnosis and Monitoring of Renal Disease

Proteinuria and abnormal urine sediment are the first signs of renal damage. Renal involvement, although often subclinical, is already present at the time of diagnosis of SLE in 25 – 50% of patients, while another 60% of patients will develop it during the course of the disease [76]. These Figures underscore the necessity of vigilance in searching for early signs of renal injury by the use of urinalysis followed by urine sediment analysis (at a dedicated laboratory), even in patients with subtle low-grade abnormalities (hematuria or proteinuria) [77]. Subtle urinary abnormalities may either represent milder forms of nephritis or more severe nephritis modified by previous corticosteroid therapy. When in doubt, renal biopsy remains the gold standard for the diagnosis of lupus nephritis; renal biopsy should ideally be performed before initiation of treatment according to widely accepted indications for this procedure. Progression of the disease from a mild form to a severe one may also occur even in patients under treatment, emphasizing the need for close monitoring.

Patients with LN should be classified by their kidney biopsy results, including an assessment of segmental or global involvement of the glomeruli and a measure of chronicity. Renal function and other measures of glomerular injury should be monitored. Serological markers should only be used as supplementary markers of disease activity. Patients should be categorised according to whether they are experiencing a first attack or a flare [78].

Prognostic Factors and Outcome Measures

Working definitions for terms regarding disease severity (mild, moderate or severe) depending on histopathological classes, degree of proteinuria and kidney functions. Although not formally validated in controlled studies, this classification is based on individual parameters which have been shown to be significant predictors of response to therapy and kidney outcome, and therefore may be a useful tool in understanding differences between trials and in determining optimal therapy for the patient [79].

Laboratory parameters such as elevated serum creatinine, severe anemia (Hb < 8 g/100 ml), low serum C3 and C4 (the last especially among African–Americans) and high anti-ds DNA titres at diagnosis; and finally concomitant involvement of other major organs, presence of antiphospholipid syndrome [80] and pregnancy are all predictors of severe disease and adverse renal outcome. Poor compliance and late response to therapy are additional risk factors for adverse renal outcome [75, 81].

TREATMENT OF LUPUS NEPHRITIS

Introduction

Ideally, the optimal treatment of lupus nephritis should result in lifelong remission with minimal toxicity, prolong life expectancy, and is cost effective. Various therapeutic regimens including corticosteroids, cyclophosphamide (CY), azathioprine (AZA), mycophenolate mofetil (MMF), methotrexate (MTX), ciclosporin A (CsA), tacrolimus, immunoglobulins (IVIG), anti-TNF and anti-CD20 agents, plasmapheresis, and angiotensin-converting enzyme inhibitors (ACEIs) are currently used or are under investigation towards this goal [82].

Terminology used in the management of lupus nephritis [83]:
Induction is a period of intensive therapy with the aim of achieving a clinically meaningful and sustained response in a patient with active disease. It would normally involve the use of intravenous and/or oral corticosteroids and either intravenous CY or oral MMF for patients with class III and IV LN. The duration of the induction period varies depending on disease severity, but it should usually be continued for at least 3 months and may be extended to 6 months or more if the patient still has active disease. Where significant proteinuria is present, the addition of an ACE inhibitor or ARB should always be considered to reduce urine protein excretion and protect renal function.

The term ***'response'*** is preferable to 'remission'. A complete response is demonstrated by an inactive urinary sediment, a decrease in proteinuria to ≤0.2 g/day and normal or stable (within 10% of normal GFR if previously abnormal) renal function. Partial response is a level of improvement usually defined as an inactive sediment proteinuria ≤0.5 g/day, with normal (GFR > 90 mL/min) or stable (<10% deterioration from baseline if GFR was previously abnormal) renal function. A sustained response of at least 3 to 6 months can be regarded as a remission but cannot be judged to be a complete remission in the absence of a biopsy.

A flare is defined as an increase in disease activity requiring more intensive therapy. It is indicated by an increase in proteinuria or serum creatinine, an abnormal urinary sediment or a reduction in creatinine clearance due to active disease. Three types of flare can be defined: a proteinuric flare is characterised by a persistent increase in proteinuria to values higher than 0.5–1.0 g/day after a complete response is achieved or a doubling of proteinuria, with values higher than 1.0 g/day, after achieving a partial response. Nephritic flare is an increase or recurrence of active urinary sediment (increased haematuria with or without reappearance of cellular casts) with or without a concomitant increase in proteinuria. Nephritic flares are usually associated with a decline in renal function. A severe nephritic flare is an increase or recurrence of active urinary sediment with an increase ≥25% in serum creatinine, an extrarenal flare affects one or more extrarenal systems in patients with LN and may require a change in therapy. Repeat biopsy is considered as the 'gold standard' for assessing renal activity.

Maintenance is a period of less intensive therapy following a period of induction therapy that has achieved a partial or complete response, with the aim of keeping the patient free of disease activity. Maintenance therapies are usually administered orally (corticosteroids, MMF or azathioprine) at the lowest possible dose to maintain response. Maintenance therapy should also involve the treatment of concurrent conditions, such as hypertension, diabetes and hyperlipidaemia.

Targets of Treatment Strategies in LN

We agree with the view that treatment of lupus nephritis should aim the following targets

1. Obtain a complete remission
2. Maintenance of renal function
3. Reduction of renal flares
4. Control of proteinuria
5. Control of blood pressure
6. Control of vascular risk factors
7. Identification and treatment of antiphospholipid syndrome nephropathy
8. Minimisation of treatment-related toxicity
9. Assessment of infection risk
10. Bone protection
11. Optimization of adjunctive therapies
12. Encourage patient's compliance
13. Overall reduction of mortality

Treatment Paradigm

The current treatment paradigm for lupus nephritis consists of initial induction therapy followed by maintenance therapy. The former is usually an aggressive treatment with a rather short duration (3 – 6 months) and aims to control the disease activity and achieve remission, while the later is less intense but more prolonged and aims to sustain remission and prevent the flares of the disease.

Corticosteroids

Corticosteroids, in various compounds, doses and route of administration, are widely prescribed both for induction and maintenance therapy of lupus nephritis. However, they exhibit major adverse/side effects, including growth retardation in children, diabetes mellitus, arterial hypertension, hyperlipidemia, atherosclerosis, depression, osteoporosis, avascular bone necrosis and immunosuppression. Adjunct therapy with calcium salts, vitamin D supplements and biphosphonates prevents osteoporosis. Modest salt and glucose restriction are necessary for the prevention of hypertension and corticosteroid-induced diabetes mellitus, respectively.

Intravenous administration of methylprednisolone

Pulse methylprednisolone (MP) therapy involves the intravenous administration of 1 g (or 1 g/m^2) MP over a short period of time (20 – 60 min) in order to rapidly suppress inflammation in severe lupus nephritis [84]. Intravenous pulses of methylprednisolone (IV-MP) are usually administered for 3 consecutive days followed by a single pulse every month, alone or in combination with cytotoxic agents such as CY. Corticosteroids are administered orally in between the pulses, at the lowest possible dose, starting with 0.5 – 0.6 mg/kg once a day of prednisolone or equivalent dose of MP followed by gradual tapering to 0.25 mg/kg every other day within 3 months.

It was shown that IV-MP is inferior to IV-CY for severe lupus nephritis and that IV-MP when combined with IV-CY provides additional benefit without increasing toxicity [85, 86]. More recently, Grootscholten *et al* [87] found that corticosteroids in combination with CY were more effective in hindering the progression of chronic lesions and preventing flares than corticosteroids in combination with AZA.

Oral administration of corticosteroids

A number of trials have shown that oral prednisone alone is inferior to a combination of prednisone with cytotoxic agents for induction of remission of active lupus nephritis [88]. Patients treated with prednisone alone were more likely to experience renal flares, progression of renal scarring and develop end stage renal disease (ESRD). Thus, current treatment of class III, IV and V lupus nephritis consists of oral corticosteroids in combination with other immunosuppressive and cytotoxic agents. The usual starting dose of prednisone is 0.5 – 1 mg/kg/day or its equivalent of methylprednisolone, followed by tapering of the dose after the initial 4 – 6 weeks. The maximum dose of prednisone recommended for maintenance therapy is 0.25 mg/kg on alternate days (15 mg of prednisone every other day for the average adult).

Cyclophosphamide

Cyclophosphamide as induction therapy for proliferative lupus nephritis

Cyclophosphamide and corticosteroids have been compared in randomized controlled trials (RCTs) with long-term follow-up periods (4 – 11 years) and these studies demonstrated that renal function was significantly better preserved, and the risk of ESRD and clinical recurrence of class IV were significantly reduced [89, 90] in the CY group. The advantage of treatment with IV-CY (National Institutes of Health therapy: NIH protocol) was particularly apparent in the high-risk subgroup of patients who had chronic histological changes in renal biopsy at study entry [88].

Combination with IV-MP appeared to provide additional benefit over IV-MP alone and did not confer additional risk for adverse events [86]. The dose of IV-CY was $0.5 - 1$ g/m^2, given every month, which is lower than the cumulative dose when CY is administered orally. The efficacy of IV-CY or oral CY has also been demonstrated in several populations [91]. Concerns about toxicity by the NIH protocol led to the development of the European Lupus Nephritis Trial (ELNT), during which a less intensive regimen of IV-CY was tested as induction therapy. In brief, two groups of European patients with proliferative lupus nephritis were studied. The dose of corticosteroids was the same for both groups of patients (three 750 mg IV-MP pulses on days $1 - 3$ followed by 0.5 mg/kg/day prednisolone for 4 weeks and gradual tapering to maintain $5 - 7.5$ mg of prednisolone/day). That dose was lower compared with that used in the NIH protocol. The low IV-CY group of patients received 500 mg IV-CY every 2 weeks (3 g cumulative dose of IV-CY/patient). The other group received the NIH dose of IV-CY. After 7 years of follow-up, the low dose IV-CY therapy achieved clinical results comparable to those obtained with a high-dose regimen in European patients with SLE. Low-dose IV-CY may be a good alternative therapy for selected, white European patients who are known to exhibit a milder form of lupus nephritis. In the same study, early response to therapy at 6 months was the best predictor of good long-term renal outcome [92]. After 10 years of follow up of 90 patients randomized in the ELNT; it was reorted that death, sustained doubling of serum creatinine and end-stage renal disease rates did not differ between the LD and HD group (11% *vs* 4%, 14% *vs* 11% and 5% *vs* 9%, respectively) nor did mean serum creatinine, 24-h proteinuria and damage score at last followup. Most patients in both groups were still treated with glucocorticoids, other immunosuppressants and blood pressure lowering drugs. These data confirm that a LD IVCY regimen followed by AZA – the "Euro-Lupus regimen" – achieves good clinical results in the very long-term [93]. Very high doses of IV-CY have also been used as part of an experimental immunoablation stem cell transplantation regimen for the treatment of resistant lupus nephritis [94].

Cyclophosphamide as maintenance therapy of proliferative lupus nephritis

It was reported that prolonged courses (2.5 years) of high-dose IV-CY (1 g/m^2) are more efficacious than 6 months of IV-CY in preserving renal function and in reducing the rate of flares in patients with severe lupus nephritis, thus documenting the need for maintenance therapy following initial induction. However, long courses of IV-CY are associated with increased rates of gonadal toxicity and thus the use of IV-CY as a maintenance therapy is decreasing. Additionally, IV-CY may be associated with more deaths compared with the IV-MP group [85, 86].

Cyclophosphamide for the treatment of membranous lupus nephritis

In a randomized controlled trial from the NIH; three different therapies were administered for 12 months. The first group of patients received IV-CY, the second oral CsA and the third oral prednisolone. Although both CY and CsA were more effective than prednisolone, IV-CY led to more sustained remission [95].

The major drawbacks after CY therapy were toxicity especially gonadal toxicity and relapse after discontinuation of treatment. Avascular necrosis of the bone, osteoporosis, bacterial infections necessitating hospitalization, hypertension, hyperlipidemia, valvular heart disease and premature amenorrhoea did not differ significantly among the three groups of patients treated either with an extended course of high-dose IV-CY, or with pulses of IV-MP, or with a combination of IV-CY and IV-MP [86].

MYCOPHENOLATE MOFETIL (MMF) AND MYCOPHENOLATE SODIUM

MMF is a prodrug, with the active agent being mycophenolic acid (MPA). MMF inhibits both B- and T-lymphocyte proliferation. Lymphocytes, unlike other eukaryotic cells, depend on the de novo synthetic pathway of purine nucleotides. MPA reversibly and non-competitively inhibits inosine monophosphate dehydrogenase (IMP-DH), which catalyses a rate-limiting step in this pathway, therefore having a relatively lymphocyte-specific effect. Also, MMF is 5 folds more potently inhibits the type II isoform of IMP-DH expressed in stimulated lymphocytes [96]. MMF also decreases glomerular, tubular and interstitial cellular proliferation in the rat remnant kidney model and reduces mesangial cell proliferation in experimental systems [97]. MMF has been used in lupus nephritis, both in induction and maintenance treatment of Classes III, IV and V LN disease. In general, it is thought to represent an effective alternative therapy for proliferative lupus nephritis with normal renal function in low to medium-risk patients. Two metanalyses of randomizes controlled trials (RCTs) by Moore and Derry [98] and Walsh et al [99] claimed superiority of MMF in terms of efficacy. However, the strength of the metanalysis is influenced by biases of the included studies. Thus any claims for the superiority of MMF need additional documentation.

Ginzler et al [100] reported a comparison of induction therapy with MMF with the IV-CY NIH regimen. MMF regimen was associated with increased complete remission rate, fewer severe infections and hospitalizations. Patients receiving MMF developed more diarrhoea. However, a large randomized controlled study of 370 patients comparing MMF with CY has failed to demonstrate the superiority of MMF versus CY [101]. In this trial response rates to MMF and CY were similar in Caucasian (56 versus 54%) and Asian patients (53 versus 64%), but in a post-hoc analysis, Hispanic patients responded more to MMF than to CY (61 versus 39%, $p < 0.05$), a finding that requires confirmation.

Taken together, these data suggest that MMF may be considered as a first-line induction therapy for the treatment of lupus nephritis in patients without severe renal dysfunction [99]. However, the efficacy of MMF for the treatment of refractory lupus nephritis or with abnormal renal function requires further documentation [102].

Chan et al [103] reported an extended long-term study, with median follow-up of 63 months looking at MMF as continuous induction-maintenance treatment for Class IV lupus nephritis. Thirty-three patients were randomized to receive MMF, and 31 were randomized to cyclophosphamide and then AZA treatment arm, both together with prednisolone. Doubling of baseline creatinine, relapse-free survival and the hazard ratio for relapse were similar between the two groups during follow-up (P=0.667). MMF treatment was associated with fewer infections and infections requiring hospital admission (P=0.013 and 0.014, respectively).

In a randomized study of 59 patients with DPLN, following induction, the MMF dose (2 g/day for 6 months) was reduced by 25% (i.e., to 750 mg twice daily) after the first 6 months and continued after the first year at a dose of 500 mg twice daily for at least another year before further tapering in stable patients. In the other arm, oral CY was replaced by oral AZA 1.5 – 2 mg/kg/day at 6 months. Contreras *et al* [104] reported that either MMF (0.5 – 3 g/day for 1 – 3 years) or AZA (1 – 3 mg/kg/day for 1 – 3 years) appeared more efficacious and safer than quarterly pulse CY in a US population with a high prevalence of African–Americans, Hispanics, and patients with class IV lupus nephritis. The follow-up period was 34 months. One death was reported in the MMF and four in the IV-CY group.

The suboptimal dose of CY combined with the unusually high doses of corticosteroids used in this trial may explain the lower efficacy and the higher rates of adverse events observed in the CY group Longer follow-up beyond the 5-year time point is essential establish the efficacy-to-toxicity ratio of this therapy.

It is important to educate patients not to get pregnancy while receiving MMF therapy based on toxicity in animal studies and uncontrolled human data [105, 106].

As so many lupus patients are young women of child-bearing age, the risk of ovarian toxicity with NIH-regimen cyclophosphamide is of major concern. MMF use is not associated with a significant risk of ovarian toxicity. The role of MMF and of low dose cyclophosphamide regimens may change in the light of the above trials, and as patient choice regarding their treatment increases.

MMF has also been successfully used in a number of other complications of SLE, such as thrombocytopenia [107], and haemolytic anaemia [108].

Azathioprine

The efficacy of AZA in inducing remission of proliferative lupus nephritis was evaluated in two different studies carried out by the NIH [109] and in the Netherlands [110]. Both of them reported that CY was superior to AZA in preserving renal function. AZA has mainly been used as a corticosteroid-sparing drug achieving maintenance of remission in several trials. AZA was used as maintenance therapy in both arms of the ELNT, which showed that its sequential use (at a dose of 2 mg/kg/day for at least 30 months) after the induction of remission reduced toxicity of induction therapy without compromising the overall efficacy [92, 111]. In a prospective cohort study on class IV, the sequential use of AZA (1.5 mg/kg/day and gradual dose tapering for at least 24 months), after induction treatment with oral CY (2.5 mg/kg/day for 6 months), was effective in preserving renal function in a Chinese population after 10 years of follow-up [91].

Calcineurine Inhibitors (Cyclosporine A/Tacrolimus)

CsA is usually administered for a period of 12 – 43 months in a low dose (1.5 – 5 mg/kg/day divided in two doses). Cyclosporine has a beneficial effect on proteinuria, on histology, on severity status of the disease, but also high rates of disease relapse after discontinuation of therapy [112-114]. The most frequent side effects of CsA are hypertension, hirsutism, gingival hyperplasia, and most importantly, the acute reversible and chronic irreversible nephrotoxicity.

Recently, the safety and efficacy of CsA towards AZA as maintenance treatment of class IV were evaluated in a multicenter, randomized trial. Seventy-five patients initially treated with IV-MP (0.5 – 1 g/day) for 3 consecutive days, followed by oral prednisolone (1 mg/kg/day for 15 consecutive days followed by tapering of the dose) in combination with oral CY (1 – 2 mg/kg) for 3 months. Subsequently, patients were randomly assigned for 2 years either to CsA (4 mg/kg/day and adjusted so that the trough levels are maintained at 75 – 200 ng/ml if proteinuria was less than 1 g/day) or to AZA (2 mg/kg/day). Treatment continued for up to 4 years (follow-up study). The authors concluded that for patients with class IV, AZA or CsA combined with low-dose corticosteroids demonstrated equal efficacy in the prevention of flares [115].

The administration of low-dose CsA may be an acceptable adjunctive agent for induction or maintenance treatment of class IV with normal renal function and proteinuria of less than 3 g/day and membranous lupus nephritis, especially for patients contemplating childbearing or during pregnancy. Side effects are minor and can be further minimized with careful monitoring. The optimum dose and the value of trough blood levels have not been determined. An important limitation for the administration of calcineurin inhibitors is their chronic irreversible nephrotoxicity. Successful treatment of isolated lupus nephritis cases with tacrolimus led to the conduction of small open-label studies with promising results. Tacrolimus was administered as induction therapy at a dose of 0.1 mg/kg/day up to 3 mg/day in patients with class III, IV and V lupus nephritis, with normal renal function. The authors concluded that it was an effective option for selected patients with lupus nephritis [116, 117].

The ongoing randomized clinical trials will help to clarify the role of tacrolimus in the treatment of lupus nephritis.

Plasmapheresis (Plasma Exchange Therapy)

A beneficial effect of plasmapheresis in the treatment of severe lupus nephritis combined with immunosuppressive therapy has been demonstrated in an open-label trial [118]. However, a randomized control study showed no additional benefit from combining plasmaphresis and standard therapy compared with standard therapy alone [119]. Additionally, in another retrospective control study a higher mortality and frequency of bacterial and viral infection was exhibited in the plasmapheresis compared with the IV-CY group [120]. In our opinion and practice, we reserved plasmapheresis for refractory lupus nephritis with evident severe active vasculitis with manifest skin necrosis.

The Role of Antimalarial Drugs

The use of antimalarials has been reviewed. It has been shown that such therapy may influence mortality rate in SLE. Sisó, et al [121] studied the effect of exposure to antimalarial drugs at diagnosis of lupus nephritis on the outcome of disease in a cohort of 206 consecutive patients with lupus nephritis. They showed that exposure to antimalarials before the diagnosis of lupus nephritis was negatively associated with the development of renal failure, hypertension, thrombosis and infection, and with a better survival rate at the end of the follow-up. Withdrawal of antimalarials increases the risk of flare in lupus nephritis. There has been a revival in the use of antimalarials in SLE, and we would recommend continuing rather than stopping these drugs in patients who develop nephritis. It is important to focus on overall mortality, as well as renal survival. The data with antimalarials is interesting when one considers that cyclophosphamide has been reported not to influence overall mortality.

Kasitanon, et al [122] reported that patients with membranous lupus nephritis treated with hydroxychloroquine did better compared with the control.

Management of Chronic Kidney Disease in Lupus Nephritis

We stress on application of the same standard of care for chronic kidney disease through detection and management of reversible causes like gastrointestinal losses, encourage renoprotective strategic measures through salt restriction and the use of angiotensin converting enzyme inhibitors or angiotensin receptors blockers, use of lipid lowering agents and advocate the management of complications like anemia, acidosis, metabolic bone disease and renal replacement therapy whenever indicated.

ERYTHROPOIETIN (EPO)

Anemia is common in SLE, usually in the form of anemia of chronic disease (ACD). Anti-EPO antibodies are rather common and EPO response seems to be blunted in anemic SLE patients [123, 124]. Data regarding the correlation between immune response and recombinant human erythropoetin (rHuEPO) therapy are controversial, ranging from no correlation to a beneficial immune modulatory effect of rHuEPO in lupus nephritis [125]. However, at present, there is little rationale for the widespread use of rHuEPO in lupus nephritis. We advocate its use of hemoglobin is below 10 gm/dl aiming a target hemoglobin of 11-12 gm/dl.

INFECTION RISK AND VACCINATION

Infection is an important cause of early mortality in LN. It is important to take an infection history to assess the nature of previous infections. Infections may relate to immunosuppressive therapy or to a number of immune defects associated with SLE. Such defects include congenital or acquired immunoglobulin deficiency, complement deficiency, mannose binding lectin deficiency, impaired splenic function and an increased risk of salmonella infections [126]. It is likely that further predisposing factors for infection in lupus will be identified in the future. The issue of vaccination is important as this may help to reduce the risk of infection. However, it is also recognised that vaccinations in some instances can trigger lupus flares. It may be that the risk might vary with the nature of the vaccine, being highest with live vaccines. Pneumovax and influenza vaccination would be reasonable, as these are subunit and inactivated vaccines respectively. Live vaccines would be

IMMUNOTHERAPY

Novel immunotherapies are often initially trialled in patients with resistant lupus, hence encountering the most difficult group of patients. This can be justified as physicians will of course initially turn to currently proven medications. However, currently effective drugs, such as corticosteroids and cyclophosphamide, have significant toxicities. Standard immunosuppressive therapies have a number of risks that are common to nearly all drugs in this group including cytopenias, increased risk of infection and in the long term increased risk of malignancy. It is therefore important that new immunotherapeutic agents are designed to try and reduce some of the well-known risks associated with current immunosuppressive drugs.

Novel immunosuppressive/modulatory therapies for SLE

B-cell depletion therapy

Anti-CD20. Rituximab is a chimeric anti-CD20 monoclonal antibody, which depletes B cells from the peripheral circulation, but allows regeneration from stem cells. Several groups have published uncontrolled studies regarding the use of rituximab treatment in SLE with positive results. Leandro et al [127] reported that SLE patients treated with rituximab as two pulses of 1 gm 2 weeks apart, in most cases, together with cyclophosphamide, and methylprednisolone showed marked improvement. B-cell depletion lasted for 3-8 months, though one patient remained depleted beyond 4 yrs. Only 1 out of 24 did not deplete the B cells. Twenty-two patients were able to stop immunosuppressive medication, with 13 remaining without immunosuppressives for mean follow-up of 23 months.

Looney et al [128] reported a Phase I/II dose escalation trial in 18 SLE patients of rituximab added to ongoing immunosuppressive therapy (patients who received cyclophosphamide were excluded). There were three regimens: low dose (single infusion of 100 mg/m2), intermediate dose (single infusion of 375 mg/m2) and high dose (4 weekly infusions of 375 mg/m2). Rituximab was generally well tolerated with no major adverse events thought to be rituximab-related (three serious adverse events in total). Looking at those patients who intensely depleted their B-cell population (11/17 patients), the Systemic Lupus Activity Measure (SLAM) score was decreased significantly at 2 and 3 months. Six patients developed human anti-chimeric antibodies (HACAs) at 5100 ng/ml. No consistent changes in anti-dsDNA antibodies were seen in this study, but 6 of 17 patients did not achieve B-cell depletion, and dsDNA levels were reduced in four of the eight patients that depleted.

Vigna-Perez et al [129] reported 22 patients with lupus nephritis treated with rituximab (0.5 to 1.0 g at Days 1 and 15) added to their immunosuppressive treatment that included different combinations of AZA, MMF, cyclophosphamide and corticosteroids. Significant reduction of disease activity and proteinuria was noted (P<0.05), 20/22 patients achieved B-cell depletion. There were no significant changes in the levels of dsDNA antibodies and complement fractions at 30, 60 and 90 days after rituximab. One patient died at Day 70 from invasive histoplasmosis.

An open trial of 10 patients with active proliferative LN (Classes III and IV) was conducted using 4 weekly rituximab intravenous infusions of 375 mg/m2, combined with oral prednisolone [130]. Eight out of 10 patients had partial remission by a median of 2 months, with five of these achieving complete remission by 3 months, defined as normal serum albumin creatinine, urinary sediment and <500 mg/24 h urine protein excretion. Four patients had sustained complete remission for 12 months with no other immunosuppressive drugs other than low-dose oral steroids. Two patients were considered treatment failures. Thrombocytopenia and cutaneous involvement also showed improvement in the responder group. One of the patients who achieved complete remission had a relapse at the fifth month. One patient developed an allergic infusion reaction, and one patient developed pneumococcal meningitis at the time B cells were recovering. All patients, except the case of allergic reaction, achieved complete B-cell depletion. There was no correlation between the degree of depletion and the outcome. The duration of B-cell depletion was variable lasting from 1 month to 7 months.

While the bulk of clinical information regarding rituximab has come from open studies with small patient numbers, randomized clinical trials have now been commenced. The EXPLORER trial was a multicentre, randomized, placebo-controlled Phase II/III and Phase III clinical trial of rituximab in SLE, which planned to recruit 250 patients with moderate to severe disease, as determined by the BILAG index (patients with active moderate or severe glomerulonephritis were excluded). It aimed to assess the clinical response to rituximab in combination with an immunosuppressive medication, compared with placebo. A recent press release from Genentech and Biogen Idec announced that the study was terminated because the primary and secondary end-points were not achieved [131].

The most common side effects observed in patients treated with rituximab were infections (viral, bacterial and fungal), infusion reactions, skin rash and pruritus, nausea and abdominal pain. HACA responses can be produced, though as yet have not caused major clinical problem. The HACA response has theoretical potential to cause problems in re-treatments. There are not yet available results from randomized controlled trials in SLE to estimate the true incidence of all of the above complications. Recently, the development of PML has been noted in SLE patients treated with rituximab. PML has also been reported in other immunocompromised patients, including HIV positive patients, cancer patients, transplant patients and patients with SLE not treated with rituximab. The incidence of PML in autoimmune diseases is not known; however, there are a number of cases reported in the literature. PML has been reported in patients with SLE receiving prednisone, AZA, cyclophosphamide and MMF. There are reports of PML in rituximab-treated NHL patients, but not RA treated with rituximab. PML seemed to occur as a result of the combination of the disease itself and the effects of immunosuppression by the drug [132].

B-Cell Tolerization

LJP-394 (abetimus). LJP-394 (La Jolla Pharmaceuticals, San Diego, USA) or abetimus consists of four double-stranded oligodeoxyribonucleotides attached to non-immunogenic polyethylene glycol as a carrier. It is a synthetic B-cell toleragen molecule, which acts as an 'anti-anti DNA', by cross-linking surface anti-dsDNA antibody molecules, with consequent decrease in anti-dsDNA antibody production. One drawback is the frequency of administration—as a weekly infusion over a period of over 4 months—but no major toxicity has been shown in almost 1000 patients [133].

A total of 230 SLE patients were included in a randomized double-blind placebo-controlled trial [134]. LJP-394 decreased levels of anti-dsDNA antibodies, with complement C3 levels tending to increase. Overall results showed no effect on time to renal flare. However, the LJP-394 group took longer to treatment with high-dose corticosteroids or high-dose cyclophosphamide, and also received 41% less high-dose cyclophosphamide treatments. There was no increase in serious adverse events observed in the LJP-394 group. However, results in a subpopulation with high-affinity antidsDNA antibodies are worth mentioning (189 out of 213 patients tested, 89% LJP-394, 90% placebo). In this subgroup, there were 67% less renal flares, and 62% less high-dose cyclophosphamide treatments. In patients with renal impairment (serum creatinine 51.5 mg/dl), renal flares fell by 50% in the overall LJP-394 group, with no renal flares in the high-affinity subgroup.

Modulation of Costimulatory Molecules

CD40L is over-expressed in autoimmune diseases, such as SLE and murine lupus and may contribute to disease pathology [135]. It is probably premature at this stage to comment on the efficacy of anti-CD40L in SLE patients, but safety issues regarding thromboembolism are of concern [136].

Anti-Cytokine Therapies

In our view, therapies targeting anti-interleukin 10, anti- TNF, or anti-complement are limited, still experimental.

Non-specific immunotherapies

Intravenous immunoglobulin
Since one decade, Boletis, et al [137] reported through their RCT in lupus nephritis that a beneficial effect of monthly IVIG of 0.4gm/kg/ dose. Levy et al. [138] reported improvement in proteinuria in six out of seven patients treated with IVIG. It is worth noting that there may be an increased risk of renal dysfunction with high-dose IVIG. Sucrose containing IVIg may be a risk factor for osmotic nephrosis. Other risk factors for toxicity include pre-existing renal disease, volume depletion and old age [139].

A variety of other features of SLE have been treated with IVIG including cytopenias, neurological involvement, cerebritis and secondary APS. Seventeen (85%) of 20 patients responded to treatment with a 5-day high dose regime [140].

PERIPHERAL BLOOD STEM CELL TRANSPLANTATION

The concept underlying this strategy is to try to 'reset' the aberrant immune system. The survey from the European Blood and Marrow Transplant and European League against Rheumatism (EBMT/EULAR) registry [141] included 53 patients, treated in 23 centers, with 66% having kidney involvement. Conditioning regimes varied, but most commonly mobilization of peripheral blood stem cells involved cyclophosphamide and G-CSF. In 33/50 patients, disease activity remitted by 6 months, but 10/31 relapsed after 6 months. Twelve deaths occurred, seven being procedure related.

Lisukov et al. [142] reported that three out of six SLE patients from one centre treated with autologous PBSCT died due to transplant-related complications. The American experience reported by Traynor et al [143] was more encouraging with 15 SLE patients treated with no procedure-related mortality. Ten out of 12 patients followed up for over 1 yr stopped immunosuppressive therapy. Two patients showed evidence of relapse, one requiring treatment.

Patient selection is the key, given the risk–benefit ratio of undergoing PBSCT. There are no easy predictors to assess which are the best patients to transplant, and Jayne et al [144] suggested that outcome could be improved by better selection of patients and conditioning regimes. The longer the delay, the more likely organ failure from the disease, thereby increasing procedure related mortality, or leading to PBSCT being contra-indicated.

Against the use of PBSCT in SLE is that renal failure (a major organ affected) can be treated effectively with dialysis or renal transplantation. The latter procedure is highly successful, with a low risk of lupus nephritis recurrence, though aPL-positive patients do worse.

Submaximal (non-myeloablative) immunotherapy without stem cell rescue has also been tried, Burt et al. [145] reported a study enrolling 50 patients, of whom 48 underwent autologous non-myeloablative stem cell transplantation. Mortality was 2/50 by intention to treat. Overall 5-yr survival was 84%, with 50% probability of disease-free survival at 5 years.

Treatment of Membranous Lupus Nephritis (MLN)

Data from uncontrolled studies indicate that a combined regimen consisting of corticosteroids and ciclosporin, MMF or cyclophosphamide as initial therapy is effective in inducing a complete renal response in most patients with membranous nephritis [146-148]. In a study of 38 patients with membranous lupus nephritis, Mok et al. [146] found that one-third of patients did not respond completely to 12 months' treatment with prednisone and azathioprine. Four patients, who were refractory to treatment, responded completely to rescue therapy with cyclophosphamide, MMF or ciclosporin. After a mean observation period of more than 7 years, only 13% of patients had a deterioration in their creatinine clearance rate of more than 20%. More aggressive and costly regimens, therefore, should be reserved for patients who have truly refractory disease, persistent nephrotic syndrome, or declining renal function. In one trial from the NIH, 42 patients with WHO class V lupus nephritis were randomly assigned to receive intravenous cyclophosphamide, ciclosporin or oral prednisone for 12 months. Based on the results published in an abstract [95]. Intravenous cyclophosphamide and ciclosporin were more effective than prednisone alone in inducing remission of proteinuria, but intravenous cyclophosphamide resulted in more sustained remissions. The role of MMF therapy in membranous nephritis requires further investigation. Austin et al [149] present data from their prospective study of immunosuppressive therapy in 42 patients with nephrosis and pure MLN (patients with evidence of proliferative lupus nephritis were excluded). The number of patients enrolled in this study is relatively small; however, this sample is larger than in many of the other retrospective and/or uncontrolled articles about treatment of MLN. The patients were randomly assigned to a 1-yr treatment phase that involved high-dosage alternate-day prednisone alone (PRED) or adjunctive therapy with either six doses of alternate-month intravenous cyclophosphamide (IVCY) or 11 mo of daily cyclosporine started at approximately 5mg/kg per d (CsA). The primary end point was time to complete or partial remission during this 1-yr treatment protocol. As a secondary measure, the patients were assessed for relapse in a follow-up phase with a median duration of 60 months after the end of treatment. Their data demonstrate 1-yr rates of combined complete and partial remissions of 27, 60, and 83% in the PRED, IVCY, and CsA groups, respectively. Two thirds of the remissions in both the IVCY and CsA treatment groups were complete. Consistent with previous therapeutic trials using CsA, however, the authors found a significant relapse rate in the CsA group, with proteinuria often rebounding to severely nephrotic levels within 1 yr of stopping therapy. CsA was started at a fixed dosage in this study and was adjusted in response to a rise in creatinine or the development of hypertension, which occurred in nine of 12 patients. No data are provided on the final dosage or CsA levels achieved in this study. Of note, patients who had not entered a remission by 12 mo or who had experienced relapse were eligible for entry into an uncontrolled observational trial with IVCY. Eight of these 10 patients subsequently experience remission with this further therapy. It is clear from these data that, as in idiopathic membranous nephropathy, corticosteroids are not sufficient to induce a remission in most cases and adjunctive treatment with either CsA or cyclophosphamide is required. Tacrolimus therapy was evaluated in six patients with membranous/inactive lupus nephritis and persistent proteinuria, despite angiotensin–aldosterone axis blockade [150]. Tacrolimus treatment significantly reduced proteinuria and increased serum albumin levels. The efficacy was most pronounced in the four patients with membranous lupus nephritis, whose proteinuria improved by over 80%. The advantages of tacrolimus over ciclosporin in the treatment of lupus nephritis are lower incidences of blood pressure elevation, hyperlipidemia and adverse cosmetic effects. However, patients must be closely monitored for neurotoxicity and adverse metabolic effects. As with ciclosporin, relapse of proteinuria is common after discontinuation of tacrolimus.

A number of nonimmunosuppressive strategies can help to reduce proteinuria in MLN [151] and should, therefore, be instituted early in all cases. These strategies include the use of angiotensin-converting-enzyme inhibitors or angiotensin II receptor blockers (or both), titrated up to the maximal tolerated dose, and tight control of cardiovascular risk factors such as hyperlipidemia and hypertension. The 3-hydroxy-3-methyl-glutaryl-CoA reductase inhibitors (statins) are useful for their dual effects of assuaging hyperlipidemia and reducing urinary protein excretion [152]. Prophylactic low-dose aspirin or anticoagulation should be considered in patients who have multiple vascular risk factors and persistent, heavy proteinuria.

End-Stage Renal Disease and Systemic Lupus Erythematosus

About 20% of patients progressing to ESRD require maintenance dialysis or renal transplantation within ten years [153]. The activity of SLE after the development of ESRD has been reported [154]. The activity of SLE after the development of ESRD tends to decline as reflected by the clinical and serological features. Cheigh et al [5] reported that lupus activity was clinically apparent in 55.4% of patients with ESRD during the first year and in 6.5% during the fifth year. It was believed that the disease became inactive within ten years of the development of ESRD. This so-called "burn-out" phenomenon was first described by Fries et al [155]. However, SLE flare during dialysis is also not rare. Some investigators reported that several risk factors could predict the persistence of activity of SLE [3, 156, 157]. On the other hand, it is still uncertain whether the "burn-out" phenomenon is dependent on the uremic state or on treatment by dialysis. Moreover, the lupus activity may reflect the natural disease course of SLE, which seems to show a gradual wane [158]. There are exceptions however. Some patients may show frequent flares of SLE during dialysis and require an aggressive treatment with corticosteroid and immunosuppressive agents [159].

Renal Transplantation and Systemic Lupus Erythematosus

When to transplant

There are no firm rules regarding the optimal timing of renal transplantation in SLE. Roth et al, [160] proposed a minimum dialysis period of 1 year, to permit patients' SLE to `burn out'. This recommendation was based only on the post-transplant serum creatinine levels of a small number of SLE patients (n=15) and has not been supported by subsequent studies. Indeed, some patients with living-related donors proceed successfully straight to transplantation, with no intervening dialysis period. In many cases, however, a 3-month dialysis period to ensure that spontaneous renal recovery will not occur is prudent. Kimberly et al [161] reported that 17 of 41 SLE patients reaching ESRD were able to discontinue dialysis (at least temporarily), and noted that rapid loss of renal function predicted those patients who were most likely to recover.

At most transplant centers, demonstration of serological quiescence is an important (if not absolute) criterion for transplantation. However, just as serological parameters (double-stranded DNA antibody titers and complement levels) frequently fail to predict SLE flares [162], serology is imperfect guides to the appropriate timing of renal transplantation. In some SLE patients e.g. those with heritable deficiencies of complement proteins, serum complement levels may never normalize. Among Caucasian SLE patients, 37% have at least one C4A null allele [163]. Thus, decisions about when to transplant patients with SLE must be made on an individual basis, considering all clinical and serological data. Ideally, the rheumatologist, transplant nephrologist, and transplant surgeon all participate in such discussions. However, in the more recent reports [164, 165]. it was shown that patients with ESRD and who have potential living donors may have the opportunity to undergo pre-emptive living donor kidney transplantation, in contrast to the near universal timing of cadaveric kidney transplantation after the initiation of chronic dialysis. Moreover, pre emptive live-related transplantation is associated with a greater rate of allograft survival than transplantation from living donors after the commencement of chronic dialysis [164].

Selection and preparation

Most patients with SLE are suitable candidates for renal transplantation. However, a number of them may present some disease-related problems. A major issue for SLE candidates for transplantation may be the presence of extrarenal complications related either to the disease itself or to previous steroid and/or immunosuppressive therapy. Cardiovascular disease frequently occurs in SLE patients and represents a leading cause of morbidity and mortality [166]. In addition to these risk factors, SLE patients are often carriers of antiphospholipid antibodies which increase the risk of cardiac and cerebral complications [167]. Pretransplant and post-transplant corticosteroid therapy may further exacerbate cardiovascular complications, as well as produce severe osteoporosis, diabetes mellitus, myopathy, and cataracts. Also, infections are more frequent and severe in SLE patients, particularly in those who have received long-term and/or vigorous immunosuppression before transplantation [168], and also represent the major cause of death in children [169]. Finally, patients with SLE might be exposed to an increased risk of malignancy, although it is difficult to interpret the available data definitively [170].

The work-up for the transplant candidate does not differ from the general guidelines recommended by the American Society of Transplantation [171] and by the European Best Practice Guidelines for Renal Transplantation [172]. However, for the reasons already mentioned, cardiac evaluation requires a careful preoperative screening. Besides electrocardiogram and echocardiography, exercise thallium testing, sestamibi testing, exercise echocardiography, and/or dipyridamole echocardiography are all recommended. Patients at high risk (such as heavy smokers, those with severe left ventricular hypertrophy, severe hypertension, diabetes, previous cardiovascular events, and/ or long-term dialysis) should undergo a coronary angiography and should be treated with revascularization when needed. A Magnetic Resonance Image is indicated for patients who suffered from lupus cerebritis.

The presence of anti-phospholipid syndrome (aPL) should be evaluated, as the risk for the development of thrombotic microangiopathy in the renal allograft and for transplant vessel thrombosis is increased. It has been shown that thrombotic events are much more frequent in renal transplant recipients with anticardiolipin antibodies [173]. Stone *et al* [174] followed a group of 85 transplanted SLE patients. Fifteen of the 25 patients with aPL suffered from associated clinical events, while only 5 of the patients without aPL had such an event ($P < 0.0001$). Another retrospective study showed the presence of aPL in 57% of 56 primary nonfunctioning transplanted kidneys. Early graft failure was particularly frequent in patients on peritoneal dialysis [175].

On the basis of the few data available, a pretransplant screening of aPL before transplantation is strongly recommended both to forewarn the risk of early graft failure and to indicate which patient may benefit from an early anticoagulation. Whether aPL positive patients should be treated peri- and postoperatively with anti-coagulants is not known yet. Moreover, anticoagulation perioperatively can lead to serious bleeding complications. In one unit, they treat all renal transplant recipients with prophylactic doses of low molecular-weight heparin during the first week after transplantation [176].

Lupus patients have a high prevalence (30–90%) of anti-lymphocyte antibodies [177]. This may cause positive cross-matches. Therefore, during the pre-transplant workup cross-matches should be performed with autologous lymphocytes. These results can be taken into account when cross-matching with donor lymphocytes is performed. Also, particular attention should be paid to the disease activity and its treatment. The results of renal transplantation are poor in patients whose conditions necessitated steroids on dialysis, as well as for those showing poor clinical conditions due to previous immunosuppression. It is reasonable to recommend a one to two year waiting period before transplantation to try and attain stabilization and recovery from the metabolic and toxic effects of steroids and cytotoxic agents. Also for patients with rapid progression to renal failure we would suggest waiting at least three months before transplantation, in order to evaluate a possible recovery of renal function [178]. With the exception of these cases, patients should receive renal transplantation as soon as possible, as there is now convincing evidence that the longer the time on dialysis the worse the results, the most successful strategy being represented by a preemptive transplantation [179].

Most lupus patients are extensively treated with corticosteroids for their disease. Therefore, bone mineral density should be assessed before transplantation to guide post-transplant prophylaxis for osteoporosis with additional calcium, vitamin D and eventually bisphosphonates [176].

Risk of Recurrence

The extent of the risk of recurrence of lupus nephritis after renal transplantation is still a controversial issue. A number of retrospective studies have reported a recurrence rate ranging between 2 and 4% [180, 181]. However, in a large series of cyclosporine-treated SLE patients, Stone et al. [174] found that recurrence occurred in 9% of cases. In a smaller group of SLE transplant patients, Goral et al [182] reported recurrence in 30% of cases. At least in part, these discrepancies may be accounted for by the different indications for biopsy and by the different ethnicities. However, there is agreement that the histological lesions in grafts with recurrence are usually not severe. Most cases show mesangial glomerulonephritis or mild focal proliferative lesions. Diffuse proliferative glomerulonephritis and membranous nephropathy are rare. Recurrence is diagnosed in mean after three years, but cases have been reported five days or 13 years after transplantation [174, 183].

There is little information about the impact of recurrence on the outcome of renal transplant. In a wide French series no patient lost the kidney graft because of recurrence; [180] in a retrospective analysis of Stone et al [174] four patients out of 97 had a graft failure attributed to SLE recurrence. A case of one patient in whom recurrence of lupus nephritis caused the loss of the kidney both in the first and in the second allograft has been reported [184]. Thus it seems that recurrence is relatively rare and does not affect the outcome of the transplanted kidney in most cases, but in some particular patients recurrence may lead to severe renal dysfunction.

Immunosuppressive Therapy

The basic immunosuppression for SLE transplant patients does not differ from that normally used. Among the drugs used for transplant immunosuppression, MMF, azathioprine, tacrolimus and cyclosporine have also been employed successfully to treat lupus nephritis. There are no prospective studies in lupus patients comparing the effects of the various immunosuppressive drugs. special attention should be given to the impact of immunosuppressives on cardiovascular risk factors. It becomes clear that during maintenance immunosuppression other drugs (i.e. MMF or azathioprine) should be used preferentially. Especially MMF is a good candidate because it could have anti-atherogenic properties [185]. The ultimate choice of the maintenance immunosuppressive regimen in the individual lupus patient after renal transplantation should be guided by the individual characteristics of the patient.

Results of Renal Transplantation

SLE patients that undergo renal transplantation might be different from non-SLE recipients in many respects. They are generally younger, with fewer co morbidities; a majority of them are women with a greater percentage of African-American patients. SLE patients might have a unique immunological profile, they are more likely to have received blood transfusions and their PRA levels are higher than non-SLE recipients. They also have higher than average theoretical risk of allograft failure due to recurrence of SLE activity and thrombosis [174, 175]. In addition to cardiovascular disease, infections are a common cause of morbidity and mortality in SLE patients and may contribute to poor allograft and recipient outcomes [186].

General speaking, the results reported in the literature are controversial, with some studies showing poor allograft survival associated with SLE, whereas others reported allograft and recipient survival rates comparable with non-SLE recipients. There is agreement that in SLE patients, living transplantation offers better results than cadaveric transplantation [187]. Instead, divergent results were reported when SLE patients were compared to renal transplant recipients with other diseases. Some reports outlined that patient and graft survival rates of patients with lupus nephritis were similar to those of patients with other primary renal diseases [180, 181]. However, Ponticelli, et al reported a worse graft survival in SLE patients [188].

It should be pointed out, however, that none of these studies had adequate controls. Usually the outcome of SLE patients was compared with that of other renal transplant recipients without taking into account the criteria of inclusion, the period of transplantation, the available treatments at that time, and so on. The clinical conditions of the recipient at the time of transplantation are very important, an issue often neglected in the published reports. It is a common experience that some patients are devastated by the prolonged administration of corticosteroid, or by a full blown nephrotic syndrome, or by severe extrarenal complications. Clearly, poor clinical conditions can have a deleterious impact on the graft and patient survival after transplantation. Another factor influencing the outcome is the compliance of the patient, which is poorer in adolescents, in patients with poor socioeconomic conditions, and in women with esthetic disfiguration. These aspects are difficult to analyze in large retrospective surveys. It should be pointed out, however, that there a trend to postpone the transplant in high-risk patients, namely those with poor clinical conditions, those who developed renal failure after a rapidly progressive course, and those who received a vigorous long-term immunosuppression. These criteria of selection may have influenced the results.

Cadaveric renal transplantation

An analysis performed by Nossent *et al.* on behalf of the Dutch Working Party on SLE showed that patient survival after renal transplantation at 1 year and another for 5 years was 86.5% and graft survival was 67.6% and 54.1%, respectively [189]. The single-centre study of Stone *et al* [174] corrected for confounding factors by using a control group of patients that was transplanted in the same period, treated with either cyclosporine A or tacrolimus and matched for age, sex, race, type of allograft, number of previous transplants and year of transplantation. In this analysis the outcome for lupus patients was less favorable. The allograft survival for lupus patients versus controls was at 1 year: 81.7% versus 88.2%; at 2 years 74.7% versus 84.4%; at 5 years 45.9% versus 75% and at 10 years 18.5% versus 34.8%. The relative hazard ratio of allograft loss in lupus patients was 2.1 (95% CI: 1.06–4.06; $P < 0.04$). The reasons for this increased allograft loss in lupus patients was recurrence of LN leading to graft loss (3.8%) and thrombosis or thrombotic microangiopathy attributed to aPL (15.4%). These less favorable results were not confirmed in an analysis using data from the United States Renal Data System (USRDS). Ward [190] reported that the hazard ratio adjusted for confounding factors for graft loss in 772 lupus patients undergoing first cadaveric renal transplantation was 1.08 (95% CI: 0.94–1.23; $P = 0.28$) compared to 32 644 control patients. Also, mortality did not differ between the groups. An analysis of the United Network of Organ Sharing (UNOS) database [175] also did not show a difference in patient and graft survival between SLE patients and non-lupus patients after transplantation with kidneys from either living (SLE: 789; nonlupus: 21 228) or cadaveric donors (SLE 1170; non-lupus: 42 651). However, a recent large follow-up study using data from both the USRDS and UNOS registry compared 2886 SLE recipients with 89 958 non-SLE recipients [191]. Lupus patients showed a worse transplant (HR 1.09, 95% CI: 1.02–1.15, $P < 0.05$) and patient survival (HR 1.18, $P < 0.05$) compared to diabetes patients if corrected for many confounding factors. There were no significant differences when kidneys from living donors were transplanted. These aggregated data, indicate that graft survival and patient survival in lupus patients are more or less comparable to other patient groups.

Living donor transplantation

Initial single centre reports indicated, as for transplantation in other diseases, that results in lupus patients for living donor transplantation (LDTx) were superior to cadaveric donor transplantation. Bumgardner et al reported living-related graft survival among patients with ESRD caused by lupus nephritis to be comparable to that of the comparison group, but cadaveric graft survival at one year was 60% among patients with ESRD caused by lupus nephritis ($N\ 5\ 10$) and 90% among patients in the comparison group ($N\ 5\ 20$) [192]. In 390 lupus patients undergoing LDTx, 5-year graft and patient survival were 77 and 94.4%, respectively, compared to 58.1% and 83.3% in 772 lupus patients receiving CADTx. Similar results were obtained in additional analyses [191]. Therefore, LDTx is the preferred treatment for SLE patients with ESRF. If a living donor is available, the possibility of a pre-emptive transplantation should be considered, since the results of such an approach are superior in terms of graft and patient survival, irrespective of the cause of the original kidney disease [164]. This will prevent dialysis-associated morbidity, mortality, costs and loss of quality of life. However, we are convinced that pre-emptive transplantation should not be pursued in those patients with ongoing disease activity or severe iatrogenic morbidity. A waiting period before transplantation to obtain decreased disease activity and to improve clinical condition might then be a better solution.

Renal Transplantation and SLE Summary

Most patients with lupus nephritis are suitable candidates for kidney transplantation. However, patients who have received vigorous and prolonged immunosuppression and/or corticosteroid therapy, patients with Anti-Phospholipid (aPL) syndrome, and those with an aggressive disease need a careful work-up and adequate preparation before being admitted to receive transplantation. With the exception of these cases, the results of renal transplantation are quite good in SLE patients. Lupus nephritis may recur after transplantation, but in most cases recurrence neither causes severe histologic lesions nor has any clinical impact on the long-term outcome. The possibility of minimizing the use of corticosteroids after transplantation may reduce the risk of iatrogenic morbidity and improve the compliance of the patient.

Lupus Nephritis in Children

Lupus nephritis is one of the main clinical presentations (up to 80%) of childhood SLE and it determines the course and outcome of the disease [193]. Clinically overt nephropathy is more often a presenting clinical manifestation of SLE in children than in adults. Overall 60–80% of children with SLE have abnormalities of the urinary tests or of renal function early in the course of the disease. In 90% of patients renal disease occurs within two years from disease onset [193, 194]. Clinically significant renal involvement ranges from asymptomatic urinary findings to nephrotic syndrome and renal failure [195].

In a 1994 review of the presentation of lupus nephritis from different studies involving 208 children, 55% presented with nephrotic syndrome and 43% with proteinuria of lesser degrees. Most children had microscopic hematuria while relatively few (1.4%) presented with macroscopic hematuria. Fifty percent of the children had impaired renal function at onset, while only 1.4% had acute renal failure requiring renal replacement therapy. A small proportion presented with a rapidly progressive glomerulonephritis with biopsy-proven crescentic glomerulonephritis. Hypertension was found in 40% of children [196].

Pathological findings may not always correlate with clinical manifestations, so performing a renal biopsy is crucial for planning effective therapy [197]. An analysis of nine investigations on renal biopsy findings in childhood SLE (comprising 365 children and adolescents) showed that 25% had WHO class I-II, and 65% had class III or IV, supporting a high frequency of severe renal involvement in childhood SLE [196]. Class V accounted for

9% of patients, an incidence lower with respect to that observed in adults. However, an increased incidence of class V has been reported in childhood SLE [198]. According to ISN/RPS classification, Mark et al [199] provide evidence that up to half of children have the most severe class (class IV or diffuse LN).

Clinicopathological correlation has been evaluated in children according to different histopathological classification. At disease onset, more severe proteinuria, more hematuria, a lower serum albumin and the need for antihypertensive drugs were all associated with a higher class of lupus nephritis [200]. The new ISN/RPS classification demonstrated that subgroup IV-G LN is associated with the worst clinical outcome in children with LN [199]. Sumboondonda et al [201] found that renal function (urinalysis and serum creatinine) correlated with the activity index but not the chronicity index at the initial biopsy. However, neither index predicted long-term renal outcome. Rush et al [202] examined only those patients with class IV disease and found a significant correlation between the AI and the CI and renal function at the initial biopsy. In addition they found that a high CI score at diagnosis predicted a poor renal outcome at the four-year follow-up. In another pediatric study, McCurdy et al [203] reported that AI and CI in the initial biopsy did correlate with progression to renal failure on follow-up.

Treatment

Treatment of children with SLE is challenging. The therapeutic issues, risks and balances faced by adult patients are further complicated by an unpredictable disease course and long requirement for therapy in children with SLE. Further, non-compliance is a major obstacle to satisfactory outcome which must be recognized and dealt with in every adolescent in our efforts to attain optimal outcome [204]. Unfortunately, there have been no randomized controlled trials in children to assess the drugs currently used in the treatment of pediatric SLE. Data therefore, come from uncontrolled studies, case reports, and extrapolation from the experience with adults with SLE.

Therapeutic options for patients with LN are depending on the histological lesions observed on renal biopsy. Patients with class II LN do not need specific therapy, as there is little probability of progression [205]. Nevertheless, careful follow-up of the patient is necessary, as transformation to a more severe renal disease is possible. For patients with suspected class III at the time of diagnosis, but with normal renal function, blood pressure (BP) and proteinuria below the nephrotic range, oral prednisone should be started at 1mg/kg/day in a single daily dose. Others also recommend to add Hydroxychloroquine at the initiation of steroid therapy because of its role as a steroid sparing agent and because it has been shown to reverse the changes in plasma lipids induced by steroids [206, 207]. WHO class III with high activity should be considered on a spectrum with class IV, with a significant risk of progression [208]. Currently, most nephrologists adopt the philosophy of separating the treatment of these patients into induction and maintenance. Three consecutive days of methyl prednisolone 30mg/kg (up to 1g) pulses followed by oral prednisone in combination with 6 monthly doses of CY (500mg/m^2/dose) is the standard induction therapy for these patients with gradual tapering of corticosteroid, three maintenance protocols have been advocated, quarterly intravenous CY, oral AZA and MMF [208].

There is no consensus on the optimal dose of oral prednisone and how the dosage should be decreased. The optimal duration of maintenance therapy is not known and there is no study comparing different durations of treatment. Some authors maintain the treatment for 18-24 months while others propose a longer duration up to 5-8 years [110, 209].

Corticosteroid therapy's impact on body image and stature compounded by the impact of SLE on school function frequently lead to anger and depression. The result is often both overt and covert non-compliance [205].

Actually, the IV CY experience is the only published series describing successful long term regiment of childhood SLE [210, 211]. A major concern regarding the use of CY in young patients is gonadal toxicity. There are no published data on the long-term gonadal toxicity of CY pulses given to prepubertal girls. The gonadal toxicity of pulse CY in men has not been studied. However, studies in children with idiopathic nephrotic syndrome indicate that toxicity may occur if the cumulative dosage is higher than 200mg/kg [212].

In children, AZA is traditionally used as the initial second-line agent. Its efficacy as a first line treatment has been suggested, but the study was uncontrolled [213]. The long-term safety profile of AZA in dose of 2-2.5mg/kg/day has proven to be good. Although it is associated with an increased risk of infection, other side effects are mild, including reversible hematologic and hepatic side effects and occasional nausea and diarrhea. Moreover, it does not have the clearly documented gonadal toxicity seen with CY.

The experience with MMF in children with LN is contradictory. Some describe good results in some lupus children [214-216]. Adam's et al [217] conclude that MMF (22mg/kg/day) has been less effective and is complicated by more adverse effects than quarterly IV CY. This may be the result of poor compliance by children and adolescents, which is primarily related to adverse gastrointestinal effects.

Indeed in children prospective studies are needed to compare MMF to AZA in terms of efficacy and safety as maintenance therapy in children with severe LN, as well as to investigate whether MMF could replace CY or could be used as a good corticosteroids sparing agent.

In children with CY-refractory or relapsed class IV LN in which the maximum dosage of CY has already been administered, there are no clear guidelines for treatment. In one report, five children with recurrent class IV LN were treated with combination CY and methotrexate. Nine monthly doses of IV CY (750-1000mg/m²/dose) and IV methotrexate (50-300mg/m²/month) were given on the same day. Although this study represents only a small number of patients, all five experienced long-term remission [218].

Marks et al [219] demonstrate that children with refractory LN respond well to the combination of rituximab and CY. They used a regimen of rituximab 750mg/m² (maximum dose of 1g) on days 1 and 15, with a pre-medication of methyl prednisolone, chlorpheniramine and paracetamol (acetaminophen) each at 100mg, followed by CY 750mg or 500mg if the patient's dry weight was <50kg on days 2 and 16. Oral prednisolone in tapering doses was given on days 2,3,4,16,17 and 18. Although this is a small study (seven children), significant improvements were seen in both systemic disease activity and renal parameters.

Information on the use of plasmaphersis, IVIG, autologous stem cell transplantation and therapies directed to T and B cells or complement are sparse and recruited from case reports.

Outcome of LN in Children

In spite of improvement in care of children with SLE we and others reported high mortality rates at 10-20% and 10 year renal survival at 75-90% [220, 221].

Of equal concern is the fact that a large percentage of patients with LN need to continue on therapy for prolonged periods of time, exposing them to detrimental effects of immunosuppressive agents and adding to their disease-related morbidity. Similar to adult studies, pediatric studies have also demonstrated poorer renal survival in children of male gender [222], those with HTN [223], nephrotic syndrome [199] and those who fail to achieve remission with therapy [223]. African-American ethnicity in some studies has also been shown to adversely affect renal outcome [224]. While poorer renal survival in children with class IV is expected [199], others have not found histological class to be predictive of outcome [225].

We have the impression that predictors of mortality include HTN, hematuria, impaired renal function, lack of remission of renal disease, low total hemolytic complement, class IV nephritis, and the non-use of IV CY.

With ESRD, theses patients do as well as non-lupus patients. Clinical and biological symptoms of the disease most often improve in patients on chronic dialysis, thus allowing stopping of corticosteroids and immunosuppressive therapy, however, clinical manifestations can persist or even appear at this stage [226].

Renal transplantation in children with LN encompasses some particular concerns. These children have extra-renal organ involvement, which impacts on their suitability for surgery and recovery. Activity of the SLE in other organs, corticosteroid effects and marked immune suppression must all be considered when evaluating the suitability of these children for transplantation. These patients have an increased incidence of diabetes, atherosclerosis and antiphospholipid syndrome, as well as an increased risk of infection. All of these factors pose increased risk at the time of renal transplantation and increased risk of ultimate complications or graft rejection [178].

Lupus Nephritis and Pregnancy

To discuss the issues related to LN and pregnancy is out the scope of this chapter, but in a summary, pregnancy may affect kidney disease and vice versa kidney disease may affect pregnancy. Renal function may decline as a result of pregnancy among patients with renal disease, determined in part by the severity of underlying renal disease. In general, patients without significant chronic renal disease (serum creatinine less than 1.4 mg/100 ml or 124 μmol/l) who are in remission have an excellent outcome. Among those with an initial value between 1.4 and 1.9 mg/100 ml (124 and 168 μmol/l), the risk of exacerbation of renal dysfunction is significant. The risk of acceleration is even higher among those with an initial plasma creatinine concentration above 2.0 mg/100 ml (177 μmol/l) [227].

Patients with renal disease should be monitored jointly by a nephrologist and by an obstetrician familiar with the effects of renal disease on pregnancy. Monitoring should include increased frequency of prenatal visits; early detection and treatment. of asymptomatic bacteriuria; serial monitoring (at least monthly) of maternal renal function; close monitoring for the development of pre-eclampsia; fetal surveillance with ultrasound and fetal heart rate monitoring to assess fetal growth and well-being; and treatment of maternal hypertension (maintaining diastolic levels between 90 and 110 mmHg) [228].

Pregnancy may increase lupus disease activity but these flares are usually mild; for renal disease flares, corticosteroids are the drugs of choice. Prednisone, hydroxychloroquine, AZA, CsA, NSAIDs and aspirin may be used during pregnancy if needed to control manifestations of SLE (small risk of causing fetal harm). Their administration is permitted throughout pregnancy, in the usually prescribed dose. Methotrexate, MMF and CY are contra-indicated during pregnancy and lactation.

DRUG-INDUCED LUPUS ERYTHEMATOSUS AND LN

Drug-induced lupus erythematosus (DIL or DILE) is a rare adverse reaction to a large variety of drugs with features resembling those of idiopathic SLE. It usually develops only after months and, quite commonly, years of treatment with the offending agent, although latencies of days or weeks have been described in some instances [229]. There are some indications that the risk of DIL can increase with higher daily and cumulative doses and with longer duration of therapy.

Although as many as 100 drugs have been reported to cause DRL, most cases are related to procainamide, hydralazine, minocycline, and quinidine [230, 231]. It usually takes several months or even years of continuous therapy with the medication before symptoms appear. For the high-risk drugs such as procainamide and hydralazine, only 5-20 % of people treated for one to two years at currently used doses will develop drug-induced lupus. With most of the other drugs, the risk is less than 1 % that those taking the medication will develop DILE. Risk factors that have been linked to hydralazine-induced SLE are high daily doses, slow acetylator and HLA-DRw4 phenotypes, therapy longer than 3 months, female gender and a family history of autoimmune disease [232].

It seems that the pathophysiological mechanisms for the occurrence of DIL are unclear, it may be due to drug interaction with formation of reactive metabolites that directly affect lymphocyte function [230], the presence of autoreactive lymphocytes with subsequent antibody formation [233] or generation of toxic metabolites that may facilitate autoimmunity [234]. Usually, there is no renal involvement in DIL. However, hydralazine-induced DILE may be associated with glomerulonephritis in 5-10 % of affected patients [235]. Most people with drug-induced lupus develop antinuclear antibodies, or ANAs, although those with a form of drug-induced lupus related to quinidine often are ANA-negative. The ANAs in drug-induced lupus are primarily autoantibodies that are able to react with a histone-DNA complex, which is the major component of the nucleus of all cells Patients with DRL rarely have antibodies to double-stranded (ds) DNA, whereas in SLE, antibodies to ds-DNA are common [230].

Drug-induced lupus erythematosus is usually not as severe as SLE. Usually, the symptoms go away within a few days to weeks after stopping the medication. However, the complete disappearance of symptoms can sometimes take months, and the disappearance of abnormal autoantibodies may take a few years. Patients should avoid the medication in the future, or symptoms usually return [229].

Death from DILE is extremely rare and may result from renal involvement. In diagnosing DILE, first excluding the possibility of renal idiopathic lupus rather than DILE is extremely crucial [236].

SLE and DILE

There is no evidence that people with SLE are more likely to develop drug-induced lupus. The use of procainamide, hydralazine, isoniazid, or various anticonvulsants has not been associated with an increase in SLE disease activity or onset of flares. The major risk factor for developing drug-induced lupus is chronic, long-term use of a drug known to cause this problem. Usually DILE occurs in males over 50 years old, because they have a higher chance of developing chronic diseases that require this type of continuous medication: procainamide or quinidine is prescribed for cardiac arrhythmias, and hydralazine is prescribed for hypertension. The high female-to-male ratio associated with SLE is not a distinguishing feature of drug-induced lupus [230]. Usually, symptoms of DIL resolve within several days to weeks after stopping the medication that caused the condition [236]. In rare occasions, high doses of prednisolone and other immunosuppressive drugs are indicated to treat persons with severe drug-induced lupus that affects the heart, kidney, and neurological system [237].

ACKNOWLEGEMENT

The authors would like to express deep gratitude to professor Fatma Moustaf, professor of pathology for her permission to use all the Figures besides writing the nephropathology sector. All the Figures are belonging to her archive and also will be included in her Nephropathology Atlas (in processing).

REFERENCES

[1] Cervera, R., Khamashta, M. A., Font, J., et al (1993). Systemic lupus erythematosus: clinical and immunologic patterns of disease expression in a cohort of 1000 patients. *Medicine*, (Baltimore); *72*, 113-24.

[2] Klippel, J. H. (1990). Systemic lupus erythematosus. Treatment-related complications superimposed on chronic disease., *JAMA; 263*, 1812-5.

[3] MacGowan, J. R., Ellis, S., Griffiths, M. & Isenberg, D. A. (2002). *Retrospective analysis of outcome in a cohort of patients with lupus nephritis treated between*, 1977 and 1999. Rheumatology, *41*, 981-7.

[4] Ward, M. M. (2000). Changes in the incidence of end-stage renal disease due to lupus nephritis, 1982-1995. *Arch Intern Med*, *160*, 3136-40.

[5] Cheigh, J. S., Kim, H., Stenzel, K. H., et al. (1990). Systemic lupus erythematosus in patients with end-stage renal disease: long-term follow-up on the prognosis of patients at the evolution of lupus activity. *Am J Kidney Dis*, *16*, 189-195.

[6] Szeto, C., Li, P. K., Wong, T. Y., Leung, C. & Lui, S. (1998). Factors associated with active lupus erythematosus after end-stage renal disease. *J Rheum, 25*, 1520-5.

[7] Tang, S., Lui, S. L. & Lai, K. N. (2005). Pathogenesis of lupus nephritis: an update. *Nephrology*, (Carlton). 10(2), 174-9.

[8] Holborow, E. J., Weir, D. M. & Johnson, G. D. (1957). A serum factor in lupus erythematosus with affinity for tissue nuclei. *Br Med J, 13*, 732-4.

[9] Hahn, B. H. (1998). Antibodies to DNA. *N Engl J Med, 338*, 1359-68.

[10] Winfield, J. B., Faiferman, I. & Koffler, D. (1977). Avidity of anti-DNA antibodies in serum and IgG glomerular eluates from patients with systemic lupus erythematosus. Association of high avidity antinative DNA antibody with glomerulonephritis. *J Clin Invest, 59*, 90-96.

[11] Bootsma, H., Spronk, P., Derksen, R. et al (1995). Prevention of relapses in systemic lupus erythematosus. *Lancet, 345*, 1595-9.

[12] Diamond, B., Katz, J. B., Paul, E., et al (1992) The role of somatic mutation in the pathogenic anti-DNA response. *Annu Rev Immunol, 10*, 731-57.

[13] Fournie, G. J. (1988). Circulating DNA and lupus nephritis. *Kidney Int., 33*, 487-97.

[14] Rekvig, O. P., Kalaaji, M. & Nossent, H. (2004). Anti-DNA antibody subpopulations and lupus nephritis. *Autoimmun Rev, 3*, 1-6.

[15] Madaio, M. P., Fabbi, M., Tiso, M., Daga, A. & Puccetti, A. (1996). Spontaneously produced anti-DNA/DNase I autoantibodies modulate nuclear apoptosis in living cells. *Eur J Immunol, 26*, 3035-41.

[16] Hsieh, S. C., Sun, K. H., Tsai, C. Y. et al (2001). Monoclonal anti-double stranded DNA antibody is a leucocyte-binding protein to up-regulate interleukin-8 gene expression and elicit apoptosis of normal human polymorphonuclear neutrophils. *Rheumatology*, (Oxford), *40*, 851-8.

[17] Kubota, T., Watanabe, N., Kanai, Y. & Stollar, B. D. (1996). Enhancement of oxidative cleavage of DNA by the binding sites of two anti-double-stranded DNA antibodies. *J Biol Chem., 271*, 6555-61.

[18] Lai, K. N., Leung, J. C., Lai, K. B., Lai, F. M. & Wong, K. C. (1996). Increased release of von Willebrand factor antigen from endothelial cells by anti-DNA autoantibodies. *Ann Rheum Dis, 55*, 57-62.

[19] Lai, K. N., Leung, J. C., Lai, K. B., Wong, K. C. & Lai, C. K. (1996). Upregulation of adhesion molecule expression on endothelial cells by anti-DNA autoantibodies in systemic lupus erythematosus. *Clin Immunol Immunopathol, 81*, 229-38.

[20] Lai, K. N., Leung, J. C., Lai, K. B. & Lai, C. K. (1997). Effect of anti-DNA autoantibodies on the gene expression of interleukin 8, transforming growth factor-beta, and nitric oxide synthase in cultured endothelial cells. Scand. *J Rheumatol, 26*, 461-7.

[21] Lai, K. N., Leung, J. C., Lai, K. B., Li, P. K. & Lai, C. K. (1996). Anti-DNA autoantibodies stimulate the release of interleukin-1 and interleukin-6 from endothelial cells. *J. Pathol, 178*, 451-7.

[22] Sabry et al [Sabry A., sheashaa H., El-husseini A (2006). Proinflammatory cytokines (TNF-a and IL-6) in Egyptian patients with SLE: *Its correlation with disease activity*. *Cytokine, 35*, 148-153.

[23] Sabry, A., sheashaa, H. & El-husseini, A. (2007). Intercellular adhesion molecules in systemic lupus erythematosus patients with lupus nephritis. *Clin Rheumatol, Nov, 26(11)*, 1819-23.

[24] Amoura, Z., Piette, J. C., Bach, J. F. & Koutouzov, S. (1999). The key role of nucleosomes in lupus. *Arthritis Rheum*, *42*, 833-43.
[25] Berden, J. H. (1997). *Lupus nephritis. Kidney Int.*, *52*, 538-58.
[26] Berden, J. H., Licht, R., van Bruggen, M. C. & Tax, W. J. (1999). Role of nucleosomes for induction and glomerular binding of autoantibodies in lupus nephritis. *Curr Opin. Nephrol Hypertens*, *8*, 299-306.
[27] Tax, W. J., Kramers, C., van Bruggen, M. C. & Berden, J. H. (1995). Apoptosis, nucleosomes, and nephritis in systemic lupus erythematosus. *Kidney Int.*, *48*, 666-73.
[28] Mevorach, D., Zhou, J. L., Song, X. & Elkon, K. B. (1998). Systemic exposure to irradiated apoptotic cells induces autoantibody production. *J. Exp. Med.*, *188*, 387-92.
[29] van Bruggen, M. C., Kramers, C., Walgreen, B., (1997). et al. Nucleosomes and histones are present in glomerular deposits in human lupus nephritis. *Nephrol. Dial. Transplant. 12*, 57-66.
[30] Kamradt, T. & Mitchison, N. A. (2001). Tolerance and autoimmunity. *N. Engl. J. Med.*, *344*, 655-64.
[31] Nagata, S. & Golstein, P. (1995). *The Fas death factor. Science*, *267*, 1449-56.
[32] Hengartner, M. O. (2000). *The biochemistry of apoptosis. Nature*, *407*, 770-76.
[33] Reilly, C. M., Farrelly, L. W., Viti, D. (2002). et al. Modulation of renal disease in MRL/lpr mice by pharmacologic inhibition of inducible nitric oxide synthase. *Kidney Int. 61*, 839-46.
[34] Chan, T. M., Li, F. K., Tang, C. S. et al. (2000). Efficacy of mycophenolate mofetil in patients with diffuse proliferative lupus nephritis. Hong Kong- Guangzhou Nephrology Study Group. *N. Engl. J. Med.*, *343*, 1156-62.
[35] Yu, C. C., Yang, C. W., Wu, M. S. et al. (2001). Mycophenolate mofetil reduces renal cortical inducible nitric oxide synthase mRNA expression and diminishes glomerulosclerosis in MRL/lpr mice. *J. Lab. Clin. Med.*, *138*, 69-77.
[36] Lui, S. L., Tsang, R., Wong, D. et al. (2002). Effect of mycophenolate mofetil on severity of nephritis and nitric oxide production in lupus-prone MRL/lpr mice. *Lupus*, *11*, 411-18.
[37] Davidson, A., Aranow, C. (2006). Pathogenesis and treatment of systemic lupus erythematosus nephritis. *Curr Opin Rheumatol.*, Sep; *18(5)*, 468-75.
[38] Waldman, M. & Madaio, M. P. (2005). Pathogenic autoantibodies in lupus *nephritis. Lupus*, *14*, 19-24.
[39] Kashgarian., M. (1994). Lupus nephritis: *Lessons from the path lab. Kidney Int*, *45*, 928.
[40] Fries, J. W., Mendrick, D. L. & Rennke, H. G. (1988). Determinants of immune complex-mediated glomerulonephritis. *Kidney Int*, *34*, 333.
[41] Lefkowith, J. B. & Gilkeson, G. S. (1996). Nephritogenic autoantibodies in lupus. Current concepts and continuing controversies. *Arthritis Rheum*, *39*, 894.
[42] Vlahakos, D. V., Foster, M. H., Adams, S., et al. (1992). Anti-DNA antibodies form immune deposits at distinct glomerular and vascular sites. *Kidney Int*, *41*, 1690.
[43] D'Andrea, D. M., Coupaye-Gerard, B., Kleyman, T. R., et al. (1996). Lupus autoantibodies interact directly with distinct glomerular and vascular cell surface antigens. *Kidney Int*, *49*, 1214.
[44] Schur, P. H. (1987). IgG subclasses — A review. *Ann Allergy*, *58*, 89.

[45] Schur, P. H., Monroe, M. & Rothfield, N. (1972). The gammaG subclass of antinuclear and antinucleic acid antibodies. *Arthritis Rheum, 15*, 174.

[46] Lewis, E. J., Busch, G. J. & Schur, P. H. (1970). Gamma G globulin subgroup composition of the glomerular deposits in human renal diseases. *J Clin Invest, 49*, 1103.

[47] Dei, R., Marmo, F., Corte, D., et al (1982). Age-related changes in the prevalence of precipitating antibodies to BK virus in infants and children. *J Med Microbiol Aug, 15(3)*, 285-91.

[48] Taguchi, F., Hara, K. & Nagaki, D. (1978). BK papovavirus in urine of a patient with systemic lupus erythematosus. *Acta Virol.*, Nov; *22(6)*, 513.

[49] Van Ghelue, M., Moens, U., Bendiksen, S. & Rekvig, O. P. (2003). Autoimmunity to nucleosomes related to viral infection: a focus on hapten-carrier complex formation. *J Autoimmun, 20(2)*, 171-82.

[50] Andreassen, K., Bredholt, G., Moens, U., et al, (1999), T cell lines specific for polyomavirus T-antigen recognize T-antigen complexed with nucleosomes: a molecular basis for anti-DNA antibody production. *Eur J Immunol, 29*, 2715-2728.

[51] Flaegstad, T., Fredriksen, K., Dahl, B., et al, (1988). Inoculation with BK virus may break immunological tolerance to histone and DNA antigens. *Proc Natl Acad Sci U S A*; *85(21)*, 8171-5.

[52] Moens, U., Seternes, O. M., Hey, A. W., et al (1995). Johansen *et al.*, In vivo expression of a single viral DNA-binding protein generates systemic lupus erythematosus-related autoimmunity to double-stranded DNA and histones. *Proc Natl Acad Sci USA*; *92*, 12393-12397.

[53] Rekvig, O. P., Moens, U., Sundsfjord, A., Bredholt, G., Osei, A., et al, (1997). Experimental expression in mice and spontaneous expression in human SLE of polyomavirus T-antigen: a molecular basis for induction of antibodies to DNA and eukaryotic transcription factors. *J Clin Invest, 99*, 2045-2054.

[54] Fredriksen, K., Skogsholm, A., Flaegstad, T., et al (1993). Antibodies to dsDNA are produced during primary BK virus infection in man, indicating that anti-dsDNA antibodies may be related to virus replication in vivo. *Scand J Immuno., 38(4)*, 401-6.

[55] Sundsfjord, A., Osei, A., Rosenqvist, H., et al. (1999). BK and JC viruses in patients with systemic lupus erythematosus: prevalent and persistent BK viruria, sequence stability of the viral regulatory regions, and nondetectable viremia. *J Infect Dis, 180(1)*, 1-9.

[56] Arthur, R. R. & Shah, K. V. (1989). Occurrence and significance of papovaviruses BK and JC in the urine. *Prog Med Virol, 36*, 42-61.

[57] Bendiksen, S., Rekvig, O. P., Van Ghelue, M., et al (2000). VP1 DNA sequences of JC and BK viruses detected in urine of systemic lupus erythematosus patients reveal no differences from strains expressed in normal individuals. *J Gen Virol, 81(Pt 11)*, 2625-33.

[58] Colla, L., Mesiano, P., Morellini, V., et al. (2007). Human polyomavirus BK in patients with lupus nephritis: clinical and histological correlations. *Lupus, 16(11)*, 881-6.

[59] Chabre, H., Amoura, Z., Piette, J. C., et al. (1995) Presence of nucleosome-restricted antibodies in patients with SLE. *Arthritis Rheum, 38*, 1485.

[60] Hahn, B. H. (1998). Antibodies to DNA. *N Engl J Med, 338*, 1359-1368.

[61] Appel, G. B. & Cameron, J. S. (2007). *Lupus nephritis*. In: Johnson RJ., Feehaly J., Floege J., ed. *Comprehensive Clinical Nephrology*, 3rd ed. St. Louis: Mosby, 291-305.

[62] Weening, J. J., D'Agati, V. D., Schwartz, M. M., Seshan, S. V., et al. (2004). The classification of glomerulonephritis in systemic lupus erythematosus revisited. *J Am Soc Nephrol, 15(2)*, 241-50.
[63] Corwin, H. L., Schwartz, M. M. & Lewis, E (1988). The importance of sample size in the interpretation of the renal biopsy. *Am J Nephrol, 8*, 85-93.
[64] Austin, H. A., Muenz, L. R., Joyce, K. M., et al (1983). Prognostic factors in lupus nephritis: Contribution of renal histologic data. *Am J Med, 75*, 382.
[65] Balow, J. E. & Austin, H. A. (1988). Renal disease in systemic lupus erythematosus. *Rheum Dis Clin North Am, 14*, 117.
[66] Austin, H. A., Muenz, L. R., Joyce, K. M., et al. (1984). Diffuse proliferative lupus nephritis: Identification of specific pathologic features affecting renal outcome. *Kidney Int, 25*, 689.
[67] Martins, L., Rocha, G., Rodrigues, A., et al (2002). Lupus nephritis: a retrospective review of 78 cases from a single center. *Clin Nephrol, 57*, 114-119.
[68] Highson, M. D., Nadasdy, T., McCarty, G. A., Sholer, C., Min, K. W. & Silva, F. (1992). Renal thrombotic microangiopathy in patients with systemic lupus erythematosus and the antiphospholipid syndrome. *Am J Kidney Dis, 2*, 150-158.
[69] Schwartz, M. M., Kawala, K. S., Corwin, H. L. & Lewis, E. J. (1987). The prognosis of segmental glomerulonephritis in systemic lupus erythematosus. *Kidney Int, 32(2)*, 274-9.
[70] Appel, G. B., Cohen, D. J., Pirani, C. L., Meltzer, J. I. & Estes, D. (1987). Long-term follow-up of patients with lupus nephritis. A study based on the classification of the World Health Organization. *Am J Med Nov, 83(5)*, 877-85.
[71] Schwartz, M. M., Lan, S. P., Bonsib, S. M., Gephardt, G. N. & Sharma, H. M. (1989). Clinical outcome of three discrete histologic patterns of injury in severe lupus glomerulonephritis. *Am J Kidney Dis, 13(4)*, 273-83.
[72] Lloyd, W. & Schur, P. H. (1981) Immune complexes, complement, and anti-DNA in exacerbations of systemic lupus erythematosus (SLE). *Medicine (Baltimore), 60(3)*, 208-17.
[73] Jennette, J. C., Iskandar, S. S. & Dalldorf, F. G. (1983). Pathologic differentiation between lupus and nonlupus membranous glomerulopathy. *Kidney Int Sep, 24(3)*, 377-85.
[74] Baldwin, D. S., Gluck, M. C., Lowenstein, J. & Gallo, G. R. (1977). Lupus nephritis. Clinical course as related to morphologic forms and their transitions. *Am J Med, 62*, 12.
[75] Austin, H. A., III, Boumpas, D. T., Vaughan, E. M., et al. (1994). Predicting renal outcomes in severe lupus nephritis: Contributions of clinical and histologic data. *Kidney Int, 45*, 544-550.
[76] Cameron, J. S. (1999). Lupus nephritis. *J Am Soc Nephrol, 10*, 413 -24.
[77] Renal Disease Subcommittee Of The American College Of Rheumatology Ad Hoc Committee On Systemic Lupus Erythematosus Response Criteria (2006). The American College of Rheumatology response criteria for proliferative and membranous renal disease in systemic lupus erythematosus clinical trials. *Arthritis Rheum, 54*, 421-32.
[78] Gordon, C., Jayne, D., Pusey, C., et al. (2009). European consensus statement on the terminology used in the management of lupus glomerulonephritis. *Lupus, 18*, 257-263.

[79] Dooley, M. A., Hogan, S., Jennett, C., et al. (1997). Cyclophosphamide therapy for lupus nephritis: poor renal survival in black Americans. Glomerular Disease Collaborative Network. *Kidney Int*, *51*, 1188 -95.

[80] Tektonidou, M. G., Sotsiou, F., Nakopoulou, L., et al. (2004). Antiphospholipid syndrome nephropathy in patients with systemic lupus erythematosus and antiphospholipid antibodies: prevalence, clinical associations, and long-term outcome. *Arthritis Rheum*, *50*, 2569-79.

[81] Manger, K., Manger, B., Repp, R., et al. (2002). Definition of risk factors for death, end stage renal disease, and thromboembolic events in a monocentric cohort of 338 patients with systemic lupus erythematosus. *Ann Rheum Dis*, *61*, 1065 -70.

[82] Perysinaki, G., Panagiotakis, S., Bertsias, G. & Boumpas, D. T. (2008): Pharmacotherapy of lupus nephritis: time for a consensus? *Expert Opin Pharmacother*, *9(12)*, 2099-2115.

[83] Gordon, C., Jayne, D., Pusey, C., et al. (2009). European consensus statement on the terminology used in management of lupus glomerulonephritis. *Lupus*, *18*, 257-263.

[84] Ponticelli, C. (1990). Current treatment recommendations for lupus nephritis. *Drugs*, *40*, 19-30.

[85] Boumpas, D. T., Austin, III H. A., Vaughn, E. M., et al (1992). Controlled trial of pulse methylprednisolone versus two regimens of pulse cyclophosphamide in severe lupus nephritis. *Lancet*, *340*, 741-5.

[86] Illei, G. G., Austin, H. A. III., Crane, M., et al (2001). Combination therapy with pulse cyclophosphamide plus pulse methylprednisolone improves long-term renal outcome without adding toxicity in patients with lupus nephritis. *Ann Intern Med*, *135*, 248 -57.

[87] Grootscholten, C., Bajema, I. M., Florquin, S., et al (2007). Treatment with cyclophosphamide delays the progression of chronic lesions more effectively than does treatment with azathioprine plus methylprednisolone in patients with proliferative lupus nephritis. *Arthritis Rheum*, *56*, 924 -37.

[88] Austin, H. A. III., Klippel, J. H., Balow, J. E., et al. (1986). Therapy of lupus nephritis: controlled trial of prednisone and cytotoxic drugs. *N Engl J Med*, *314*, 614 -9.

[89] Donadio, J. V. Jr., Holley, K. E., Ferguson, R. H., et al. (1978). Treatment of diffuse proliferative lupus nephritis with prednisone and combined prednisone and cyclophosphamide. *N Engl J Med*, *299*, 1151 -5.

[90] Balow, J. E., Austin, H. A. III., Muenz, L. R., et al (1984). Effect of treatment on the evolution of renal abnormalities in lupus nephritis. *N Engl J Med*, *311*, 491-5.

[91] Chan, T. M., Tse, K. C., Tang, C. S., et al. (2005). Long-term outcome of patients with diffuse proliferative lupus nephritis treated with prednisolone and oral cyclophosphamide followed by azathioprine., *Lupus*, *14*, 265 -72.

[92] Houssiau, F. A., Vasconcelos, C., Cruz, D. D., et al. (2004). Early response to immunosuppressive therapy predicts good renal outcome in lupus nephritis: lessons from long-term follow up of patients in the *Euro-Lupus Nephritis Trial. Arthritis Rheum*, 50, 3934 -40.

[93] Houssiau, F. A., Vasconcelos, C., Cruz, D. D., et al. (2009). The 10-year follow-up data of the Euro-Lupus Nephritis Trial comparing low-dose *versus* high-dose intravenous cyclophosphamide *Ann Rheum Dis* published, 2009.

[94] Petri, M., Brodsky, R. (2006). High-dose cyclophosphamide and stem cell transplantation for refractory systemic lupus erythematosus., *Jama*, *295*, 559 -60.

[95] Austin, H., Vaughn, E. M., Balow, J. E., et al. (2004). Lupus membranous nephropathy: controlled trial of prednisone, pulse cyclophosphamide and cyclosporine [abstract]. AJ Am Soc Nephrol, 2004, 15, 54A

[96] Allison, A. C. & Eugui, E. M. (2000). Mycophenolate mofetil and its mechanisms of action. *Immunopharmacology, 47*, 85-118.

[97] Adu, D., Cross, J. & Jayne, D. R. (2001). Treatment of systemic lupus erythematosus with mycophenolate mofetil. *Lupus, 10*, 203-8.

[98] Moore, R. A. & Derry, S. (2006). Systematic review and meta-analysis of randomised trials and cohort studies of mycophenolate mofetil in lupus nephritis. *Arthritis Res Ther, 8*, R182.

[99] Walsh, M., James, M., Jayne, D., et al. (2007). Mycophenolate mofetil for induction therapy of lupus nephritis: a systematic review and meta-analysis. *Clin J Am Soc Nephrol, 2*, 968-75.

[100] Ginzler, E. M., Dooley, M. A., Aranow, C., et al. (2005). Mycophenolate mofetil or intravenous cyclophosphamide for lupus nephritis. *N Engl J Med, 353*, 2219-28.

[101] Ginzler, E. M., Appel, G. B., Dooley, M. A., et al. (2007). Mycophenolate mofetil and intravenous cyclophosphamide in the Aspreva Lupus Management Study (ALMS): efficacy by racial group. Arthritis American College of Rheumatology *Meeting, Boston, USA*; 6-11 November.

[102] Mok, C. C. (2006). Therapeutic options for resistant lupus nephritis. *Semin Arthritis Rheum, 36*, 71-81.

[103] Chan, T. M., Tse, K. C., Tang, C. S., Mok, M. Y. & Li, F. K. (2005). Hong Kong Nephrology Study Group. Long-term study of mycophenolate mofetil as continuous induction and maintenance treatment for diffuse proliferative lupus nephritis. *J Am Soc Nephrol, 16*, 1076-84.

[104] Contreras, G., Pardo, V., Leclercq, B., et al. (2004). Sequential therapies for proliferative lupus nephritis. *N Engl J Med, 350*, 971-80.

[105] Ostensen, M., Khamashta, M., Lockshin, M., et al. (2006). Anti-inflammatory and immunosuppressive drugs and reproduction. *Arthritis Res Ther, 8*, 209.

[106] Le Ray, C., Coulomb, A., Elefant, E., et al. (2004). Mycophenolate mofetil in pregnancy after renal transplantation: a case of major fetal malformations. *Obstet Gynecol, 103*, 1091-4.

[107] Vasoo, S., Thumboo, J. & Fong, K. Y. (2003). Refractory immune thrombocytopenia in systemic lupus erythematosus: response to mycophenolate mofetil. *Lupus, 12*, 630-2.

[108] Mak, A. & Mok, C. C. (2005). Mycophenolate mofetil for refractory haemolytic anemia in systemic lupus erythematosus. *Lupus, 14*, 856-8.

[109] Steinberg, A. D. & Steinberg, S. C. (1991). Long-term preservation of renal function in patients with lupus nephritis receiving treatment that includes cyclophosphamide versus those treated with prednisone alone. *Arthritis Rheum, 34*, 945-50.

[110] Grootscholten, C., Ligtenberg, G., Hagen, E. C., etal. (2006). Azathioprine/methylprednisolone versus cyclophosphamide in proliferative lupus nephritis. A randomized controlled trial. *Kidney Int, 70*, 732-42.

[111] Houssiau, F. A., Vasconcelos, C., Cruz, D. D., et al. (2002). Immunosuppressive therapy in lupus nephritis: the Euro-Lupus Nephritis Trial, a randomized trial of low-dose versus high-dose intravenous cyclophosphamide. *Arthritis Rheum, 46*, 2121-31.

[112] Caccavo, D., Lagana, B., Miiterhofer, A. P., et al. (1997). Long-term treatment of systemic lupus erythematosus with cyclosporin A. *Arthritis Rheum*, *40*, 27-35.

[113] Ogawa, H., Kameda, H., Nagasawa, H., et al. (2007). Prospective study of low-dose cyclosporine A in patients with refractory lupus nephritis. *Mod Rheumatol*, *17*, 92-7.

[114] Hu, W., Liu, Z., Shen, S., et al. (2003). Cyclosporine A in treatment of membranous lupus nephropathy. *Chin Med J.* (England), *116*, 1827-30.

[115] Moroni, G., Doria, A., Mosca, M., et al. (2006). A randomized pilot trial comparing cyclosporine and azathioprine for maintenance therapy in diffuse lupus nephritis over four years. *Clin J Am Soc Nephrol*, *1*, 925 -32.

[116] Maruyama, M., Yamasaki, Y., Sada, K., et al. (2006). Good response of membranous lupus nephritis to tacrolimus. *Clin Nephrol*, *65*, 276 -9.

[117] Mok, C. C., Tong, K. H., To, C. H., et al. (2005). Tacrolimus for induction therapy of diffuse proliferative lupus nephritis: an open-labeled pilot study. *Kidney Int*, *68*, 813-7.

[118] Euler, H. H., Schroeder, J. O., Harten, P., et al. (1994). Treatment-free remission in severe systemic lupus erythematosus following synchronization of plasmapheresis with subsequent pulse cyclophosphamide. *Arthritis Rheum*, *37*, 1784.

[119] Lewis, E. J., Hunsicker, L. G., Lan, S. P., et al. (1992). A controlled trial of plasmapheresis therapy in severe lupus nephritis. The Lupus Nephritis Collaborative Study Group. *N Engl J Med*, *326*, 1373.

[120] Smith, J. W. & Weinstein, R. Hillyer (2003). Therapeutic apheresis: a summary of current indication categories endorsed by the AABB and the American Society for Apheresis. *Transfusion*, *43*, 820.

[121] Sisó, A., Ramos-Casals, M., Bové, A., et al. (2008). Previous antimalarial therapy in patients diagnosed with lupus nephritis: influence on outcomes and survival. *Lupus*, *17*, 281-288.

[122] Kasitanon, N., Fine, D. M., Haas, M., Magder, L. S. & Petri, M. (2006). Hydroxychloroquine use predicts complete renal remission within 12 months among patients treated with mycophenolate mofetil therapy for membranous lupus nephritis. *Lupus*, *15*, 366-370.

[123] Voulgarelis, M., Kokori, SIG., Ioannidis, J. P. A., et al. (2000). Anaemia in systemic lupus erythematosus: aetiological profile and the role of erythropoietin. *Ann Rheum Dis*, *59*, 217 -22.

[124] Schett, G., Fibras, U., Fureder, W., et al. (2001). Decreased serum erythropoietin and its relation to anti-erythropoetin antibodies in anaemia of systemic lupus erythematosus. *Rheumatology*, (Oxford), *40*, 424 -31.

[125] Kiss, E., Kávai, M., Csipõ, I., et al. (1998). Recombinant human erythropoietin modulates erythrocyte complement receptor 1 functional activity in patients with lupus nephritis. *Clin Nephrol*, *49*, 364 -9.

[126] Zandman-Goddard, G., Shoenfeld, Y. (2005). Infections and SLE. *Autoimmunity*, *38*, 473-485

[127] Leandro, M. J., Cambridge, G., Edwards, J. C., et al. (2005). B-cell depletion in the treatment of patients with systemic lupus erythematosus: a longitudinal analysis of 24 patients. *Rheumatology*, *44*, 1542-5.

[128] Looney, R. J., Anolik, J. H., Campbell, D. et al. (2004). B cell depletion as a novel treatment for systemic lupus erythematosus: a phase I/II dose-escalation trial of rituximab. *Arthritis Rheum*, *50*, 2580-9.

[129] Vigna-Perez, M., Hernandez-Castro, B., Paredes-Saharopulos, O., et al. (2006). Clinical and immunological effects of rituximab in patients with lupus nephritis refractory to conventional therapy: a pilot study. *Arthritis Res Ther*, *8*, R83.
[130] Sfikakis, P. P., Boletis, J. N., Lionaki, S. et al (2005). Remission of proliferative lupus nephritis following B cell depletion therapy is preceded by down-regulation of the T cell costimulatory molecule CD40 ligand. *Arthritis Rheum*, *52*, 501-13.
[131] Genentech and Biogen Idec. (2008). http://www.gene.com/gene/news/press-releases/dis (19 December, date last accessed).
[132] Calabrese, L. H., Molloy, E. S., Huang, D. & Ransohoff, R. M. (2007). Progressive multifocal leukoencephalopathy in rheumatic diseases: evolving clinical and pathologic patterns of disease. *Arthritis Rheum*, *56*, 2116-28.
[133] Wallace, D. J. & Tumlin, J. A. (2004). LJP 394 (abetimus sodium, Riquent) *in the management of systemic lupus erythematosus.*, Lupus, *13*, 323-27.
[134] Alarcon-Segovia, D., Tumlin, J. A., Furie, R. A. et al. (2003). LJP 394 for the prevention of renal flare in patients with systemic lupus erythematosus: results from a randomized, double-blind, placebo-controlled study. *Arthritis Rheum*, *48*, 442-54.
[135] Huang, W., Sinha, J., Newman, J., et al. (2002). The effect of anti-CD40 ligand antibody on B cells in human systemic lupus erythematosus. *Arthritis Rheum*, *46*, 1554-62.
[136] Boumpas, D. T., Furie, R., Manzi, S., et al. (2003). A short course of BG9588 (anti-CD40 ligand antibody) improves serologic activity and decreases hematuria in patients with proliferative lupus glomerulonephritis. *Arthritis Rheum*, *48*, 719-27.
[137] Boletis, J. N., Ioannidis, J. P., Boki, K. A., et al. (1999). Intravenous immunoglobulin compared with cyclophosphamide for proliferative lupus nephritis. Lancet, *354*, 569-70.
[138] Levy Y., Sherer Y., George J et al (2000). Intravenous immunoglobulin treatment of lupus nephritis. Semin *Arthritis Rheum*, *29*, 321-7.
[139] Orbach, H., Tishler, M. & Shoenfeld, Y. (2004). Intravenous immunoglobulin and the kidney— a two-edged sword. *Semin Arthritis Rheum*, *34*, 593-601.
[140] Levy, Y., Sherer, Y., Ahmed, A., et al. (1999). A study of 20 SLE patients with intravenous immunoglobulin—clinical and serologic response. *Lupus*, *8*, 705-12.
[141] Jayne, D., Passweg, J., Marmont, A., et al. (2004). Autologous stem cell transplantation for systemic lupus erythematosus. *Lupus*, *13*, 168-76.
[142] Lisukov, I. A., Sizikova, S. A., Kulagin, A. D., et al. (2004). High-dose immunosuppression with autologous stem cell transplantation in severe refractory systemic lupus erythematosus. *Lupus*, *13*, 89-94.
[143] Traynor, A. E., Barr, W. G., Rosa, R. M., et al. (2002). Hematopoietic stem cell transplantation for severe and refractory lupus. Analysis after five years and fifteen patients. *Arthritis Rheum*, *46*, 2917-23.
[144] Jayne, D., Passweg, J., Marmont, A., et al. (2004). Autologous stem cell transplantation for systemic lupus erythematosus. *Lupus*, *13*, 168-76.
[145] Burt, R. K., Traynor, A., Statkute, L., et al. (2006). Non myeloablative hematopoietic stem cell transplantation for systemic lupus erythematosus. *J Am Med Assoc*, *295*, 527-35.
[146] Mok, C. C., *et al.* (2004). Treatment of pure membranous lupus nephropathy with prednisone and azathioprine: an open-label trial. *Am J Kidney Dis, 43*, 269-276.

[147] Moroni, G. et al. (1998). Treatment of membranous lupus nephritis. *Am J Kidney Dis 31*, 681-686.

[148] Spetie, D. N., et al. (2004). Mycophenolate therapy of SLE membranous nephropathy. *Kidney Int, 66*, 2411-2415.

[149] Austin, H. A., Illei, G. G., Braun, M. J. & Balow, J. E. (2009). Randomized, controlled trial of prednisone, cyclophosphamide, and cyclosporine in lupus membranous nephropathy. *J Am Soc Nephrol, 20*, 901-911.

[150] Tse, K. C., Lam, M. F., Tang, S. C., et al. (2007). A pilot study on tacrolimus treatment in membranous or quiescent lupus nephritis with proteinuria resistant to angiotensin inhibition or blockade. *Lupus,* 16, 46-51.

[151] schieppati, A., ruggenenti, P., Perna, A., et al. (2003). Nonimmunosuppressive therapy of membranous nephropathy. *Semin. Nephrol., 23*, 333-339.

[152] Lee, T. M., su, S. F. & Tsai, C. H. (2002). effect of pravastatin on proteinuria in patients with well controlled hypertension. *Hypertension, 40*, 67-73

[153] Stone, J. H. (1998). End-stage renal disease in lupus: disease activity, dialysis, and the outcome of transplantation. *Lupus, 7*, 654-9.

[154] Okano, K., Yumura, W., Nitta, K. et al. (2001). Analysis of lupus activity in end-stage renal disease treated by hemodialysis. *Intern Med*, 2001, *40*, 598-602.

[155] Fries, J. F., Powers, R. & Kempson, R. (1974). Late stage lupus nephropathy. *J Rheum, 1*, 166-75.

[156] Nossent, H. C., Swaak, T. J. G. & Berden, J. M. (1990). Systemic lupus erythematosus: analysis of disease activity in 55 patients with end-stage renal failure treated with hemodialysis or continuous ambulatory peritoneal dialysis. *Am J Med, 89*, 169-74.

[157] Shafi, S. T. & Gupta, M. (2007). Risk of vascular access thrombosis in patients with systemic lupus erythematosus on hemodialysis. *J Vasc Access, 8*, 103-108.

[158] Coplon, N. S., Diskin, C. J., Petersen, J. & Swenson, R. S. (1983). The long-term clinical course of systemic lupus erythematosus in end-stage renal disease. *N Engl J Med, 308*, 186-90.

[159] Cheigh, J. S. & Stenzel, K. H. (1993). End-stage renal disease in systemic lupus erythematosus. *Am J Kidney Dis*, *21*, 2-8.

[160] Roth, D. et al (1987). Renal transplantation in systemic lupus erythematosus: one center's experience. *Am J Nephrol, 7*, 367-374.

[161] Kimberly, R. (1983). Reversible `end-stage' lupus nephritis: analysis of patients able to discontinue dialysis. *Am J Med, 74*, 361- 368.

[162] Esdaile, J. (1996). Laboratory tests as predictors of disease exacerbations in systemic lupus erythematosus: why some tests fail. *Arthritis Rheum, 39*, 370-378.

[163] Howard, P., Bias, W., Arnett, F. & McLean, R. (1986). Relationship between C4 null genes, HLA-D region antigens, and genetic susceptibility to systemic lupus erythematosus in Caucasian and Black Americans. *Am J Med, 81*, 187- 193.

[164] Mange, K. C., Joffe, M. M. & Feldman, H. I. (2001). The effect of the use or nonuse of long-term dialysis on the subsequent survival of renal transplants from living donors. *N Eng J Med, 344*, 726-731.

[165] Mange, K. C., Joffe, M. M. & Feldman, H. I. (2003). Dialysis prior to living donor kidney transplantation and rates of acute rejection. *Nephrol Dial Transplant, 18*, 172-177.

[166] Moroni, G., La Marchesina, U., Banfi, G., et al. (1995). Cardiologic abnormalities in patients with long-term lupus nephritis. *Clin Nephrol, 43*, 20-28.
[167] Brey, R. L., Stallworth, C. L. & McGlasson, D. L. et al (2002). Antiphospholipid and stroke in young women. *Stroke, 33*, 2396-2401.
[168] Altieri, P., Sau, G., Cao, R., et al. (2002). Immunosuppressive treatment in dialysis patients. Nephrol Dial Transplant, 17 (suppl. 8), S2-S9.
[169] Bartosh, S. M., Fine, R. N. & Sullivan, E. K. (2001). Outcome after transplantation of young patients with systemic lupus erythematosus: a report of the North American pediatric renal transplant cooperative study. *Transplantation, 72*, 973-978.
[170] Bernatsky, S., Clarke, A. & Ramsey-Goldman, R. (2002). Malignancy and systemic lupus erythematosus. *Curr Rheumatol Rep, 4*, 351-358.
[171] Kasiske, B. L., Vazquez, M. A., Harmon, W. E., et al. (2000). Recommendations for the outpatient surveillance of renal transplant recipients. American Society of Transplantation. *J Am Soc Nephrol, 11*, (suppl. 15), S1-S8.
[172] Berthoux, F., Abramowicz, D., Bradley, B., et al. (2000). European best practice guidelines for renal transplantation. *Nephrol Dial Transplant, 15*, (suppl. 7): 1-85.
[173] Moroni, G., Ventura, D., Riva, P., et al. (2004). Antiphospholipid antibodies are associated with an increased risk for chronic renal insufficiency in patients with lupus nephritis. *Am J Kidney Dis, 43*, 28-36.
[174] Stone, J. H., Millward, C. L., Olson, J. L., et al. (1998). Frequency of recurrent lupus nephritis among ninety-seven renal transplant patients during the cyclosporine era. *Arthritis Rheum, 41*, 678-686.
[175] Bunnapradist, S., Chung, P., Peng, A., et al. (2006). Outcomes of renal transplantation for recipients with lupus nephritis: analysis of the organ procurement and transplantation network database. *Transplantation, 82*, 612-618.
[176] Rietveld, A. & Berden, Jo H. M. (2008). Renal replacement therapy in lupus nephritis. *Nephrol Dial Transplant, 23*, 3056-3060.
[177] Osman, C. & Swaak, A. (1994). Lymphocytotoxic antibodies in SLE: a review of the literature. *Clin Rheumatol, 13*, 21-27.
[178] Moroni, G., Tantardini, F. & Ponticelli, C. (2003). Renal replacement therapy in lupus nephritis. *J Nephrol, 16*, 787-791.
[179] Wolfe, R. A., Ashby, V. B., Milford, E. L., et al. (1999). Comparison of mortality in all patients on dialysis., patients on dialysis awaiting transplantation and recipients of a first cadaveric transplant. *N Engl J Med, 341*, 1725-1730.
[180] Grimbert, P., Frappier, J., Bedrossian, J., et al. (1998). Long-term outcome of kidney transplantation in patients with systemic lupus erythematosus: a multicenter study. Groupe Cooperatif de Transplantation d'Ile de France. *Transplantation, 66*, 1000-1003.
[181] Deegens, J. K., Artz, M. A., Hoijtsma, A. J., et al. (2003). Outcome of renal transplantation in patients with systemic lupus erythematosus. *Transplant Int, 16*, 411-418.
[182] Goral, S., Ynares, C., Shappell, S. B. et al (2003). Recurrent lupus nephritis in renal transplant recipients revisited: it is not rare. *Transplantation, 75*, 651-656.
[183] Ahuya, T. S., Boughton, J., Weiss, V., et al. (2001). Late recurrence of lupus nephritis in a renal transplant recipient: response to mycophenolate mofetil. *Am J Med Sci, 322*, 166-169.

[184] Isaac, I. & Shihab, F. S. (2002). Recurrent lupus nephritis in the second allograft of a patient with systemic lupus erythematosus. *Nephron, 92*, 947-949.

[185] Leuven, S. I van., Kastelein, J. J. P., Allison, A. C., et al. (2006). Mycophenolate mofetil (MMF): firing at the atherosclerotic plaque from different angles? *Cardiovasc Res, 69*, 341-347.

[186] Zandman-Goddard, G. & Shoenfeld, Y. (2003). SLE and infections. *Clin Rev Allergy Immunol, 25*, 29-40.

[187] Magee, J. C., Leichtman, A. B. & Merion, R. M. (1998). Renal transplantation for systemic lupus erythematosus: excellent long-term results with both living and cadaveric donors. *Transplant Proc, 30*, 1798-1799.

[188] Ponticelli, C. & Moroni, G. (2005). Renal transplantation in lupus nephritis. *Lupus, 14*, 95-8.

[189] Nossent, H. C., Swaak, T. J. & Berden, J. H. (1991). For the Dutch Working Party on Systemic Lupus Erythematosus. Systemic lupus erythematosus after renal transplantation: patient and graft survival and disease activity. *Ann Int Med, 114*, 183-188.

[190] Ward, M. M. (2000). Outcomes of renal transplantation among patients with end-stage disease caused by lupus nephritis. *Kidney Int, 57*, 2136-2143.

[191] Chelamcharla, M., Javaid, B., Baird, B., et al. (2007). The outcome of renal transplantation among systemic lupus erythematosus patients. *Nephrol Dial Transplant, 22*, 3623-3630.

[192] Bumgardner, G. L., Mauer, S. M., Payne, W., et al. (1988). Single-center 1-15 year results of renal transplantation in patients with systemic lupus erythematosus. *Transplantation, 46*, 703-709.

[193] Bogdanovic, R., Nikolic, V., Pasic, S., et al. (2004) Lupus nephritis in childhood: a review of 53 patients followed at a single center. *Pediatr Nephrol, 19*, 36-44.

[194] Font, J., Cervera, R., Espinosa, G., et al. (1998) . Systemic lupus erythematosus (SLE) in childhood: analysis of clinical and immunological findings in 34 patients and comparison with SLE characteristics in adults. *Ann Rheum Dis, 57*, 456-9.

[195] Perfumo, F. & Martini, A. (2005). Lupus nephritis in children. *Lupus, 14*, 83-88.

[196] Cameron, J. S. (1994). Lupus nephritis in childhood and adolescence, *Pediatr Nephrol, 8(2)*, 230-249.

[197] Bakkaloglu, A. (2001). Lupus nephropathy in children. *Nephrol Dial Transplant, 16,* (Suppl 6), 126-28.

[198] Sorof, J. M., Perez, M. D., Brewer, E. D., et al. (1998). Increasing incidence of childhood class V lupus nephritis. *J Rheumatol, 25*, 1413-18.

[199] Marks, S. D., Sebire, N. J., Pilkington, C. & Tullus, K. (2007). Clinicopathological correlations of pediatric lupus nephritis. *Pediatr Nephrol, 22(1)*, 77-83.

[200] Zappitelli, M., Duffy, C., Bernard, C., et al. (2004). Clinicopathological study of the WHO classification in childhood lupus nephritis. *Pediatr Nephrol, 19*, 503-10.

[201] Sumboonnanonda, A., Suntornpoch, V., Parichatikanond, P., et al. (1998). Renal pathology and long-term outcome in childhood SLE. *J Med Assoc Thai, 81*, 830-34.

[202] Rush, P. J., Baumal, R., Shore, A., et al. (1986). Correlation of renal histology with outcome in children with lupus nephritis. *Kidney Int, 29*, 1066-71.

[203] McCurdy, D. K., Lehman, T. J. A., Bernstein, B., et al. (1992). Lupus nephritis: prognostic factors in children. *Pediatrics, 89*, 240-46.

[204] Macdermott, E. J., Adams, A. & Lehman, T. J. A. (2007) Systemic lupus erythematosus in children: current and emerging therapies. *Lupus, 16,* 677-683.
[205] Lee, H. S., Mujais, S. K., Kasinath, B. S., Spargo, B. H. & Katz, A. I. (1984) Course of renal pathology in patients with systemic lupus erythematosus. *Am J Med, 77(4),* 612-620.
[206] Wallace, D. J., Metzger, A. L.,Stecher, V. J., Turnbull, B. A. & Kern, P. A. (1990). Cholesterol-lowering effect of hydroxychloroqine in patients with rheumatic disease: reversal of deleterious effects of steroids on lipids. *Am J Med, 89,* 322-326.
[207] Hodis, H. N., Quismorio, F. P. Jr., Wickham, E. & Blankenhorn, D. H. (1993). The lipid, lipoprotein and apolipoprotein effects of Hydroxychloroquine in patients with systemic lupus erythematosus. *J Rheumatol, 20,* 661-665.
[208] Adams, A., MacDermott, E. J., Lehman, T. J. A. (2006) Pharmacotherapy of lupus nephritis in children. *Drugs, 66(9),* 1191-1207.
[209] Grootscholten, C. & Berden, J. H. (2006). Discontinuation of immunosuppression in proliferative lupus nephritis: is it possible? *Nephrol Dial Transplant, 21(6),* 1465-1469.
[210] Tucker, L. R., Menon, S., Schaller, J. G., et al. (1995). Adult and childhood onset systemic lupus erythematosus: a comparison of onset, clinical features, serology and outcome. *Br J Rheumatol, 34,* 866-72.
[211] Al Salloum, A. A. (2003). Cyclophosphamide therapy for lupus nephritis: poor renal survival in Arab children. *Pediatr Nephrol, 18,* 357-361.
[212] Niaudet, P. (2000). Treatment of lupus nephritis. *Pediatr Nephrol, 14,* 158-166.
[213] Donadio, J. V. Jr., Holley, K. E., Wagnoer, R. D., Ferguson, R. H., McDuffie, F. C. (1974). Further observations on the treatment of lupus nephritis with prednisone and combined prednisone and azathioprine. *Arthritis Rheum, 17,* 573-581.
[214] Filler, G., Hansen, M., LeBlance, C., Lepage, N., Franke, D., Mai, I., et al. (2003). Pharmacokinetice of mycophenolate mofetil for autoimmune disease in children. *Pediatr Nephrol, 18,* 445-449.
[215] Buratti, S., Szer, I. S., Spencer, C. H., Bartosh, S. & Reiff, A. (2001). Mycophenolate Mofetil treatment of severe renal disease in pediatric onset systemic lupus erythematosus. *J Rheumatol, 28,* 2103-2108.
[216] Fu, Y. F. & Liu, G. L. (2001). Mycophenolate mofetil therapy for children with lupus nephritis refractory to both intravenous cyclosphamide and cyclosporine. *Clin Nephrol, 55,* 318-321.
[217] Adams, A., MacDermott, E. J. & Lehman, T. J. A. (2006) Pharmacotherapy of lupus nephritis in children. *Drugs, 66(9),* 1191-1207.
[218] Lehman, T. J., Edelheit, B. S. & Onel, K. B. (2004). Combined intravenous methotrexate and Cyclophosphamide for refractory childhood lipus nephritis. *Ann Rheum Dis, 63,* 321-323.
[219] Marks, S. D., Patey, S., Brogan, P. A., et al. (2005). B lymphocyte depletion therapy in children with refractory systemic lupus erythematosus. *Arthritis Rheum, 52(10),* 3168-3174.
[220] Bakr, A. (2005). Epidemiology treatment and outcome of children systemic lupus erythematosus in Egypt. *Pediatr Nephrol, 20,* 1081-1086.
[221] Perfumo, F. & Martini, A. (2005). Lupus nephritis in children. Lupus *14,* 83-88. Sorof JM., Perez MD., Brewer ED., et al. (1998) Increasing incidence of childhood class V lupus nephritis. *J Rheumatol, 25,* 1413-18.

[222] Lee, B. S., Cho, H. Y., Kim, E. J., et al. (2007). Clinical outcomes of childhood lupus nephritis: a single center's experience. *Pediatr Nephrol, 22*, 222-231.

[223] Wang, L. C., Yang, Y. H., Lu, M. Y., Chiang, B. L. (2004). Retrospective analysis of the renal outcome of pediatric lupus. *Clin Rheumatol, 23*, 318-323.

[224] Hagelberg, S., Lee, Y., Bargman, J. et al. (2002). Longterm followup of childhood lupus nephritis. *J Rheumatol, 29*, 2635-2642.

[225] Pattaragarn, A., Sumboonnanonda, A., Parichatikanond, P. et al. (2005). Systemic lupus erythematosus in Thai children: clinicopathologic findings and outcome in 82 patients. J Med Assoc Thai 88 *Suppl, 8*, S232-241.

[226] Niudat, P. & Salmon, R. (2009). Lupus nephritis in Pediatric Nephrology (Sixth edition) Ellis D. Avner., William E. Harmon, Patrick Niaudet, Norishige Yoshikawa (Eds.) Springer-Verlag *Berlin Heidelberg*, 1123-1153.

[227] Jones, D. C. & Hayslett, J. C. (1996). Outcome of pregnancy in women with moderate or severe renal insuffi ciency. *N Engl J Med, 335*, 226 -32.

[228] Chobanian, A. V., Bakris, G. L., Black, H. R., et al. (2003). Seventh Report of the Joint National Committee on prevention, detection, evaluation, and treatment of high blood pressure. *Hypertension, 42*, 1206 -52.

[229] Borchers, A. T., Keen, C. L. & Gershwin, M. E. (2007). Drug-induced lupus. *Ann N Y Acad Sci*, 1108, 166-82.

[230] Antonov, D., Kazandjieva, J., Etugov, D., et al. (2004). Drug-induced lupus erythematosus. *Clin Dermatol, 22(2)*, 157-66.

[231] Bannwarth, B. (2007). Drug-induced musculoskeletal disorders. *Drug Saf., 30(1)*, 27-46

[232] Finks, S. W., Finks, A. L. & Self, T. H. (2006). Hydralazine-induced lupus; Maintaining vigilance with increased use in patients with heart failure. *South Med J, 99*, 18-22.

[233] Yung, R., Powers., D., Johnson, K., et al (1996). Mechanism of drug-induced lupus II. T cells overexpressing lymphocyte function-associated antigen 1 become autoreactive and induce a lupus like disease in syngeneic mice. *J Clin Invest, 97*, 2866-71.

[234] Berning, S. E. & Iseman, M. D. (1997). Rifamycin-induced lupus syndrome. *Lancet.* May, 24, *349(9064)*, 1521-2.

[235] Shapiro, K. S., Pinn, V. W., Harrington, J. T., et al. (1984). Immune complex glomerulonephritis in hydralazine-induced SLE. *Am J Kidney Dis, 3,* 270.

[236] Dedeoglu, F. (2009). Drug-induced autoimmunity. *Curr Opin Rheumatol, 21(5)*, 547-51.

[237] Uz, E., Bavbek, N., Turgut, F. H., et al. (2007). Cefuroxime-induced lupus. *J Natl Med Assoc, 99(9)*, 1066-7.

In: Autoimmune Diseases: Symptoms, Diagnosis and Treatment   ISBN: 978-1-61668-007-7
Editor: Kyle J. Brenner, pp. 167-208   © 2010 Nova Science Publishers, Inc.

Chapter 3

FROM IMMUNOBIOLOGY TO GENETICS: IN SEARCH OF A CURE FOR AUTOIMMUNITY

Sylvie Lesage[1*], Erin E. Hillhouse[1], Véronique Dugas[1], Geneviève Chabot-Roy[2], Adam-Nicolas Pelletier[1], Marie Vilquin[3] and Fanny Guimont-Desrochers[1]

[1]University of Montreal, Department of Microbiology and Immunology, Montreal, Quebec, Canada, Maisonneuve-Rosemont Hospital Research Center, Cellular Immunogenetics Unit, Montreal, Quebec, Canada
[2]Maisonneuve-Rosemont Hospital Research Center, Cellular Immunogenetics Unit, Montreal, Quebec, Canada
[3]Maisonneuve-Rosemont Hospital Research Center, Cellular Immunogenetics Unit, Montreal, Quebec, Canada, Lille University of Sciences and Technologies, Villeneuve d'Ascq, France

ABSTRACT

The Human Genome Project has facilitated the identification of various genetic regions associated with disease susceptibility. This identification step is important as it yields clues into the pathways implicated in defining disease susceptibility and may uncover important therapeutic targets. Indeed, by performing genome-wide scans, one can identify many genetic loci associated with autoimmune disease susceptibility. However, the odds ratio of each locus is relatively low. Therefore, the limitation of these studies is in the biological translation of the data. This raises the question of how one validates the contribution of all of these genetic variations to human disease.

An alternative strategy for the identification of various genetic regions associated with disease susceptibility is to compare genetically resistant and susceptible individuals for biological variations. The subsequent challenge is then to demonstrate that the biological variations are causal to disease. For instance, autoimmune diseases are thought

---

[*] Corresponding author: Maisonneuve-Rosemont Hospital, Research Center, 5415, boul de l'Assomption, Montréal, Québec, CANADA

to arise as a consequence of disturbances in self-tolerance. Herein, the various mechanisms of self-tolerance, with particular emphasis on the defects potentially contributing to the onset of autoimmune diabetes, will be described. Specifically, this chapter will focus on the contribution of the acquired immune system and the innate immune system, including T and B cell tolerance, dendritic cells, macrophages and NK cells, as well as the potential interplay between these distinct phenotypes in defining the genetic predisposition to autoimmune diseases.

INTRODUCTION

Various biological processes collectively make up the immune system, which protects us from disease through the recognition and killing of foreign agents and tumor cells. However, during abnormal circumstances, the immune system mounts a hyperactive immune response against the organism's own healthy cells and tissues resulting in inflammation and tissue damage, which leads to an autoimmune disease. An autoimmune response can be specific for a particular cell type, such as pancreatic β cells in type 1 diabetes (T1D) or oligodendrocytes in multiple sclerosis (MS), but it can also target a broader range of cell types and tissues, such as nuclear antigens in systemic lupus erythematosus (SLE). Extended research throughout the years has established that both environmental and genetic factors play a role in the development of autoimmune diseases. Moreover, most autoimmune diseases are defined as complex genetic traits, since the susceptibility to disease involves a multitude of low risk factor genes.

This chapter will describe the technical advances in genetic studies, which have resulted in the identification of genetic regions associated with disease susceptibility. First, we will present an overview of the execution of genetic studies as well as the advantages and disadvantages of using the genome-wide association study approach, a novel technology allowing the rapid identification of genetic loci associated with disease susecptibility. Next, we will present the current understanding of the immune system and its role in preventing autoimmune disease development and progression. Lastly, we will also describe various defects in immune tolerance mechanisms as well as linkage analyses of these phenotypes and their contribution to autoimmune disease susceptibility.

DETERMINING GENETIC SUSCEPTIBILITY

Mouse models have been most useful in delineating the genetic factors involved in defining susceptibility to complex traits. Indeed, mice share approximately 99% of their genome with humans. Moreover, with a century of mouse genetics [1], we now have hundreds of inbred and mutant mouse strains, which have deficiencies ranging from different stages of embryology to adulthood to a vast array of biological systems, such as the immune system, the endocrine tissues as well as the neurons. Having these various mouse strains, as well as a dense genetic map at our disposal, has facilitated the study of the mammalian biological system and its relevance to human conditions. A key advantage of using a live animal model is the full accessibility to affected tissue throughout progression of disease as well as prior to onset of clinical symptoms; an accomplishment which cannot be achieved in humans.

Because of the various benefits involved, classical genetic approaches have relied on the comparison of inbred strains to identify genetic loci associated with disease. More recently, two methods of experimentation have dominated the study of mammalian biology: reverse and forward genetics. While reverse genetics aims to define the biological function of a known gene, forward genetics describes the genes associated with a biological phenotype or function. A variety of different molecular genetic approaches can be used for either strategy. Common techniques used for reverse genetics include the use of various mouse strains to study the function of the gene in the context of a whole animal model. In particular, these include transgenic, knockout, knockdown and congenic mouse strains as well as inducible gene expression mouse models [2]. Similar strategies are applied to cell lines in order to determine the cell specific effect of eliminating or over-expressing a specific gene. Alternatively, forward genetic approaches have been extensively used in Drosophila and have been more recently applied to the mammalian system [3-5]. Indeed, mutagen-induced point mutations which are randomly distributed throughout the genome have allowed the identification of many intracellular signalling components associated with specific phenotypes [3-5]. Therefore, both reverse and forward genetics have their independent merits, where one determines the function of a defined gene while the other uncovers the genetic description of a given phenotype. Yet, neither of these approaches efficiently identifies the genetic susceptibility of complex traits.

Nonetheless, the success of forward genetics heavily relies on the knowledge of the mouse genomic sequence and the advent of new technologies facilitating genome-wide analyses. Indeed, the availability of human genomic sequences has facilitated the development of a novel technology, which is commonly referred to as a genome-wide association study (GWAS). The GWAS approach has been applied to large human cohorts and has completely revolutionized this field of research, allowing for the characterization of multiple genetic complex traits. This technique is undeniably responsible for significantly increasing the discovery rate of risk loci for many human traits and diseases, including inflammatory and autoimmune diseases [6]. Due to the prominent impact of this approach, a brief description of the strategy is provided below.

Because of the genetic heterogeneity found in humans, as opposed to inbred mice, the identification of loci that are significantly associated with a given trait of disease requires a sizeable number of patients in order to complete the study. For a GWAS, two groups are required: test subjects with the disease (cases) and similar subjects without (controls). Essentially, the genome of each individual is analysed for selected markers of genetic variation, usually for a single DNA base change, which are called single nucleotide polymorphisms (SNPs). Each SNP is linked to a known allele in the examined population and, thus, they are used as markers to define the allelic genotype of each individual. Various quantifiable phenotypes can then be correlated with the SNP results. The frequency of a given genotype is compared between cases and controls and, depending on the observed frequency of these variations in the subjects with disease, the variations may or may not be found to be "associated" with the disease. The associated genetic variations are then considered as indicators of disease susceptibility regions [7]. These regions can vary both in size, depending on the extent of the linkage disequilibrium, and in gene content [8], where the number of genes within the region can range from several to none. Moreover, a SNP located outside a coding sequence might be correlated to the causal variant located within a coding sequence, which can lead to a functional or structural modification of the protein (protein quality). It can also be associated with a regulatory variant, therefore modifying the gene expression (protein quantity). In all cases, *functional studies are needed to characterize the actual effect of the variant.*

In order to determine the significance of the genetic variation to susceptibility, a GWAS utilizes a classical logarithm of odds (LOD) score linkage analysis, where the probability of linkage between disease and marker loci is compared to the probability of no linkage. This odds ratio is then taken to determine the LOD ratio. Currently, genetic association p-values smaller than 5×10^{-8} are the accepted measure of significant association to disease [9]. Nevertheless, many factors contribute to a given susceptibility locus, making the validation of significance quite difficult and new statistical validation approaches are constantly being revised to increase the sensitivity of the GWAS [10].

In complex genetic traits, most loci will confer low risk to disease. However, in some instances, a single locus is highly associated with, and significantly contributes to, disease predisposition. In such cases, it becomes very difficult to identify other loci conferring a relatively low risk. The HLA (Human Leukocyte Antigen) in humans, or the MHC (Major Histocompatibility Complex) in mice, is a perfect example of a locus strongly associated with autoimmune disease predisposition. Although the exact association between the HLA and autoimmunity remains unclear, a common view suggests that a breakdown occurs in the immunological tolerance to self-antigens through aberrant class I and class II presentation of self or foreign peptides to autoreactive lymphocytes [11-14]. Indeed, the HLA is one of the most extensively studied regions in the human genome because of the contribution of multiple variants at this locus towards multiple diseases. Indeed, the HLA has been associated with susceptibility to MS, T1D, SLE, ulcerative colitis (UC), Crohn's disease (CD), as well as rheumatoid arthritis (RA) [15] and has the greatest and/or most consistent genetic risk associated with these diseases in comparison to other loci linked to disease susceptibility [6]. For example, *HLA* (located on human chromosome 6) has the most significant linkage to T1D with a LOD score of 213.2 and accounts for approximately 50% of the inheritable susceptibility [12]. After the HLA, the next suggestive evidence of linkage to T1D is located near *CTLA4* and *INS* (insulin gene) with a LOD score of 3.28 and 3.16, respectively [15]. Thus, it is clear that the remaining susceptibility genes have much lower overall contributions to diabetes risk compared to the collective contribution of HLA genes. Nevertheless, *variation within the HLA locus does not explain autoimmune disease development for all subjects*, therefore, it remains important to identify and understand how susceptibility genes with lower LOD scores influence disease development. We must bear in mind that the ultimate aim of these investigations is to provide a sufficient understanding of the pathways contributing to autoimmune disease to facilitate the design of new specific therapeutic approaches related to the genotype of the patient.

Genetic association studies are limited in part by the occurrence of linkage disequilibrium (LD), where combinations of alleles at two or more loci, not necessarily found on the same chromosome, occur more or less frequently in a population than would be expected. Thus, LD measures the non-random associations between polymorphisms at different loci. As a result, if one identifies a variant that is associated with disease, it will be *difficult to determine whether the variant is causal of disease or whether its association simply reflects LD with the true causal variant.* Indeed, HLA haplotypes demonstrate strong LD. Hence, the causal HLA variants have remained vague for the great majority of diseases [12].

Regardless of advances in genetics and the increasing availability of novel genetic tools, we have yet to identify the causal gene or genes for >75% of the newly identified susceptibility loci [6]. Indeed, at least 17 genetic regions associate with lupus predisposition and each of these genetic intervals potentially represent causal genetic variants that largely remain to be discovered [16]. Moreover, of the 421 genes within the HLA, only 40% are known to be expressed, while fewer than one third of these genes have a defined biological function [12]. Clearly, *identifying a susceptibility region does not readily define the causal gene or mechanism*. Extensive studies are needed in order to first determine which genetic variants actually contribute to disease susceptibility followed by how these variants affect biological function and increase susceptibility to disease [17]. This task will require very strong collaborations between human geneticists and experimental biologists if we are to understand how these sequence variants influence disease pathogenesis.

Prior to the development of the GWAS, a major limitation of human genetic studies was that the technology relied on testing a small number of variants across the genome, with each study using a different set of variants and/or typing methodology. This problem has resulted in a literature base that can be complex and at times conflicting. In order to differentiate the effects of tightly linked loci, a dense map of variation is needed in *large cohorts of ethnically diverse populations*, so that rare, distinguishing recombination events can be identified [12]. Particularly, a large number of DNA markers (> 100 000 SNPs) from clinically well-defined patients and matched controls need to be genotyped. Using larger cohorts for all studies including replication studies facilitates the identification of most of the genetic variation in the human genome [6]. It should be noted that large inbred families could unexpectedly highlight the major effect of a susceptibility gene, which in a heterogeneous sample of small families displays only a minor overall effect [18].

Another limitation, which also applies to the current GWAS technology, is the *inability to replicate genetic associations in some or all subsequent studies*. This could be due to sampling variation (different samples of families from a same population containing different frequencies of susceptibility genes), population genetic variation (ethnic groups), population environmental factors leading to different levels of penetrance of interacting susceptibility genotypes, combinations of the above, or no true linkage (false positive) [18]. Indeed, a common limitation of the GWAS approach is the high potential for false-positives given the massive number of statistical tests performed. Consequently, there is a greater requirement for reproduction of results and a higher threshold of statistical significance [19].

The analysis of a GWAS must take into account that weak linkage associations could be attributed to 2 key possibilities:

1. The *susceptibility gene occurs in only a small proportion of patients*, or
2. The *susceptibility gene produces only a slight increase in risk*, suggesting the possibility that the gene acts concurrently with other genes to cause disease.

Therefore, in a given individual, the combination of these minor genes could have a stronger effect on disease development and susceptibility. Nevertheless, *weak linkage association to a particular region means that the gene itself will be difficult to locate, difficult to confirm* in independent studies and *difficult to isolate* by genetic procedures.

Finally, identification of genetic variants and molecular pathways associated with disease susceptibility through linkage analysis studies in mice compared to data obtained in humans shows that an interesting parallel can be made, at least for autoimmune diabetes, where common genes and pathways contribute to disease predisposition [20]. There are also significant advantages to using mouse models rather than humans. Mouse genetic studies take advantage of established inbred strains which simplify the genetic approach and reduce the cost. As opposed to humans, where thousands of individuals need to be genotyped to identify significant linkages, a few hundred mice are sufficient to identify multiple genetic loci associated with disease. For this approach, highly significant differences must be observed for a given phenotype upon comparison between two independent inbred strains. These strains are then interbred for two generations (F2), where these F2 generation offspring exhibit random recombination events between the two parental strains. Subsequently, the linkage analysis of the phenotype and genotype allows for the rapid identification of genetic loci, as well as interacting loci, involved in determining the phenotype. Thus, the combination of the human GWAS approach and mouse genetics may rapidly help identify key pathways regulating immune tolerance and preventing autoimmune disease progression.

In conclusion, the introduction of the GWAS approach has had an extraordinary impact on our knowledge of the genetics of many autoimmune diseases, bringing to light many unexpected candidate genes and biological pathways [6]. The GWAS facilitates the discovery of susceptibility genes for a given disease, where clinicians may then use these susceptibility genes to assess the likelihood of an individual in developing the disease. More importantly, identification of causal genes will increase the understanding of the disease process, which will ultimately lead to the creation of preventative therapies. However, many susceptibility loci remain to be discovered and may necessitate the generation of new tools in order to access the more infrequent variants [21]. Identification of the variants causal to disease will also require extensive investigations. Furthermore, designing methods for prevention will require that we also understand the mechanisms through which genetic susceptibility occurs and how these interact with non-genetic factors. Therefore, although genetic studies are part of the answer to developing new therapies, determining the absolute susceptibility to disease will depend on establishing the contribution of both genetic and non-genetic factors.

Hereafter, we discuss the contribution of variations in immune tolerance to autoimmune disease susceptibility and the implication of genetic studies in understanding biological pathways associated with autoimmune diseases.

T Cells

T cells are necessary and sufficient for the progression of various autoimmune pathologies, such as T1D, RA and thyroiditis. For instance, transfer of T cells from a diabetic mouse to an otherwise healthy mouse is sufficient to induce autoimmune diabetes progression [22]. Also, in individuals affected by SLE, T cells are known to be hyperactive and resistant to apoptosis [23]. Moreover, patients suffering from RA show elevated amounts of the inflammatory cytokine IL-17, a cytokine produced by a subset of CD4 T cells [24]. Clearly, T lymphocytes are implicated in the susceptibility of these diseases as well as other autoimmune pathologies. The defects in T cell function that lead to autoimmune pathologies can result from various immune check points involved in imposing T cell tolerance to self-tissues. Some critical events in the control of T cell tolerance will be discussed below. Moreover, we will describe how defects in T cell tolerance induction may contribute to autoimmune disease susceptibility and progression.

Overview of T Cell Differentiation and Function

The thymus, a primary lymphoid organ, is the siege of thymocytes' early education events. Here, thymocytes which recognize self-peptides with low affinity in the context of MHC class I or II molecules will differentiate into naïve T cells expressing CD8 or CD4 co-receptor, respectively. These T lymphocytes will then exit the thymus, migrate to the periphery and travel through secondary lymphoid organs in search of a pathogen. Defects in a T cell's ability to recognize pathogens and mount an efficient response leads to an impaired ability to fight infections, which can result in deleterious consequences for the host. Consequently, the T cell responses must be intricately tuned to allow adequate recognition of pathogenic antigens, all the while precluding T cell activation upon binding to self-antigens. Both central and peripheral tolerance mechanisms are responsible for establishing this balance.

Central Tolerance

The role of the thymus is to generate functional T cells, while eliminating autoreactive T cells. This is achieved by way of positive and negative thymic selection processes, which collectively are commonly referred to as "central tolerance". During positive selection, immature T cells, hereafter referred to as thymocytes, with a low affinity for self-MHC peptide complexes are allowed to mature. This ensures that thymocytes which emigrate from the thymus will sufficiently recognize both self-peptide/MHC complexes, which will promote T cell survival, and pathogenic-peptide/MHC complexes presented at the surface of a professional Antigen-Presenting Cell (APC), namely dendritic cells, macrophages and B cells, which will induce an efficient immune response. On the other hand, T cell discrimination between self and non-self proteins is critical in the prevention of autoimmune reactions. Negative selection is the process that entails the elimination of thymocytes exhibiting a strong affinity or avidity for self-peptides before they escape from the thymus. Indeed, thymic dendritic cells (tDC) and medullary thymic epithelial cells (mTEC) constitutively process and present self-peptides to thymocytes. If the strength of the interaction between the T cell receptor (TCR) on the thymocyte and the peptide/MHC complex on the APC exceeds a certain threshold, the T cell will be subject to apoptosis, a tightly regulated cell death process that does not lead to inflammation. Therefore, negative selection should allow for the efficient elimination of most autoreactive T cells. Nevertheless, defects in the negative selection process will enhance susceptibility to autoimmune diseases.

In this regard, a defect in the induction of the Bcl-2 family member Bim, a pro-apoptotic mediator, correlates with impaired negative selection [25]. As suggested, $Bim^{-/-}$ animals show an increase in susceptibility to autoimmune diseases and develop severe kidney autoimmune disease [24]. Moreover, Bim expression is dysregulated in autoimmune diabetes-prone NOD mice [26], a commonly used murine model that is also susceptible to other autoimmune deficiencies, such as thyroiditis and SLE [27, 28]. Moreover, abnormally low and high thresholds for positive and negative thymocyte selections, respectively, are also responsible for an increased proportion of autoreactive T cells in the NOD mouse and possibly in other mouse strains, as well [29-31].

Negative selection is also dependent on the efficiency of antigen presentation by tDC and mTECs. tDCs present ubiquitously expressed self-antigens to immature thymocytes resulting in the apoptosis of thymocytes which have a high affinity to self-antigens. Consequently, this limits the export of autoreactive T cells from the thymus into the periphery. However, not all antigens are expressed by DCs circulating in the thymus. Some tissue-specific antigens (TSA) remain sequestered within organs such as the skin, eyes, brain, pancreas, etc. It has recently been shown that mTECs specialize in the presentation of TSA to thymocytes, a mechanism regulated by Aire (autoimmune regulator) [32]. Indeed, Aire is mainly expressed by mTECs [33]. Therefore, defects in Aire should lead to an increase in autoimmune susceptibility to specific organs. Indeed, Aire-deficient mice develop autoimmune responses to a limited set of antigens, where the antigenic specificity is conferred by the genetic background of the mouse strain being studied [32, 34]. More importantly, mutations in *AIRE* are responsible for causing the autosomal recessive Autoimmune Polyendocrinopathy-Candidiasis-Ectodermal Dystrophy (APECED) pathology, where patients develop massive lymphocytic infiltrations and produce multiple autoantibodies to various tissues [35-37]. Finally, Aire-deficient mice have facilitated the identification of the biological role of this protein in the induction of negative selection and tolerance to tissue-specific self-antigens [32, 38-40]. In summary, negative selection generally induces apoptosis of thymocytes that are specific for ubiquitously or ectopically expressed self-antigens. As a result, reported defects in negative selection processes have been associated with a direct increase in susceptibility to autoimmune disease progression.

Peripheral Tolerance

Although thymic selection processes promote the maturation of T cells that are not self-reactive, a sizeable proportion of autoreactive T cells can be found in periphery. In an attempt to control autoimmune responses in the periphery, some T cells with a relatively high affinity for self-peptide/MHC complexes are spared from negative selection and undergo a distinct differentiation programme which leads to immune regulation [41]. The most studied regulatory T cell population is defined as "natural" (ie: originating from the thymus) lymphocytes which express both the CD4 co-receptor and the activation marker CD25 (nTregs). In humans, as in mice, the up-regulation of the transcription factor FOXP3 is a requisite step for the differentiation and function of nTregs [42]. However, FOXP3 expression is not limited to nTregs as is also expressed by CD4 T cells which acquire their regulatory phenotype and function in the periphery, giving rise to the term "inducible" Tregs (iTregs). Indeed, in the presence of IL-2 and TGF-β and in the absence of inflammatory cytokines, naïve CD4 T cells up-regulate the expression of FOXP3 and become potent regulators [43]. Importantly, when Tregs encounter an APC presenting a peptide for which they are specific, they become activated and abrogate the proliferation of surrounding T cells via IL-2 deprivation, cell-to-cell contact and secretion of immunoregulatory cytokines, such as IL-10 [44]. Clearly, Tregs play a prominent role in peripheral tolerance mechanisms [45].

As Tregs are central to the maintenance of peripheral tolerance, it is not surprising to find that genetic defects in *FOXP3*, which precludes the appropriate generation and function of Tregs, are associated with autoimmune diseases in both humans and mice. In humans, individuals bearing mutations in the *FOXP3* gene develop a multi-organ autoimmune disease that is usually lethal before the age of 2 [46]. Similarly, the Scurfy mouse model, which carries a mutation in *Foxp3,* also presents a severe autoimmune phenotype comparable to the disease observed in humans [47]. Together, these data demonstrate that a defect in the regulation of Tregs is sufficient to confer an increased risk of developing an autoimmune disease. Despite the lack of a clear association between Treg number and the prevalence of any given autoimmune disease, several different groups have highlighted functional defects in Tregs from patients suffering from relapsing-remitting MS [42]. Moreover, many pathways associated with type 1 diabetes predisposition might affect Treg function, such as the CTLA-4 and the IL-2/CD25 pathways. In particular, the insulin-dependent diabetes 3 *(Idd3)* locus, which defines a susceptibility region for autoimmune diabetes in NOD mice, encompasses the *Il2* gene, where genetic variants of this gene have been identified [48, 49]. Although it is tempting to suggest that the biological contribution of *Il2* genetic variants alters Treg function and, thus, increases autoimmune susceptibility, the mechanism of action of the *Il2* variants has not been fully determined and is subject to debate [48-53]. Finally, even though CD4+CD25+ FOXP3+ Tregs are the most extensively studied, other subtypes of immunoregulatory T cells have also been identified for their role in tolerance maintenance, such as CD8αα intraepithelial lymphocytes [54] and Double Negative (DN) T lymphocytes [55]. However, their role in the prevention of autoimmune disease progression remains to be fully established.

As discussed above, mechanisms involved in the presentation of TSA are present in the thymus. Indeed, AIRE has proven to be a requisite for an efficient selection of non-autoreactive thymocytes. However, it has recently been proposed that AIRE could also be expressed in the periphery in order to further delete self-specific T cells. For instance, extrathymic Aire-expressing cells (eTACs) reside mainly in T-cell zones located in secondary lymphoid organs [56]. These stromal cells are positive for MHC class II expression and are, thus, presumably capable of antigen presentation [56, 57]. Even though it has been demonstrated that eTACs can directly interact with and delete autoreactive T cells, their precise role in autoimmune disease prevention remains to be established.

Another key mechanism which limits aberrant autoreactive T cell responses in the periphery is the "two signal model". This model illustrates the intrinsic activation requirement of naïve T cells to receive both a TCR signal (recognition of a peptide-MHC complex) as well as co-stimulation signals. More specifically, after emigrating from the thymus, naïve T lymphocytes circulate within lymphoid organs aiming to encounter an APC presenting an antigen for which they exhibit sufficient affinity. However, the interaction between the TCR and a peptide-MHC complex alone is insufficient to induce the full T cell activation necessary to provoke an immune response. Consequently, APCs upregulate co-stimulatory molecules, such as CD80 and CD86, only in presence of inflammation [58]. Naïve T cells, which constitutively express the counter-ligand, CD28, can, thus, be fully activated to induce an immune response. In absence of this co-stimulatory signal, the T cell will become non-responsive or will become subject to apoptosis, two other mechanisms of peripheral tolerance that are respectively referred to as anergy and activation-induced cell death (AICD). As a result, in the absence of inflammation, a potentially autoreactive T cell will either become unresponsive or will be removed from the circulation. Interestingly, deletion of co-stimulatory molecules, such as CD80 and CD86 or CD28 in NOD mice accelerates the onset and severity of autoimmune diabetes [59, 60], further highlighting the importance of tight regulation of co-stimulation for the prevention of autoimmune disease. The loss of CD80 and CD86 co-stimulatory proteins also leads to a dramatic decrease in Treg numbers in the thymus and periphery [61], which may explain part of the mechanism by which these molecules contribute to the maintenance of immune tolerance. Moreover, it should be noted that activated T cells up-regulate the expression of CTLA-4, an inhibitor of T cell activation which competes with CD28 for binding to CD80 and CD86 [62] and is directly involved in anergy induction as well as the control of Treg function [63, 64]. The expression of CTLA-4 is crucial in order to avoid lymphoproliferative disorders, as its signalling leads to cell cycle arrest, inhibition of CD25 and CD69 up-regulation, decreased IL-2 production as well as an increased threshold for subsequent activation [56]. Indeed, CTLA-4 deficiency leads to massive lymphoproliferation and multi-organ tissue infiltration leading to death within 3 to 4 weeks of age [65, 66]. This fulminant immune response to multiple tissues underlines the critical role of CTLA-4 in the induction of immune tolerance. The contribution of CTLA-4 genetic variants to autoimmune susceptibility has been confirmed in both mice and humans [67, 68]. Specifically, in NOD mice, the *Idd5.1* autoimmune diabetes susceptibility locus includes *Ctla-4* as a candidate gene. Furthermore, through recent GWAS, genetic variants of *CTLA-4* have been associated with susceptibility to numerous autoimmune diseases, including SLE, RA, Grave's and celiac diseases [69]. The biological implications for different CTLA-4 genetic variants are under current investigation [70-73].

Finally, other defects in co-stimulation pathways have been associated with autoimmunity. Indeed, PD-1 (Programmed Death 1) also acts as a negative regulator expressed on the surface of activated T and B cells. PD-1 is thought to be responsible for the maintenance of long term tolerance following activation, mainly by limiting T cell function [74]. Deficiencies in PD-1 are known to induce spontaneous autoimmunity in different mouse strains, notably autoimmune cardiomyopathy in BALB/c mice [75] and a lupus-like disease in C57BL/6 mice, an otherwise auto-immune resistant strain [76]. Moreover, polymorphisms in PD-1 have been associated with various autoimmune pathologies in numerous human cohorts, pinpointing its role in tolerance induction [74].

Peripheral tolerance is also maintained by immune-regulation of the Th1/Th2/Th17 pathways. Indeed, in 1986, Mosmann showed that CD4 T cells can be separated into two distinct populations according to their cytokine production profile, namely Th1 and Th2 [77]. Th1 cells produce IL-2 and IFN-γ pro-inflammatory cytokines and promote cytotoxic and inflammatory responses, while Th2 cells secrete IL-4 and IL-10, both of which are associated with immune deviation and tolerance induction. Another pro-inflammatory subset of CD4 T cells has recently been identified and is designated Th17 for its prominent potential at producing the IL-17 cytokine, a chemotactic cytokine facilitating the recruitment of neutrophils [78]. Other than IL-17, Th17 cells also produce a vast array of pro-inflammatory cytokines, including IL-1, IL-6, IL-8, IL-22 and TNFα, which are known to recruit and activate monocytes, macrophages, neutrophils and other innate immune cells. In particular,

Th17 cells have been associated with MS and RA pathologies, while Th1 contribute to T1D and MS [79-82]. Evidence that Th17 contribute to autoimmune progression has been recently revealed by various genetic deletions in molecules contributing to Th17 differentiation, such as IL-12, IL-23 and IL-25 [83, 84].

Alterations in the balance of immune-regulation in favor of Th1 or Th17 immune responses may promote autoimmunity. IL-12 and IL-21 are cytokines which respectively promote Th1 and Th17 differentiation [85-87]. Genetic variants of both of these cytokines are included within autoimmune diabetes susceptibility regions, where *Il12* is located within *Idd4* and *Il21* is included within the *Idd3* interval [88, 89]. Interestingly, the IL-12p40 gene product can pair with IL-12p35 to form the Th1 promoting IL-12 cytokine or with IL-23p19 to create the Th17 promoting IL-23 cytokine [90]. Therefore, understanding the biological role of IL12p40 genetic variants may generate interesting therapeutic targets playing a central role in both Th1 and Th17 phenotypes. In contrast, IL-21 specifically impacts Th17, not Th1, differentiation. IL-21 is also implicated in chronic infections and the generation of memory T cells [91-93], which may contribute to autoimmune progression. In autoimmune prone NOD mice, pancreatic levels of IL-21 increase during diabetes development whereas the genetic ablation of the IL-21 pathway prevents autoimmune diabetes progression [89, 94]. Together, these results suggest that an intricate balance of the immune regulation of Th subsets is at play in defining the susceptibility to autoimmune diseases.

In summary, T cells, which develop in the thymus, must recognize self-peptide/MHC proteins with sufficient affinity in order to promote their maturation and survival. Yet, they must not recognize self-peptide/MHC complexes with ample affinity to induce an immune response. This dichotomy between self/non-self recognition has been a central theme in trying to understand the role of the immune response. Other than central tolerance, which is mostly mediated by negative selection, potentially autoreactive T cells are also subject to peripheral tolerance mechanisms, such as inhibition by Tregs, anergy, AICD and immune-regulation of the various Th pathways. Both co-stimulatory molecules and cytokines are key players in the regulation of the majority of the pathways involved in peripheral tolerance induction. Here, we have highlighted evidence demonstrating that alterations in any of these pathways which facilitate T cell activation are sufficient to increase the susceptibility to autoimmune disease progression. However, it should be noted that autoimmune diseases are multi-factorial. Essentially, although genetic ablation leads to severe phenotypes, the role of subtle genetic variants encoded within the genome only slightly increases the risk of developing autoimmunity. We will now describe how another major cellular subset, namely B cells, contributes to autoimmune disease progression.

B Cells

B lymphocytes are an important part of our adaptive immune system. The principal functions of B cells are to act as Antigen Presenting Cells (APCs), produce antibodies, and develop into memory B cells after activation. Activation of the B cell occurs when the B cell receptor (BCR), which is a membrane-bound immunoglobulin, binds with sufficient affinity to extracellular antigen. Upon activation, the B cell can further differentiate into either a plasma B cell or a memory B cell, both of which will maintain their antigenic-specificity and increase their affinity towards the antigen. Affinity maturation contributes to the enhanced immune response, which occurs upon antigen re-encounter.

B Cell Tolerance

The BCR itself recognizes not only foreign, but also self-antigens. To prevent destructive autoimmune responses, B cells are subject to various immune tolerance mechanisms [95-97]. Indeed, it has been suggested that up to 75% of newly produced B cells carry BCRs that are highly autoreactive [98-100]. Therefore, immune tolerance must be tightly regulated. The first mechanisms of B cell immune tolerance take place as B cells are maturing in the bone marrow and are thus collectively referred to as central tolerance. Indeed, if immature B cells recognize self-antigens with high avidity, they are eliminated by a process known as clonal deletion, which results in apoptosis. Yet, potentially autoreactive immature B cells that recognize self-antigens are not always eliminated. For one, surface IgM expression may be sufficiently down-regulated to allow maturation of the B cell. Secondly, intracellular signalling pathways may be altered to decrease their potential to respond towards self-antigen. This process leads to B cell anergy and allows maturation of unresponsive B cells. Finally, central tolerance mechanisms are not fail-safe allowing some autoreactive B cells that recognize low avidity self-antigens to survive and make their way into the periphery. Here, peripheral tolerance mechanisms will further restrict autoreactive B cells through clonal deletion, anergy, receptor editing and extrinsic suppression [101]. Nevertheless, a defect in any of the various mechanisms involved in immune tolerance would increase the pool of autoreactive B cells and facilitate the progression of autoimmune diseases.

Autoreactive B Cell Activation

For autoimmune disease progression, it is not sufficient to carry a high number of potentially autoreactive B cells; these cells must also recognize their cognate antigen and be fully activated in order to contribute to autoimmunity. Indeed, cytokines play an important role in the activation of autoreactive B cells. Type I interferon (IFN) has both direct and indirect effects on B cells [102-105]. Type I IFN can indirectly enhance B cell responses through the activation of dendritic cells, which will then secrete cytokines, such as IFN and BAFF, which can then directly stimulate B cell responses [104, 105]. BAFF, also known as a B cell activating factor, is a member of the tumour necrosis factor (TNF) family that induces B cell proliferation and promotes B cell survival [106]. In fact, peripheral B cell survival depends on the ability of the cells to compete for BAFF [107]. Under normal circumstances, autoreactive B cells will die in the periphery due to the limited availability of BAFF paired with their reduced responsiveness to this cytokine [108]. However, elevated levels of BAFF are often characteristic of B cell-induced autoimmune diseases [106] where increased levels of this cytokine will result in the rescue of autoreactive B cells that would have normally been deleted. Therefore, B cell-activating cytokines play an important role in the development of autoimmune diseases since they do not neglect autoreactive B cells of their stimulatory effect.

Toll-like receptors (TLRs) can also activate autoreactive B cells and therefore are directly involved in the break in B cell tolerance. TLRs, which are also known as pattern recognition receptors (PRR), are expressed by a multitude of cells, including monocytes, macrophages, dendritic cells and B cells, and recognize pathogen-associated molecular patterns (PAMPs). Amongst the cells that express TLRs, B cells exhibit a unique status as they also express an antigen-specific receptor, the BCR. In fact, TLR expression is upregulated in B cells after BCR activation [109]. It is the simultaneous activation of TLRs and the BCR on autoreactive B cells that induces their proliferation, up-regulation of co-stimulatory molecules, secretion of pro-inflammatory cytokines and the differentiation into plasma cells that produce high levels of autoantibodies [110]. Consequently, TLR activation has a direct effect on autoreactive B cell activation, but also indirectly activates autoreactive T cells as the up-regulation of co-stimulatory molecules on autoreactive B cells results in more efficient antigen-presentation. More specifically, TLR-activated B cells are known to play an important role in the development of various autoimmune diseases such as arthritis [111], experimental autoimmune encephalomyelitis (EAE) [112], which is a model of MS, as well as T1D [113]. Therefore, TLRs are clearly involved in autoimmune disease development.

A Preventive Role for B Cells

Autoreactive B cells promote autoimmune disease progression by secreting pathogenic autoantibodies and presenting autoantigens to T cells. Yet, B cells can also play an essential role in impeding autoimmune disease development. For instance, IL-10-producing B cells have been suggested to resolve or completely inhibit disease development for EAE, arthritis, chronic intestinal inflammation as well as MS [114-118]. In fact, B cells critically depend on TLR to produce IL-10 in order to suppress inflammation [119]. Therefore, B cells themselves can have diverse effects on the outcome of autoimmunity.

Autoreactive B Cells in Disease

Nonetheless, autoreactive B cells clearly play an important role in the development of autoimmunity. Autoreactive B cells promote disease not only by the production of autoantibodies, but also by serving as APCs for autoreactive T cells [110]. More specifically, B cells are known to play a role in the development of several autoimmune diseases, such as RA, SLE, Sjogren's syndrome, Autoimmune Thyroiditis and others [110]. A major challenge has been to determine what leads to the break in B cell tolerance resulting in disease progression. Defects in B cell tolerance mechanisms lead to increased frequencies of autoreactive B cells in the periphery where the over-expression of B cell-activating cytokines and TLR signalling evidently contribute to disease progression.

B Cells and Genetics

As mentioned above, autoreactive B cells are a part of the normal naïve B cell repertoire in the periphery. However, most autoreactive B cells remain functionally naïve for autoantibody production by differential peripheral checkpoints, such as receptor editing, clonal deletion, and anergy. Therefore, the presence of autoreactive B cells does not always signify disease, which is mediated through the regulation of their activation and function. Nevertheless, the existence of pathogenic autoantibodies is indicative of a break in B cell tolerance and autoimmune disease development.

Recent studies have significantly advanced our understanding of the mechanisms by which autoreactive B cells escape tolerance. A large number of loci and candidate genes have been shown to be associated with susceptibility to the development of autoimmune diseases, in particular SLE, which is a multigenic autoimmune disease characterized by the production of autoantibodies due to a breakdown in tolerance [120-124]. Among these, defects in the inhibitory Fc receptor (FcγRIIB), a component of the inhibitory signalling pathway that is important for the maintenance of B cell tolerance, has been shown to be genetically associated with the development of autoimmunity. Indeed, the partial restoration of FcγRIIB levels on B cells from lupus-prone mouse strains is sufficient to prevent disease development [125]. However, the precise mechanism by which FcγRIIB expression on B cells contributes to B cell tolerance maintenance is still under investigation. Moreover, a Y chromosome-linked "autoimmune accelerator" locus (Yaa), in combination with the FcγRIIB gene, significantly increases the onset and severity of lupus development in non-autoimmune-prone C57BL/6 mice [126]. Interestingly, B cells containing the Yaa locus exhibit increased TLR7 expression, which responds to RNA-related antigen stimulation, resulting in increased B cell sensitivity to RNA-containing self-antigens and their subsequent activation [127]. In addition, TLR7 translocation has shown to accelerate SLE autoimmunity [128]. Thus, both the FcγRIIB gene and Yaa locus have been associated with SLE susceptibility.

Genetic studies have also highlighted Ly108, a glycoprotein expressed by B cells belonging to the signalling lymphocytic activation molecule (SLAM) family, as a lupus susceptibility gene [120]. Ly108 is located on murine chromosome 1 and is associated with the production of autoantibody to chromatin. Thus, autoreactive B cells with an elevated level of expression of the Ly108.1 isoform escape multiple B cell tolerance mechanisms such as deletion, receptor revision, and anergy induction by tuning down BCR signalling at the immature stage of B cell development. Therefore the Ly108 gene plays a pivotal role in the regulation of autoreactive B cell checkpoints.

Using a GWAS approach, an association between BANK1 (B cell scaffold protein with ankyrin repeats 1) and SLE was identified. BANK1 variants affect the regulatory sites and key functional domains of the gene [129], which may contribute to sustained B cell receptor signalling and B cell hyperactivity, both of which are characteristic of the disease.

Finally, a GWAS mapped the control of marginal zone (MZ) B cell expansion to a region on chromosome 4, which includes the *Idd11* diabetes susceptibility loci, with a LOD score of 4.4 [130]. Interestingly, MZ B cells are expanded 2- to 3-fold in NOD mice compared with non-diabetic C57BL/6 (B6) mice by 3 weeks of age, the time when autoreactive T cells are first activated. This supports the hypothesis that this B cell trait is related to the development of diabetes in the NOD mouse.

Altogether, our increased understanding of how autoreactive B cells are activated and regulated has led to the emergence of several therapeutic approaches that focus on the blockade of co-stimulatory signals, the specific targeting of the BCR and the depletion of B cells altogether [131]. Indeed, impressive results have been obtained using rituximab, an antibody to CD20 that specifically depletes B cells [132]. However, as mentioned above, B cells can also prevent autoimmune disease progression and, thus, depletion of B cells may not always be beneficial. Consequently, none of these therapies are perfect and they will inevitably affect other aspects of the immune system. Therefore, further investigation is necessary in order to advance our knowledge of immune dysregulation and to enhance the design of autoimmune disease therapies. We will now illustrate how another key APC, namely the dendritic cell, contributes to autoimmune disease progression.

DENDRITIC CELLS

Dendritic cells (DCs), which were only described quite recently relative to other immune cell types [133-137], compose approximately 1% of the immune cells found in the spleen. Despite their limited proportions, they entice immunologists due to their prominent antigen presenting potential [138]. Indeed, they are considered as the professional APC with the highest proficiency for activating naïve T cells, which places them at the bridge between innate and adaptive immunity. This central position within the immune response suggests that the modulation of this cell type may provide new therapeutic approaches in cancer, autoimmunity and vaccination. Consequently, DCs have been extensively studied since their initial description and are now known to include many distinct subsets with unique phenotypes that carry out a multitude of immune functions.

Apart from their role in activating the adaptive arm of the immune system, DCs significantly contribute to immune tolerance mechanisms. Indeed, DCs clearly impact both central and peripheral induction of T cell tolerance. Thus, a better understanding of the underlying mechanism of tolerance induction may provide clues regarding how defects in this pathway may favour the development of autoimmunity.

T Cell Tolerance as Mediated by Dendritic Cells

Central tolerance is mostly mediated by the process of negative selection of potentially autoreactive clones. DCs contribute to this process by presenting self-antigens to T cells [139]. Thymic dendritic cell subsets include $CD8\alpha^+CD172a^-$ DC, $CD8\alpha^-CD172a^+$ DC, and plasmacytoid DC (pDC) [140, 141], where the role of pDC in thymic tolerance has yet to be examined. The $CD8\alpha^+CD172a^-$ DCs differentiate from thymic precursors while the $CD8\alpha^-CD172a^+$ DCs recirculate from the periphery [142, 143]. Therefore, $CD8\alpha^+CD172a^-$ DCs present thymic self-antigens while $CD8\alpha^-CD172a^+$ DCs present peripheral self-antigens to thymocytes. Thus, together, these DC subsets allow for the efficient deletion of thymocytes expressing a potentially autoreactive TCR. Most recently, it has been suggested that $CD8\alpha^-CD172a^+$ DCs also contribute to T cell tolerance processes by promoting the differentiation of Tregs [143, 144]. As thymic DCs play a key role in mediating central tolerance, defects in thymic subsets should, thus, have dire consequences and promote autoimmune progression. However, negative selection processes are not affected in mice deficient for CD47, the counter-ligand of CD172a necessary for transmigration of CD172a$^+$ cells [145-149], where the proportion of CD8α$^-$CD172a$^+$ thymic DCs is significantly reduced [149]. Therefore, additional studies are required to determine the exact contribution of thymic DCs to central tolerance mechanisms.

DCs are also known to participate in peripheral immune tolerance. For instance, increasing the number of DCs in NOD mice completely abrogates autoimmune disease onset [150]. Moreover, ablation of DCs in mice results in the induction of an autoimmune phenotype, demonstrating that the presence of DCs at steady state contributes to immune tolerance [151]. Yet, it should be noted that a fine balance exists between the role of DCs in tolerance induction and immune activation. Indeed, promoting DC survival also favours autoimmune progression [152]. Therefore, understanding how DCs function is crucial for the development of appropriate therapeutic approaches.

Specific Role of Dendritic Cell Subsets in Immune Tolerance

In recent years, many DC subsets have been described [153]. In mice, the so-called conventional DC (cDC) expresses high levels of CD11c and can be further segregated into two functionally distinct subsets according to the expression of CD8α, where CD8α+ DCs appear to contribute more extensively to tolerance induction than the CD8α- counterpart. Specifically, the CD8α- DCs have been reported to contribute to the pathogenesis of T1D, where they transport β cell antigens from the islets to the pancreatic lymph node, which promotes autoreactive T cell activation facilitating insulitis development [154]. Moreover, specific ablation of CD8α- DCs results in the absence of insulitis and diabetes [155]. However, these results should be interpreted with caution, as CD8α- DCs define two functionally distinct subsets, namely monocyte-derived DCs, which arise in response to inflammation, or a steady state population, which exhibits low levels of co-stimulatory molecules. Clear phenotypic differences between these two subsets have yet to be resolved and, thus, preclude their distinction particularly in an inflammatory context where the inflammatory DC subset predominates. In contrast, the CD8α+ DCs contribute to tolerance induction. In the spleen, CD8α+ DCs specifically express the DEC-205 endocytic receptor. Anti-DEC-205 antibodies directly coupled to antigen can be used to efficiently target CD8α+ DCs *in vivo* without activating DCs. Using this strategy, it was demonstrated that CD8α+ DCs specifically induce T cell tolerance [156, 157]. Interestingly, the lymphoid cDC subset has recently been divided into 2 new subsets in the spleen depending on the expression of the CD103 integrin [158]. The CD103$^+$ subset has been shown to induce tolerance, as it exhibits an increased potential of cross-presentation relative to the CD103$^-$ counterpart [158]. Indeed, the ability of CD8α+ DCs to cross-present antigen on MHC class I, which is essential for the tolerization of autoreactive CD8 T cells [159], can now be entirely attributed to the CD103+ subset. Finally, deficiencies in CD8α+ or CD8α- DC subsets by genetic ablation of various transcription factors, such as RelB, IRF-2, IRF-4, IRF8, TRAF6 and PU.1, have been reported to favour autoimmune pathologies [160-167]. Yet, these transcription factors do not exclusively affect the differentiation of these DC subsets, thus, more work is required to determine the specific contribution of DC subset deletion to promoting inflammatory responses and contributing to autoimmune progression.

Although the conventional DC subsets have been more extensively characterized, other DC subsets are emerging as important players in either tolerance or activation mechanisms. One such subset would be the $CD11c^{low}$ $B220^+$ $PDCA-1^+$ plasmacytoid DCs (pDC) [155]. They are generally known for their great capacity to secrete type I IFN in response to viral infections and tumours. However, pDCs express low levels of MHC class II, a characteristic associated with CD4 T cell tolerance induction [168]. Moreover, pDCs have recently been shown to induce the generation of $CD4^+CD25^+$ regulatory T cells [169]. Finally, elimination of pDCs accelerates insulitis onset and diabetes progression [155]. Together, these results suggest that pDCs are important players in preventing autoimmune disease progression.

Recently, a new DC subset named interferon-producing killer dendritic cell (IKDC) has been identified (1). This novel cell type shares phenotypic and functional characteristics of Natural Killer cells and DCs, as they can produce impressive amounts of IFN-γ and exhibit cytotoxic activity as well as process and present antigen to naïve T cells [170-173]. Because IKDCs are phenotypically similar to pDCs (low levels of MHC and co-stimulatory molecules), which are known to confer tolerance, IKDCs may play a role in tolerance [4-5]. Indeed, low IKDC number is associated with autoimmune diabetes susceptibility when comparing autoimmune-diabetes prone and resistant murine models [6]. In order to identify the genetic regions regulating their proportion, a linkage analysis using SNPs (Single Nucleotide Polymorphism) was performed and showed that the distal arm of chromosome 7 regulated IKDC number. Moreover, NOD.Lc7 congenic mice, for which the distal arm of chromosome 7 has been replaced by that of the C57L mouse strain, carry high numbers of IKDCs, thus, confirming that this genetic interval does indeed regulate IKDC number. Interestingly, NOD.Lc7 mice no longer develop diabetes [7], further supporting the association between IKDC number and autoimmune diabetes resistance.

Although the Lc7 interval regulates IKDC number and confers protection from diabetes progression, much more work is needed to provide a direct link between these two phenotypes. Indeed, the Lc7 interval is involved in preventing islet β cell apoptosis. However, the Lc7 interval encodes for more than 500 genes making it difficult to determine which genes are causal to this phenotype. As a result, diabetes resistance may be due to the β cells' increased resistance to apoptosis, increased IKDC number, other yet undiscovered phenotypes defined by Lc7, or a combination of the effects of many genes within this interval.

Linkage analysis of phenotypic traits results in the identification of genes regulating this trait, but does not directly associate the phenotypic traits with disease susceptibility. Therefore, until the biological function of IKDCs is fully elucidated, these results simply suggest that IKDCs may be involved in tolerance. Hence, further cellular and functional studies are needed to demonstrate a *bona fide* role of the IKDC subset in tolerance. Still, the identification of the particular genes regulating IKDC number on chromosomes 7 may prove useful in defining the contribution of IKDCs to autoimmune diabetes susceptibility.

Whether the subset is beneficial or detrimental to immune tolerance, it is clear that DCs hold a vital importance in immune tolerance. The various mechanisms that modulate the autoimmune response and tolerance induction constitute potential interesting treatment methods. It has been shown in NOD mice that T1D can be prevented upon dendritic cell transfer [174], which is a sign that such treatments are promising. There is, however, a need for further characterization of most DC subsets, whether it be regarding their function, proportion or link to autoimmunity. Furthermore, the recent discovery of IKDCs demonstrates that there might be other unknown subtypes of DCs with unique phenotypes that have yet to be revealed that could help explain current issues.

In summary, although dendritic cells are present in low number, they clearly play a predominant role in immune tolerance. However, genetic variants involved in defining DC subsets or function have not yet been underlined. This may be a direct consequence of the multiple DC lineages as well as the rarity of this cell type. Still, the modulation of DC number and function may prove critical in the prevention of autoimmune diseases. We will now illustrate how another component of the APC family, namely macrophages, contributes to autoimmune disease development.

MACROPHAGES

Macrophages represent a heterogeneous population of mononuclear leukocytes that originate from circulating monocytes to become tissue-resident. However, during the course of infection, monocytes can directly differentiate into activated macrophages and are recruited to sites of inflammation. They recognize pathogens via several receptors specific for antibodies or foreign antigens, such as Fc receptors or Toll Like Receptors (TLRs), respectively. Upon stimulation, macrophages phagocytose the pathogen and present the antigens to the adaptive immune system, after which a full blown immune response ensues.

Macrophages in Tolerance

Other than their role in phagocytosis of pathogens, macrophages are certainly important mediators of tolerance induction. This leukocyte of the innate immune system is involved in the efficient removal of apoptotic cells, a process known to contribute to the maintenance of immune tolerance. Indeed, perpetual tissue turnover generates a high number of apoptotic cells, which must be rapidly removed in order to prevent inflammation [175]. Moreover, defects in apoptotic cell clearance are thought to be implicated in autoimmune pathologies such as SLE, where autoantibodies specific for intracellular proteins are responsible for inflammation [176]. Furthermore, removal of apoptotic cells by macrophages, as well as other phagocytes, leads to the secretion of anti-inflammatory cytokines and contributes to the maintenance of immune tolerance [177]. Finally, apoptotic cell uptake allows the presentation of self-antigens by macrophages to T cells in the absence of co-stimulatory molecules, thereby inducing T cell anergy of potentially autoreactive T cells.

Macrophages eliminate apoptotic cells through other mechanisms in addition to phagocytosis. They are also responsible for the main production of the C1q complement component, which is known to opsonize apoptotic cells, thereby facilitating their uptake by macrophages, as well as other cells [178]. In addition, C1q binding on apoptotic cells induces TGF-β production by macrophages, which in turn facilitates conversion of naïve CD4 T cells into Tregs [179]. Interestingly, C1q-deficient mice have increased tissue apoptotic bodies, and are prone to autoimmunity [180]. Thus, macrophages are important contributors to induction of immune tolerance, in particular via the clearance of apoptotic cells.

Macrophages and T cell Tolerance

Macrophages can also participate in immune tolerance induction upon interacting with T lymphocytes. On the one hand, macrophages have the capacity to suppress T cell proliferation via the induction of two enzymes involved in amino acid catabolism, IDO (indoleamine 2,3-dioxygenase) and iNOS (inducible nitric oxide synthase) [181]. For instance, IDO is associated with T cell suppression via tryptophan depletion and generation of pro-apoptotic metabolites [182]. Moreover, it has been proposed that NO production is implicated in reducing inflammatory T cell expansion, which is associated with autoimmune diseases [183, 184]. Indeed, EAE remission phases are markedly reduced in mice deficient for *NOS2*, for which NO production is significantly decreased [185]. On the other hand, macrophages are potent inducers of regulatory T cells. Indeed, human monocyte-derived macrophages induce the differentiation of IL-10-producing T cells [186]. IL-10 is a potent immunosuppressive cytokine which in turn leads to generalized T cell anergy. Moreover, it has been shown that TGF-β treated macrophages can induce the development of various Treg subsets *in vivo* [187, 188]. Therefore, macrophages significantly contribute to the induction of peripheral T cell tolerance mechanisms.

Macrophages in Autoimmunity

With the description provided above, macrophages clearly contribute to various immune tolerance mechanisms. Therefore, defects in macrophage functions may be associated with autoimmune disease pathogenesis. For instance, autoimmune diabetes-susceptible NOD mice show significant defects in their macrophage functions when compared to autoimmune diabetes resistant strains [189-191]. Specifically, macrophages from NOD mice show an increase in IL-12 production when co-cultured with T cells, which may lead to an amplification of pathogenic T cells in these mice [191]. Therefore, the association of macrophage function with various autoimmune disease models, such as EAE and autoimmune diabetes, highly suggests a contribution of these professional phagocytes in human autoimmune pathologies.

Macrophages and Genetics

Genetic studies comparing diabetes-resistant and –susceptible mouse strains have revealed a candidate gene, Nramp1, situated within the Idd5.2 region. Nramp, mainly expressed by macrophages, has been identified for its role in resistance to intracellular pathogens, such as *Mycobacterium* or *Salmonella* [192, 193]. It has been demonstrated that Nramp is recruited to the phagosomal membrane following phagocytosis, where it impacts on the pathogen's replication [194]. Moreover, Nramp1 is necessary for efficient recycling of iron from senescent erythrocytes following phagocytosis by macrophages [195]. Recent work has validated Nramp as an important player in autoimmune disease susceptibility, as silencing the Nramp protein *in vivo* in mice that carried the autoimmune-susceptibility alleles led to a decreased incidence of diabetes [190]. These results provide an interesting example of where cellular biology meets genetics to validate genes involved in disease susceptibility and progression.

In conclusion, macrophages significantly contribute to immune tolerance induction and modulation of their functions may help prevent autoimmune disease progression. Consequently, more work is needed to better understand the biology and genetics of macrophages to establish them as potential therapeutic targets. Finally, we will illustrate how Natural Killer cells are involved in autoimmune disease development.

NATURAL KILLER CELLS

Over 30 years ago, large granular lymphocytes were identified and designated "Natural Killer" (NK) cells in light of their ability to spontaneously eliminate tumour cells without prior sensitization. Today, the tumour immunosurveillance capacity of NK cells is a well documented and accepted function of these cells [196]. Indeed, an increase in the incidence of leukemia has been observed in patients exhibiting dysfunctional NK cells, highlighting the importance of NK cells in the prevention of tumours [197]. In this section, we will define the unique differentiation pathway of NK cells, elaborate on their ability to discriminate between self-tissue and infected or cancerous cells, address their role in the prevention and promotion of autoimmune disease progression and discuss the genetic associations of the NK cell phenotype and function with autoimmune disease susceptibility.

Differentiation of NK cells

As opposed to T and B lymphocytes, NK cells are a minor lymphocyte population (2-10% of total lymphocytes) that do not express antigen specific receptors, posing additional challenges to the delineation of their differentiation from the bone marrow. It has now been established that NK cells arise from hematopoietic precursors, specifically the early lymphoid progenitors (ELP) and the common lymphoid progenitors (CLP) subsets [198, 199]. Interestingly, NK cells appear to be close relatives of T cells since they can differentiate from the thymic bipotent T/NK cell progenitor [200, 201]. CD122 expression, a component of the IL-15R, is essential for NK cell maturation [202], since IL-15 induces the proliferation and differentiation of NK cells [203] as well as the up-regulation of Gata-3, IRF-2 and T-bet, which are all lineage and function determining transcription factors [204].

Most recently, a maturation and developmental relationship between various NK cell phenotypes has been clearly depicted. Indeed, phenotypic characterization has allowed for the identification of 4 distinct subsets exhibiting different functions, which can be distinguished according to CD11b and CD27 expression in mice, or CD56 and CD27 expression in humans [205-208]. $CD11b^{low}CD27^{low}$ describes the most immature of the NK cell subsets [206]. These immature cells subsequently undergo the following sequential differentiating steps from $CD11b^{low}CD27^{hi}$ to $CD11b^{hi}CD27^{hi}$ and finally to mature and activated $CD11b^{high}CD27^{low}$ NK cells [206]. In agreement with this maturation scenario, the $CD11b^{low}CD27^{hi}$ subset composes the majority of the NK cell population in foetal and neonatal mice [209]. Moreover, the $CD11b^{high}$ cells express higher levels and a broader variety of NK receptors, such as the Ly49 receptors, are found at peripheral sites in adult mice and show more potent effector NK cell functions [210].

The Biological Function of NK Cells

As their name indicates, NK cells are mostly known for their ability to kill target cells. Indeed, upon efficient stimulation, NK cells have the capacity to eliminate tumours and virally-infected cells. They carry out their cytotoxic function through various, non-redundant mechanisms, where their cytotoxic capacity differs depending on the particular NK cell subset and their variegated expression of NK receptors [211]. NK cells can spontaneously lyse their targets by releasing perforin and granzyme granules [212, 213], or induce apoptosis of target cells through their expression of death ligands, such as FASL, TNF-α and TRAIL [214-216].

In addition to their killing potential, NK cells can modulate the outcome of adaptive immune responses through cytokine production. In fact, activated NK cells rapidly produce vast amount of cytokines, including IFN-γ, GM-CSF and TNF-α, to promote inflammation and secrete chemokines, such as MIP-1a MIP-1b, CCL1 and RANTES [217-219], to recruit lymphocytes and amplify the inflammatory response. Cytokines released by NK cells will also promote the maturation of DCs and influence T cell polarization [220]. Therefore, through cytokine production, NK cells create a bridge between innate an adaptive immunity.

NK Cells and Target Recognition

Mature NK cells play an important role in immunosurveillance. The "missing-self" hypothesis was originally put forth to explain how NK cells recognize targets lacking MHC class I expression [221]. However, it is now well understood that NK cells recognize their targets by integrating the responses of both inhibitory and activating receptors, which signal respectively through immunoreceptor tyrosine-based inhibitory motif (ITIM) and activation motif (ITAM). Generally, inhibitory receptors bind to self-MHC class I molecules thereby preventing the NK cell response towards healthy self-tissue but not towards infected or cancerous cells, where the MHC class I expression is often down-regulated [222]. In addition, ligands for NK cell activating receptors are seldom expressed in healthy tissue, while these ligands are often upregulated in cancers. Therefore, by integrating the signalling responses of both inhibitory and activating receptors, NK cells do not lyse healthy tissue but do specifically eliminate tumour cells.

Inhibitory receptors include a family of Ly49 molecules in mice and killer inhibitory receptors (KIR) in humans [223-225]. Both of these families of receptors contain more than 10 members, each of which confers a unique MHC class I binding specificity [226]. The NK cell population expresses different combinations of inhibitory receptors with different specificity, generating a broad NK cell repertoire to generate an adequate recognition of the highly polymorphic MHC class I haplotypes *[227, 228]*. For instance, the Ly49 gene cluster is a large family of highly related genes and is also quite polymorphic between various inbred strains of mice. Consequently, NK cells from the 129 as well as the inbred C57BL/6 strains respond differently to intracellular infections, tumour induction and bone marrow transplantation [229-231]. In addition, the NOD strain has allelic variants of both the 129 and C57BL/6 mouse strains as well as the unique Ly49w gene, again conferring a unique NK cell specificity [232]. These genetic variations have been proposed to contribute to the variability in susceptibility to disease among the different strains [233].

Other than the Ly49 family, NK cells express a variety of immunoreceptors which can modulate their function. By far, NKGD2 is the most extensively studied activating receptor. NKG2D ligands, such as MICA, MICB, Rae1 and H60, are normally absent or expressed at a very low level in healthy tissue, but their expression is strongly induced in various pathological conditions [234, 235]. Other NK receptors have also been characterized and include the natural cytotoxicity receptors NKp30, NKp44 and NKp46 [236-238], the CD94/NKG2A receptor [239], the inhibitory receptor for non-MHC molecules, NKR-P1B [240], and the 2B4 (CD244) activating receptor [241].

In summary, upon maturation, NK cells acquire the expression of several activating and inhibitory receptors, which is dictated both by its genome as well as the environment in which the NK cells differentiate [228]. NK cells, thus, compose a heterogeneous population, where each cell type expresses a distinct set and level of activating and inhibitory receptors.

NK Cells in Autoimmunity

Because of their capacity to respond promptly, NK cells needs to be carefully regulated to prevent damage to healthy tissues which could lead to autoimmunity. Interestingly, under distinct circumstances, NK cells have been shown to either prevent or promote the development of autoimmune responses.

On the one hand, NK cells have been proposed to play an immunoregulatory protective function, since their numbers and functions are decreased in patients afflicted with MS, SLE, RA or T1D [242-245]. In addition, depletion of NK cells in mouse and rat models of MS increases disease severity [246-248]. In one of these studies, it was suggested that NK cells prevent MS development through the elimination of the pathogenic CD4+ effector T cells [247]. Moreover, others have demonstrated that NK cells inhibit the proliferation of auto-reactive T cells [249]. NK cells have also been proposed to control autoimmunity by killing activated autologous macrophages [250]. The observations that NK cells prevent autoimmune progression have not been limited to models of MS. Indeed, autoimmune diabetes-susceptible NOD mice are protected from disease progression by the activation of NK cells through the administration of complete Freund's adjuvant (CFA). Interestingly, depletion of NK cells prior to CFA injection abolishes the protective effect [251]. Finally, NK cells also produce Th2 cytokines, such as IL-5, IL-10 and IL-13, which counterbalances the effect of the pro-inflammatory IFNγ Th1 cytokine, and, thus, prevents autoimmunity [252-254].

On the other hand, NK cells are cytopathic and induce inflammation and, as such, may contribute to autoimmune disease progression. Evidence in support of their contribution to autoimmunity has been presented in various models. For instance, in a model of myasthenia gravis, NK cell depletion during the priming phase prevents disease onset. In this setting, NK cells are required to mount a Th1 response facilitating the production of pathogenic autoantibodies [255]. NK cells also eliminate pancreatic β cells in a virally-induced model of autoimmune diabetes [256]. Moreover, NK cells have been associated with aggressive insulitis where NK cell depletion reduced the incidence of autoimmune diabetes in NOD mice [257]. In further support of a role for NK cells in autoimmune diabetes progression, NK cells from recently diagnosed diabetic patients showed a high level IFN-γ expression. Interestingly, the NK cell activation state is reduced in long standing patients [258], suggesting that NK cells could participate in the initiation of the disease and become non-functional or exhausted upon chronic stimulation.

Altogether, these reports suggest that NK cells may prevent or promote autoimmunity depending on the disease state, the cytokine milieu, the type of NK cell subset as well as many other parameters. More work will be needed to decipher the exact contribution of NK cells and their various subsets to autoimmune disease progression.

NK Cells and Genetics

Genetic variations in NK cell function or receptor expression are associated with autoimmune disease progression. For instance, NK cells from autoimmune-prone NOD mice have poor effector function, supporting the view that adequate NK cell function protects from autoimmune disease progression [259-261]. Moreover, NOD mice overexpress the NKG2D activating ligand, Rae-1, and this phenotype associates with altered NKG2D functions [262]. Similarly, a study on human diabetic patients has also noted a reduced expression of NKG2D as well as a genetic association between a specific allele of MICA, a non-classical MHC class I molecule, and disease susceptibility [258]. Together, these results suggest an important role for NKGD2 and its ligands in contributing to autoimmune susceptibility.

Genetic susceptibility to autoimmune diseases has been extensively studied using NOD mice and has revealed many genetic loci associated with disease predisposition [263]. At least one of two loci identified, namely the *Idd6* and the *Idd19* loci, is highly relevant to NK cell function. The genetic interval containing both of these loci is located on chromosome 6 and includes the NK receptor complex which encodes for the NK receptors genes [264]. Further studies are needed to determine the genetic polymorphism(s) within this interval which directly promote susceptibility to disease. Finally, DAP12, DAP10 and Flt3L, which are important at defining NK cell as well as DC function, are located in the proximal region of chromosome 7, an interval associated with disease susceptibility. Moreover, these genes are differentially expressed between the autoimmune-prone NOD and the autoimmune-resistant C57BL/6 strains [257]. Future work is needed to establish their exact role in autoimmune susceptibility.

In conclusion, the contribution of the various facets of NK cells, such as their function, receptors, phenotype, subset, maturation, differentiation, and cytokine production, to autoimmune disease susceptibility remains to be fully elucidated. Until then, this fascinating cell type will continue to intrigue us.

CONCLUSION

Autoimmune susceptibility is multigenic and is determined by the sum of genetic variants found within an individual. These genetic variants have most probably been selected over time by natural selection processes, as they enhance the individual's protection against specific pathogens. Genetic variants may, therefore, increase the reactivity of the immune system and it is the accumulation of these genetic variants within a given person which increases their risk of developing an autoimmune syndrome. As a result, the immune system must find a balance between tolerance to self and reactivity to non-self. This balance is interdependent on the environment, i.e. pathogens, where stronger immune responses promote survival of the individual but may also lead to autoimmune diseases, whereas weaker immune responses may result in inefficient elimination of pathogens, which can be fatal.

Finally, we are entering an interesting era where genetics meets biology and biology meets genetics in the attempt to decipher the susceptibility to complex disease traits. Collaboration between geneticists and immunobiologists should help unravel the mysteries behind susceptibility to autoimmune diseases. The specific contribution of given cellular pathways to disease susceptibility will most certainly reveal new drug targets in the modulation of responses. An integration of the whole systems biology approaches and genetic information will most certainly prove useful. It should be noted, however, that in developed countries the incidence of autoimmune diseases is rising faster than can be simply explained by the natural selection of genetic variants. This suggests that environmental factors are most probably at play. Therefore, not only should we focus on defining the contribution of each genetic factor associated with disease susceptibility, but it will also be imperative to examine their interaction with environment.

REFERENCES

[1] Paigen, K. (2003). One hundred years of mouse genetics: an intellectual history. I. The classical period (1902-1980). *Genetics, 163*, 1-7.

[2] Paigen, K. (2003). One hundred years of mouse genetics: an intellectual history. II. The molecular revolution (1981-2002). *Genetics, 163*, 1227-1235.

[3] Hoyne, G. F. & Goodnow, C. C. (2006). The use of genomewide ENU mutagenesis screens to unravel complex mammalian traits: identifying genes that regulate organ-specific and systemic autoimmunity. *Immunol Rev, 210*, 27-39.

[4] Kile, B. T. & Hilton, D. J. (2005). The art and design of genetic screens: mouse. *Nat Rev Genet, 6*, 557-567.

[5] St Johnston, D. (2002). The art and design of genetic screens: Drosophila melanogaster. *Nat Rev Genet, 3*, 176-188.

[6] Lettre, G. & Rioux, J. D. (2008). Autoimmune diseases: insights from genome-wide association studies. *Hum Mol Genet, 17*, R116-121.

[7] Pearson, T. A. & Manolio, T. A. (2008). How to interpret a genome-wide association study. *JAMA, 299*, 1335-1344.

[8] Barrett, J. C., Hansoul, S., Nicolae, D. L., Cho, J. H., Duerr, R. H., Rioux, J. D., Brant, S. R., Silverberg, M. S., Taylor, K. D., Barmada, M. M., Bitton, A., Dassopoulos, T.,

Datta, L. W., Green, T., Griffiths, A. M., Kistner, E. O., Murtha, M. T., Regueiro, M. D., Rotter, J. I., Schumm, L. P., Steinhart, A. H., Targan, S. R., Xavier, R. J., Libioulle, C., Sandor, C., Lathrop, M., Belaiche, J., Dewit, O., Gut, I., Heath, S., Laukens, D., Mni, M., Rutgeerts, P., Van Gossum, A., Zelenika, D., Franchimont, D., Hugot, J. P., de Vos, M., Vermeire, S., Louis, E., Cardon, L. R., Anderson, C. A., Drummond, H., Nimmo, E., Ahmad, T., Prescott, N. J., Onnie, C. M., Fisher, S. A., Marchini, J., Ghori, J., Bumpstead, S., Gwilliam, R., Tremelling, M., Deloukas, P., Mansfield, J., Jewell, D., Satsangi, J., Mathew, C. G., Parkes, M., Georges, M. & Daly, M. J. (2008). Genome-wide association defines more than 30 distinct susceptibility loci for Crohn's disease. *Nat Genet, 40*, 955-962.

[9] Risch, N. & Merikangas, K. (1996). The future of genetic studies of complex human diseases. *Science, 273*, 1516-1517.

[10] Jacobs, K. B., Yeager, M., Wacholder, S., Craig, D., Kraft, P., Hunter, D. J., Paschal, J., Manolio, T. A., Tucker, M., Hoover, R. N., Thomas, G. D., Chanock, S. J. & Chatterjee, N. (2009). A new statistic and its power to infer membership in a genome-wide association study using genotype frequencies. *Nat Genet.*

[11] Muller-Hilke, B. (2009). HLA class II and autoimmunity: epitope selection vs differential expression. *Acta Histochem, 111*, 379-381.

[12] Fernando, M. M., Stevens, C. R., Walsh, E. C., De Jager, P. L., Goyette, P., Plenge, R. M., Vyse, T. J. & Rioux, J. D. (2008). Defining the role of the MHC in autoimmunity: a review and pooled analysis. *PLoS Genet, 4*, e1000024.

[13] Harbo, H. F., Lie, B. A., Sawcer, S., Celius, E. G., Dai, K. Z., Oturai, A., Hillert, J., Lorentzen, A. R., Laaksonen, M., Myhr, K. M., Ryder, L. P., Fredrikson, S., Nyland, H., Sorensen, P. S., Sandberg-Wollheim, M., Andersen, O., Svejgaard, A., Edland, A., Mellgren, S. I., Compston, A., Vartdal, F. & Spurkland, A. (2004). Genes in the HLA class I region may contribute to the HLA class II-associated genetic susceptibility to multiple sclerosis. *Tissue Antigens, 63*, 237-247.

[14] Horton, R., Wilming, L., Rand, V., Lovering, R. C., Bruford, E. A., Khodiyar, V. K., Lush, M. J., Povey, S., Talbot, C. C., Jr., Wright, M. W., Wain, H. M., Trowsdale, J., Ziegler, A. & Beck, S. (2004). Gene map of the extended human MHC. *Nat Rev Genet, 5*, 889-899.

[15] Concannon, P., Chen, W. M., Julier, C., Morahan, G., Akolkar, B., Erlich, H. A., Hilner, J. E., Nerup, J., Nierras, C., Pociot, F., Todd, J. A. & Rich, S. S. (2009). Genome-wide scan for linkage to type 1 diabetes in 2,496 multiplex families from the Type 1 Diabetes Genetics Consortium. *Diabetes, 58*, 1018-1022.

[16] Harley, J. B., Kelly, J. A. & Kaufman, K. M. (2006). Unraveling the genetics of systemic lupus erythematosus. *Springer Semin Immunopathol, 28*, 119-130.

[17] Rioux, J. D., Goyette, P., Vyse, T. J., Hammarstrom, L., Fernando, M. M., Green, T., De Jager, P. L., Foisy, S., Wang, J., de Bakker, P. I., Leslie, S., McVean, G., Padyukov, L., Alfredsson, L., Annese, V., Hafler, D. A., Pan-Hammarstrom, Q., Matell, R., Sawcer, S. J., Compston, A. D., Cree, B. A., Mirel, D. B., Daly, M. J., Behrens, T. W., Klareskog, L., Gregersen, P. K., Oksenberg, J. R. & Hauser, S. L. (2009). Mapping of multiple susceptibility variants within the MHC region for 7 immune-mediated diseases. *Proc Natl Acad Sci, U S A, 106*, 18680-18685.

[18] Field, L. L. (2002). Genetic linkage and association studies of Type I diabetes: challenges and rewards. *Diabetologia 45*, 21-35.

[19] Hunter, D. J. & Kraft. P. (2007). Drinking from the fire hose--statistical issues in genomewide association studies. *N Engl J Med, 357,* 436-439.

[20] Maier, L. M. & Wicker, L. S. (2005). Genetic susceptibility to type 1 diabetes. *Curr Opin Immunol, 17,* 601-608.

[21] Manolio, T. A., Collins, F .S., Cox, N. J., Goldstein, D. B., Hindorff, L. A., Hunter, D. J., McCarthy, M. I., Ramos, E. M., Cardon, L. R., Chakravarti, A., Cho, J. H., Guttmacher, A. E., Kong, A., Kruglyak, L., Mardis, E., Rotimi, C. N., Slatkin, M., Valle, D., Whittemore, A. S., Boehnke, M., Clark, A. G., Eichler, E. E., Gibson, G., Haines, J. L., Mackay, T. F., McCarroll, S. A. & Visscher, P. M. (2009). Finding the missing heritability of complex diseases. *Nature, 461,* 747-753.

[22] Haskins, K. (2005). Pathogenic T-cell clones in autoimmune diabetes: more lessons from the NOD mouse. *Advances in immunology, 87,* 123-162.

[23] La Cava, A. (2009). Lupus and T cells. *Lupus, 18,* 196-201.

[24] Chabaud, M., Durand, J. M., Buchs, N., Fossiez, F., Page, G., Frappart, L. & Miossec. P. (1999). Human interleukin-*17,* A T cell-derived proinflammatory cytokine produced by the rheumatoid synovium. *Arthritis Rheum, 42,* 963-970.

[25] Bouillet, P., Purton, J. F., Godfrey, D. I., Zhang, L. C., Coultas, L., Puthalakath, H., Pellegrini, M., Cory, S., Adams, J. M. & Strasser, A. (2002). BH3-only Bcl-2 family member Bim is required for apoptosis of autoreactive thymocytes. *Nature, 415,* 922-926.

[26] Liston, A., Lesage, S., Gray, D. H., O'Reilly, L. A., Strasser, A., Fahrer, A. M., Boyd, R. L., Wilson, J., Baxter, A. G., Gallo, E. M., Crabtree, G. R., Peng, K., Wilson, S. R. & Goodnow, C. C. (2004). Generalized resistance to thymic deletion in the NOD mouse; a polygenic trait characterized by defective induction of Bim. *Immunity, 21,* 817-830.

[27] Many, M. C., Maniratunga, S. & Denef, J. F. (1996). The non-obese diabetic (NOD) mouse: an animal model for autoimmune thyroiditis. *Exp Clin Endocrinol Diabetes* 104 Suppl 3, 17-20.

[28] Silveira, P. A. & A. G. Baxter. (2001). The NOD mouse as a model of SLE. *Autoimmunity 34,* 53-64.

[29] Kwon, H., H. S. Jun, Y. Yang, C. Mora, S. Mariathasan, P. S. Ohashi, R. A. Flavell, & J. W. Yoon. (2005). Development of autoreactive diabetogenic T cells in the thymus of NOD mice. *J Autoimmun 24,* 11-23.

[30] Kishimoto, H. & J. Sprent. (2001). A defect in central tolerance in NOD mice. *Nature immunology* 2, 1025-1031.

[31] Lesage, S., Hartley, S. B., Akkaraju, S., Wilson, J., Townsend, M. & Goodnow, C. C. (2002). Failure to censor forbidden clones of CD4 T cells in autoimmune diabetes. *The Journal of experimental medicine, 196,* 1175-1188.

[32] Anderson, M. S., Venanzi, E. S., Klein, L., Chen, Z., Berzins, S. P., Turley, S. J., von Boehmer, H., Bronson, R., Dierich, A., Benoist, C. & Mathis, D. (2002). Projection of an immunological self shadow within the thymus by the aire protein. *Science, 298,* 1395-1401.

[33] Hubert, F. X., Kinkel, S. A., Webster, K. E., Cannon, P., Crewther, P. E., Proeitto, A. I., Wu, L., Heath, W. R. & Scott, H. S. (2008). A specific anti-Aire antibody reveals aire expression is restricted to medullary thymic epithelial cells and not expressed in periphery. *J Immunol, 180,* 3824-3832.

[34] Jiang, W., Anderson, M. S., Bronson, R., Mathis, D. & Benoist, C. (2005). Modifier loci condition autoimmunity provoked by Aire deficiency. *J Exp Med, 202,* 805-815.

[35] Peterson, P., Org, T. & Rebane, A. (2008). Transcriptional regulation by AIRE: molecular mechanisms of central tolerance. *Nature reviews, 8,* 948-957.

[36] 1997. An autoimmune disease, Apeced, caused by mutations in a novel gene featuring two PHD-type zinc-finger domains. *Nature genetics, 17,* 399-403.

[37] Mathis, D. & Benoist, C. (2009). Aire. *Annual review of immunology, 27,* 287-312.

[38] Anderson, M. S., Venanzi, E. S., Chen, Z., Berzins, S. P., Benoist, C. & Mathis, D. (2005). The cellular mechanism of Aire control of T cell tolerance. *Immunity, 23,* 227-239.

[39] Liston, A., Lesage, S., Wilson, J., Peltonen, L. & Goodnow, C. C. (2003). Aire regulates negative selection of organ-specific T cells. *Nat Immunol, 4,* 350-354.

[40] Liston, A., Gray, D. H., Lesage, S. Fletcher, A. L., Wilson, J., Webster, K. E., Scott, H. S., Boyd, R. L., Peltonen, L. & Goodnow, C. C. (2004). Gene dosage--limiting role of Aire in thymic expression, clonal deletion, & organ-specific autoimmunity. *J Exp Med, 200,* 1015-1026.

[41] Andre, S., Tough, D. F., Lacroix-Desmazes, S., Kaveri, S. V. & Bayry, J. (2009). Surveillance of antigen-presenting cells by CD4+ CD25+ regulatory T cells in autoimmunity: immunopathogenesis and therapeutic implications. *The American journal of pathology, 174,* 1575-1587.

[42] Brusko, T. M., Putnam, A. L. & Bluestone, J. A. (2008). Human regulatory T cells: role in autoimmune disease and therapeutic opportunities. *Immunological reviews, 223,* 371-390.

[43] Chen, W., Jin, W., Hardegen, N., Lei, K. J., Li, L., Marinos, N., McGrady, G. & Wahl. S. M. (2003). Conversion of peripheral CD4+CD25- naive T cells to CD4+CD25+ regulatory T cells by TGF-beta induction of transcription factor Foxp3. *The Journal of experimental medicine, 198,* 1875-1886.

[44] Vignali, D. A., Collison, L. W. & Workman, C. J. (2008). How regulatory T cells work. *Nat Rev Immunol.*

[45] Sakaguchi, S., Yamaguchi, T., Nomura, T. & Ono, M. (2008). Regulatory T cells and immune tolerance. *Cell, 133,* 775-787.

[46] Bussone, G. & Mouthon, L. (2009). Autoimmune manifestations in primary immune deficiencies. *Autoimmunity reviews, 8,* 332-336.

[47] Bennett, C. L., Christie, J., Ramsdell, F., Brunkow, M. E., Ferguson, P. J., Whitesell, L., Kelly, T. E., Saulsbury, F. T., Chance, P. F. & Ochs, H. D. (2001). The immune dysregulation, polyendocrinopathy, enteropathy, X-linked syndrome (IPEX) is caused by mutations of FOXP3. *Nature genetics, 27,* 20-21.

[48] Yamanouchi, J., Rainbow, D., Serra, P., Howlett, S., Hunter, K., Garner, V. E., Gonzalez-Munoz, A., Clark, J., Veijola, R., Cubbon, R., Chen, S. L., Rosa, R., Cumiskey, A. M., Serreze, D. V., Gregory, S., Rogers, J., Lyons, P. A., Healy, B., Smink, L. J., Todd, J. A., Peterson, L. B., Wicker, L. S. & Santamaria, P. (2007). Interleukin-2 gene variation impairs regulatory T cell function and causes autoimmunity. *Nat Genet, 39,* 329-337.

[49] Kamanaka, M., Rainbow, D., Schuster-Gossler, K., Eynon, E. E., Chervonsky, A. V., Wicker, L. S. & Flavell, R. A. (2009). Amino acid polymorphisms altering the

[50] Anderson, A. C., Chandwaskar, R., Lee, D. H. & Kuchroo, V. K. (2008). Cutting Edge, The Idd3 Genetic Interval Determines Regulatory T Cell Function through CD11b+CD11c- APC. *J Immunol, 181,* 7449-7452.

[51] Sgouroudis, E., Albanese, A. & Piccirillo, C. A. (2008). Impact of protective IL-2 allelic variants on CD4+ Foxp3+ regulatory T cell function in situ and resistance to autoimmune diabetes in NOD mice. *J Immunol, 181,* 6283-6292.

[52] Tang, Q., Adams, J. Y., Penaranda, C., Melli, K., Piaggio, E., Sgouroudis, E., Piccirillo, C. A., Salomon, B. L. & Bluestone, J. A. (2008). Central Role of Defective Interleukin-2 Production in the Triggering of Islet Autoimmune Destruction. *Immunity.*

[53] McGuire, H. M., Vogelzang, A., Hill, N., Flodstrom-Tullberg, M., Sprent, J. & King, C. (2009). Loss of parity between IL-2 and IL-21 in the NOD Idd3 locus. *Proc Natl Acad Sci U S A.*

[54] Lambolez, F., Kronenberg, M. & Cheroutre, H. (2007). Thymic differentiation of TCR alpha beta(+) CD8 alpha alpha(+) IELs. *Immunological reviews, 215,* 178-188.

[55] Ford, M. S., Chen, W., Wong, S., Li, C., Vanama, R., Elford, A. R., Asa, S. L., Ohashi, P. S. & Zhang, L. (2007). Peptide-activated double-negative T cells can prevent autoimmune type-1 diabetes development. *European journal of immunology, 37,* 2234-2241.

[56] Gardner, J. M., Devoss, J. J., Friedman, R. S., Wong, D. J., Tan, Y. X., Zhou, X., Johannes, K. P., Su, M. A., Chang, H. Y., Krummel, M. F. & Anderson, M. S. (2008). Deletional tolerance mediated by extrathymic Aire-expressing cells. *Science, 321,* 843-847.

[57] Lee, J. W., Epardaud, M., Sun, J., Becker, J. E., Cheng, A. C., Yonekura, A. R., Heath, J. K. & Turley, S. J. (2007). Peripheral antigen display by lymph node stroma promotes T cell tolerance to intestinal self. *Nature immunology, 8,* 181-190.

[58] Linsley, P. S. & Ledbetter, J. A. (1993). The role of the CD28 receptor during T cell responses to antigen. *Annual review of immunology, 11,* 191-212.

[59] Lesage, S. & Goodnow, C. C. (2001). Organ-specific autoimmune disease: a deficiency of tolerogenic stimulation. *J Exp Med, 194,* F31-36.

[60] Salomon, B., Lenschow, D. J., Rhee, L., Ashourian, N., Singh, B., Sharpe, A. & Bluestone. J. A. (2000). B7/CD28 costimulation is essential for the homeostasis of the CD4+CD25+ immunoregulatory T cells that control autoimmune diabetes. *Immunity, 12,* 431-440.

[61] Zeng, M., Guinet, E. & Nouri-Shirazi, M. (2009). B7-1 and B7-2 differentially control peripheral homeostasis of CD4(+)CD25(+)Foxp3(+) regulatory T cells. *Transplant immunology, 20,* 171-179.

[62] Greenwald, R. J., Freeman, G. J. & Sharpe, A. H. (2005). The B7 family revisited. *Annu Rev Immunol, 23,* 515-548.

[63] Greenwald, R. J., Boussiotis, V. A., Lorsbach, R. B., Abbas, A. K. & Sharpe, A. H. 2001. CTLA-4 regulates induction of anergy in vivo. *Immunity, 14,* 145-155.

[64] Wing, K., Onishi, Y., Prieto-Martin, P., Yamaguchi, T., Miyara, M., Fehervari, Z., Nomura, T. & Sakaguchi, S. (2008). CTLA-4 control over Foxp3+ regulatory T cell function. *Science, 322,* 271-275.

[65] Chambers, C. A., Cado, D., Truong, T. & Allison, J. P. (1997). Thymocyte development is normal in CTLA-4-deficient mice. *Proc Natl Acad Sci U S A, 94,* 9296-9301.

[66] Tivol, E. A., Borriello, F., Schweitzer, A. N., Lynch, W. P., Bluestone, J. A. & Sharpe. A. H. (1995). Loss of CTLA-4 leads to massive lymphoproliferation and fatal multiorgan tissue destruction, revealing a critical negative regulatory role of CTLA-4. *Immunity, 3,* 541-547.

[67] Hill, N. J., Lyons, P. A., Armitage, N., Todd, J. A., Wicker, L. S. & Peterson, L. B. (2000). NOD Idd5 locus controls insulitis and diabetes and overlaps the orthologous CTLA4/IDDM12 and NRAMP1 loci in humans. *Diabetes, 49,* 1744-1747.

[68] Ueda, H., Howson, J. M., Esposito, L., Heward, J., Snook, H., Chamberlain, G., Rainbow, D. B., Hunter, K. M., Smith, A. N., Di Genova, G., Herr, M. H., Dahlman, I., Payne, F., Smyth, D., Lowe, C., Twells, R. C., Howlett, S., Healy, B., Nutland, S., Rance, H. E., Everett, V., Smink, L. J., Lam, A. C., Cordell, H. J., Walker, N. M., Bordin, C., Hulme, J., Motzo, C., Cucca, F., Hess, J. F., Metzker, M. L., Rogers, J., Gregory, S., Allahabadia, A., Nithiyananthan, R., Tuomilehto-Wolf, E., Tuomilehto, J., Bingley, P., Gillespie, K. M., Undlien, D. E., Ronningen, K. S., Guja, C., Ionescu-Tirgoviste, C., Savage, D. A., Maxwell, A. P., Carson, D. J., Patterson, C. C., Franklyn, J. A., Clayton, D. G., Peterson, L. B., Wicker, L. S., Todd, J. A. & Gough, S. C. (2003). Association of the T-cell regulatory gene CTLA4 with susceptibility to autoimmune disease. *Nature, 423,* 506-511.

[69] Maier, L. M. & Hafler, D. A. (2009). Autoimmunity risk alleles in costimulation pathways. *Immunological reviews, 229,* 322-336.

[70] Vijayakrishnan, L., Slavik, J. M., Illes, Z., Greenwald, R. J., Rainbow, D., Greve, B., Peterson, L. B., Hafler, D. A., Freeman, G. J., Sharpe, A. H., Wicker, L. S. & Kuchroo. V. K. (2004). An autoimmune disease-associated CTLA-4 splice variant lacking the B7 binding domain signals negatively in T cells. *Immunity, 20,* 563-575.

[71] Anjos, S. M. & Polychronakos, C. (2006). Functional evaluation of the autoimmunity-associated CTLA4 gene, The effect of the (AT) repeat in the 3'untranslated region (UTR). *J Autoimmun.*

[72] Chen, Z., Stockton, J., Mathis, D. & Benoist, C. (2006). Modeling CTLA4-linked autoimmunity with RNA interference in mice. *Proc Natl Acad Sci U S A 103,* 16400-16405.

[73] Araki, M., Chung, D., Liu, S., Rainbow, D. B., Chamberlain, G., Garner, V., Hunter, K. M., Vijayakrishnan, L., Peterson, L. B., Oukka, M., Sharpe, A. H., Sobel, R., Kuchroo, V. K. & Wicker, L. S. (2009). Genetic evidence that the differential expression of the ligand-independent isoform of CTLA-4 is the molecular basis of the Idd5.1 type 1 diabetes region in nonobese diabetic mice. *J Immunol, 183,* 5146-5157.

[74] Fife, B. T. & Bluestone, J. A. (2008). Control of peripheral T-cell tolerance and autoimmunity via the CTLA-4 and PD-1 pathways. *Immunological reviews, 224,* 166-182.

[75] Nishimura, H., Okazaki, T., Tanaka, Y., Nakatani, K., Hara, M., Matsumori, A., Sasayama, S., Mizoguchi, A., Hiai, H., Minato, N. & Honjo, T. (2001). Autoimmune dilated cardiomyopathy in PD-1 receptor-deficient mice. *Science (New York, N.Y, 291,* 319-322.

[76] Nishimura, H., Nose, M., Hiai, H., Minato, N. & Honjo, T. (1999). Development of lupus-like autoimmune diseases by disruption of the PD-1 gene encoding an ITIM motif-carrying immunoreceptor. *Immunity, 11,* 141-151.

[77] Steinman, L. (2007). A brief history of T(H)17, the first major revision in the T(H)1/T(H)2 hypothesis of T cell-mediated tissue damage. *Nat Med, 13,* 139-145.

[78] Weaver, C. T., Hatton, R. D., Mangan, P. R. & Harrington, L. E. (2007). IL-17 family cytokines and the expanding diversity of effector T cell lineages. *Annu Rev Immunol, 25,* 821-852.

[79] Kroenke, M. A., Carlson, T. J., Andjelkovic, A. V. & Segal, B. M. (2008). IL-12- and IL-23-modulated T cells induce distinct types of EAE based on histology, CNS chemokine profile, & response to cytokine inhibition. *J Exp Med, 205,* 1535-1541.

[80] Ogura, H., Murakami, M., Okuyama, Y., Tsuruoka, M., Kitabayashi, C., Kanamoto, M., Nishihara, M., Iwakura, Y. & Hirano, T. (2008). Interleukin-17 promotes autoimmunity by triggering a positive-feedback loop via interleukin-6 induction. *Immunity, 29,* 628-636.

[81] Rabinovitch, A., Suarez-Pinzon, W. L., Sorensen, O., Bleackley, R. C. & Power, R. F. (1995). IFN-gamma gene expression in pancreatic islet-infiltrating mononuclear cells correlates with autoimmune diabetes in nonobese diabetic mice. *J Immunol, 154,* 4874-4882.

[82] Korn, T., Bettelli, E., Oukka, M. & Kuchroo, V. K. (2009). IL-17 and Th17 Cells. *Annu Rev Immunol.*

[83] Kleinschek, M. A., Owyang, A. M., Joyce-Shaikh, B., Langrish, C. L., Chen, Y., Gorman, D. M., Blumenschein, W. M., McClanahan, T., Brombacher, F., Hurst, S. D., Kastelein, R. A. & Cua, D. J. (2007). IL-25 regulates Th17 function in autoimmune inflammation. *J Exp Med, 204,* 161-170.

[84] Cua, D. J., Sherlock, J., Chen, Y., Murphy, C. A., Joyce, B., Seymour, B., Lucian, L., To, W., Kwan, S., Churakova, T., Zurawski, S., Wiekowski, M., Lira, S. A., Gorman, D., Kastelein, R. A. & Sedgwick, J. D. (2003). Interleukin-23 rather than interleukin-12 is the critical cytokine for autoimmune inflammation of the brain. *Nature, 421,* 744-748.

[85] Adorini, L. (2001). Interleukin 12 and autoimmune diabetes. *Nat Genet, 27,* 131-132.

[86] Zhou, L., Ivanov, II, Spolski, R., Min, R., Shenderov, K., Egawa, T., Levy, D. E., Leonard, W. J. & Littman, D. R. (2007). IL-6 programs T(H)-17 cell differentiation by promoting sequential engagement of the IL-21 and IL-23 pathways. *Nat Immunol, 8,* 967-974.

[87] Huber, M., Brustle, A., Reinhard, K., Guralnik, A., Walter, G., Mahiny, A., von Low, E. & Lohoff, M. (2008). IRF4 is essential for IL-21-mediated induction, amplification, & stabilization of the Th17 phenotype. *Proc Natl Acad Sci U S A, 105,* 20846-20851.

[88] Simpson, P. B., Mistry, M. S., Maki, R. A., Yang, W., Schwarz, D. A., Johnson, E. B., Lio, F. M. & Alleva, D. G. (2003). Cutting edge: diabetes-associated quantitative trait locus, Idd4, is responsible for the IL-12p40 overexpression defect in nonobese diabetic (NOD) mice. *J Immunol, 171,* 3333-3337.

[89] Spolski, R., Kashyap, M., Robinson, C., Yu, Z. & Leonard, W. J. (2008). IL-21 signaling is critical for the development of type I diabetes in the NOD mouse. *Proc Natl Acad Sci U S A.*

[90] Oppmann, B., Lesley, R., Blom, B., Timans, J. C., Xu, Y., Hunte, B., Vega, F., Yu, N., Wang, J., Singh, K., Zonin, F., Vaisberg, E., Churakova, T., Liu, M., Gorman, D., Wagner, J., Zurawski, S., Liu, Y., Abrams, J. S., Moore, K. W., Rennick, D., de Waal-Malefyt, R., Hannum, C., Bazan, J. F. & Kastelein, R. A. (2000). Novel p19 protein engages IL-12p40 to form a cytokine, IL-23, with biological activities similar as well as distinct from IL-12. *Immunity, 13,* 715-725.

[91] Elsaesser, H., Sauer, K. & Brooks, D. G. (2009). IL-21 is required to control chronic viral infection. *Science, 324,* 1569-1572.

[92] Frohlich, A., Kisielow, J., Schmitz, I., Freigang, S., Shamshiev, A. T., Weber, J., Marsland, B. J., Oxenius, A. & Kopf, M. (2009). IL-21R on T cells is critical for sustained functionality and control of chronic viral infection. *Science, 324,* 1576-1580.

[93] Yi, J. S., Du, M. & Zajac, A. J. (2009). A vital role for interleukin-21 in the control of a chronic viral infection. *Science, 324,* 1572-1576.

[94] Sutherland, A. P., Van Belle, T., Wurster, A. L., Suto, A., Michaud, M., Zhang, D., Grusby, M. J. & von Herrath, M. (2009). Interleukin-21 is required for the development of type 1 diabetes in NOD mice. *Diabetes, 58,* 1144-1155.

[95] Gay, D., Saunders, T., Camper, S. & Weigert, M. (1993). Receptor editing: an approach by autoreactive B cells to escape tolerance. *J Exp Med, 177,* 999-1008.

[96] Goodnow, C. C., Crosbie, J., Adelstein, S., Lavoie, T. B., Smith-Gill, S. J., Brink, R. A., Pritchard-Briscoe, H., Wotherspoon, J. S., Loblay, R. H., Raphael, K., et al. (1988). Altered immunoglobulin expression and functional silencing of self-reactive B lymphocytes in transgenic mice. *Nature, 334,* 676-682.

[97] Nemazee, D. A. & Burki, K. (1989). Clonal deletion of B lymphocytes in a transgenic mouse bearing anti-MHC class I antibody genes. *Nature, 337,* 562-566.

[98] Merrell, K. T., Benschop, R. J., Gauld, S. B., Aviszus, K., Decote-Ricardo, D., Wysocki, L. J. & Cambier, J. C. (2006). Identification of anergic B cells within a wild-type repertoire. *Immunity, 25,* 953-962.

[99] Wardemann, H., Yurasov, S., Schaefer, A., Young, J. W., Meffre, E. & Nussenzweig. M. C. (2003). Predominant autoantibody production by early human B cell precursors. *Science, 301,* 1374-1377.

[100] Novobrantseva, T., Xu, S., Tan, J. E., Maruyama, M., Schwers, S., Pelanda, R. & Lam. K. P. (2005). Stochastic pairing of Ig heavy and light chains frequently generates B cell antigen receptors that are subject to editing in vivo. *Int Immunol, 17,* 343-350.

[101] Goodnow, C. C., Sprent, J., Fazekas de St Groth, B. & Vinuesa, C. G. (2005). Cellular and genetic mechanisms of self tolerance and autoimmunity. *Nature, 435,* 590-597.

[102] Braun, D., Caramalho, I. & Demengeot, J. (2002). IFN-alpha/beta enhances BCR-dependent B cell responses. *Int Immunol, 14,* 411-419.

[103] Coro, E. S., Chang, W. L. & Baumgarth, N. (2006). Type I IFN receptor signals directly stimulate local B cells early following influenza virus infection. *J Immunol, 176,* 4343-4351.

[104] Jego, G., Palucka, A. K., Blanck, J. P., Chalouni, C., Pascual, V. & Banchereau, J. (2003). Plasmacytoid dendritic cells induce plasma cell differentiation through type I interferon and interleukin 6. *Immunity, 19,* 225-234.

[105] Le Bon, A., Schiavoni, G., D'Agostino, G., Gresser, I., Belardelli, F. & Tough, D. F. (2001). Type i interferons potently enhance humoral immunity and can promote isotype switching by stimulating dendritic cells in vivo. *Immunity, 14,* 461-470.

[106] Mackay, F. & Schneider, P. (2009). Cracking the BAFF code. *Nat Rev Immunol, 9*, 491-502.

[107] Stadanlick, J. E. & Cancro, M. P. (2008). BAFF and the plasticity of peripheral B cell tolerance. *Curr Opin Immunol, 20*, 158-161.

[108] Brink, R. (2006). Regulation of B cell self-tolerance by BAFF. *Semin Immunol, 18*, 276-283.

[109] Bernasconi, N. L., Onai, N. & Lanzavecchia, A. (2003). A role for Toll-like receptors in acquired immunity: up-regulation of TLR9 by BCR triggering in naive B cells and constitutive expression in memory B cells. *Blood, 101*, 4500-4504.

[110] Meyer-Bahlburg, A. & Rawlings, D. J. (2008). B cell autonomous TLR signaling and autoimmunity. *Autoimmun Rev, 7*, 313-316.

[111] Deng, G. M., Nilsson, I. M., Verdrengh, M., Collins, L. V. & Tarkowski, A. (1999). Intra-articularly localized bacterial DNA containing CpG motifs induces arthritis. *Nat Med, 5*, 702-705.

[112] Segal, B. M., Chang, J. T. & Shevach, E. M. (2000). CpG oligonucleotides are potent adjuvants for the activation of autoreactive encephalitogenic T cells in vivo. *J Immunol, 164*, 5683-5688.

[113] Lang, K. S., Recher, M., Junt, T., Navarini, A. A., Harris, N. L., Freigang, S., Odermatt, B., Conrad, C., Ittner, L. M., Bauer, S., Luther, S. A., Uematsu, S., Akira, S., Hengartner, H. & Zinkernagel, R. M. (2005). Toll-like receptor engagement converts T-cell autoreactivity into overt autoimmune disease. *Nat Med, 11*, 138-145.

[114] Fillatreau, S., Sweenie, C. H., McGeachy, M. J., Gray, D. & Anderton, S. M. (2002). B cells regulate autoimmunity by provision of IL-10. *Nat Immunol, 3*, 944-950.

[115] Mauri, C., Gray, D., Mushtaq, N. & Londei, M. (2003). Prevention of arthritis by interleukin 10-producing B cells. *J Exp Med, 197*, 489-501.

[116] Mizoguchi, A., Mizoguchi, E., Takedatsu, H., Blumberg, R. S. & Bhan. A. K. (2002). Chronic intestinal inflammatory condition generates IL-10-producing regulatory B cell subset characterized by CD1d upregulation. *Immunity, 16*, 219-230.

[117] Duddy, M. E., Alter, A. & Bar-Or, A. (2004). Distinct profiles of human B cell effector cytokines, a role in immune regulation? *J Immunol, 172*, 3422-3427.

[118] Duddy, M., Niino, M., Adatia, F., Hebert, S., Freedman, M., Atkins, H., Kim, H. J. & Bar-Or, A. (2007). Distinct effector cytokine profiles of memory and naive human B cell subsets and implication in multiple sclerosis. *J Immunol, 178*, 6092-6099.

[119] Lampropoulou, V., Hoehlig, K., Roch, T., Neves, P., Calderon Gomez, E., Sweenie, C. H., Hao, Y., Freitas, A. A., Steinhoff, U., Anderton, S. M. & Fillatreau, S. (2008). TLR-activated B cells suppress T cell-mediated autoimmunity. *J Immunol, 180*, 4763-4773.

[120] Kumar, K. R., Li, L., Yan, M., Bhaskarabhatla, M., Mobley, A. B., Nguyen, C., Mooney, J. M., Schatzle, J. D., Wakeland, E. K. & Mohan, C. (2006). Regulation of B cell tolerance by the lupus susceptibility gene Ly108. *Science, 312*, 1665-1669.

[121] Morel, L., Croker, B. P., Blenman, K. R., Mohan, C., Huang, G., Gilkeson, G. & Wakeland. E. K. (2000). Genetic reconstitution of systemic lupus erythematosus immunopathology with polycongenic murine strains. *Proc Natl Acad Sci U S A, 97*, 6670-6675.

[122] Morel, L. & Wakeland, E. K. (2000). Lessons from the NZM2410 model and related strains. *Int Rev Immunol, 19*, 423-446.

[123] Vyse, T. J. & Kotzin, B. L. (1998). Genetic susceptibility to systemic lupus erythematosus. *Annu Rev Immunol, 16,* 261-292.

[124] Vyse, T. J., Rozzo, S. J., Drake, C. G., Appel, V. B., Lemeur, M., Izui, S., Palmer, E. & Kotzin, B. L. (1998). Contributions of Ea(z) and Eb(z) MHC genes to lupus susceptibility in New Zealand mice. *J Immunol, 160,* 2757-2766.

[125] McGaha, T. L., Sorrentino, B. & Ravetch, J. V. (2005). Restoration of tolerance in lupus by targeted inhibitory receptor expression. *Science, 307,* 590-593.

[126] Bolland, S., Yim, Y. S., Tus, K., Wakeland, E. K. & Ravetch, J. V. (2002). Genetic modifiers of systemic lupus erythematosus in FcgammaRIIB(-/-) mice. *J Exp Med 195,* 1167-1174.

[127] Pisitkun, P., Deane, J. A., Difilippantonio, M. J., Tarasenko, T., Satterthwaite, A. B. & Bolland, S. (2006). Autoreactive B cell responses to RNA-related antigens due to TLR7 gene duplication. *Science, 312,* 1669-1672.

[128] Subramanian, S., Tus, K., Li, Q. Z., Wang, A., Tian, X. H., Zhou, J., Liang, C., Bartov, G., McDaniel, L. D., Zhou, X. J., Schultz, R. A. & Wakeland, E. K. (2006). A Tlr7 translocation accelerates systemic autoimmunity in murine lupus. *Proc Natl Acad Sci U S A 103,* 9970-9975.

[129] Kozyrev, S. V., Abelson, A. K., Wojcik, J., Zaghlool, A., Linga Reddy, M. V., Sanchez, E., Gunnarsson, I., Svenungsson, E., Sturfelt, G., Jonsen, A., Truedsson, L., Pons-Estel, B. A., Witte, T., D'Alfonso, S., Barizzone, N., Danieli, M. G., Gutierrez, C., Suarez, A. Junker, P., Laustrup, H., Gonzalez-Escribano, M. F., Martin, J., Abderrahim, H. & Alarcon-Riquelme, M. E. (2008). Functional variants in the B-cell gene BANK1 are associated with systemic lupus erythematosus. *Nat Genet, 40,* 211-216.

[130] Rolf, J., Motta, V., Duarte, N., Lundholm, M., Berntman, E., Bergman, M. L., Sorokin, L., Cardell, S. L. & Holmberg, D. (2005). The enlarged population of marginal zone/CD1d(high) B lymphocytes in nonobese diabetic mice maps to diabetes susceptibility region Idd11. *J Immunol, 174,* 4821-4827.

[131] Blank, M. & Shoenfeld, Y. (2007). B cell targeted therapy in autoimmunity. *J Autoimmun, 28,* 62-68.

[132] Perosa, F., Favoino, E., Caragnano, M. A., Prete, M. & Dammacco, F. (2005). CD20, a target antigen for immunotherapy of autoimmune diseases. *Autoimmun Rev, 4,* 526-531.

[133] Steinman, R. M. & Cohn, Z. A. (1973). Identification of a novel cell type in peripheral lymphoid organs of mice. I. Morphology, quantitation, tissue distribution. *J Exp Med, 137,* 1142-1162.

[134] Steinman, R. M. & Cohn, Z. A. (1974). Identification of a novel cell type in peripheral lymphoid organs of mice. II. Functional properties in vitro. *J Exp Med, 139,* 380-397.

[135] Steinman, R. M., Lustig, D. S. & Cohn, Z. A. (1974). Identification of a novel cell type in peripheral lymphoid organs of mice. 3. Functional properties in vivo. *J Exp Med, 139,* 1431-1445.

[136] Steinman, R. M., Adams, J. C. & Cohn, Z. A. (1975). Identification of a novel cell type in peripheral lymphoid organs of mice. IV. Identification and distribution in mouse spleen. *J Exp Med, 141,* 804-820.

[137] Steinman, R. M., Kaplan, G., Witmer, M. D. & Cohn, Z. A. (1979). Identification of a novel cell type in peripheral lymphoid organs of mice. V. Purification of spleen dendritic cells, new surface markers, & maintenance in vitro. *J Exp Med, 149,* 1-16.

[138] Steinman, R. M., Gutchinov, B., Witmer, M. D. & Nussenzweig. M. C. (1983). Dendritic cells are the principal stimulators of the primary mixed leukocyte reaction in mice. *J Exp Med, 157,* 613-627.

[139] Goldschneider, I. & Cone, R. E. (2003). A central role for peripheral dendritic cells in the induction of acquired thymic tolerance. *Trends Immunol, 24,* 77-81.

[140] Vremec, D., Pooley, J., Hochrein, H., Wu, L. & Shortman, K. (2000). CD4 and CD8 expression by dendritic cell subtypes in mouse thymus and spleen. *J Immunol, 164,* 2978-2986.

[141] Lahoud, M. H., Proietto, A. I., Gartlan, K. H., Kitsoulis, S., Curtis, J., Wettenhall, J., Sofi, M., Daunt, C., O'Keeffe, M., Caminschi, I., Satterley, K., Rizzitelli, A., Schnorrer, P., Hinohara, A., Yamaguchi, Y., Wu, L., Smyth, G., Handman, E., Shortman, K. & Wright, M. D. (2006). Signal regulatory protein molecules are differentially expressed by CD8- dendritic cells. *J Immunol, 177,* 372-382.

[142] Donskoy, E. & Goldschneider, I. (2003). Two developmentally distinct populations of dendritic cells inhabit the adult mouse thymus: demonstration by differential importation of hematogenous precursors under steady state conditions. *J Immunol, 170,* 3514-3521.

[143] Proietto, A. I., van Dommelen, S. & Wu, L. (2009). The impact of circulating dendritic cells on the development and differentiation of thymocytes. *Immunol Cell Biol, 87,* 39-45.

[144] Proietto, A. I., van Dommelen, S., Zhou, P., Rizzitelli, A., D'Amico, A., Steptoe, R. J., Naik, S. H., Lahoud, M. H., Liu, Y., Zheng, P., Shortman, K. & Wu, L. (2008). Dendritic cells in the thymus contribute to T-regulatory cell induction. *Proc Natl Acad Sci U S A, 105,* 19869-19874.

[145] Lindberg, F. P., Bullard, D. C., Caver, T. E., Gresham, H. D., Beaudet, A. L. & Brown. E. J. (1996). Decreased resistance to bacterial infection and granulocyte defects in IAP-deficient mice. *Science, 274,* 795-798.

[146] Liu, Y., Buhring, H. J., Zen, K., Burst, S. L., Schnell, F. J., Williams, I. R. & Parkos. C. A. (2002). Signal regulatory protein (SIRPalpha), a cellular ligand for CD47, regulates neutrophil transmigration. *J Biol Chem, 277,* 10028-10036.

[147] Hagnerud, S., Manna, P. P., Cella, M., Stenberg, A., Frazier, W. A., Colonna, M. & Oldenborg. P. A. (2006). Deficit of CD47 Results in a Defect of Marginal Zone Dendritic Cells, Blunted Immune Response to Particulate Antigen and Impairment of Skin Dendritic Cell Migration. *J Immunol, 176,* 5772-5778.

[148] Van, V. Q., Lesage, S., Bouguermouh, S., Gautier, P., Rubio, M., Levesque, M., Nguyen, S., Galibert, L. & Sarfati, M. (2006). Expression of the self-marker CD47 on dendritic cells governs their trafficking to secondary lymphoid organs. *Embo J, 25,* 5560-5568.

[149] Guimont-Desrochers, F., Beauchamp, C., Chabot-Roy, G., Dugas, V., Hillhouse, E. E., Dusseault, J., Langlois, G., Gautier-Ethier, P., Darwiche, J., Sarfati, M. & Lesage, S. (2009). Absence of CD47 in vivo influences thymic dendritic cell subset proportions but not negative selection of thymocytes. *Int Immunol, 21,* 167-177.

[150] O'Keeffe, M., Brodnicki, T. C., Fancke, B., Vremec, D., Morahan, G., Maraskovsky, E., Steptoe, R., Harrison, L. C. & Shortman, K. (2005). Fms-like tyrosine kinase 3 ligand administration overcomes a genetically determined dendritic cell deficiency in NOD mice and protects against diabetes development. *Int Immunol, 17,* 307-314.

[151] Ohnmacht, C., Pullner, A., King, S. B. S., Drexler, I., Meier, S., Brocker, T. & Voehringer, D. (2009). Constitutive ablation of dendritic cells breaks self-tolerance of CD4 T cells and results in spontaneous fatal autoimmunity. *J Exp Med, 206,* 549-559.

[152] Chen, M., Wang, Y. H., Wang, Y., Huang, L., Sandoval, H., Liu, Y. J. & Wang, J. (2006). Dendritic cell apoptosis in the maintenance of immune tolerance. *Science 311,* 1160-1164.

[153] Shortman, K. & Naik, S. H. (2007). Steady-state and inflammatory dendritic-cell development. *Nat Rev Immunol, 7,* 19-30.

[154] Turley, S., Poirot, L., Hattori, M., Benoist, C. & Mathis, D. (2003). Physiological beta cell death triggers priming of self-reactive T cells by dendritic cells in a type-1 diabetes model. *J Exp Med, 198,* 1527-1537.

[155] Saxena, V., Ondr, J. K., Magnusen, A. F., Munn, D. H. & Katz, J. D. (2007). The countervailing actions of myeloid and plasmacytoid dendritic cells control autoimmune diabetes in the nonobese diabetic mouse. *J Immunol, 179,* 5041-5053.

[156] Hawiger, D., Inaba, K., Dorsett, Y., Guo, M., Mahnke, K., Rivera, M., Ravetch, J. V., Steinman, R. M. & Nussenzweig, M. C. (2001). Dendritic cells induce peripheral T cell unresponsiveness under steady state conditions in vivo. *J Exp Med, 194,* 769-779.

[157] Bonifaz, L., Bonnyay, D., Mahnke, K., Rivera, M., Nussenzweig, M. C. & Steinman. R. M. (2002). Efficient targeting of protein antigen to the dendritic cell receptor DEC-205 in the steady state leads to antigen presentation on major histocompatibility complex class I products and peripheral CD8+ T cell tolerance. *J Exp Med, 196,* 1627-1638.

[158] Qiu, C. H., Miyake, Y., Kaise, H., Kitamura, H., Ohara, O. & Tanaka, M. (2009). Novel Subset of CD8 + Dendritic Cells Localized in the Marginal Zone Is Responsible for Tolerance to Cell-Associated Antigens. *The Journal of Immunology, 182,* 4127-4136.

[159] Belz, G. T., Behrens, G. M. N., Smith, C. M., Miller, J. F. A. P., Jones, C., Lejon, K., Fathman, C. G., Mueller, S. N., Shortman, K., Carbone, F. R. & Heath, W. R. (2002). The CD8alpha(+) dendritic cell is responsible for inducing peripheral self-tolerance to tissue-associated antigens. *J Exp Med, 196,* 1099-1104.

[160] Wu, L., D'Amico, A., Winkel, K. D., Suter, M., Lo, D. & Shortman, K. (1998). RelB is essential for the development of myeloid-related CD8alpha- dendritic cells but not of lymphoid-related CD8alpha+ dendritic cells. *Immunity, 9,* 839-847.

[161] Weih, F., Carrasco, D., Durham, S. K., Barton, D. S., Rizzo, C. A., Ryseck, R. P., Lira, S. A. & Bravo, R. (1995). Multiorgan inflammation and hematopoietic abnormalities in mice with a targeted disruption of RelB, a member of the NF-kappa B/Rel family. *Cell, 80,* 331-340.

[162] Ichikawa, E., Hida, S., Omatsu, Y., Shimoyama, S., Takahara, K., Miyagawa, S., Inaba, K. & Taki, S. (2004). Defective development of splenic and epidermal CD4+ dendritic cells in mice deficient for IFN regulatory factor-2. *Proc Natl Acad Sci U S A, 101,* 3909-3914.

[163] Schiavoni, G., Mattei, F., Sestili, P., Borghi, P., Venditti, M., Morse, H. C., 3rd, Belardelli, F. & Gabriele, L. (2002). ICSBP is essential for the development of mouse type I interferon-producing cells and for the generation and activation of CD8alpha(+) dendritic cells. *J Exp Med, 196,* 1415-1425.

[164] Aliberti, J., Schulz, O., Pennington, D. J., Tsujimura, H., Reis e Sousa, C., Ozato, K. & Sher, A. (2003). Essential role for ICSBP in the in vivo development of murine CD8alpha + dendritic cells. *Blood, 101,* 305-310.

[165] Suzuki, S., Honma, K., Matsuyama, T., Suzuki, K., Toriyama, K., Akitoyo, I., Yamamoto, K., Suematsu, T., Nakamura, M., Yui, K. & Kumatori, A. (2004). Critical roles of interferon regulatory factor 4 in CD11bhighCD8alpha- dendritic cell development. *Proc Natl Acad Sci U S A, 101*, 8981-8986.

[166] Tamura, T., Tailor, P., Yamaoka, K., Kong, H. J., Tsujimura, H., O'Shea, J. J., Singh, H. & Ozato, K. (2005). IFN regulatory factor-4 and -8 govern dendritic cell subset development and their functional diversity. *J Immunol, 174*, 2573-2581.

[167] Kobayashi, T., Walsh, P. T., Walsh, M. C., Speirs, K. M., Chiffoleau, E., King, C. G., Hancock, W. W., Caamano, J. H., Hunter, C. A., Scott, P., Turka, L. A. & Choi, Y. (2003). TRAF6 is a critical factor for dendritic cell maturation and development. *Immunity, 19*, 353-363.

[168] Ochando, J. C., Homma, C., Yang, Y., Hidalgo, A., Garin, A., Tacke, F., Angeli, V., Li, Y., Boros, P., Ding, Y., Jessberger, R., Trinchieri, G., Lira, S. A., Randolph, G. J. & Bromberg. J. S. (2006). Alloantigen-presenting plasmacytoid dendritic cells mediate tolerance to vascularized grafts. *Nat Immunol, 7*, 652-662.

[169] Chen, W., Liang, X., Peterson, A. J., Munn, D. H. & Blazar. B. R. (2008). The indoleamine 2,3-dioxygenase pathway is essential for human plasmacytoid dendritic cell-induced adaptive T regulatory cell generation. *J Immunol, 181*, 5396-5404.

[170] Chan, C., Crafton, E., Fan, H., Flook, J., Yoshimura, K., Skarica, M., Brockstedt, D., Dubensky, T., Stins, M., Lanier, L., Pardoll, D. & Housseau, F. (2006). Interferon-producing killer dendritic cells provide a link between innate and adaptive immunity. *Nat Med, 12*, 207-213.

[171] Himoudi, N., Yan, M., Bouma, G., Morgenstern, D., Wallace, R., Seddon, B., Buddle, J., Eddaoudi, A., Howe, S. J., Cooper, N. & Anderson, J. (2009). Migratory and antigen presentation functions of IFN-producing killer dendritic cells. *Cancer Res, 69*, 6598-6606.

[172] Pletneva, M., Fan, H., Park, J. J., Radojcic, V., Jie, C., Yu, Y., Chan, C., Redwood, A., Pardoll, D. & Housseau, F. (2009). IFN-producing killer dendritic cells are antigen-presenting cells endowed with T-cell cross-priming capacity. *Cancer Res, 69*, 6607-6614.

[173] Terme, M., Mignot, G., Ullrich, E., Bonmort, M., Minard-Colin, V., Jacquet, A., Schultze, J. L., Kroemer, G., Leclerc, C., Chaput, N. & Zitvogel, L. (2009). The dendritic cell-like functions of IFN-producing killer dendritic cells reside in the CD11b+ subset and are licensed by tumor cells. *Cancer Res, 69*, 6590-6597.

[174] Clare-Salzler, M. J., Brooks, J., Chai, A., Van Herle, K. & Anderson, C. (1992). Prevention of diabetes in nonobese diabetic mice by dendritic cell transfer. *J Clin Invest 90*, 741-748.

[175] Schulze, C., Munoz, L. E., Franz, S., Sarter, K., Chaurio, R. A., Gaipl, U. S. & Herrmann, M. (2008). Clearance deficiency--a potential link between infections and autoimmunity. *Autoimmunity reviews, 8*, 5-8.

[176] Wermeling, F., Karlsson, M. C. & McGaha, T. L. (2009). An anatomical view on macrophages in tolerance. *Autoimmunity reviews, 9*, 49-52.

[177] Lleo, A., Selmi, C., Invernizzi, P., Podda, M. & Gershwin, M. E. (2008). The consequences of apoptosis in autoimmunity. *Journal of autoimmunity, 31*, 257-262.

[178] Lu, J. H., Teh, B. K., Wang, L., Wang, Y. N., Tan, Y. S., Lai, M. C. & Reid. K. B. (2008). The classical and regulatory functions of C1q in immunity and autoimmunity. *Cellular & molecular immunology, 5,* 9-21.

[179] Gershov, D., Kim, S., Brot, N. & Elkon, K. B. (2000). C-Reactive protein binds to apoptotic cells, protects the cells from assembly of the terminal complement components, & sustains an antiinflammatory innate immune response, implications for systemic autoimmunity. *The Journal of experimental medicine, 192,* 1353-1364.

[180] Botto, M., Dell'Agnola, C., Bygrave, A. E., Thompson, E. M., Cook, H. T., Petry, F., Loos, M., Pandolfi, P. P. & Walport, M. J. (1998). Homozygous C1q deficiency causes glomerulonephritis associated with multiple apoptotic bodies. *Nature genetics, 19,* 56-59.

[181] Matlack, R., Yeh, K., Rosini, L., Gonzalez, D., Taylor, J., Silberman, D., Pennello, A. & Riggs, J. (2006). Peritoneal macrophages suppress T-cell activation by amino acid catabolism. *Immunology, 117,* 386-395.

[182] Gajewski, T. F., Meng, Y. & Harlin. H. (2006). Immune suppression in the tumor microenvironment. *J Immunother, 29,* 233-240.

[183] Wei, X. Q., Charles, I. G., Smith, A., Ure, J., Feng, G. J., Huang, F. P., Xu, D., Muller, W., Moncada, S. & Liew, F. Y. (1995). Altered immune responses in mice lacking inducible nitric oxide synthase. *Nature, 375,* 408-411.

[184] Kahl, K. G., Schmidt, H. H., Jung, S., Sherman, P., Toyka, K. V. & Zielasek, J. (2004). Experimental autoimmune encephalomyelitis in mice with a targeted deletion of the inducible nitric oxide synthase gene: increased T-helper 1 response. *Neuroscience letters, 358,* 58-62.

[185] Fenyk-Melody, J. E., Garrison, A. E., Brunnert, S. R., Weidner, J. R., Shen, F., Shelton, B. A. & Mudgett. J. S. (1998). Experimental autoimmune encephalomyelitis is exacerbated in mice lacking the NOS2 gene. *J Immunol, 160,* 2940-2946.

[186] Hoves, S., Krause, S. W., Schutz, C., Halbritter, D., Scholmerich, J., Herfarth, H. & Fleck, M. (2006). Monocyte-derived human macrophages mediate anergy in allogeneic T cells and induce regulatory T cells. *J Immunol, 177,* 2691-2698.

[187] Kosiewicz, M. M., Alard, P., Liang, S. & Clark, S. L. (2004). Mechanisms of tolerance induced by transforming growth factor-beta-treated antigen-presenting cells, CD8 regulatory T cells inhibit the effector phase of the immune response in primed mice through a mechanism involving Fas ligand. *International immunology, 16,* 697-706.

[188] Alard, P., Clark, S. L. & Kosiewicz, M. M. (2004). Mechanisms of tolerance induced by TGF beta-treated APC: CD4 regulatory T cells prevent the induction of the immune response possibly through a mechanism involving TGF beta. *European journal of immunology, 34,* 1021-1030.

[189] Shultz, L. D., Schweitzer, P. A., Christianson, S. W., Gott, B., Schweitzer, I. B., Tennent, B., McKenna, S., Mobraaten, L., Rajan, T. V., Greiner, D. L. et al. (1995). Multiple defects in innate and adaptive immunologic function in NOD/LtSz-scid mice. *J Immunol, 154,* 180-191.

[190] Kissler, S., Stern, P., Takahashi, K., Hunter, K., Peterson, L. B. & Wicker. L. S. (2006). In vivo RNA interference demonstrates a role for Nramp1 in modifying susceptibility to type 1 diabetes. *Nature genetics, 38,* 479-483.

[191] Marleau, A. M., Summers, K. L. & Singh, B. (2008). Differential Contributions of APC Subsets to T Cell Activation in Nonobese Diabetic Mice. *J Immunol, 180,* 5235-5249.

[192] Vidal, S. M., Malo, D., Vogan, K., Skamene, E. & Gros, P. (1993). Natural resistance to infection with intracellular parasites: isolation of a candidate for Bcg. *Cell, 73,* 469-485.

[193] Gruenheid, S., Pinner, E., Desjardins, M. & Gros, P. (1997). Natural resistance to infection with intracellular pathogens: the Nramp1 protein is recruited to the membrane of the phagosome. *The Journal of experimental medicine, 185,* 717-730.

[194] Gruenheid, S. & Gros, P. (2000). Genetic susceptibility to intracellular infections: Nramp1, macrophage function and divalent cations transport. *Current opinion in microbiology, 3,* 43-48.

[195] Soe-Lin, S., Apte, S. S., Andriopoulos, B., Jr., Andrews, M. C., Schranzhofer, M., Kahawita, T., Garcia-Santos, D. & Ponka, P. (2009). Nramp1 promotes efficient macrophage recycling of iron following erythrophagocytosis in vivo. *Proceedings of the National Academy of Sciences of the United States of America, 106,* 5960-5965.

[196] Raulet, D. H. & Guerra, N. (2009). Oncogenic stress sensed by the immune system: role of natural killer cell receptors. *Nat Rev Immunol, 9,* 568-580.

[197] Smith, B. R., Rosenthal, D. S. & Ault, K. A. (1985). Natural killer lymphocytes in hairy cell leukemia: presence of phenotypically identifiable cells with defective functional activity. *Exp Hematol, 13,* 189-193.

[198] Igarashi, H., Gregory, S. C., Yokota, T., Sakaguchi, N. & Kincade, P. W. (2002). Transcription from the RAG1 locus marks the earliest lymphocyte progenitors in bone marrow. *Immunity, 17,* 117-130.

[199] Kondo, M., Weissman, I. L. & Akashi, K. (1997). Identification of clonogenic common lymphoid progenitors in mouse bone marrow. *Cell, 91,* 661-672.

[200] Carlyle, J. R., Michie, A. M., Cho, S. K. & Zuniga-Pflucker, J. C. (1998). Natural killer cell development and function precede alpha beta T cell differentiation in mouse fetal thymic ontogeny. *J Immunol, 160,* 744-753.

[201] Spits, H., Lanier, L. L. & Phillips, J. H. (1995). Development of human T and natural killer cells. *Blood, 85,* 2654-2670.

[202] Di Santo, J. P. (2006). Natural killer cell developmental pathways: a question of balance. *Annu Rev Immunol, 24,* 257-286.

[203] Rosmaraki, E. E., Douagi, I., Roth, C., Colucci, F., Cumano, A. & Di Santo, J. P. (2001). Identification of committed NK cell progenitors in adult murine bone marrow. *Eur J Immunol, 31,* 1900-1909.

[204] Di Santo, J. P. & Vosshenrich, C. A. (2006). Bone marrow versus thymic pathways of natural killer cell development. *Immunol Rev, 214,* 35-46.

[205] Vossen, M. T., Matmati, M., Hertoghs, K. M., Baars, P. A., Gent, M. R., Leclercq, G., Hamann, J., Kuijpers, T. W. & van Lier, R. A. (2008). CD27 defines phenotypically and functionally different human NK cell subsets. *J Immunol, 180,* 3739-3745.

[206] Chiossone, L., Chaix, J., Fuseri, N., Roth, C., Vivier, E. & Walzer, T. (2009). Maturation of mouse NK cells is a 4-stage developmental program. *Blood, 113,* 5488-5496.

[207] Hayakawa, Y. & Smyth, M. J. (2006). CD27 dissects mature NK cells into two subsets with distinct responsiveness and migratory capacity. *J Immunol, 176,* 1517-1524.

[208] Silva, A., Andrews, D. M., Brooks, A. G., Smyth, M. J. & Hayakawa, Y. (2008). Application of CD27 as a marker for distinguishing human NK cell subsets. *Int Immunol, 20,* 625-630.

[209] Takeda, K., Cretney, E., Hayakawa, Y., Ota, T., Akiba, H., Ogasawara, K., Yagita, H., Kinoshita, K., Okumura, K. & Smyth, M. J. (2005). TRAIL identifies immature natural killer cells in newborn mice and adult mouse liver. *Blood, 105,* 2082-2089.

[210] Kim, S., Iizuka, K., Kang, H. S., Dokun, A., French, A. R., Greco, S. & Yokoyama. W. M. (2002). In vivo developmental stages in murine natural killer cell maturation. *Nat Immunol, 3,* 523-528.

[211] Hayakawa, Y., Huntington, N. D., Nutt, S. L. & Smyth, M. J. (2006). Functional subsets of mouse natural killer cells. *Immunol Rev, 214,* 47-55.

[212] Roder, J. C., Argov, S., Klein, M., Petersson, C., Kiessling, R., Andersson, K. & Hansson, M. (1980). Target-effector cell interaction in the natural killer cell system. V. Energy requirements, membrane integrity, & the possible involvement of lysosomal enzymes. *Immunology, 40,* 107-116.

[213] Dean, J. H., Silva, J. S., Mc, C. J., Leonard, C. M., Cannon, G. B. & Herberman, R. B. (1975). Functional activities of rosette separated human peripheral blood leukocytes. *J Immunol, 115,* 1449-1455.

[214] Liu, C. C., Walsh, C. M., Eto, N., Clark, W. R. & Young, J. D. (1995). Morphologic and functional characterization of perforin-deficient lymphokine-activated killer cells. *J Immunol, 155,* 602-608.

[215] Arase, H., Arase, N. & Saito, T. (1995). Fas-mediated cytotoxicity by freshly isolated natural killer cells. *J Exp Med, 181,* 1235-1238.

[216] Kashii, Y., Giorda, R., Herberman, R. B., Whiteside, T. L. & Vujanovic, N. L. (1999). Constitutive expression and role of the TNF family ligands in apoptotic killing of tumor cells by human NK cells. *J Immunol, 163,* 5358-5366.

[217] Cooper, M. A., Fehniger, T. A. & Caligiuri, M. A. (2001). The biology of human natural killer-cell subsets. *Trends Immunol, 22,* 633-640.

[218] Robertson, M. J. (2002). Role of chemokines in the biology of natural killer cells. *J Leukoc Biol, 71,* 173-183.

[219] Cosman, D., Mullberg, J., Sutherland, C. L., Chin, W., Armitage, R., Fanslow, W., Kubin, M. & Chalupny, N. J. (2001). ULBPs, novel MHC class I-related molecules, bind to CMV glycoprotein UL16 and stimulate NK cytotoxicity through the NKG2D receptor. *Immunity, 14,* 123-133.

[220] Strowig, T., Brilot, F. & Munz, C. (2008). Noncytotoxic functions of NK cells: direct pathogen restriction and assistance to adaptive immunity. *J Immunol, 180,* 7785-7791.

[221] Karre, K., Ljunggren, H. G., Piontek, G. & Kiessling, R. (1986). Selective rejection of H-2-deficient lymphoma variants suggests alternative immune defence strategy. *Nature, 319,* 675-678.

[222] Garcia-Lora, A., Algarra, I. & Garrido, F. (2003). MHC class I antigens, immune surveillance, & tumor immune escape. *J Cell Physiol, 195,* 346-355.

[223] Karlhofer, F. M., Ribaudo, R. K. & Yokoyama, W. M. (1992). MHC class I alloantigen specificity of Ly-49+ IL-2-activated natural killer cells. *Nature, 358,* 66-70.

[224] Colonna, M. & Samaridis, J. (1995). Cloning of immunoglobulin-superfamily members associated with HLA-C and HLA-B recognition by human natural killer cells. *Science, 268,* 405-408.

[225] D'Andrea, A., Chang, C., Franz-Bacon, K., McClanahan, T., Phillips, J. H. & Lanier, L. L. (1995). Molecular cloning of NKB1. A natural killer cell receptor for HLA-B allotypes. *J Immunol, 155,* 2306-2310.

[226] Yokoyama, W. M. & Seaman, W. E. (1993). The Ly-49 and NKR-P1 gene families encoding lectin-like receptors on natural killer cells: the NK gene complex. *Annu Rev Immunol, 11,* 613-635.

[227] Brennan, J., Mager, D., Jefferies, W. & Takei, F. (1994). Expression of different members of the Ly-49 gene family defines distinct natural killer cell subsets and cell adhesion properties. *J Exp Med, 180,* 2287-2295.

[228] Raulet, D. H., Held, W., Correa, I., Dorfman, J. R., Wu, M. F. & Corral, L. (1997). Specificity, tolerance and developmental regulation of natural killer cells defined by expression of class I-specific Ly49 receptors. *Immunol Rev, 155,* 41-52.

[229] Mo, X. Y., Sangster, M., Sarawar, S., Coleclough, C. & Doherty, P. C. (1995). Differential antigen burden modulates the gamma interferon but not the immunoglobulin response in mice that vary in susceptibility to Sendai virus pneumonia. *J Virol, 69,* 5592-5598.

[230] Mayer, A., Lilly, F. & Duran-Reynals, M. L. (1980). Genetically dominant resistance in mice to 3-methylcholanthrene-induced lymphoma. *Proc Natl Acad Sci U S A, 77,* 2960-2963.

[231] Lotzova, E., Dicke, K. A., Trentin, J. J. & Gallagher, M. T. (1977). Genetic control of bone marrow transplantation in irradiated mice: classification of mouse strains according to their responsiveness to bone marrow allografts and xenografts. *Transplant Proc, 9,* 289-292.

[232] Silver, E. T., Gong, D., Hazes, B. & Kane, K. P. (2001). Ly-49W, an activating receptor of nonobese diabetic mice with close homology to the inhibitory receptor Ly-49G, recognizes H-2D(k) and H-2D(d). *J Immunol, 166,* 2333-2341.

[233] Makrigiannis, A. P. & Anderson, S. K. (2003). Regulation of natural killer cell function. *Cancer Biol Ther, 2,* 610-616.

[234] Groh, V., Rhinehart, R., Secrist, H., Bauer, S., Grabstein, K. H. & Spies, T. (1999). Broad tumor-associated expression and recognition by tumor-derived gamma delta T cells of MICA and MICB. *Proc Natl Acad Sci U S A, 96,* 6879-6884.

[235] Diefenbach, A., Jensen, E. R., Jamieson, A. M. & Raulet, D. H. (2001). Rae1 and H60 ligands of the NKG2D receptor stimulate tumour immunity. *Nature, 413,* 165-171.

[236] Pende, D., Parolini, S., Pessino, A., Sivori, S., Augugliaro, R., Morelli, L., Marcenaro, E., Accame, L., Malaspina, A., Biassoni, R., Bottino, C., Moretta, L. & Moretta, A. (1999). Identification and molecular characterization of NKp30, a novel triggering receptor involved in natural cytotoxicity mediated by human natural killer cells. *J Exp Med, 190,* 1505-1516.

[237] Vitale, M., Bottino, C., Sivori, S., Sanseverino, L., Castriconi, R., Marcenaro, E., Augugliaro, R., Moretta, L. & Moretta, A. (1998). NKp44, a novel triggering surface molecule specifically expressed by activated natural killer cells, is involved in non-major histocompatibility complex-restricted tumor cell lysis. *J Exp Med, 187,* 2065-2072.

[238] Sivori, S., Vitale, M., Morelli, L., Sanseverino, L., Augugliaro, R., Bottino, C., Moretta, L. & Moretta, A. (1997). p46, a novel natural killer cell-specific surface molecule that mediates cell activation. *J Exp Med, 186,* 1129-1136.

[239] Moretta, A., Vitale, M., Sivori, S., Bottino, C., Morelli, L., Augugliaro, R., Barbaresi, M., Pende, D., Ciccone, E., Lopez-Botet, M. & Moretta, L. (1994). Human natural

killer cell receptors for HLA-class I molecules. Evidence that the Kp43 (CD94) molecule functions as receptor for HLA-B alleles. *J Exp Med, 180,* 545-555.

[240] Carlyle, J. R., Martin, A., Mehra, A., Attisano, L., Tsui, F. W. & Zuniga-Pflucker, J. C. (1999). Mouse NKR-P1B, a novel NK1.1 antigen with inhibitory function. *J Immunol 162,* 5917-5923.

[241] Brown, M. H., Boles, K., van der Merwe, P. A., Kumar, V., Mathew, P. A. & Barclay, A. N. (1998). 2B4, the natural killer and T cell immunoglobulin superfamily surface protein, is a ligand for CD48. *J Exp Med, 188,* 2083-2090.

[242] Grunebaum, E., Malatzky-Goshen, E. & Shoenfeld, Y. (1989). Natural killer cells and autoimmunity. *Immunol Res, 8,* 292-304.

[243] Baxter, A. G. & Smyth, M. J. (2002). The role of NK cells in autoimmune disease. *Autoimmunity, 35,* 1-14.

[244] Shibatomi, K., Ida, H., Yamasaki, S., Nakashima, T., Origuchi, T., Kawakami, A., Migita, K., Kawabe, Y., Tsujihata, M., Anderson, P. & Eguchi, K. (2001). A novel role for interleukin-18 in human natural killer cell death, high serum levels and low natural killer cell numbers in patients with systemic autoimmune diseases. *Arthritis Rheum, 44,* 884-892.

[245] Grom, A. A., Villanueva, J., Lee, S., Goldmuntz, E. A., Passo, M. H. & Filipovich, A. (2003). Natural killer cell dysfunction in patients with systemic-onset juvenile rheumatoid arthritis and macrophage activation syndrome. *J Pediatr, 142,* 292-296.

[246] Hammarberg, H., Lidman, O., Lundberg, C., Eltayeb, S. Y., Gielen, A. W., Muhallab, S., Svenningsson, A., Linda, H., van Der Meide, P. H., Cullheim, S., Olsson, T. & Piehl, F. (2000). Neuroprotection by encephalomyelitis: rescue of mechanically injured neurons and neurotrophin production by CNS-infiltrating T and natural killer cells. *J Neurosci, 20,* 5283-5291.

[247] Zhang, B., Yamamura, T., Kondo, T., Fujiwara, M. & Tabira, T. (1997). Regulation of experimental autoimmune encephalomyelitis by natural killer (NK) cells. *J Exp Med, 186,* 1677-1687.

[248] Matsumoto, Y., Kohyama, K., Aikawa, Y., Shin, T., Kawazoe, Y., Suzuki, Y. & Tanuma, N. (1998). Role of natural killer cells and TCR gamma delta T cells in acute autoimmune encephalomyelitis. *Eur J Immunol, 28,* 1681-1688.

[249] Smeltz, R. B., Wolf, N. A. & Swanborg, R. H. (1999). Inhibition of autoimmune T cell responses in the DA rat by bone marrow-derived NK cells in vitro: implications for autoimmunity. *J Immunol, 163,* 1390-1397.

[250] Nedvetzki, S., Sowinski, S., Eagle, R. A., Harris, J., Vely, F., Pende, D., Trowsdale, J., Vivier, E. Gordon, S. & Davis, D. M. (2007). Reciprocal regulation of human natural killer cells and macrophages associated with distinct immune synapses. *Blood, 109,* 3776-3785.

[251] Lee, I. F., Qin, H., Trudeau, J., Dutz, J. & Tan, R. (2004). Regulation of autoimmune diabetes by complete Freund's adjuvant is mediated by NK cells. *J Immunol, 172,* 937-942.

[252] Colucci, F., Di Santo, J. P. & Leibson, P. J. (2002). Natural killer cell activation in mice and men: different triggers for similar weapons? *Nat Immunol, 3,* 807-813.

[253] Loza, M. J., Zamai, L., Azzoni, L., Rosati, E. & Perussia, B. (2002). Expression of type 1 (interferon gamma) and type 2 (interleukin-13, interleukin-5) cytokines at distinct stages of natural killer cell differentiation from progenitor cells. *Blood, 99,* 1273-1281.

[254] Lauwerys, B. R., Garot, N., Renauld, J. C. & Houssiau, F. A. (2000). Cytokine production and killer activity of NK/T-NK cells derived with IL-2, IL-*15,* or the combination of IL-12 and IL-18. *J Immunol, 165,* 1847-1853.

[255] Shi, F. D., Wang, H. B., Li, H., Hong, S., Taniguchi, M., Link, H., Van Kaer, L. & Ljunggren, H. G. (2000). Natural killer cells determine the outcome of B cell-mediated autoimmunity. *Nat Immunol, 1,* 245-251.

[256] Flodstrom, M., Maday, A., Balakrishna, D., Cleary, M. M., Yoshimura, A. & Sarvetnick, N. (2002). Target cell defense prevents the development of diabetes after viral infection. *Nat Immunol, 3,* 373-382.

[257] Poirot, L., Benoist, C. & Mathis, D. (2004). Natural killer cells distinguish innocuous and destructive forms of pancreatic islet autoimmunity. *Proc Natl Acad Sci* U S A, *101,* 8102-8107.

[258] Rodacki, M., Svoren, B., Butty, V., Besse, W., Laffel, L., Benoist, C. & Mathis, D. (2007). Altered natural killer cells in type 1 diabetic patients. *Diabetes, 56,* 177-185.

[259] Carnaud, C., Gombert, J., Donnars, O., Garchon, H. & Herbelin, A. (2001). Protection against diabetes and improved NK/NKT cell performance in NOD.NK1.1 mice congenic at the NK complex. *J Immunol, 166,* 2404-2411.

[260] Poulton, L. D., Smyth, M. J., Hawke, C. G., Silveira, P., Shepherd, D., Naidenko, O. V., Godfrey, D. I. & Baxter, A. G. (2001). Cytometric and functional analyses of NK and NKT cell deficiencies in NOD mice. *Int Immunol, 13,* 887-896.

[261] Johansson, S. E., Hall, H., Bjorklund, J. & Hoglund, P. (2004). Broadly impaired NK cell function in non-obese diabetic mice is partially restored by NK cell activation in vivo and by IL-12/IL-18 in vitro. *Int Immunol, 16,* 1-11.

[262] Ogasawara, K., Hamerman, J. A., Hsin, H., Chikuma, S., Bour-Jordan, H., Chen, T., Pertel, T., Carnaud, C., Bluestone, J. A. & Lanier, L. L. (2003). Impairment of NK cell function by NKG2D modulation in NOD mice. *Immunity, 18,* 41-51.

[263] Wicker, L. S., Todd, J. A. & Peterson, L. B. (1995). Genetic control of autoimmune diabetes in the NOD mouse. *Annu Rev Immunol, 13,* 179-200.

[264] Rogner, U. C., Boitard, C., Morin, J., Melanitou, E. & Avner, P. (2001). Three loci on mouse chromosome 6 influence onset and final incidence of type I diabetes in NOD.C3H congenic strains. *Genomics, 74,* 163-171.

In: Autoimmune Diseases: Symptoms, Diagnosis and Treatment   ISBN: 978-1-61668-007-7
Editor: Kyle J. Brenner, pp. 209-231   © 2010 Nova Science Publishers, Inc.

Chapter 4

CENTRAL NERVOUS SYSTEM MANIFESTATIONS IN SYSTEMIC LUPUS ERYTHEMATOSUS: DIAGNOSIS TO TREATMENT

Simone Appenzeller[*,1,2] *and Mariana Postal*[3]

[1]Rheumatology Unit - State University of Campinas, Brazil
[2] Rheumatology Lab-State University of Campinas, Brazil
[3] Department of Neurology, State University of Campinas, Brazil

ABSTRACT

Systemic lupus erythematosus (SLE) is an autoimmune disease with central nervous system (CNS) involvement occurring in up to 75% of the patients. However the frequency of these manifestations in SLE studies varies widely, depending on the type of manifestations included and the method used for evaluation. CNS involvement may be considered primary if directly related to SLE activity in the CNS or secondary when related to treatment, infections, metabolic abnormalities or other systemic manifestations such as uremia and hypertension. The involvement may vary from subtle signs such as headache and mood disorders to severe, and life threatening conditions, such as stroke, myelopathy and acute confusionalstate. Any part of the peripheral or CNS may be affected by the disease. The diagnosis of primary CNS involvement by SLE is often difficult, as both focal and diffuse manifestations may occur and there is no gold standard for diagnosis. In this paper we review the main clinical manifestations of CNS in SLE, possible etiological mechanisms and neuroimaging features associated with these manifestations. We further analyze the most important tools that can help bedside diagnosis and discuss current treatment options.

---

[*] Corresponding author: Department of Medicine, Faculty of Medical Science, State University of Campinas (UNICAMP), Cidade Universitaria Zeferino Vaz, CEP 13083970 Campinas-SP-Brazil, Tel: +55 1937887734, Fax: +55 19 32891818, E-mail: appenzellersimone@yahoo.com

INTRODUCTION

Systemic lupus erythematosus (SLE) is an autoimmune disease of unknown etiology which affects different organs, such as the skin, kidney, brain and joints [1]. Neuropsychiatric (NP) manifestations occur in up to 75% of the patients. However the frequency of these manifestations in SLE studies varies widely, depending on the type of manifestations included and the method used for evaluation [1-3]. NP involvement may be considered primary if directly related to SLE activity in the central nervous system (CNS) or peripheral nervous system (PNS) or secondary when related to treatment, infections, metabolic abnormalities or other systemic manifestations such as uremia and hypertension [4].

The involvement is heterogeneous and may vary from subtle signs such as headache and mood disorders to severe, and life threatening conditions, such as stroke, myelopathy and acute confusional state. Any part of the peripheral or CNS may be affected by the disease [5]. The diagnosis of primary NP involvement by SLE is often difficult, as both focal and diffuse manifestations may occur and a gold standard for diagnosis is still absent [4].

The aim of this study is to review the main clinical manifestations of NP involvement in SLE, possible etiological mechanisms and neuroimaging features associated with these manifestations. We further analyze the most important tools that can help bedside diagnosis and discuss current treatments.

Classification Criteria

The large number of papers published about NP manifestations in SLE evidence more manifestations attributable to SLE than seizures and psychosis described in the original classification criteria by Tan et al. [7]. In addition, the several distinct pathologic mechanisms of NP damage in SLE predispose to different central and peripheral presentations, including focal and diffuse disease. The lack of definitions of individual manifestations and the absence of standardization for investigation were reflected in the prevalence and frequency of NP manifestations in different reports, varying from 24-74% of SLE patients [1, 3, 4, 9-19].

In 1999, the American College of Rheumatology developed case definitions that included appropriate terminology, classification criteria and complementary examinations for 19 NP syndromes (Table 1) [6].

These criteria were a result of a consensus meeting of experts of several subspecialties (rheumatology, neurology, immunology, and psychiatry). Furthermore, in 2001, these criteria have been validated in a cross-sectional study with a specificity of 46% [8]. Several studies have used these classification criteria in order to determine frequency and prevalence of CNS involvement in SLE population [9-19]. Although these studies show a substantial variability between the frequency of CNS manifestations, suggesting differences between cohorts or bias in data acquisition, this classification allows us to compare the results across cohorts (Tables 2,3) [4].

Table 1. Central nervous system manifestation following ACR case definitions

Central nervous system manifestations	Peripheral nervous system manifestations
Aseptic meningitis	Acute Inflammatory Demyelinating Polyradiculoneuropathy
Acute Confusional State	Autonomic Disorders
Anxiety Disorder	Cranial Neuropathy
Cerebrovascular Disease	Mononeuropathy
Cognitive Dysfunction	Myasthenia Gravis
Demyelinating Syndrome	Plexopathy
Headache	Polyneuropathy
Movement Disorder	
Mood Disorders	
Myelopathy	
Psychosis	
Seizures	

Addapted from ACR Ad hoc Committee on Neuropsychiatric Lupus Nomenclature (6).

Clinical Relevance

The clinical relevance of NP manifestations in SLE has been determined by analyzing the impact of these manifestations in mortality, quality of life, overall damage scores and working disability [16, 17, 20-32].

Using mortality as indicative for poor outcome in NP manifestations, there are studies suggesting that patients with NP have increased mortality when compared to SLE patients without these manifestations [20-24]. Although some studies did not find an increased mortality among patients with CNS manifestations when compared to SLE patients without CNS manifestations and controls [24-28], the presence of CNS manifestations, independently of its etiology, seems to have a negative impact in quality of life [32], overall damage scores [15, 16, 28], higher fatigue scores [15, 31] and unemployment [28, 29, 31].

The association of lower quality of life with NP events over time, independent of progression in cumulative organ damage, emphasizes the persistent negative effect of NP events in the lives of patients with SLE [32].

The ACR damage score (ACR/SLICC-DI) has been developed to determine irreversible damage in SLE patients, irrespectively if attributed to disease itself or secondary to comorbidities or medications. In the ACR/SLICC-DI seizures, psychosis, mood disorders, cerebrovascular disease, neuropathy, mononeuritis multiplex, acute confusional state and myelopathy are scored in addition to several other clinical manifestations in order to determine the global damage score. Using the items of NP in order to create a NP damage score, the strongest risk factors for the development of significant NP damage was the presence of greater disease activity at the time of CNS involvement onset and the presence of antiphospholipid antibodies [16]. Cumulative organ damage was higher in patients with NP disease because they were more likely to have received corticosteroids or immunosuppressive drugs [15].

Table 2. SLE: Classification criteria of neuropsychiatric manifestations: Analysis of CNS

Authors/year	No of patients	Prevalence NP (%)	Headache (%)	Seizure disorder (%)	Anxiety disorder (%)	Mood disorder (%)	Movement disorder (%)	Cognitive dysfunction (%)	Cerebrovascular disease (%)	Acute confusion (%)	Aseptic meningitis (%)	Myelopathy (%)	Psychosis (%)	Demyelinating syndrome (%)
Ainiala et al., 2001	46	91	54	9	13	44	2	80	15	7	2	0	0	2
Costallat et al., 2001	527	34	3*	7,4	0,8*	3,0*	0,8	1,3*	2,5	3	0,4	1	5,3	0,2
Mok et al., 2001	518	19	4	28	1,5	6	2	NR	19	14	1	8	11	1,5
Brey et al, 2002	128	80	57	16	24	23,0	1	79	2	0	0	5,0	6,5	0
Alfreta et al., 2003	61	72	21	11	6	27	0	52	24	0	0	0	0	3
Sanna et al., 2003	323	57,3	24	8,3	7,4	16,7	1,2	10,8	17,6	3,7	0	1,2	7,7	0,9
Hanly et al., 2004	111	37	24,4	2,4	2,4	9,8	0	7,3	9,8	7,0	2,4	0	7,3	2,4
Mikdashi et al., 2004	130	56,9	NR	7,6	0	NR	0	27,3	25,7	0	0	6,1	15,1	0
Appenzeller et al., 2205	72	NR	30	11,3	NR	10,5	0,8	27,1	NR	7,5	0,8	2,3	4,5	NR
Hanly et al., 2005	53	31	9,4	0	0	0	0	1,9	0	3,8	0	0	0	1,9
Shimojima et al., 2005	25	100	12	36	0	0	0	12	24	0	0	4	32	0
Robert et al, 2006	50	78	55,6	20,5	0	0	23,1	18	16,2	16,2	0	0	16,2	0
Hanly J et al., 2009	209	NR	32,1	6,7	8	23,4	0,3	8,4	5,7	3,7	0,3	0,3	1,7	2

Table 3. SLE: Classification criteria of neuropsychiatric manifestations: analysis of peripheral nervous system

Authors/Year	No of patients	Autonomic neuropathy (%)	Myasthenia gravis (%)	Mononeuropathy (%)	Cranial neuropathy (%)	Plexopathy (%)	Polyneuropathy (%)	Guillain-Barré syndrome (%)
Ainiala et al., 2001	46	0	2	0	7	0	28	2
Costallat et al., 2001	527	0	0,2	1,3	1,5	0	4	0,2
Mok et al., 2001	518	0	0	1,5	3	0	1	0
Brey et al., 2002	128	0	0	8	2	0	22	0
Alfreta et al., 2003	61	3	0	0	4	0	13	0
Sanna et al., 2003	323	0	1,5	1,8	1,5	0	2,8	0,6
Hanly et al., 2004	111	0	0	0	4,9	0	4,9	0
Mikdashi et al, 2004	130	0	0	0	0	0	18,2	0
Appenzeller et al., 2005	72	NR	NR	3	2,3	NR	NR	NR
Hanly et al., 2005	53	0	0	0	0	0	0	0
Shimojima et al.,2005	25	0	0	0	0	0	12	0
Robert et al., 2006	50	NR	0	7,9	0	0	0	0
Hanly J et al., 2009	209	0	0,7	1	3,3	0,3	2	0
Appenzeller et al., 2005								

NR: Not rated
No: Number

Fatigue is also an important aspect of life in SLE patients. A recent study [31] shows the main reasons for being unemployed were fatigue, hours of work missed, pain, and cognitive impairment. Another study [15] in the same area proved that patients with NP disease reported more fatigue and had significantly lower scores on 7 of 8 subscales of the SF-36 (Short form 36 health survey questionnaire) [15].

Working disability has been studied in NP in several studies [28, 29, 31]. The number of cognitive spheres, and especially attention, memory, and executive functions, were important factors associated with unemployment in patients with SLE [31]. The association between memory function and employment status in patients with SLE underscores the need for judicious assessment of cognitive function and for the development of appropriate strategies that will either reverse cognitive impairment or help patients overcome obstacles they may face in daily life. Pertaining to employment, persons with cognitive impairment may benefit from specific training programs [29].

Furthermore it is necessary to determine the course of NP manifestations. There are only a limited amount of follow-up studies evaluating NP manifestations in SLE patients [33-38]. CNS involvement seems to have a general good prognosis, with improvement or stabilization of symptoms in most of the patients [33]. The presence of antiphospholipid antibodies, higher number of NP events and hippocampal atrophy were negative prognostic factors [33,35]. Furthermore, the progression of hippocampal atrophy was a predictor for progressive cognitive impairment [35]. Perhaps the absence of abnormalities on MRI may suggest reversibility or stabilization of NP manifestations, whereas the presence of progressive atrophy may be related to worse prognosis over time. The presence of brain abnormalities at or around the diagnosis of SLE may indicate that the clinical diagnosis of SLE is preceded by the presence of lupus autoantibodies for many years and that the brain is particularly vulnerable early in the disease course. These findings indicate that the brain may be affected extremely early in the disease course, even before the clinical diagnosis of SLE is made [39].

These findings were consistent with the hypothesis of subclinical CNS functional involvement, as suggested by magnetic resonance spectroscopy studies [40, 41].

Pathology

The rationale for identifying the etiology and pathogenic mechanisms underlying NP disease in SLE is to facilitate the logical development of appropriate and effective therapies [4, 42].

Histopathological studies of brains of SLE patients with and without CNS manifestations revealed a predominant small vessel infarction, with little signs of true vasculitis [4, 43-46]. Multiple microinfarcts, noninflammatory thickening of small vessels with intimae proliferation, small-vessel occlusion, and intracranial embolism or hemorrhage have all been shown in SLE patients [43-46]. Although small vessel vasculopathy is frequently found in autopsy findings, a parallel between these and CNS symptoms was not always evident. Therefore, in addition to vasculopathy, autoantibodies and inflammatory mediators may be involved in different disease expression in CNS SLE.

Autoantibodies directed against neurons, ribosomes and phospholipids-associated proteins have been associated with CNS manifestations and may be locally produced or cross the blood-brain barrier [43, 47]. Antineuronal antibodies have been shown to induce memory deficits, seizures and neuropathological changes in animal models [48, 49]. In SLE patients, the presence of antineuronal antibodies has been increased in patients with NP manifestations, although no clinical manifestations and no diagnostic specificity could be identified [42]. The N-methyl-D-aspartate receptors (NMDA), NR2a and NR2b have been shown to occur in patients with NP manifestations and appear to have a functional consequence leading to neuronal injury. Although anti-NR2 antibodies have been studied in SLE patients, only Anti-NR2 antibodies in cerebrospinal fluid (CSF), not in the serum, are associated with diffuse neuropsychiatric manifestations in NPSLE [50]. These antibodies have been shown to be involved in learning, memory [51] and psychosis [52]. Anti-ribosomal P (anti-P) antibodies have a limited sensitivity and specificity for NP SLE with a prevalence of 13–20%, depending on the ethnic group [53-55]. Clinically they are associated with psychosis and depression [56-58]. Others have not confirmed an association of the presence of these antibodies with these neuropsychiatric disorders [59]. Antiphospholipid antibodies are associated with predominantly focal manifestations of NP-SLE. The most common neurological disorders are those of vascular origin, such as transient cerebral ischemia or stroke, but other associations include seizures, chorea, transverse myelitis, thrombosis, chorea, transverse myelitis and cerebrovascular events, cerebral venous thrombosis and cognitive dysfunction [11, 60-63]. Two studies investigated the role of anti-endothelial antibodies (AECA) in CNS SLE and found a higher prevalence and concentration in patients with NP manifestations than without. The results of these studies suggest a relationship between AECA and a biological origin of NP manifestations [64,65].

More recently, serum S100B protein level have been shown to be increased in patients with SLE. S100B levels were significantly higher in patients with defined NP syndromes than in controls and non-NPSLE patients, reflecting continuing neurological damage. This data also suggest that S100B protein levels may be a useful test in the diagnosis of NPSLE, particularly in acute forms of this syndrome. [66].

Several studies have analyzed the role of inflammatory process in the manifestations of CNS. Interleukins [67-69], tumor necrosis factors [70] and metalloproteinase [71,72] have been shown to be increased in cerebrospinal fluid (CSF) in patients with CNS manifestations and even associated with some specific clinical manifestations and MRI findings [69, 71].

A recent multicenter retrospective study showed that CSF interleukin 6 (IL-6) might be an effective measure in diagnosing lupus psycosis (LP), although exclusion of infectious meningoencephalitis and cerebrovascular accident is necessary [73]. In this study, SLE patients with psychiatric manifestations were included. The diagnosis of LP and psychosis due to causes other than SLE (non-LP) was confirmed by retrospective review of the clinical records. Receiver operating characteristic curve analysis revealed that the sensitivity and specificity of CSF IL-6 for diagnosis of LP were high, showing the efficacy of CSF IL-6 in the diagnosis of psychosis.

Therefore the three primary immunopathogenic mechanisms involved in CNS manifestations of SLE patients seem to have a final common pathway: the involvement of the cerebral microvasculature [4, 42].

The strict exclusion of patients with other etiologies of CNS than SLE disease, in addition to the analysis of individual manifestations may provide a more homogenous clinical population and may favor elucidation of pathological mechanism involved in CNS manifestations in SLE.

Table 4. Investigation in patients presenting with CNS manifestations with suspected SLE and in patients with previous diagnosis of SLE

CNS manifestation in patients with suspected SLE	Exclude infection	e.g., CBC (white blood cell analysis, blood) and urine culture, CSF analysis, chest x-ray
	Exclude metabolic abnormalities	e.g., diabetes, renal insufficiency
	Exclude other systemic diseases	e.g., HIV, Hepatitis B and C, bacterial endocarditis
	Laboratory investigation	e.g., CBC, urine sediment analysis, complement
	Antinuclear antibodies	anti-Sm, antiphospholipid antibodies, anti DNA
	Neuroimaging investigation	
CNS manifestations in patients with previous diagnosis of SLE	Exclude infection	e.g., CBC (white blood cell analysis, blood) and urine culture, CSF analysis, chest x-ray
	Identify and treat aggravating factors	e.g., hypertension, metabolic abnormalities
	Neuroimaging investigation	

Diagnosis

The correct diagnosis of CNS manifestations in patients with previous diagnosis of SLE, attributing individual manifestations to SLE disease activity or to a secondary cause remains a challenge in clinical practice [4] (Table 4).

Because of the absence of diagnostic gold standard for most of the individual manifestations, clinical, laboratory and neuroimaging features are necessary for exclusion of alternative etiologies [4]. The approach differs according to the presence of focal manifestations or diffuse CNS involvement (Figure 1).

The ACR nomenclature provides tools for accessing these manifestations in a systematic manner [4]. Using these guidelines, Hanly et al [13] were able to determine that 41% of the CNS manifestation in their cohort was secondary to non-SLE causes. Furthermore, several studies have shown the occurrence of subclinical NP involvement, which clinical significance has still to be determined (Table 5) [35, 42].

Clinical and laboratory investigation

CNS infection should always be excluded by cerebrospinal fluid (CSF) examinations. Non-specific abnormalities may be found in the CSF of 33% of patients with NP disease and include mild pleocytosis and elevated protein levels [74]. The clinical usefulness of measuring CSF autoantibodies, cytokines and biomarkers of neurological damage [75] is still a subject of research [4, 42]. In considering circulating autoantibodies, those that are most likely to provide the greatest diagnostic yield are antiphospholipid antibodies. The value of measuring anti-P antibodies remains uncertain, given the conflicting results to date. The role of anti-NR2 antibodies in NP-SLE is currently unknown [4]. The approach in patients with CNS manifestations as initial symptoms and clinical suspicion of SLE disease includes, in addition to the investigation described above, exams that are useful for diagnosing SLE.

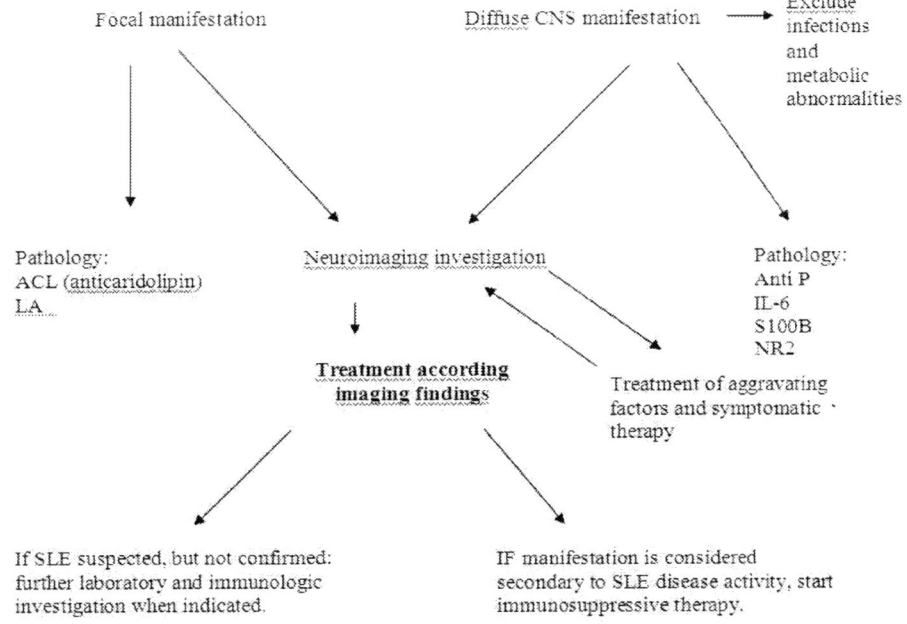

Figure 1. Suggestive investigation in a patient with CNS manifestations as initial symptom and clinical suspicion of disease and with established disease

Table 5. Differential diagnosis of CNS SLE

Differential diagnosis	Examples
Endocrine diseases	Diabetes mellitus Thyroid disorders
Medication	Antihistamines Antidepressants Antiepileptic drugs Anti-inflammatory drugs Beta blockers Statins
Metabolic abnormalities	Electrolyte disturbance (calcium, sodium, potassium) Uremia
Other primary CNS diseases	Cerebral hemorrhage (aneurism) Cerebral ischemia Parkinson disease Trauma
Other primary psychiatric illness	Anxiety Depression Psychosis
Other psychological stressors	Fatigue Pain Sleep disorders
Systemic diseases	Cardiac disease (arritmia, valvar disease) Fever Hypertension Hypoxemia Infectious disease

Neuroimaging

In SLE, both structural and functional neuroimaging methods may be useful for determine CNS abnormalities. Cranial tomography (CT) may be the preferred technique in several centers for the diagnosis of gross structural abnormalities, such as infarcts, hemorrhage, tumors and abscesses, especially because it may be used in severely ill patients and its availability in most centers around the world. However, magnetic resonance imaging (MRI) has largely replaced CT, because of the excellent soft-tissue contrast observed with MRI and the ability to acquire multiplanar images (table 6) [71].

Although MRI abnormalities may be found in 19-70% of SLE patients, its clinical significance for diagnosis of NP SLE has still to be determined, because these abnormalities may occur in both, patients with and without CNS manifestations [4, 76-78]. Atrophy was described in 6-12% of SLE patients, depending upon linear or volumetric measurements have been applied [76]. Age, disease activity, the presence of past history of CNS manifestations and the use of corticosteroid have all been associated with the occurrence of atrophy [76, 80-86]. Although most studies have analyzed cerebral atrophy as a hole, some studies [76, 87] have determined that that there are different patterns in cortical and subcortical involvement in SLE patients. The impact of cerebral atrophy has been studied, indicating that cognitive impairment may be present more frequently in both corpus callosum and hippocampal atrophy [35, 76]. In relation to different domains of cognitive dysfunction, hippocampal atrophy was associated with lower scores in general memory ($p=0.015$), verbal memory ($p=0.01$), and delayed recall ($p=0.01$) [35].

White matter lesions have been frequently detected SLE patients, but may occur in both symptomatic in asymptomatic patients. In a large prospective population-based study involving healthy individuals, the presence of these lesions were associated with cognitive impairment [88]. Fluid-attenuating inversion recovery (FLAIR) images are more sensible for detecting theses lesions than T2 images [79]. Although these white matter lesions are often considered nonspecific, they may be attributed to age, hypertension, disease duration, small vessel disease and the presence of NP manifestations [79, 82]. In the presence of larger lesions, the differential diagnosis with multiple sclerosis is mandatory [82]. Small hyperintense white matter lesions in SLE are associated with central nervous system symptoms and antiphospholipid antibodies, and progress over time in patients with more severe SLE. Therefore, in the context of SLE, these lesions are likely consequences of central nervous system damage and not mere incidental finding [89].

Magnetization transfer imaging (MTI) is particularly suited to the detection and quantification of diffuse brain damage [90, 91], but its utility in clinical practice has still to be determined. Diffusion weighted imaging (DWI) and perfusion MRI are highly effective in the detection of hyperacute and subacute brain injury, in particular acute ischemia following stroke [92].

Magnetic resonance angiography (MRA) permits visualization of cerebral blood flow, although it is not optimum for visualization of flow in small caliber vessels that are the ones primarily involved in NP-SLE [93].

Table 6. SLE. Studies using magnetic resonance imaging (MRI)

Authors/Year	No of patients	Stroke (%)	Cerebral hemorraghe (%)	Atrophy (%)	White matter lesions (WM) (%)	Associations and observations
Vermess et al., 1983	9	0	0	0	88.9	All with CNS involvement, MRI more sensitive than CT
Mc Cune et al., 1988	28	0	0	67%	53	Deficit associated with focal neurological and seizures; MRI important to detect brain damage
Sibbitt et al, 1989	21	47.6	4.8	33.3 Focal Edema: 38%	0	All patients had CNS involvement, MRI more sensitive than CT
Baum et al; 1993	21	-	-	52,4	57,1	More frequent changes in patients with focal symptoms
Stimmler et al., 1993	51	0	0	21,9%	15,6	All hospitalized patients; Associates hypertension and nephritis, patients with focal lesions have more changes to MRI; Suggests vasculopathy (also present in the elderly)
Cauli et al., 1994	40	-	-	-	37,5	More frequent changes in patients with organic symptoms and higher activity index
Jarek et al., 1994	32	0	0	0	16	Frequency similar to the normal population
Chinn et al., 1997	47	8,5		32,5	23	Semiautomatic segmentation, MRI shows chronic changes of ischemic origin
Kozora et al., 1998	20	0	0	35	35	Patients without neuropsychiatric manifestations; No clinical relevance
Sanna et al.; 2000	68	4,4			44	SLICC with abnormal MRI; WM more frequent in patients with neuropsychiatric manifestations
Walecki et al.; 2002	50	20	2	54	54	Association between severity of symptoms and MRI findings, association between Antiphospholipid syndrome and WM lesions
Oku et al., 2003	44	0	0	42	84	Correlation of MRI findings with clinical symptoms
Cotton et al., 2004	58	6,9	0	37,9	59	70% of patients with MRI changes, independent of the presence of neuropsychiatric manifestations
Abreu et al., 2005	23	13	0	0	65,2	More frequent changes in patients with NP manifestations
Ainialia et al; 2005	43	present	present	present	present	Association with permanent damage (SLICC-ACR/DI) Atrophy associated with corticosteroids
Sundgren et al., 2005	15	18	9	54,5	81,8	MRI is important to define the etiology of acute ischemic events

CNS: Central nervous system CT: Cranial tomography MRI: Magnetic Resonance Imaging No: number NP: Neuropsychiatric SLICC-ACR/DI: The Systemic Lupus International Collaborating Clinics/American College of rheumatology WM: White matter

Functional studies may be performed using different methods. Positron emission tomography (PET) scanning is sensitive, but practical considerations limit its applicability [4]. Single photon emission computed tomography (SPECT) scanning provides semi-quantitative analysis of regional cerebral blood flow and metabolism. SPECT studies in SLE patients have identified both diffuse and focal deficits which may be fixed or reversible [94-

98]. Magnetic resonance spectroscopy (MRS) allows the identification and quantification of brain metabolites, which reflect the quantity and integrity of neuronal cells, is reduced in SLE patients [41, 42, 99]. Several studies suggest that the peak of n-acetyl groups, at 2.0 parts per million (ppm), which originates largely from N-acetylaspartate (NAA) can be used as a neuronal marker since NAA it is found exclusively in neurons and their processes in the mature brain [100]. In human brain spectra NAA is reduced in situations known to be associated with neuronal loss, such as in neuronal degenerative disorders, stroke and glial tumors [101]. When decrease in the relative NAA signal arises from neuronal or axonal degeneration, irreversible changes are expected. Several studies observed that CNS manifestations in SLE are associated with reduction in NAA/Cr ratios and NAA/Cho ratios, not only in lesions, but also in normal appearing white matter (WM) when compared to controls [41, 42, 99].

Treatment of primary CNS manifestations

Due to the large number of CNS manifestations and the great spectra of differential diagnoses, individual approach is necessary for each patient. It is necessary first to identify and treat potential aggravating factors such as hypertension, infection and metabolic abnormalities and second, symptomatic therapy should be considered, such as anticonvulsants, antidepressants and antipsychotic medications, when necessary [4].

Immunosuppressive therapies with high-dose corticosteroids, azathioprine and cyclophosphamide, mycophenolate mofetil and rituximab have all been used in association with corticosteroids (oral or intravenous pulse therapy) in SLE patients with CNS involvement [102-115]. There are only a few controlled studies for treatment of CNS manifestations in SLE, therefore treatment should be admisteted on a patients basis (costs, comorbidities, severity) [100-111].

Corticosteroids

For diffuse neuropsychiatric lupus with inflammatory CNS disease corticosteroids have been the mainstay of treatment [116-118]. Although the approach to corticosteroid therapy for CNS lupus remains largely empirical, corticosteroids continue to represent the first line of treatment for SLE with suspected diffuse CNS involvement [116]. High dose oral prednisolone (1–2mg/kg/daily) or intravenous methylprednisolone infusions (500mg–1g daily for three days), with oral prednisolone to follow, are indicated for acute severe CNS manifestations [117]. The use of high dose corticosteroids is also recommended during the early phases of myelitis, especially during the first week of onset of symptoms [118]. Corticosteroid have also shown efficacy in mild neuropsychiatric symptoms and inactive SLE, showing that improvement in cognition and mood can be observed relatively low doses of corticosteroids (0.5mg/kg of prednisone daily for 6 months) [102]. Corticosteroids have also been used for the treatment of aseptic meningitis [117] and psychosis not responsive to antipsychotic treatment [120]. Furthermore intrathecal corticosteroids may also be an option in patients with severe diffuse involvement and without response to systemic corticosteroid administration [121].

Cyclophosphamide

The use of intravenous cyclophosphamide is currently recommended for acute severe CNS disease, in those refractory to corticosteroids or when a steroid-sparing effect is desired [106-110, 113, 117, 118, 123-125]. There are only a few controlled studies for treatment of CNS manifestations in SLE There is only one controlled trial to support the therapeutic regimen with cyclophosphamide [100-111], but animal studies have shown that immunosuppression with cyclophosphamide in autoimmune MRL/lpr mice prevents neuronal atrophy [126], reduces levels of autoantibodies and attenuates leukocytes in. ltration in the brain [127] while improving behavioral abnormalities [128]. However, in the absence of randomized controlled trials comparing the effectiveness and safety of cyclophosphamide to other immunosuppressive drugs in the treatment of severe CNS disease, the use of cyclophosphamide in severe CNS lupus continues to be based on clinical experience.

Plasmapheresis

Plasmapheresis is useful to remove free antibodies, complement components and circulating immune complexes [117]. It seems that patients who respond better to plasmapheresis are those with more severe illness, refractory to corticosteroids and cyclophosphamide therapy, and with the highest levels of circulating immune complexes. Combination therapy with synchronized plasmapheresis and subsequent cyclophosphamide in severe SLE has been proposed by some authors [129].

Intravenous immunoglobulin

Intravenous immunoglobulin (IVIg) has proved useful in the treatment of autoimmune neurological diseases such as peripheral neuropathy, myasthenia gravis, MS and Guillain–Barre´ syndrome [130,131], but there are few reports of the use of IVIg in CNS lupus, including acute severe diffuse CNS disease and psychosis [132,133].

Intrathecal methotrexate

Intrathecal administration of methotrexate has been reported as a possible treatment for SLE CNS involvement, patients not responsive to conventional steroid therapy [134,135]. Side effects including itching sensation of lower limbs, headache and incontinence were mild and transient, suggesting that this therapeutic approach may represent a promising method for treating severe CNS lupus in selected cases and deserves further investigation [117].

Other agents

Azathioprine is used for the treatment of a wide spectrum of SLE manifestations and its use as a steroid sparing agent is widely accepted. Reports using azathioprine in NP SLE have shown beneficial effects, especially in patients unable to tolerate cyclophosphamide [136-138]. Mycophenolate mofetil has also been used in the treatment of NPSLE. Clinical improvement of neuropsychiatric symptoms and improvement in brain SPECT hypoperfusion patterns were reported in more than two thirds of the patients when 1g/day mycophenolate was given for 12 months [139]. Ilioprost has been used in one SLE patient for Raynaud's, who also presented severe cognitive dysfunction and hypoperfusion detected by SPECT, with normalization of perfusion abnormalities [140].

Most recently, B-lymphocyte function has been recognized as a major component in the pathogenesis of autoimmune diseases. Rituximab, a chimeric monoclonal antibody directed against CD20 lymphocytes (commonly called B-cells), was developed as a primary treatment against B-cell lymphoma and is now approved for use in the treatment of rheumatoid arthritis. Besides, Rituximab therapy offers a potential innovation in the current treatment regimens for children with aggressive SLE that includes both renal and extra-renal manifestations [141].

Rituximab has been reported in NPSLE by several authors [141,142]. Treatment with rituximab resulted in rapid improvement of central nervous system-related manifestations, particularly acute confusional state. It also improved cognitive dysfunction, psychosis and seizure and reduced the SLEDAI score. The down regulation of functional molecules on B and T cells suggests that rituximab modulates the interaction of activated B and T cells through co-stimulatory molecules [142].

Anticoagulation

Anticoagulation is indicated for focal disease when antiphospholipid antibodies are implicated [114,115]. The presence of antiphospholipid antibodies is strongly associated with thrombotic CNS events (including transient ischemic attacks, ischemic stroke, amaurosis fugax, and cerebral venous thrombosis), chorea, dementia, headache, transverse myelitis and seizures [11, 13, 60-63, 140, 143-146]. Many SLE patients with focal neurological manifestations and aPL, who would have previously received a high dose of corticosteroids and/or immunosuppression, are today being successfully treated with anticoagulation [114]. Corticosteroids do not seem to be helpful for the treatment of focal/thrombotic CNS disease [116].

REFERENCES

[1] West, SG. Neuropsychiatric lupus. *Rheum Dis Clin North Am*, 1994, 20, 129-158.
[2] Hanly, JG; Walsh, NM; Sangalang, V. Brain pathology in systemic lupus erythematosus. *J Rheumatol*, 1992, 19, 732-741.
[3] Johnson, RT; Richardson, EP. The neurological manifestations of systemic lupus erythematosus. *Medicine*, (Baltimore), 1968, 47, 337-369.
[4] Hanly, JG. Neuropsychiatric lupus. *Rheum Dis Clin North Am.*, 2005, 31, 273-98
[5] Kozora, E; Arciniegas, DB; Filley, CM; et al. Cognition, MRS neurometabolites, and MRI volumetrics in non-neuropsychiatric systemic lupus erythematosus: preliminary data. *Cogn Behav Neurol.*, 2005, 18, 159-62.
[6] American College of Rheumatology (ACR) nomenclature and case definitions for neuropsychiatric lupus syndromes. *Arthritis and Rheumatism*, 1999, 42, 599-608.
[7] Tan, EM; Cohen, AS; Fries, JF; et al. The 1982 revised criteria for the classification of systemic lupus erythematosus. *Arthritis Rheum*, 1982, 25, 1271-7.
[8] Ainiala, H; Hietaharju, A; Loukkola, J; et al. Validity of the new American College of Rheumatology criteria for neuropsychiatric lupus syndromes: a population-based evaluation. *Arthritis Rheum*, 2001, 45, 419-423.

[9] Ainiala, H; Loukkola, J; Peltola, J; Korpela, M; Hietaharju, A. The prevalence of neuropsychiatric syndromes in systemic lupus erythematosus. *Neurology.*, 2001, 5, 496-500.

[10] Brey, RL; Holliday, SL; Saklad, AR; et al. Neuropsychiatric syndromes in lupus: prevalence using standardized definitions. *Neurology*, 2002, 58, 1214-1220.

[11] Afeltra, A; Garzia, P; Mitterhofer, AP; et al. Neuropsychiatric lupus syndromes, relationship with antiphospholipid antibodies. *Neurology.*, 2003, 61, 108-10.

[12] Hanly, JG; Fisk, JD; McCurdy, G; Fougere, L; Douglas, JA. Neuropsychiatric syndromes in patients with systemic lupus erythematosus and rheumatoid arthritis. *J Rheumatol.*, 2005, 32, 1459-6.

[13] Sanna, G; Bertolaccini, ML; Cuadrado, MJ; et al. Neuropsychiatric manifestations in systemic lupus erythematosus: prevalence and association with antiphospholipid antibodies. *J Rheumatol.*, 2003, 30, 985-92.

[14] Mok, CC; Lau, CS; Wong, RW. Neuropsychiatric manifestations and their clinical associations in southern Chinese patients with systemic lupus erythematosus. *J Rheumatol*, 2001,28, 766-71.

[15] Hanly JG; McCurdy G; Fougere L; et al. Neuropsychiatric events in systemic lupus erythematosus: attribution and clinical significance, *J Rheumatol*, 2004, 31, 2156-62.

[16] Mikdashi J; Handwerger, B. Predictors of neuropsychiatric damage in systemic lupus erythematosus: data from the Maryland lupus cohort. *Rheumatology*, (Oxford). 2004, 43, 1555-60.

[17] Robert, M; Sunitha, R; Thulaseedharan, NK. Neuropsychiatric manifestations systemic lupus erythematosus: a study from South India. *Neurol India.*, 2006, 54, 75-7.

[18] Shimojima, Y; Matsuda, M; Gono, T; Ishii, W; Ikeda, S. Relationship between clinical factors and neuropsychiatric manifestations in systemic lupus erythematosus. *Clin Rheumatol.*, 2005, 24, 469-75

[19] Estes, D; Christian, CL. The natural history of systemic lupus erythematosus by prospective analysis. *Medicine*, (Baltimore), 1971, 50, 85-95.

[20] Feng, PH; Cheah, PS; Lee, YK. Mortality in systemic lupus erythematosus: a 10-year review. *Br Med J.*, 1973, 4, 772-4.

[21] Cheatum, DE; Hurd, ER; Strunk, SW; Ziff, M. Renal histology and clinical course of systemic lupus erythematosus. A prospective study. *Arthritis Rheum.*, 1973, 16, 670-6.

[22] Lee, P; Urowitz, MB; Bookman, AA; et al. Systemic lupus erythematosus. A review of 110 cases with reference to nephritis, the nervous system, infections, aseptic necrosis and prognosis. *Q J Med.*, 1977, 46, 1-32.

[23] Ginzler, EM; Diamond, HS; Weiner, M; et al. A multicenter study of outcome in systemic lupus erythematosus. I. Entry variables as predictors of prognosis. *Arthritis Rheum*, 1982, 25, 601-611.

[24] Sibley, JT; Olszynski, WP; Decoteau, WE; Sundaram, MB. The incidence and prognosis of central nervous system disease in systemic lupus erythematosus. *J Rheumatol*, 1992, 19, 47-52.

[25] Sergent, JS; Lockshin, MD; Klempner, MS; Lipsky, BA. Central nervous system disease in systemic lupus erythematosus. Therapy and prognosis. *Am J Med.*, 1975, 58, 644-54.

[26] Feinglass, EJ; Arnett, FC; Dorsch, CA; Zizic, TM; Stevens, MB. Neuropsychiatric manifestations of systemic lupus erythematosus: diagnosis, clinical spectrum, and relationship to other features of the disease. *Medicine*, (Baltimore). 1976, 55, 323-39.

[27] Kovacs, JA; Urowitz, MB; Gladman DD. Dilemmas in neuropsychiatric lupus. *Rheum Dis Clin North Am.*, 1993, 19, 795-814.

[28] Jonsen, A; Bengston, AA; Nived, O; Rayberg, B; Sturfelt, G. Outcome of neuropsychiatric systemic lupus erythematosus within a defined Swedish population: increased morbidity but low mortality. *Rheumatology*, 2002, 41, 1308-12.

[29] Panopalis, P; Julian, L; Yazdany, J; Gillis, JZ; Trupin, L; Hersh, A; Criswell, LA; Katz, P; Yelin, E. Impact of memory impairment on employment status in persons with systemic lupus erythematosus. *Arthritis Rheum.*, 2007, 57, 1453-60.

[30] Baker, K; Pope, J. Employment and work disability in systemic lupus erythematosus: a systematic review. Rheumatology (Oxford). 2009, 48, 281-4.

[31] Appenzeller, S; Cendes, F; Costallat, LT. Cognitive impairment and employment status in systemic lupus erythematosus: a prospective longitudinal study. *Arthritis Rheum.*, 2009, 61, 680-7

[32] Hanly, JG; Su, L; Farewell, V; et al. Prospective study of neuropsychiatric events in systemic lupus erythematosus. *J Rheumatol.*, 2009, 36, 1449-59.

[33] Carlomagno, S; Migliaresi, S; Ambrosone, L; Sannino, M; Sanges, G; Di Iorio, G. Cognitive impairment in systemic lupus erythematosus: a follow-up study. *J Neurol.*, 2000, 247, 273-9.

[34] Karassa, FB; Ioannidis, JP; Boki, KA; et al. Predictors of clinical outcome and radiologic progression in patients with neuropsychiatric manifestations of systemic lupus erythematosus. *Am J Med.*, 2000, 109, 628-34.

[35] Appenzeller, S; Carnevalle, AD; Li, LM; Costallat, LT; Cendes F. Hippocampal atrophy in Systemic lupus erythematosus. *Ann Rheum Dis.*, 2006, 65, 1585-9.

[36] Hanly, JG; Fisk, JD; Sherwood, G; Eastwood, B. Clinical course of cognitive dysfunction in systemic lupus erythematosus. *J Rheumatol*, 1994, 2, 1825-31

[37] Hay, EM; Huddy, A; Black, D; et al. A prospective study of psychiatric disorder and cognitive function in systemic lupus erythematosus. *Ann Rheum Dis*, 1994, 53, 298-303

[38] Waterloo, K; Omdal, R; Husby, G; Mellgren, SI. Neuropsychological function in systemic lupus erythematosus: a five-year longitudinal study. *Rheumatology*, (Oxford), 2002, 41, 411-415.

[39] Petri, M; Naqibuddin, M; Carson, KA; et al. Brain magnetic resonance imaging in newly diagnosed systemic lupus erythematosus. *J Rheumatol.*, 2008, 35, 2348-54

[40] Brooks, WM; Jung, RE; Ford, CC; et al. Relationship between neurometabolite derangement and neurocognitive dysfunction in systemic lupus erythematosus. *J Rheumatol*, 1999, 26, 81-85.

[41] Appenzeller, S; Li, LM; Costallat, LT; Cendes, F. Evidence of reversible axonal dysfunction in systemic lupus erythematosus: a proton MRS study. *Brain.*, 2005, 128, 2933-40.

[42] Hanly, JG; Harrison, MJ. Management of neuropsychiatric lupus. *Best Pract Res Clin Rheumatol.*, 2005, 19, 799-821.

[43] Devinsky, O; Petito, CK; Alonso, DR. Clinical and neuropathological findings in systemic lupus erythematosus, the role of vasculitis, heart emboli, and thrombotic thrombocytopenic purpura. *Ann Neurol*, 1988, 23, 380-384.

[44] Ellis, SG; Verity, MA. Central nervous system involvement in systemic lupus erythematosus: a review of neuropathologic findings in 57 cases, 1955-1977. *Sem Arthritis Rheum*, 1979, 8, 212-221.

[45] Zvaifler, NJ; Bluestein, HG. The pathogenesis of central nervous system manifestations of systemic lupus erythematosus. *Arthritis Rheum*, 1982, 25, 862-866.

[46] Abbott, NJ; Mendonca, LL; Dolman, DE. The blood-brain barrier in systemic lupus erythematosus. *Lupus.*, 2003, 12, 908-15.

[47] Karpiak, SE; Graf, L; Rapport, MM. Antiserum to brain gangliosides produces recurrent epileptiform activity. *Science.*, 1976, 194, 735-7.

[48] Kobiler, D; Allweis, C. The effect of antisynaptosomal plasma membrane antibodies on memory. *Brain Res.*, 1976, 115, 129-38.

[49] Morris, RG; Anderson, E; Lynch, GS; Baudry, M. Selective impairment of learning and blockade of long-term potentiation by an Nmethyl- D-aspartate receptor antagonist, AP5. *Nature*, 1986, 319, 774-776.

[50] Arinuma, Y; Yanagida, T; Hirohata, S. Association of cerebrospinal fluid anti-NR2 glutamate receptor antibodies with diffuse neuropsychiatric systemic lupus erythematosus. *Arthritis Rheum.*, 2008, 58, 1130-5.

[51] Akbarian, S; Sucher, NJ; Bradley, D; et al. Selective alterations in gene expression for NMDA receptor subunits in prefrontal cortex of schizophrenics. *J Neurosci.*, 1996, 16, 19-30.

[52] Teh, LS; Isenberg, DA. Antiribosomal, P protein antibodies in systemic lupus erythematosus. A reappraisal. *Arthritis Rheum*, 1994, 37, 307-315.

[53] Arnett, FC; Reveille, JD; Moutsopoulos, HM; Georgescu, L; Elkon, KB. Ribosomal P autoantibodies in systemic lupus erythematosus. Frequencies in different ethnic groups and clinical and immunogenetic associations. *Arthritis Rheum*, 1996, 39, 1833-1839.

[54] Bonfa, E; Golombek, SJ; Kaufman, LD; et al. Association between lupus psychosis and anti-ribosomal P protein antibodies. *N Engl J Med*, 1987, 317, 265-271.

[55] Karassa, FB; Afeltra, A; Ambrozic, A; et al. Accuracy of anti-ribosomal P protein antibody testing for the diagnosis of neuropsychiatric systemic lupus erythematosus: an international meta-analysis. *Arthritis Rheum.*, 2006, 54, 312-24.

[56] Tzioufas, AG; Tzortzakis, NG; Panou-Pomonis, E; et al. The clinical relevance of antibodies to ribosomal-P common epitope in two targeted systemic lupus erythematosus populations: a large cohort of consecutive patients and patients with active central nervous system disease. *Annals of Rheum Diseases*, 2000, 59, 99-104.

[57] Zandman-Goddard, G; Chapman, J; Shoenfeld, Y. Autoantibodies involved in neuropsychiatric SLE and antiphospholipid syndrome. *Semin Arthritis Rheum.*, 2007, 36, 297-315

[58] Hanly, JG. Antiphospholipid syndrome: an overview. *Cmaj*, 2003, 168, 1675-1682.

[59] Gerli, R; Caponi, L; Tincani, A; et al. Clinical and serological associations of ribosomal P autoantibodies in systemic lupus erythematosus: prospective evaluation in a large cohort of Italian patients. *Rheumatology*, (Oxford). 2002, 41, 1357-66.

[60] Love, PE; Santoro, SA. Antiphospholipid antibodies: anticardiolipin and the lupus anticoagulant in systemic lupus erythematosus (SLE) and in non-SLE disorders. Prevalence and clinical significance. *Ann Intern Med*, 1990, 112, 682-698.

[61] Menon, S; Jameson-Shortall, E; Newman, SP; Hall-Craggs, MR; Chinn, R; Isenberg, DA. A longitudinal study of anticardiolipin antibody levels and cognitive functioning in systemic lupus erythematosus. *Arthritis Rheum*, 1999, 42, 735-741.

[62] Chapman, J; Cohen-Armon, M; Shoenfeld, Y; Korczyn, AD. Antiphospholipid antibodies permeabilize and depolarize brain synaptoneurosomes. *Lupus*, 1999, 8, 127-133.

[63] Appenzeller, S; Zeller, CB; Annichino-Bizzachi, JM; et al. Cerebral venous thrombosis: influence of risk factors and imaging findings on prognosis. *Clinical Neurol and Neurourg*, 2005, 107, 371-378.

[64] Conti, F; Alessandri, C; Bompane, D; et al. Autoantibody profile in systemic lupus erythematosus with psychiatric manifestations: a role for antiendothelial-cell Abs. *Arthritis Res Ther*, 2004, 6, 366-72.

[65] Song, J; Park, YB; Lee, WK; Lee, KH; Lee, SK. Clinical associations of anti-endothelial cell Abs in patients with systemic lupus erythematosus. *Rheumatol Int*, 2000, 20, 1-7.

[66] Schenatto, CB; Xavier, RM; Bredemeier M; et al. Raised serum S100B protein levels in neuropsychiatric lupus. *Ann Rheum Dis.*, 2006, 65, 829-31

[67] Hirohata, S; Miyamoto, T. Elevated levels of interleukin-6 in cerebrospinal fluid from patients with systemic lupus erythematosus and central nervous system involvement. *Arthritis Rheum*, 1990, 33, 644-649.

[68] Jara, LJ; Irigoyen, L; Ortiz, MJ; Zazueta, B; Bravo, G; Espinoza, LR. Prolactin and interleukin-6 in neuropsychiatric lupus erythematosus. *Clin Rheumatol*, 1998, 17, 110-114.

[69] Trysberg, E; Carlsten, H; Tarkowski, A. Intrathecal cytokines in systemic lupus erythematosus with central nervous system involvement. *Lupus*, 2000, 9, 498-503.

[70] Shiozawa, S; Kuroki, Y; Kim, M; Hirohata, S; Ogino, T. Interferon-alpha in lupus psychosis. *Arthritis Rheum*, 1992, 35, 417-422.

[71] Faber-Elmann, A; Sthoeger, Z; Tcherniack, A; Dayan, M; Mozes, E. Activity of matrix metalloproteinase-9 is elevated in sera of patients with systemic lupus erythematosus. *Clin Exp Immunol.*, 2002, 127, 393-398.

[72] Ainiala, H; Hietaharju, A; Dastidar, P; et al. Increased serum matrix metalloproteinase 9 levels in systemic lupus erythematosus patients with neuropsychiatric manifestations and brain magnetic resonance imaging abnormalities. *Arthritis and Rheum*, 2004, 50, 858-65.

[73] Hirohata, S; Kanai, Y; Mitsuo, A; Tokano, Y; Hashimoto, H. NPSLE Research Subcommittee. Accuracy of cerebrospinal fluid IL-6 testing for diagnosis of lupus psychosis. A multicenter retrospective study. *Clin Rheumatol.*, 2009 Jul 12. [Epub ahead of print]

[74] Small, P; Mass, MF; Kohler, PF; Harbeck, RJ. Central nervous system involvement in SLE. Diagnostic profile and clinical features. *Arthritis Rheum*, 1977, 20, 869-878.

[75] Trysberg, E; Nylen, K; Rosengren, LE; Tarkowski, A. Neuronal and astrocytic damage in systemic lupus erythematosus patients with central nervous system involvement. *Arthritis and Rheum*, 2003, 48, 2881-87.

[76] Appenzeller, S; Rondina, JM; Li, LM; Costallat, LT; Cendes, F. Cerebral and corpus callosum atrophy in systemic lupus erythematosus. *Arthritis Rheum.*, 2005, 52, 2783-9.

[77] McCune, WJ; MacGuirre, A; Aisen, A; Gebarski, S. Identification of brain lesions in neuropsychiatric systemic lupus erythematosus by magnetic resonance scanning. *Arthritis Rheum*, 1988, 31, 159-166.

[78] Rovaris, M; Viti, B; Ciboddo, G; et al. Brain involvement in systemic immune mediated diseases: magnetic resonance and magnetisation transfer imaging study. *J Neurol Neurosurg Psychiatry.*, 2000, 68, 170-7.

[79] Sibbitt, WL; Jr; Schmidt, PJ; Hart, BL; Brooks, WM. Fluid attenuated inversion recovery (FLAIR) imaging in neuropsychiatric systemic lupus erythematosus. *J Rheumatol.*, 2003, 30, 1983-9.

[80] Cotton, F; Bouffard-Vercelli, J; Hermier, M; et al. MRI of central nervous system in a series of 58 systemic lupus erythematosus (SLE) patients with or without overt neuropsychiatric manifestations. *Rev Med Interne*, 2004, 25, 8-15.

[81] Peterson, PL; Howe, FA; Clark, CA; Axford, JS. Quantitative magnetic resonance imaging in neuropsychiatric systemic lupus erythematosus. *Lupus*, 2003, 12, 897-902.

[82] Graham, JW; Jan, W. MRI and the brain in systemic lupus erythematosus. *Lupus*, 2003, 12, 891-6.

[83] Csepany, T; Bereczki, D; Kollar, J; Sikula, J; Kiss, E; Csiba, L. MRI findings in central nervous system systemic lupus erythematosus are associated with immunoserological parameters and hypertension. *J Neurol*, 2003, 250, 1348-54.

[84] Jennings, JE; Sundgren, PC; Attwood, J; McCune, J; Maly, P. Value of MRI of the brain in patients with systemic lupus erythematosus and neurologic disturbance. *Neuroradiology*, 2004, 46, 15-21.

[85] Oku, K; Atsumi, T; Furukawa, S; et al. Cerebral imaging by magnetic resonance imaging and single photon emission computed tomography in systemic lupus erythematosus with central nervous system involvement. *Rheumatology*, (Oxford) 2003, 12, 773-7.

[86] Holliday, SL; Navarrete, MG; Hermosillo-Romo, D; Valdez, CR; Saklad, AR; Escalante, A; Brey, RL. Validating a computerized neuropsychological test battery for mixed ethnic lupus patients. *Lupus.*, 2003, 12, 697-703.

[87] Steens, SC; Admiraal-Behloul, F; Bosma, GP; et al. Selective gray matter damage in neuropsychiatric lupus. *Arthritis Rheum.*, 2004, 50, 2877-81.

[88] Vermeer, SE; Priens, ND; den Heijer, T; Hofman, A; Koudstaal, PJ; Breteler, MB. Silent brain infarcts and the risk of dementia and cognitive decline. *N Engl J Med*, 2003, 348, 1215-22.

[89] Appenzeller, S; Vasconcelos Faria, A; Li, LM; Costallat, LT; Cendes, F. Quantitative magnetic resonance imaging analyses and clinical significance of hyperintense white matter lesions in systemic lupus erythematosus patients. *Ann Neurol.*, 2008, 64, 635-43

[90] Bosma, GP; Rood, MJ; Huizinga, TW; de Jong, BA; Bollen, EL; van Buchem, MA. Detection of cerebral involvement in patients with active neuropsychiatric systemic lupus erythematosus by the use of volumetric magnetization transfer imaging. *Arthritis Rheum.*, 2000, 43, 2428-36.

[91] Bosma, GP; Rood, MJ; Zwinderman, AH; Huizinga, TW; van Buchem, MA. Evidence of central nervous system damage in patients with neuropsychiatric systemic lupus erythematosus, demonstrated by magnetization transfer imaging. *Arthritis Rheum.*, 2000, 43, 48-54.

[92] Moritani, T; Shrier, DA; Numaguchi, Y; et al. Diffusion-weighted echo-planar MR imaging of CNS involvement in systemic lupus erythematosus. *Acad Radiol.*, 2001, 8, 741-53.

[93] Demaerel, P; De Ruyter, N; Maes, F; Velghe, B; Wilms, G. Magnetic resonance angiography in suspected cerebral vasculitis. *Eur Radiol.*, 2004, 14, 1005-12.

[94] Hanly, JG. Single photon emission computed tomography scanning in neuropsychiatric systemic lupus erythematosus. *J Rheumatol.*, 1998, 25, 401-3.

[95] Nossent, JC; Hovestadt, A; Schonfeld, DH; Swaak, AJ. Single-photon-emission computed tomography of the brain in the evaluation of cerebral lupus. *Arthritis Rheum*, 1991, 34, 1397-403.

[96] Rubbert, A; Marienhagen, J; Pirner, K; et al. Single-photon emission computed tomography analysis of cerebral blood flow in the evaluation of central nervous system involvement in patients with systemic lupus erythematosus. *Arthritis Rheum*, 1993, 36, 1253-62.

[97] Rogers, MP; Waterhouse, E; Nagel, JS; et al. I-23 iofetamine SPECT scan in systemic lupus erythematousus with cognitive and other minor neuropsychiatric symptoms: a pilot study. *Lupus*, 1992, 1, 215-219.

[98] Kovacs, JA; Urowitz, MB; Gladman, DD; Zeman, R. The use of single photon emission computerized tomography in neuropsychiatric SLE: a pilot study. *J Rheumatol*, 1995, 22, 1247-53.

[99] Sabet, A; Sibbitt, WL; Jr; Stidley, CA; Danska, J; Brooks, WM. Neurometabolite markers of cerebral injury in the antiphospholipid antibody syndrome of systemic lupus erythematosus. *Stroke.*, 1998, 29, 2254-60.

[100] de Certaines, JD; Bovee, WMMJ; Podo, F. Magnetic resonance spectroscopy in biology and medicine: *functional and pathological tissue characterization.*, New York: Pergamon Press, 1992.

[101] Rudkin, TM; Arnold, DL. Proton magnetic resonance spectroscopy for the diagnosis and management of cerebral disorders. *Arch Neurol.*, 1999, 56, 919-26.

[102] Denburg, SD; Carbotte, RM; Denburg, JA. Corticosteroids and neuropsychological functioning in patients with systemic lupus erythematosus. *Arthritis Rheum*, 1994, 37, 1311-1320.

[103] Barile, L; Lavalle, C. Transverse myelitis in systemic lupus erythematosus—the effect of IV pulse methylprednisolone and cyclophosphamide. *J Rheumatol*, 1992, 19, 370-372.

[104] Eyanson, S; Passo, MH; Aldo-Benson, MA; Benson, MD. Methylprednisolone pulse therapy for nonrenal lupus erythematosus. *Ann Rheum Dis*, 1980, 39, 377-380.

[105] Mok, CC; Lau, CS; Wong, RW. Treatment of lupus psychosis with oral cyclophosphamide followed by azathioprine maintenance: an open-label study. *Am J Med*, 2003, 115, 59-62.

[106] Barile-Fabris, L; Ariza-Andraca, R; Olguin-Ortega, L; et al. Controlled clinical trial of IV cyclophosphamide versus IV methylprednisolone in severe neurological manifestations in systemic lupus erythematosus. *Ann Rheum Dis.*, 2005, 64, 620-5.

[107] Leung, FK; Fortin, PR. Intravenous cyclophosphamide and high dose corticosteroids improve MRI lesions in demyelinating syndrome in systemic lupus erythematosus. *J Rheumatol*, 2003, 30, 1871-73.

[108] Boumpas, DT; Yamada, H; Patronas, NJ; Scott, D; Klippel, JH; Balow, JE. Pulse cyclophosphamide for severe neuropsychiatric lupus. *Q J Med.*, 1991, 81, 975-984.

[109] Neuwelt, CM; Lacks, S; Kaye, BR; Ellman, JB; Borenstein, DG. Role of intravenous cyclophosphamide in the treatment of severe neuropsychiatric systemic lupus erythematosus. *Am J Med*, 1995, 98, 32-41.

[110] Ramos, PC; Mendez, MJ; Ames, PR; Khamashta, MA; Hughes, GR. Pulse cyclophosphamide in the treatment of neuropsychiatric systemic lupus erythematosus. *Clin Exp Rheumatol*, 1996, 14, 295-299.

[111] Mok, CC; Lau, CS; Chan, EY; Wong, RW. Acute transverse myelopathy in systemic lupus erythematosus: clinical presentation, treatment, and outcome. *J Rheumatol*, 1998, 25, 467-473.

[112] Galindo-Rodriguez, G; Avina-Zubieta, JA; Pizarro, S; et al. Cyclophosphamide pulse therapy in optic neuritis due to systemic lupus erythematosus: an open trial. *Am J Med*, 1999, 106, 65-69.

[113] McCune, WJ; Golbus, J; Zeldes, W; Bohlke, P; Dunne, R; Fox, DA. Clinical and immunologic effects of monthly administration of intravenous cyclophosphamide in severe systemic lupus erythematosus. *N Engl J Med*, 1988, 318, 1423-1431.

[114] Khamashta, MA; Cuadrado, MJ; Mujic, F; Taub, NA; Hunt, BJ; Hughes, GR. The management of thrombosis in the antiphospholipid-antibody syndrome. *N Engl J Med.*, 1995, 332, 993-7.

[115] Crowther, MA; Ginsberg, JS; Julian, J; et al. A comparison of two intensities of warfarin for the prevention of recurrent thrombosis in patients with the antiphospholipid antibody syndrome. *N Engl J Med.*, 2003, 349, 1133-38.

[116] Cuadrado, MJ; Khamashta, MA; Ballesteros, A; Godfrey, T; Simon, MJ; Hughes, GRV. Can neurologic manifestations of Hughes (antiphospholipid) syndrome be distinguished from multiple sclerosis? Analysis of 27 patients and review of the literature. *Medicine* (Baltimore), 2000, 79, 57-68.

[117] Sanna, G; Bertolaccini, ML; Mathieu A. Central nervous system lupus: a clinical approach to therapy, *Lupus*, 2003, 12, 935-942.

[118] Baca, V; Lavalle, C; Garcia, R; et al. Favorable response to intravenous methylprednisolone and cyclophosphamide in children with severe neuropsychiatric lupus. *J Rheumatol*, 1999, 26, 432-439.

[119] Harisdangkul, V; Doorenbos, D; Subramony, SH. Lupus transverse myelopathy: better outcome with early recognition and aggressive highdose intravenous corticosteroid pulse treatment. *J Neurol*, 1995, 242, 326-331.

[120] Chatham, WW; Kimberly, RP. Treatment of lupus with corticosteroids. *Lupus*, 2001, 10, 140-147.

[121] Funauchi, M; Ohno, M; Nozaki, Y; Sugiyama, M; Kinoshita, K; Kanamaru, A. Intrathecal corticosteroids for systemic lupus erythematosus with central nervous system involvement. *J Rheumatol*, 2003, 30, 207-208.

[122] Propper, DJ; Bucknall, RC. Acute transverse myelopathy complicating systemic lupus erythematosus. *Ann Rheum Dis*, 1989, 48, 512-515.

[123] Boumpas, DT; Yamada, H; Patronas, NJ; Scott, D; Klippel, JH; Balow JE. Pulse cyclophosphamide for severe neuropsychiatric lupus. *Q J Med*, 1991, 81, 975-984.

[124] Takada, K; Illei, GG; Boumpas, DT. Cyclophosphamide for the treatment of systemic lupus erythematosus. *Lupus*, 2001, 10, 154- 161.

[125] Trevisani, VF; Castro, AA; Neves Neto, JF; Atallah, AN. Cyclophosphamide versus methylprednisolone for the treatment of neuropsychiatric involvement in systemic lupus erythematosus. *Cochrane Database Syst Rev*, 2000, CD002265.

[126] Sakic, B; Kolb, B; Whishaw, IQ; Gorny, G; Szechtman, H; Denburg, JA. Immunosuppression prevents neuronal atrophy in lupus-prone mice: evidence for brain damage induced by autoimmune disease? *J Neuroimmunol*, 2000, 111, 93-101.

[127] Farrell, M; Sakic, B; Szechtman, H; Denburg, JA. Effect of cyclophosphamide on leukocytic in. ltration in the brain ofMRL/lpr mice. *Lupus*, 1997, 6, 268-274.

[128] Sakic, B; Szechtman, H; Denburg, SD; Denburg, JA. Immunosuppressive treatment prevents behavioral de. cit in autoimmune MRL-lpr mice. *Physiol Behav*, 1995, 58, 797-802.

[129] Schroeder, JO; Euler, HH. Treatment combining plasmapheresis and pulse cyclophosphamide in severe systemic lupus erythematosus. *Adv Exp Med Biol*, 1989, 260, 203-213.

[130] Kazatchkine, MD; Kaveri, SV. Immunomodulation of autoimmune and inflammatory diseases with intravenousimmune globulin. *N Engl J Med*, 2001, 345, 747-755.

[131] Hughes, RA; Raphael, JC; Swan, AV; van Doorn, PA. Intravenous immunoglobulin for Guillain-Barre syndrome. *Cochrane Database Syst Rev*, 2001, CD002063.

[132] Sherer, Y; Levy, Y; Langevitz, P; Lorber, M; Fabrizzi, F; Shoenfeld, Y. Successful treatment of systemic lupus erythematosus cerebritis with intravenous immunoglobulin. *Clin Rheumatol*, 1999, 18, 170-173.

[133] Tomer, Y; Shoenfeld, Y. Successful treatment of psychosis secondary to SLE with high dose intravenous immunoglobulin. *Clin Exp Rheumatol*, 1992, 10, 391-393.

[134] Valesini, G; Priori, R; Francia, A; et al. Central nervous system involvement in systemic lupus erythematosus: a new therapeutic approach with intrathecal dexamethasone and methotrexate. *Springer Semin Immunopathol*, 1994, 16, 313-321.

[135] Dong, Y; Zhang, X; Tang, F; Tian, X; Zhao, Y; Zhang, F. Intrathecal injection with methotrexate plus dexamethasone in the treatment of central nervous system involvement in systemic lupus erythematosus. *Chin Med J*, (Engl) 2001, 114, 764-766.

[136] Hay, EM. Psychiatric disorder and cognitive impairment in SLE. *Lupus*, 1994, 3, 145-148.

[137] Schantz, V; Oestergaard, LL; Junker, P. Shrinking spinal cord following transverse myelopathy in a patient with systemic lupus erythematosus and the phospholipid antibody syndrome. *J Rheumatol*, 1998, 25, 1425-1428.

[138] Moore, PM; Isenberg, D. Therapy of neuro-psychiatric systemic lupus erythematosus. *Rheumatol Europe*, 1997, 26, 36-39.

[139] Grisanti, M; Nader, A; Cacciuttolo, R. Central nervous system involvement due to systemic lupus erythematosus/antiphospholipid syndrome: successful treatment with mycophenolate mofetil. *Lupus*, 2001, 10, S31.

[140] Mathieu, A; Sanna, G; Mameli, A; et al. Sustained normalization of cerebral blood-flow after iloprost therapy in a patient with neuropsychiatric systemic lupus erythematosus. *Lupus*, 2002, 11, 52-56.

[141] Nwobi, O; Abitbol, CL; Chandar, J; Seeherunvong, W; Zilleruelo, G. Rituximab therapy for juvenile-onset systemic lupus erythematosus. *Pediatr Nephrol.*, 2008, 23, 413-9.

[142] Tokunaga, M; Saito, K; Kawabata, D; Imura, Y; Fujii, T; Nakayamada, S; Tsujimura, S; Nawata, M; Iwata, S; Azuma, T; Mimori, T; Tanaka, Y. Efficacy of rituximab (anti-CD20) for refractory systemic lupus erythematosus involving the central nervous system. *Ann Rheum Dis.*, 2007, 66, 470-5.

[143] Appenzeller, S; Costallat, LT. Clinical implications of migraine in systemic lupus erythematosus: relation to cumulative organ damage. *Cephalalgia.*, 2004, 24, 1024-30.

[144] Appenzeller, S; Cendes, F; Costallat, LT. Epileptic seizures in systemic lupus erythematosus. *Neurology.*, 2004, 63, 1808-12.

[145] Cimaz, R; Meroni, PL; Shoenfeld, Y. Epilepsy as part of systemic lupus erythematosus and systemic antiphospholipid syndrome (Hughes syndrome). *Lupus.*, 2006, 15, 191-7.

[146] D'Cruz, DP; Mellor-Pita, S; Joven, B; Sanna, G; Allanson, J; Taylor, J; Khamashta, MA; Hughes, GR. Transverse myelitis as the first manifestation of systemic lupus erythematosus or lupus-like disease: good functional outcome and relevance of antiphospholipid antibodies. *J Rheumatol.*, 2004, 31, 280-5.

In: Autoimmune Diseases: Symptoms, Diagnosis and Treatment   ISBN: 978-1-61668-007-7
Editor: Kyle J. Brenner, pp. 233-249   © 2010 Nova Science Publishers, Inc.

Chapter 5

EMERGING METHODS IN TYPE 1 DIABETES IMMUNOMODULATION: BEYOND THE CONVENTIONAL

Brett E. Phillips and *Nick Giannoukakis*[*]
Department of Pathology, Rangos Research Center,
Children's Hospital of Pittsburgh of UPMC,
One Children's Hospital Drive, 4401 Penn Avenue,
Pittsburgh, PA 15224, USA

ABSTRACT

Type 1 diabetes is an autoimmune disease likely initiated by stress on insulin-producing pancreatic beta cells which eventually leads to beta cell-specific pathogenic T-cell activation and the eventual eradication of significant beta cell mass. The absence of insulin therefore leads to hyperglycemia that requires replacement of the hormone for normal glucohomeostasis. Exogenous insulin replacement alone, however, is insufficient in preventing diabetes-associated complications because it is unable to match the tight metabolic control the body is able to marshal with the endogenous production of insulin. Therefore, the aim of type 1 diabetes therapy is the return of insulin production to levels that achieve normal glucose homeostasis with an abrogation of the underlying autoimmunity. Therapies that modulate and restore proper immune function before loss of the beta cell mass are key in the development of a true cure for type 1 diabetes. These immunoregulatory therapies will be discussed along with methods of early disease diagnosis.

---

[*] Corresponding author: E-mail: ngiann1+@pitt.edu

DISEASE DIAGNOSES AND PREDICTION

Type 1 diabetes is not clinically diagnosed until blood glucose levels become extremely elevated. During the asymptomatic period preceding clinical onset, a chronic and ever-increasing intensity of autoimmune infiltration occurs in the pancreatic islets of Langerhans. Infiltration first impairs the function of and then destroys as much as 80% of the beta cell mass [1]. Efforts have been made at identifying genetic susceptibility makers for type 1 diabetes, of which HLA alleles and DNA sequence variation at the insulin gene locus confer the highest genetic risk [2, 3]. It is worth noting that not all high-risk individuals progress to clinical disease, an indication that some environmental factor accelerates and/or facilitates the conversion to pathologic autoimmunity. Indeed, monozygote twins only display a 50% concordance in the development of type 1 diabetes [2]. Another strategy is to screen for the presence of autoantibodies before the clinical onset of diabetes. Autoantibodies against insulin (IAA), whole islets (ICA), glutamic acid decarboylase (GAD), and islet cell antigen 512 (IA-2) have shown clinical relavence in predicting the development of type 1 diabetes [4]. As in the case of high risk HLA and insulin gene risk alleles, the presence of one or more of these autoantibodies does not guarantee that the patient will develop diabetes [5, 6]. The detection of 3 separate antibodies is required to approach a 100% confidence that the patient will develop diabetes [7]. The predictive value of screening is further complicated since the presence of these autoantibodies changes with the patient's age. For example, while IAA antibodies are found in 70% of diabetic patients at 5 years and younger, the percentage drops to 30% in patients developing diabetes past the age of 15 [5, 6]. The uncertainty in predicting disease onset and the probability that not all patients will undergo early screening for type 1 diabetes only heightens the need for therapeutic strategies that will be effective after sustained damage to pancreatic beta cells has occurred.

RESTORING INSULIN PRODUCING CELL POPULATIONS

Restoration of insulin production through the regeneration of beta cell mass in new onset disease is a reality as shown in some recent studies [8, 9]. While the exact mechanism of regeneration of beta cells is not clear, mounting evidence indicates that differentiation of pancreatic endocrine cell progenitors is activated in response to damage (quite possibly by immune cell-produced cytokines and growth factors) [10, 11]or that existing beta cells can undergo replication in response to a loss of adjacent cells [12-14]. Indeed, a recently study demonstrated that pancreatic exocrine cells can transdifferentiate into functional beta-like cells through the expression of pancreatic specific transcription factors [15]. Additionally the presence of multipotent progenitor cells has been found to exist in the pancreas with the ability to give rise to functional beta cells [16]. What remains unclear is if sufficient beta cell regeneration will occur on its own, or if an exogenous intervention is required.

Islet transplantation is a clinical reality [17]. However, a number of technical issues as well as the obvious limitation of cadaveric donors reserves this option for instances where insulin replacement cannot achieve any degree of euglycemia. The largest hurdle to allogeneic cadaveric donor-derived islet transplantation has been the acute non-specific inflammation that is triggered at the time of pancreas procurement, throughout the islet isolation process and then at the time of transplantation [18, 19]. Added to this burden is an acute allogeneic rejection process with an underlying autoimmunity [20-22]. While rejection has been adequately controlled with recent variations of anti-rejection drug cocktails, eventually, islet transplants fail [20]. It is unclear whether the anti-rejection drugs participate or exacerbate an ongoing process of non-specific inflammation or if they impair the beta cells themselves [23]. Nevertheless, it may be possible, and the proof-of-concept has been demonstrated in many instances, to engineer islets ex vivo or in vivo at the transplantation site to make them resistant to the rapid acute inflammation and the rejection following transplantation [24-30]. Where islets may be in limited number, a number of stem cell-based approaches offer some alternative hope in identifying a reliable insulin-producing surrogate.

Stem cells are defined by their ability for nearly unlimited cell division and to differentiate into a large number of different cell types. If an efficient method of inducing beta cell differentiation can be discovered, these cells can provide an ideal source of insulin producing cells. Early attempts have produced low yields of insulin producing cells from embryonic stem cells, but insulin levels were low and insulin secretion was not coupled to glucose levels as with endogenous beta cells [31-39]. Later methods have produced glucose sensitive cells, but the yield of insulin producing cells remains low [40, 41]. The modification of adult stem cells, which may not naturally be able to give rise to beta-like cells, is also under development [42-46]. Adult stem cells can be harvested directly from the patient, eliminating the change of transplantation rejection with reintroduction of the modified cells into the body. The hurdles that remain for these promising techniques is testing safety, increasing production, and testing the ability of these cells to function in a hostile environment already targeting the destruction of endogenous beta cells.

In the absence of a method to reliably regenerate beta cells, and where lifelong insulin replacement does not prevent the complications associated with diabetes (kidney, nervous system, eye, circulation), it may be feasible to express an insulin transgene *in vivo* under the control of a glucose-responsive gene promoter, or in a secretory cell that is glucose-responsive itself. For example, enteroendocrine K cells in the stomach, duodenum, and jejunum express the gene for the glucose sensor glucokinase and the glucose-dependent insulinotropic peptide GIP (Gastric inhibitory peptide) which enhances insulin secretion in a glucose dependent manner [47]. Transgenic mice expressing human insulin under the GIP promoter in K cells produce sufficient insulin to maintain euglycema even in the instance of beta cell absence [47]. Currently Engene is nearing clinical trials with an oral drug delivery system called GEMS^{TM} (Gut Endocrine-cell Modification System) which will non-invasively deliver the insulin gene to K cells. This could offer an alternative to, and could obviate islet transplantation and perhaps stem cell-based alternatives.

IMMUNOMODULATION

There are two levels at which the immune system can be manipulated to achieve a therapeutic endpoint to prevent and treat type 1 diabetes. Intervention prior to any overt clinical hyperglycemia can be accomplished through suppression or eradication of autoreactive T-cells. This can be achieved by antigen-specific tolerance induction protocols (i.e. provision of beta cell antigens in a tolerogenic manner), or by administration of autologous suppressive cells that could be, preferentially, antigen-specific. At the overt clinical stage, there are two problems the therapist faces. Insulin levels must be restored by abrogating the impairment of insulin production and expanding existing insulin producing cells through endogenous or surrogate beta cells. To achieve this requires either beta cell regeneration or transplantation of beta cells (or their surrogates) along with immunosuppression. Immunosuppressive cells have been identified among all leukocyte subsets. T-cells and antigen-presenting cells currently offer the most promise to induce anti-diabetic immunoregulation.

Targeted Cell Ablation

Beta cell destruction is the direct result of T-cell activation specific for beta cell autoantigens. Antibodies have been developed to target CD3 and CD4 surface markers on T-cells. These two markers both assist the T-cell recepetor (TCR) in T-cell activation after antigen presentation. Antibodies against CD3 [48, 49] and CD4 [50] have been able to reverse new onset diabetes in NOD mouse models. Anti-CD3 antibodies demonstrated establishment of CD4+ CD25+ T-regulatory cell (Treg) populations in NOD mouse models [51] and humans [52]. Treg are a T-cell subpopulation that have anti-inflammatory properties and promote tolerance to autoantigens. Antibodies targeted against CD4+ T-cells produced an immunosuppressive effect without establishing regulatory T-cell populations [50]. Complications may arise from the inability to establish regulatory cell populations, with further danger to existing CD4+ regulatory cells already present. This maybe the reason humanized CD3 antibodies have been extended into clinical trials [53] while CD4 antibodies have remained at the animal level of research. In addition to establishment of Treg cell populations, patient blood sera cytokine profiles from CD3 clinical trials display a shift from the T-helper 1 (Th1) to T-helper 2 (Th2) cytokine profile [54]. T-helper cells are a T-cell subset that helps augment immune system function through the production of cytokines. Two subsets of Th cells exist: Th1 cells that produce IL-2 and cytokines that activate cytotoxic T-cells and Th2 cells that produce IL-10 and cytokines that inhibit T-cell activation. The balance between these two populations determines immune system responsiveness. Despite these promising results, these techniques were unable to restore euglycemia to diabetic patients.

B-cells are responsible for antibody production, and in part, antigen presentation to T-cells in type 1 diabetes [55-58]. In the Non-obese diabetic (NOD) mouse model which spontaneously develops type 1 diabetes, ablation of B-cells by genetic manipulations or antibody targeted destruction reduces the incidence of diabetes development [59, 60]. B-cell ablation with the anti-CD20 antibody rituximab (Rituxan) has also been shown to reverse one third of new onset diabetes in NOD mice [60]. While the exact mechanism is unclear, B-cell ablation impairs CD4+ CD8+ T-cell activation without effecting cell population size or subset distrubtion in other immune cells. Multiple human clinical trails are underway testing Rituxan ability to reverse type 1 diabetes.

Tolerance Strategies Using Diabetes-Associated Antigens and Peptides

T-cell proliferation is triggered following recognition of specific anitgens on antigen presenting cells. Subsequently, they will react to the same antigen on or expressed by targets throughout the body. In some instances, exogenous application of antigens in large concentration can induce anergy of T-cells responsive to the specific antigen. This phenomenon underlies a number of peptide- and antigen-based methods aimed at inducing silencing of autoreactive T-cells directly through anergy or indirectly via upregulating the activity of antigen-specific immunoregulatory sister T-cells. Autoantigens that have been reported include insulin, glutamic acid decarboxylase (GAD), and heat shock protein 60 (HSP60), while more remain unidentified [61-64]. T-cells responsive to insulin have been found in 92% of type 1 diabetic patients [65], with 66.7% patients showing responsiveness to GAD65 [66] and 87% to HSP60 [67]. NOD mice that range from a pre-diabetic state to overtly diabetic state similarly show a high degree of T-cell reactivity to insulin, specifically to the amino acid residues 9-23 that make up the insulin amino acid chain [68-72]. Methods of inactivation or complete elimination of activated T-cells have been tested as therapeutic strategies to restore proper immune function and balance.

Altered Peptide Ligands

T-cell specificity is based on its ability to recognize antigens it has been directed against. Binding of target antigens occurs through the TCR, with primary and secondary amino acid sequences on the recognized antigen being necessary for T-cell activation. By identifying the amino acid regions of importance for individual antigens, altered peptide ligands (APL) can be developed that have variations in these important regions. T-cells bind APL's without becoming fully activated while preventing endogenous autoantigens access to T-cells binding site [73]. This model of competitive inhibition has shown the ability to reduce or eliminate T-cell activation in the presence of beta cell antigens [73, 74].

The first APL considered for type 1 diabetes immunotherapy was an insulin analog produced and developed by Neurocrine Biosciences. T-cell activation by insulin is depended on the insulin amino acid region 9-23, and through modification of this region the analog NBI-6024 was developed [75]. NBI-6024 was able to promote a delay of diabetes onset and the incidence of occurrence in the NOD mouse model through its ability to shift T-helper cell (Th) populations to the Th2 profile promoting tolerance [75, 76]. NBI-6024 moved into phase II clinical trials after demonstrating safety over an extensive dosage range in phase I trials, but very little development has since ensued [76].

In contrast, the GAD65 analog from Diamyd [77] and the HSP60 analog DiaPep277 from DeveloGen Inc. [78, 79] have moved considerably into phase II studies. In trials of both peptides, diabetic recipients exhibited elevated insulin levels compared to controls in their respective clinical trials. DiaPep277 caused a shift from the Th1 to the Th2 profile displaying a similar mechanism of action as NBI-6024 [79]. The host's immune response still displayed reactivity to bacterial antigens [79]. Diverging from the other APL's, the Diamyd APL appears to mechanistically-involve an increase in CD4+CD25+ T regulartory cells (Treg) [77]. Unfortunately initial clinical trials with APL therapeutics, while promising, have been unable to restore euglycemia and more importantly insulin independence in diabetic patients [80].

Tolerance through Oral Administration of Diabetes-Associated Antigens

Oral administration of autoantigens has been shown to induce tolerance in a number of autoimmune diseases, including diabetes [81]. Treatment induces a shift to Th2 cytokine profiles, with large antigen doses inducing T-cell inactivity [81]. Intranasal administration of insulin to NOD mice, a related procedure, also conferred protection from diabetes [82]. These mice displayed increased IL-10 production levels suggesting a Th2 profile and expanded Treg populations [82]. The method has already completed phase I clinical trials and is moving into a phase II trial [83]. Unfortunately this technique relies on autoantibody screening to identify potential diabetic patients.

Tolerance through T Regulatory Cells

Tregs are an important regulatory subpopulation of T-cells and their recruitment and expansion is a commonly measured endpoint in various immunotherapy strategies. Expanding beyond monitoring their population size, studies have examined the ability of direct Treg administration in preventing the onset of diabetes. Studies in NOD mice have demonstrated the ability to reduce the spontaneous onset of diabetes [84-87]. Several protocols have also been establish at generating and expanding these cells *in vitro* [88-91]. While this method has yet to be applied to the treatment of diabetes, clinical trials are underway in the treatment of leukemia that will pave the way for future applications for type 1 diabetes.

DENDRITIC CELL TARGETED IMMUNOMODULATION

Dendritic cells are the sentinels and regulators of the immune system. Immature dendritic cells continuously circulate throughout the body sampling and examining their surroundings through a process of endocytosis [92]. These dendritic cells then travel to draining lymph nodes where they display captured autoantigens to T-cells promoting tolerance under normal conditions [93-98]. When confronted with exogenous antigens or tissue damage, dendritic cells mature, entering a new functional stage [99]. Mature dendritic cells shift their cytokine expression profiles to elicit pro-inflammatory signals and increase expression of their surface markers MHC class II and co-stimulatory molecules [99]. At the draining lymph node, the exogenous antigen is displayed on the dendritic cell's MHC complex to the T-cell's TCR. T-cell activation is fully consummated through dendritic cell co-stimulatory molecules interactions [100-102]. T-cells are thus activated towards specific antigens and can migrate into peripheral tissues to target specific cells or foreign bodies [103]. In this system, dendritic cells are the key regulators of T-cell activation and manage a tightly controlled process [93].

Dendritic cell-targeted therapies for immunosuppression rely on preventing dendritic cell maturation and hence antigen-specific T-cell activation. Prevention of costimulatory interactions leading to T-cell activation has shown to be reliably reproducible to induce immune hyporesponsiveness in various models [100-102, 104-109]. This concept has been used to achieve long-term allograft survival as well as to prevent autoimmunity [110-118]. Immature dendritic cells are believed to establish immune tolerance through changes in cytokine production, altered interactions with T-cells, and the upregulation of the number and activity of CD8+ Foxp3+ and/or CD25+ CD4+ Foxp3+ Treg [84, 88, 111, 119-130].

We have considered the ability of co-stimulation-impaired dendritic cells to induce immune tolerance in NOD mice. Administration of NOD dendritic cells treated in culture with short double-stranded oligonucleotide decoys specific for the NFkappaB (NFkB) transcription factor prevented the onset of diabetes [131]. These DC exhibited impaired NFkB nuclear translocation as well as downregulated cell-surface levels of CD40, CD80 and CD86. In a complementary approach, we treated NOD mice with dendritic cells treated in culture with a mixture of anitsense oligonucleotides targeting the primary transcripts of CD40, CD80 and CD86. These DC also prevented the onset of diabetes and facilitated the reversal of new onset disease in NOD mice [132, 133]. In both DC-based methods, we did not observe any reduction in overall T-cell responsiveness to alloantigens, displaying a preservation of immune system function. We have translated the antisense-treated DC approach to a phase I study in established human diabetic volunteers. Leukocytes of the patient are obtained by apheresis and dendritic cells are generated *in vitro* and engineered in GMP facilities with the addition of the mixture of CD40, CD80, CD86-targeting antisense DNA. These dendritic cells, expressing low levels of CD40, CD80, and CD86 are injected into the patient by intradermal administration at an anatomical site proximal to the pancreas. Attracted to the focus of inflammation, these treated cells are predicted to acquire apoptotic beta cells inside the islets (hence acquiring antigen specificity) and then will migrate into the pancreas-draining lymph nodes. Once where, they will deliver an anergizing signal to the T-cells they encounter and/or induce regulatory immune cells, like Foxp3+ T-cells. Through these changes, the ongoing autoimmune process of beta cell destruction though T-cell autoantigen activation will be halted allowing for recovery of beta cell function and possible beta cell regeneration. The clinical trial is ongoing and will soon move into a phase II efficacy trial to reverse new onset disease once safety has been confirmed in all recipients in the phase I study.

New approaches to confer co-stimulation impairment to dendritic cells are currently under development and testing. *In vivo* modification of dendritic cell function would eliminate the need for costly apheresis and GMP culture facilities for dendritic cell preparation. Microparticle delivery of the mixture of CD40, CD80, CD86-targeting antisense DNA has been demonstrated to modify dendritic cell functions once its contents are delivered by phagocytosis [134-136]. Specifically, we have shown that microsphere delivery of the antisense DNA into NOD mice at a physically-proximal location to the pancreas results in prevention of diabetes as well as reversal of new-onset disease. Dendritic cells acquiring the microspheres exhibited low co-stimulation in the absence of systemic and non-specific immunosuppression [136].

CONCLUSION

Conventional insulin replacement as a therapy for type 1 diabetes does not solve the almost certain complications due to non-physiological glucohomeostasis. Indeed, diabetes is more than a glucose/insulin problem, with the knowledge that insulin replacement does not address the cause or the recurrence of the autoimmune destruction of the pancreatic beta cells whether by islet transplantation or beta cell surrogates. Concurrently, immunosuppression has moved past the conventional pharmacologic chemical agents into the realm of biologics, including monoclonal antibodies and fusion proteins. Cell and antigen-based strategies can at least complement such methods, if not outright obviate them should antigen-specific tolerance be achieved in the absence of conventional immunosuppression. Ongoing cell trials promise to open up a new frontier, not only for autoimmune diseases but for other conditions where suppression of immunity is warranted. The application of these techniques in current type 1 diabetes clinical trials has shown further promise in their ability to not only affect the targeted cells, but lead to the establishment of other regulatory cell types. This restoration of regulatory cell populations may be necessary for long term restoration of proper immune function and the success of these technologies.

REFERENCES

[1] Bresson, D. & von Herrath, M. (2007). Moving towards efficient therapies in type 1 diabetes: to combine or not to combine? *Autoimmunity reviews, 6*, 315-322.

[2] Kantarova, D. & Buc, M. (2007). Genetic susceptibility to type 1 diabetes mellitus in humans. *Physiological research / Academia Scientiarum Bohemoslovaca, 56*, 255-266.

[3] Maier, L. M. & Wicker, L. S. (2005). Genetic susceptibility to type 1 diabetes. *Current opinion in immunology, 17*, 601-608.

[4] Isermann, B., Ritzel, R., Zorn, M., Schilling, T. & Nawroth, P. P. (2007). Autoantibodies in diabetes mellitus: current utility and perspectives. *Exp Clin Endocrinol Diabetes, 115*, 483-490.

[5] Verge, C. F., Howard, N. J., Rowley, M. J., Mackay, I. R., Zimmet, P. Z., Egan, M., Hulinska, H., Hulinsky, I., Silvestrini, R. A., Kamath, S., et al. (1994). Anti-glutamate decarboxylase and other antibodies at the onset of childhood IDDM: a population-based study. *Diabetologia, 37*, 1113-1120.

[6] Bingley, P. J., Bonifacio, E., Williams, A. J., Genovese, S., Bottazzo, G. F. & Gale, E. A. (1997). Prediction of IDDM in the general population: strategies based on combinations of autoantibody markers. *Diabetes, 46*, 1701-1710.

[7] Verge, C. F., Gianani, R., Kawasaki, E., Yu, L., Pietropaolo, M., Jackson, R. A., Chase, H. P. & Eisenbarth, G. S. (1996). Prediction of type I diabetes in first-degree relatives using a combination of insulin, GAD, and ICA512bdc/IA-2 autoantibodies. *Diabetes, 45*, 926-933.

[8] Wang, G. S., Rosenberg, L. & Scott, F. W. (2005). Tubular complexes as a source for islet neogenesis in the pancreas of diabetes-prone BB rats. *Laboratory investigation; a journal of technical methods and pathology, 85*, 675-688.

[9] Cano, D. A., Rulifson, I. C., Heiser, P. W., Swigart, L. B., Pelengaris, S., German, M., Evan, G. I., Bluestone, J. A. & Hebrok, M. (2007). Regulated -cell regeneration in the adult mouse pancreas. *Diabetes*.

[10] Sharma, A., Zangen, D. H., Reitz, P., Taneja, M., Lissauer, M. E., Miller, C. P., Weir, G. C., Habener, J. F. & Bonner-Weir, S. (1999). The homeodomain protein IDX-1 increases after an early burst of proliferation during pancreatic regeneration. *Diabetes*, *48*, 507-513.

[11] Lampeter, E. F., Gurniak, M., Brocker, U., Klemens, C., Tubes, M., Friemann, J. & Kolb, H. (1995). Regeneration of beta-cells in response to islet inflammation. *Exp Clin Endocrinol Diabetes*, *103*, Suppl 2, 74-78.

[12] Gershengorn, M. C., Hardikar, A. A., Wei, C., Geras-Raaka, E., Marcus-Samuels, B. & Raaka, B. M. (2004). Epithelial-to-mesenchymal transition generates proliferative human islet precursor cells. *Science (New York, N.Y, 306*, 2261-2264.

[13] Tokoro, T., Tezel, E., Nagasaka, T., Kaneko, T. & Nakao, A. (2003). Differentiation of acinar cells into acinoductular cells in regenerating rat pancreas. *Pancreatology*, *3*, 487-496.

[14] Bouwens, L. (1998). Transdifferentiation versus stem cell hypothesis for the regeneration of islet beta-cells in the pancreas. *Microscopy research and technique*, *43*, 332-336.

[15] Zhou, Q., Brown, J., Kanarek, A., Rajagopal, J. & Melton, D. A. (2008). In vivo reprogramming of adult pancreatic exocrine cells to beta-cells. *Nature*, *455*, 627-632.

[16] Xu, X., D'Hoker, J., Stange, G., Bonne, S., De Leu, N., Xiao, X., Van de Casteele, M., Mellitzer, G., Ling, Z., Pipeleers, D., Bouwens, L., Scharfmann, R., Gradwohl, G. & Heimberg, H. (2008). Beta cells can be generated from endogenous progenitors in injured adult mouse pancreas. *Cell*, *132*, 197-207.

[17] Marzorati, S., Pileggi, A. & Ricordi, C. (2007). Allogeneic islet transplantation. *Expert opinion on biological therapy*, *7*, 1627-1645.

[18] Bennet, W., Groth, C. G., Larsson, R., Nilsson, B. & Korsgren, O. (2000). Isolated human islets trigger an instant blood mediated inflammatory reaction, implications for intraportal islet transplantation as a treatment for patients with type 1 diabetes. *Ups J Med Sci*, *105*, 125-133.

[19] Moberg, L. (2005). The role of the innate immunity in islet transplantation. *Ups J Med Sci*, *110*, 17-55.

[20] Roelen, D. L., Huurman, V. A., Hilbrands, R., Gillard, P., Duinkerken, G., van der Meer-Prins, P. W., Versteeg-van der Voort Maarschalk, M. F., Mathieu, C., Keymeulen, B., Pipeleers, D. G., Roep, B. O. & Claas, F. H. (2009). Relevance of cytotoxic alloreactivity under different immunosuppressive regimens in clinical islet cell transplantation. *Clinical and experimental immunology*, *156*, 141-148.

[21] Huurman, V. A., Hilbrands, R., Pinkse, G. G., Gillard, P., Duinkerken, G., van de Linde, P., van der Meer-Prins, P. M., Versteeg-van der Voort Maarschalk, M. F., Verbeeck, K., Alizadeh, B. Z., Mathieu, C., Gorus, F. K., Roelen, D. L., Claas, F. H., Keymeulen, B., Pipeleers, D. G. & Roep, B. O. (2008). Cellular islet autoimmunity associates with clinical outcome of islet cell transplantation. *PLoS One*, *3*, e2435.

[22] Van Belle, T. & von Herrath, M. (2008). Immunosuppression in islet transplantation. *The Journal of clinical investigation*, *118*, 1625-1628.

[23] D'Amico, E., Hui, H., Khoury, N., Di Mario, U. & Perfetti, R. (2005). Pancreatic beta-cells expressing GLP-1 are resistant to the toxic effects of immunosuppressive drugs. *J Mol Endocrinol, 34*, 377-390.

[24] Jackson, A., McWilliams, C., Kaizer, E., Chaussabel, D., Glaser, C., Noguchi, H., Matsumoto, S., Levy, M. F. & Naziruddin, B. (2008). Gene expression profiling of human pancreatic islets undergoing a simulated process of instant blood-mediated inflammatory reaction. *Transplant Proc, 40*, 430-432.

[25] Qin, J., Jiao, Y., Chen, X., Zhou, S., Liang, C. & Zhong, C. (2009). Overexpression of suppressor of cytokine signaling 1 in islet grafts results in anti-apoptotic effects and prolongs graft survival. *Life Sci, 84*, 810-816.

[26] Kawamoto, K., Tanemura, M., Deguchi, T., Machida, T., Nishida, T., Sawa, Y., Doki, Y., Mori, M. & Ito, T. (2009). In vivo controlling of cellular response to pig islet xenografts by adenovirus-mediated expression of either membrane-bound human FasL or human decoy Fas. *Transplant Proc, 41*, 331-333.

[27] Kim, Y. H., Lim, D. G., Wee, Y. M., Kim, J. H., Yun, C. O., Choi, M. Y., Park, Y. H. Kim, S. C. & Han, D. J. (2008). Viral IL-10 gene transfer prolongs rat islet allograft survival. *Cell Transplant, 17*, 609-618.

[28] Yamasaki, S., Kurita, N., Hata, J., Moritani, M., Itakura, M. & Shimada, M. (2007). The effect of transgenic expression of TGF-beta1 on transplanted islet graft survival. *Hepatogastroenterology, 54*, 1617-1621.

[29] Mathe, Z., Dupraz, P., Rinsch, C., Thorens, B., Bosco, D., Zbinden, M., Morel, P., Berney, T. & Pepper, M. S. (2006). Tetracycline-regulated expression of VEGF-A in beta cells induces angiogenesis: improvement of engraftment following transplantation. *Cell Transplant, 15*, 621-636.

[30] Borjesson, A., Andersson, A. K. & Sandler, S. (2006). Survival of an islet allograft deficient in iNOS after implantation into diabetic NOD mice. *Cell Transplant, 15*, 769-775.

[31] Lumelsky, N., Blondel, O., Laeng, P., Velasco, I., Ravin, R. & McKay, R. (2001). Differentiation of embryonic stem cells to insulin-secreting structures similar to pancreatic islets. *Science (New York, N.Y, 292*, 1389-1394.

[32] Soria, B., Roche, E., Berna, G., Leon-Quinto, T., Reig, J. A. & Martin, F. (2000). Insulin-secreting cells derived from embryonic stem cells normalize glycemia in streptozotocin-induced diabetic mice. *Diabetes, 49*, 157-162.

[33] Kania, G., Blyszczuk, P. & Wobus, A. M. (2004). The generation of insulin-producing cells from embryonic stem cells--a discussion of controversial findings. *The International journal of developmental biology, 48*, 1061-1064.

[34] Ku, H. T., Zhang, N., Kubo, A., O'Connor, R., Mao, M., Keller, G. & Bromberg, J. S. (2004). Committing embryonic stem cells to early endocrine pancreas in vitro. *Stem cells (Dayton, Ohio), 22*, 1205-1217.

[35] Kubo, A., Shinozaki, K., Shannon, J. M., Kouskoff, V., Kennedy, M., Woo, S., Fehling, H. J. & Keller, G. (2004). Development of definitive endoderm from embryonic stem cells in culture. *Development (Cambridge, England), 131*, 1651-1662.

[36] D'Amour, K. A., Agulnick, A. D., Eliazer, S., Kelly, O. G., Kroon, E. & Baetge, E. E. (2005). Efficient differentiation of human embryonic stem cells to definitive endoderm. *Nature biotechnology, 23*, 1534-1541.

[37] D'Amour, K. A., Bang, A. G., Eliazer, S., Kelly, O. G., Agulnick, A. D., Smart, N. G., Moorman, M. A., Kroon, E., Carpenter, M. K. & Baetge, E. E. (2006). Production of pancreatic hormone-expressing endocrine cells from human embryonic stem cells. *Nature biotechnology*, *24*, 1392-1401.

[38] Pfendler, K. C., Catuar, C. S., Meneses, J. J. & Pedersen, R. A. (2005). Overexpression of Nodal promotes differentiation of mouse embryonic stem cells into mesoderm and endoderm at the expense of neuroectoderm formation. *Stem cells and development*, *14*, 162-172.

[39] McLean, A. B., D'Amour, K. A., Jones, K. L., Krishnamoorthy, M., Kulik, M. J., Reynolds, D. M., Sheppard, A. M., Liu, H., Xu, Y., Baetge, E. E. & Dalton, S. (2007). Activin a efficiently specifies definitive endoderm from human embryonic stem cells only when phosphatidylinositol 3-kinase signaling is suppressed. *Stem cells (Dayton, Ohio)*, *25*, 29-38.

[40] Jiang, J., Au, M., Lu, K., Eshpeter, A., Korbutt, G., Fisk, G. & Majumdar, A. S. (2007). Generation of insulin-producing islet-like clusters from human embryonic stem cells. *Stem cells (Dayton, Ohio)*, *25*, 1940-1953.

[41] Jiang, W., Shi, Y., Zhao, D., Chen, S., Yong, J., Zhang, J., Qing, T., Sun, X., Zhang, P., Ding, M., Li, D. & Deng, H. (2007). In vitro derivation of functional insulin-producing cells from human embryonic stem cells. *Cell research*, *17*, 333-344.

[42] Okita, K., Ichisaka, T. & Yamanaka, S. (2007). Generation of germline-competent induced pluripotent stem cells. *Nature*, *448*, 313-317.

[43] Park, I. H., Zhao, R., West, J. A., Yabuuchi, A., Huo, H., Ince, T. A., Lerou, P. H., Lensch, M. W. & Daley, G. Q. (2008). Reprogramming of human somatic cells to pluripotency with defined factors. *Nature*, *451*, 141-146.

[44] Takahashi, K., Tanabe, K., Ohnuki, M., Narita, M., Ichisaka, T., Tomoda, K. & Yamanaka, S. (2007). Induction of pluripotent stem cells from adult human fibroblasts by defined factors. *Cell*, *131*, 861-872.

[45] Yu, J., Vodyanik, M. A., Smuga-Otto, K., Antosiewicz-Bourget, J., Frane, J. L., Tian, S., Nie, J., Jonsdottir, G. A., Ruotti, V., Stewart, R., Slukvin, II, & Thomson, J. A. (2007). Induced pluripotent stem cell lines derived from human somatic cells. *Science (New York, N.Y*, *318*, 1917-1920.

[46] Meissner, A., Wernig, M. & Jaenisch, R. (2007). Direct reprogramming of genetically unmodified fibroblasts into pluripotent stem cells. *Nature biotechnology*, *25*, 1177-1181.

[47] Cheung, A. T., Dayanandan, B., Lewis, J. T., Korbutt, G. S., Rajotte, R. V., Bryer-Ash, M., Boylan, M. O., Wolfe, M. M. & Kieffer, T. J. (2000). Glucose-dependent insulin release from genetically engineered K cells. *Science (New York, N.Y*, *290*, 1959-1962.

[48] Chatenoud, L., Primo, J. & Bach, J. F. (1997). CD3 antibody-induced dominant self tolerance in overtly diabetic NOD mice. *J Immunol*, *158*, 2947-2954.

[49] Chatenoud, L., Thervet, E., Primo, J. & Bach, J. F. (1994). Anti-CD3 antibody induces long-term remission of overt autoimmunity in nonobese diabetic mice. *Proceedings of the National Academy of Sciences of the United States of America*, *91*, 123-127.

[50] Makhlouf, L., Grey, S. T., Dong, V., Csizmadia, E., Arvelo, M. B., Auchincloss, H., Jr., Ferran, C. & Sayegh, M. H. (2004). Depleting anti-CD4 monoclonal antibody cures new-onset diabetes, prevents recurrent autoimmune diabetes, and delays allograft rejection in nonobese diabetic mice. *Transplantation*, *77*, 990-997.

[51] Belghith, M., Bluestone, J. A., Barriot, S., Megret, J., Bach, J. F. & Chatenoud, L. (2003). TGF-beta-dependent mechanisms mediate restoration of self-tolerance induced by antibodies to CD3 in overt autoimmune diabetes. *Nature medicine, 9*, 1202-1208.

[52] Bisikirska, B., Colgan, J., Luban, J., Bluestone, J. A. & Herold, K. C. (2005). TCR stimulation with modified anti-CD3 mAb expands CD8+ T cell population and induces CD8+CD25+ Tregs. *The Journal of clinical investigation, 115*, 2904-2913.

[53] Herold, K. C., Gitelman, S. E., Masharani, U., Hagopian, W., Bisikirska, B., Donaldson, D., Rother, K., Diamond, B., Harlan, D. M. & Bluestone, J. A. (2005). A single course of anti-CD3 monoclonal antibody hOKT3gamma1(Ala-Ala) results in improvement in C-peptide responses and clinical parameters for at least 2 years after onset of type 1 diabetes. *Diabetes, 54*, 1763-1769.

[54] Herold, K. C., Burton, J. B., Francois, F., Poumian-Ruiz, E., Glandt, M. & Bluestone. J. A. (2003). Activation of human T cells by FcR nonbinding anti-CD3 mAb, hOKT3gamma1(Ala-Ala). *The Journal of clinical investigation, 111*, 409-418.

[55] Bour-Jordan, H., Salomon, B. L., Thompson, H. L., Santos, R., Abbas, A. K. & Bluestone, J. A. (2007). Constitutive expression of B7-1 on B cells uncovers autoimmunity toward the B cell compartment in the nonobese diabetic mouse. *J Immunol, 179*, 1004-1012.

[56] Falcone, M., Lee, J., Patstone, G., Yeung, B. & Sarvetnick, N. (1998). B lymphocytes are crucial antigen-presenting cells in the pathogenic autoimmune response to GAD65 antigen in nonobese diabetic mice. *J Immunol, 161*, 1163-1168.

[57] Noorchashm, H., Lieu, Y. K., Noorchashm, N., Rostami, S. Y., Greeley, S. A., Schlachterman, A., Song, H. K., Noto, L. E., Jevnikar, A. M., Barker, C. F. & Naji, A. (1999). I-Ag7-mediated antigen presentation by B lymphocytes is critical in overcoming a checkpoint in T cell tolerance to islet beta cells of nonobese diabetic mice. *J Immunol, 163*, 743-750.

[58] Silveira, P. A., Johnson, E., Chapman, H. D., Bui, T., Tisch, R. M. & Serreze, D. V. (2002). The preferential ability of B lymphocytes to act as diabetogenic APC in NOD mice depends on expression of self-antigen-specific immunoglobulin receptors. *European journal of immunology, 32*, 3657-3666.

[59] Serreze, D. V., Chapman, H. D., Varnum, D. S., Hanson, M. S., Reifsnyder, P. C., Richard, S. D., Fleming, S. A., Leiter, E. H. & Shultz, L. D. (1996). B lymphocytes are essential for the initiation of T cell-mediated autoimmune diabetes: analysis of a new "speed congenic" stock of NOD.Ig mu null mice. *The Journal of experimental medicine, 184*, 2049-2053.

[60] Xiu, Y., Wong, C. P., Bouaziz, J. D., Hamaguchi, Y., Wang, Y., Pop, S. M., Tisch, R. M. & Tedder, T. F. (2008). B lymphocyte depletion by CD20 monoclonal antibody prevents diabetes in nonobese diabetic mice despite isotype-specific differences in Fc gamma R effector functions. *J Immunol, 180*, 2863-2875.

[61] Atkinson, M. A. & Maclaren, N. K. 1994. The pathogenesis of insulin-dependent diabetes mellitus. *N Engl J Med, 331*, 1428-1436.

[62] Delovitch, T. L. & Singh, B. (1997). The nonobese diabetic mouse as a model of autoimmune diabetes: immune dysregulation gets the NOD. *Immunity, 7*, 727-738.

[63] Wicker, L. S., Todd, J. A. & Peterson, L. B. (1995). Genetic control of autoimmune diabetes in the NOD mouse. *Annual review of immunology, 13*, 179-200.

[64] Durinovic-Bello, I. (1998). Autoimmune diabetes: the role of T cells, MHC molecules and autoantigens. *Autoimmunity, 27*, 159-177.

[65] Alleva, D. G., Crowe, P. D., Jin, L., Kwok, W. W., Ling, N., Gottschalk, M., Conlon, P. J., Gottlieb, P. A., Putnam, A. L. & Gaur, A. (2001). A disease-associated cellular immune response in type 1 diabetics to an immunodominant epitope of insulin. *The Journal of clinical investigation, 107*, 173-180.

[66] Kotani, R., Nagata, M., Moriyama, H., Nakayama, M., Yamada, K., Chowdhury, S. A., Chakrabarty, S., Jin, Z., Yasuda, H. & Yokono, K. (2002). Detection of GAD65-reactive T-Cells in type 1 diabetes by immunoglobulin-free ELISPOT assays. *Diabetes care, 25*, 1390-1397.

[67] Abulafia-Lapid, R., Elias, D., Raz, I., Keren-Zur, Y., Atlan, H. & Cohen. I. R. (1999). T cell proliferative responses of type 1 diabetes patients and healthy individuals to human hsp60 and its peptides. *Journal of autoimmunity, 12*, 121-129.

[68] Haskins, K. & Wegmann, D. (1996). Diabetogenic T-cell clones. *Diabetes, 45*, 1299-1305.

[69] Wegmann, D. R., Norbury-Glaser, M. & Daniel, D. (1994). Insulin-specific T cells are a predominant component of islet infiltrates in pre-diabetic NOD mice. *European journal of immunology, 24*, 1853-1857.

[70] Daniel, D., Gill, R. G., Schloot, N. & Wegmann, D. (1995). Epitope specificity, cytokine production profile and diabetogenic activity of insulin-specific T cell clones isolated from NOD mice. *European journal of immunology, 25*, 1056-1062.

[71] Daniel, D. & Wegmann, D. R. (1996). Protection of nonobese diabetic mice from diabetes by intranasal or subcutaneous administration of insulin peptide B-(9-23). *Proceedings of the National Academy of Sciences of the United States of America, 93*, 956-960.

[72] Wong, F. S., Karttunen, J., Dumont, C., Wen, L., Visintin, I., Pilip, I. M., Shastri, N., Pamer, E. G. & Janeway, C. A. Jr. (1999). Identification of an MHC class I-restricted autoantigen in type 1 diabetes by screening an organ-specific cDNA library. *Nature medicine, 5*, 1026-1031.

[73] Sloan-Lancaster, J. & Allen, P. M. (1996). Altered peptide ligand-induced partial T cell activation: molecular mechanisms and role in T cell biology. *Annual review of immunology, 14*, 1-27.

[74] Nicholson, L. B. & Kuchroo, V. K. (1997). T cell recognition of self and altered self antigens. *Critical reviews in immunology, 17*, 449-462.

[75] Alleva, D. G., Gaur, A., Jin, L., Wegmann, D., Gottlieb, P. A., Pahuja, A., Johnson, E. B., Motheral, T., Putnam, A., Crowe, P. D., Ling, N., Boehme, S. A. & Conlon, P. J. (2002). Immunological characterization and therapeutic activity of an altered-peptide ligand, NBI-6024, based on the immunodominant type 1 diabetes autoantigen insulin B-chain (9-23) peptide. *Diabetes, 51*, 2126-2134.

[76] Alleva, D. G., Maki, R. A., Putnam, A. L., Robinson, J. M., Kipnes, M. S., Dandona, P., Marks, J. B., Simmons, D. L., Greenbaum, C. J., Jimenez, R. G., Conlon, P. J. & Gottlieb. P. A. (2006). Immunomodulation in type 1 diabetes by NBI-6024, an altered peptide ligand of the insulin B epitope. *Scandinavian journal of immunology, 63*, 59-69.

[77] Agardh, C. D., Cilio, C. M., Lethagen, A., Lynch, K., Leslie, R. D., Palmer, M., Harris, R. A., Robertson, J. A. & Lernmark, A. (2005). Clinical evidence for the safety of

GAD65 immunomodulation in adult-onset autoimmune diabetes. *Journal of diabetes and its complications*, *19*, 238-246.

[78] Raz, I., Avron, A., Tamir, M., Metzger, M., Symer, L., Eldor, R., Cohen, I. R. & Elias, D. (2007). Treatment of new-onset type 1 diabetes with peptide DiaPep277 is safe and associated with preserved beta-cell function: extension of a randomized, double-blind, phase II trial. *Diabetes/metabolism research and reviews*, *23*, 292-298.

[79] Raz, I., Elias, D., Avron, A., Tamir, M., Metzger, M. & Cohen, I. R. (2001). Beta-cell function in new-onset type 1 diabetes and immunomodulation with a heat-shock protein peptide (DiaPep277), a randomised, double-blind, phase II trial. *Lancet*, *358*, 1749-1753.

[80] Lazar, L., Ofan, R., Weintrob, N., Avron, A., Tamir, M., Elias, D., Phillip, M. & Josefsberg, Z. (2007). Heat-shock protein peptide DiaPep277 treatment in children with newly diagnosed type 1 diabetes: a randomised, double-blind phase II study. *Diabetes/metabolism research and reviews*, *23*, 286-291.

[81] Weiner, H. L., Friedman, A., Miller, A., Khoury, S. J., al-Sabbagh, A., Santos, L., Sayegh, M., Nussenblatt, R. B., Trentham, D. E. & Hafler, D. A. (1994). Oral tolerance: immunologic mechanisms and treatment of animal and human organ-specific autoimmune diseases by oral administration of autoantigens. *Annual review of immunology*, *12*, 809-837.

[82] Harrison, L. C., Dempsey-Collier, M., Kramer, D. R. & Takahashi, K. (1996). Aerosol insulin induces regulatory CD8 gamma delta T cells that prevent murine insulin-dependent diabetes. *The Journal of experimental medicine*, *184*, 2167-2174.

[83] Harrison, L. C., Honeyman, M. C., Steele, C. E., Stone, N. L., Sarugeri, E., Bonifacio, E., Couper, J. J. & Colman, P. G. (2004). Pancreatic beta-cell function and immune responses to insulin after administration of intranasal insulin to humans at risk for type 1 diabetes. *Diabetes care*, *27*, 2348-2355.

[84] Tarbell, K. V., Yamazaki, S., Olson, K., Toy, P. & Steinman, R. M. (2004). CD25+ CD4+ T cells, expanded with dendritic cells presenting a single autoantigenic peptide, suppress autoimmune diabetes. *The Journal of experimental medicine*, *199*, 1467-1477.

[85] Wu, A. J., Hua, H., Munson, S. H. & McDevitt, H. O. (2002). Tumor necrosis factor-alpha regulation of CD4+CD25+ T cell levels in NOD mice. *Proceedings of the National Academy of Sciences of the United States of America*, *99*, 12287-12292.

[86] Szanya, V., Ermann, J., Taylor, C., Holness, C. & Fathman, C. G. (2002). The subpopulation of CD4+CD25+ splenocytes that delays adoptive transfer of diabetes expresses L-selectin and high levels of CCR7. *J Immunol*, *169*, 2461-2465.

[87] Sarween, N., Chodos, A., Raykundalia, C., Khan, M., Abbas, A. K. & Walker, L. S. (2004). CD4+CD25+ cells controlling a pathogenic CD4 response inhibit cytokine differentiation, CXCR-3 expression, and tissue invasion. *J Immunol*, *173*, 2942-2951.

[88] Yamazaki, S., Iyoda, T., Tarbell, K., Olson, K., Velinzon, K., Inaba, K. & Steinman. R. M. (2003). Direct expansion of functional CD25+ CD4+ regulatory T cells by antigen-processing dendritic cells. *The Journal of experimental medicine*, *198*, 235-247.

[89] Takahashi, T., Kuniyasu, Y., Toda, M., Sakaguchi, N., Itoh, M., Iwata, M., Shimizu, J. & Sakaguchi, S. (1998). Immunologic self-tolerance maintained by CD25+CD4+ naturally anergic and suppressive T cells: induction of autoimmune disease by breaking their anergic/suppressive state. *International immunology*, *10*, 1969-1980.

[90] Thornton, A. M. & Shevach, E. M. (2000). Suppressor effector function of CD4+CD25+ immunoregulatory T cells is antigen nonspecific. *J Immunol, 164*, 183-190.

[91] Andersson, J., Stefanova, I., Stephens, G. L. & Shevach, E. M. (2007). CD4+CD25+ regulatory T cells are activated in vivo by recognition of self. *International immunology, 19*, 557-566.

[92] Hume, D. A., Ross, I. L., Himes, S. R., Sasmono, R. T., Wells, C. A. & Ravasi, T. (2002). The mononuclear phagocyte system revisited. *Journal of leukocyte biology 72*, 621-627.

[93] Shortman, K. & Naik, S. H. (2007). Steady-state and inflammatory dendritic-cell development. *Nature reviews, 7*, 19-30.

[94] Kurts, C., Cannarile, M., Klebba, I. & Brocker, T. (2001). Dendritic cells are sufficient to cross-present self-antigens to CD8 T cells in vivo. *J Immunol, 166*, 1439-1442.

[95] Randolph, G. J. (2001). Dendritic cell migration to lymph nodes: cytokines, chemokines, and lipid mediators. *Seminars in immunology, 13*, 267-274.

[96] Kurts, C., Carbone, F. R., Barnden, M., Blanas, E., Allison, J., Heath, W. R. & Miller. J. F. (1997). CD4+ T cell help impairs CD8+ T cell deletion induced by cross-presentation of self-antigens and favors autoimmunity. *The Journal of experimental medicine, 186*, 2057-2062.

[97] Lutz, M. B. & Schuler, G. (2002). Immature, semi-mature and fully mature dendritic cells: which signals induce tolerance or immunity? *Trends in immunology, 23*, 445-449.

[98] Vlad, G., Cortesini, R. & Suciu-Foca, N. (2005). License to heal: bidirectional interaction of antigen-specific regulatory T cells and tolerogenic APC. *J Immunol, 174*, 5907-5914.

[99] Mellman, I. & Steinman, R. M. (2001). Dendritic cells: specialized and regulated antigen processing machines. *Cell, 106*, 255-258.

[100] Bluestone, J. A. (1996). Costimulation and its role in organ transplantation. *Clinical transplantation, 10*, 104-109.

[101] Kishimoto, K., Dong, V. M. & Sayegh, M. H. (2000). The role of costimulatory molecules as targets for new immunosuppressives in transplantation. *Current opinion in urology, 10*, 57-62.

[102] Sayegh, M. H. & Turka, L. A. (1995). T cell costimulatory pathways: promising novel targets for immunosuppression and tolerance induction. *J Am Soc Nephrol, 6*, 1143-1150.

[103] Jenkins, M. K. & Schwartz, R. H. (1987). Antigen presentation by chemically modified splenocytes induces antigen-specific T cell unresponsiveness in vitro and in vivo. *The Journal of experimental medicine, 165*, 302-319.

[104] Clarkson, M. R. & Sayegh, M. H. (2005). T-cell costimulatory pathways in allograft rejection and tolerance. *Transplantation, 80*, 555-563.

[105] Lenschow, D. J., Herold, K. C., Rhee, L., Patel, B., Koons, A., Qin, H. Y., Fuchs, E., Singh, B., Thompson, C. B. & Bluestone, J. A. (1996. CD28/B7 regulation of Th1 and Th2 subsets in the development of autoimmune diabet)es. *Immunity, 5*, 285-293.

[106] Steinman, R. M., Inaba, K., Turley, S., Pierre, P. & Mellman, I. (1999). Antigen capture, processing, and presentation by dendritic cells: recent cell biological studies. *Human immunology, 60*, 562-567.

[107] Steinman, R. M. (2003). The control of immunity and tolerance by dendritic cell. *Pathologie-biologie, 51*, 59-60.

[108] Hackstein, H., Morelli, A. E. & Thomson, A. W. (2001). Designer dendritic cells for tolerance induction: guided not misguided missiles. *Trends in immunology, 22*, 437-442.

[109] Morelli, A. E. & Thomson, A. W. (2003). Dendritic cells: regulators of alloimmunity and opportunities for tolerance induction. *Immunological reviews, 196*, 125-146.

[110] Coates, P. T. & Thomson, A. W. (2002). Dendritic cells, tolerance induction and transplant outcome. *Am J Transplant, 2*, 299-307.

[111] Nouri-Shirazi, M. & Thomson, A. W. (2006). Dendritic cells as promoters of transplant tolerance. *Expert opinion on biological therapy, 6*, 325-339.

[112] Chen, D., Sung, R. & Bromberg, J. S. (2002). Gene therapy in transplantation. *Transplant immunology, 9*, 301-314.

[113] Giannoukakis, N., Thomson, A. & Robbins, P. (1999). Gene therapy in transplantation. *Gene therapy, 6*, 1499-1511.

[114] Bottino, R., Lemarchand, P., Trucco, M. & Giannoukakis, N. (2003). Gene- and cell-based therapeutics for type I diabetes mellitus. *Gene therapy, 10*, 875-889.

[115] Giannoukakis, N. & Trucco, M. (2005). Gene therapy for type 1 diabetes. *American journal of therapeutics, 12*, 512-528.

[116] Tarner, I. H. & Fathman, C. G. (2002). The potential for gene therapy in the treatment of autoimmune disease. *Clinical immunology (Orlando, Fla, 104*, 204-216.

[117] Tarner, I. H., Slavin, A. J., McBride, J., Levicnik, A., Smith, R., Nolan, G. P., Contag, C. H. & Fathman, C. G. (2003). Treatment of autoimmune disease by adoptive cellular gene therapy. *Annals of the New York Academy of Sciences, 998*, 512-519.

[118] Trucco, M., Robbins, P. D., Thomson, A. W. & Giannoukakis, N. (2002). Gene therapy strategies to prevent autoimmune disorders. *Current gene therapy, 2*, 341-354.

[119] Chen, W. (2006). Dendritic cells and (CD4+)CD25+ T regulatory cells: crosstalk between two professionals in immunity versus tolerance. *Front Biosci, 11*, 1360-1370.

[120] Hugues, S., Boissonnas, A., Amigorena, S. & Fetler, L. (2006). The dynamics of dendritic cell-T cell interactions in priming and tolerance. *Current opinion in immunology, 18*, 491-495.

[121] Beissert, S., Schwarz, A. & Schwarz, T. (2006). Regulatory T cells. *The Journal of investigative dermatology, 126*, 15-24.

[122] Enk, A. H. (2006). DCs and cytokines cooperate for the induction of tregs. *Ernst Schering Research Foundation workshop*, 97-106.

[123] Huber, S. & Schramm, C. (2006). TGF-beta and CD4+CD25+ regulatory T cells. *Front Biosci, 11*, 1014-1023.

[124] Lohr, J., Knoechel, B. & Abbas, A. K. (2006). Regulatory T cells in the periphery. *Immunological reviews, 212*, 149-162.

[125] Roncarolo, M. G., Gregori, S., Battaglia, M., Bacchetta, R., Fleischhauer, K. & Levings, M. K. (2006). Interleukin-10-secreting type 1 regulatory T cells in rodents and humans. *Immunological reviews, 212*, 28-50.

[126] Shevach, E. M., DiPaolo, R. A., Andersson, J., Zhao, D. M., Stephens, G. L. & Thornton, A. M. (2006). The lifestyle of naturally occurring CD4+ CD25+ Foxp3+ regulatory T cells. *Immunological reviews, 212*, 60-73.

[127] Tang, Q. & Bluestone, J. A. (2006). Regulatory T-cell physiology and application to treat autoimmunity. *Immunological reviews*, *212*, 217-237.

[128] Verhagen, J., Blaser, K., Akdis, C. A. & Akdis, M. (2006). Mechanisms of allergen-specific immunotherapy: T-regulatory cells and more. *Immunology and allergy clinics of North America*, *26*, 207-231, vi.

[129] Zhang, L., Yi, H., Xia, X. P. & Zhao, Y. (2006). Transforming growth factor-beta: an important role in CD4+CD25+ regulatory T cells and immune tolerance. *Autoimmunity*, *39*, 269-276.

[130] Marguti, I., Yamamoto, G. L., da Costa, T. B., Rizzo, L. V. & de Moraes, L. V. (2009). Expansion of CD4+ CD25+ Foxp3+ T cells by bone marrow-derived dendritic cells. *Immunology*, *127*, 50-61.

[131] Ma, L., Qian, S., Liang, X., Wang, L., Woodward, J. E., Giannoukakis, N., Robbins, P. D., Bertera, S., Trucco, M., Fung, J. J. & Lu, L. (2003). Prevention of diabetes in NOD mice by administration of dendritic cells deficient in nuclear transcription factor-kappaB activity. *Diabetes*, *52*, 1976-1985.

[132] Machen, J., Harnaha, J., Lakomy, R., Styche, A., Trucco, M. & Giannoukakis, N. (2004). Antisense oligonucleotides down-regulating costimulation confer diabetes-preventive properties to nonobese diabetic mouse dendritic cells. *J Immunol*, *173*, 4331-4341.

[133] Harnaha, J., Machen, J., Wright, M., Lakomy, R., Styche, A., Trucco, M., Makaroun, S. & Giannoukakis, N. (2006). Interleukin-7 is a survival factor for CD4+ CD25+ T-cells and is expressed by diabetes-suppressive dendritic cells. *Diabetes*, *55*, 158-170.

[134] Waeckerle-Men, Y., Allmen, E. U., Gander, B., Scandella, E., Schlosser, E., Schmidtke, G., Merkle, H. P. & Groettrup, M. (2006). Encapsulation of proteins and peptides into biodegradable poly(D,L-lactide-co-glycolide) microspheres prolongs and enhances antigen presentation by human dendritic cells. *Vaccine*, *24*, 1847-1857.

[135] Yoshida, M. & Babensee, J. E. (2006). Molecular aspects of microparticle phagocytosis by dendritic cells. *Journal of biomaterials science*, *17*, 893-907.

[136] Phillips, B., Nylander, K., Harnaha, J., Machen, J., Lakomy, R., Styche, A., Gillis, K., Brown, L., Lafreniere, D., Gallo, M., Knox, J., Hogeland, K., Trucco, M. & Giannoukakis, N. (2008). A microsphere-based vaccine prevents and reverses new-onset autoimmune diabetes. *Diabetes*, *57*, 1544-1555.

In: Autoimmune Diseases: Symptoms, Diagnosis and Treatment   ISBN: 978-1-61668-007-7
Editor: Kyle J. Brenner, pp. 251-264   © 2010 Nova Science Publishers, Inc.

Chapter 6

LUPUS NEPHRITIS: FROM DIAGNOSIS TO TREATMENT

Nailú Angélica Sinicato, Mariana Postal and Simone Appenzeller[1, 2*]

[1]Rheumatology Unit - State University of Campinas [2], Brazil
Rheumatology Lab-State University of Campinas; [3], Brazil
Department of Neurology, State University of Campinas, Brazil

ABSTRACT

Systemic lupus erythematosus (SLE) is a complex, multisystem autoimmune disorder, which often involves referral to multiple medical specialists. Lupus nephritis (LN) occurs in approximately 35% of adults with SLE and predicts poor survival. The 2003 joint International Society of Nephrology and Renal Pathology Society (ISN/RPS) histological classification improved the characterization of the biopsies of patients with lupus nephritis, to provide additional prognostic information and enhance guidance for therapy. Understanding of the value of partial remission, and the prognosis for certain socio economic and ethnic groups in lupus nephritis has also improved. Despite this progress, however, therapy is still not optimal. Although effective immunosuppressive therapies are available for many patients with SLE, some patients do not respond to initial treatment, and others have a relapsing course of disease after remission. The optimal maintenance immunosuppressive treatment and the duration of therapy for patients with lupus nephritis are not entirely clear. Immunosuppressive regimens for severe lupus nephritis can also be associated with a variety of major adverse effects, which include an increased risk of infection, infertility, bone damage, bladder lesions, and cosmetic changes (such as cushingoid appearance or alopecia).These adverse reactions harm patients and limit the potential for future therapy.In this chapter we will review clinical manifestations, histology correlation, and treatment options in SLE nephritis.

---

[*] Corresponding author: Department of Medicine, Faculty of Medical Science, State University of Campinas (UNICAMP), Cidade Universitaria Zeferino Vaz, CEP 13083970 Campinas-SP-Brazil, Tel: +55 1937887734, Fax: +55 19 32891818, E-mail: appenzellersimone@yahoo.com

INTRODUCTION

Systemic lupus erythematosus (SLE) is a disorder linked to loss of immune tolerance to self-antigens and the production of a variety of autoantibodies [1].

Renal involvement is present at diagnosis in approximately 25% of SLE patients, depending on the cohort. In most cases, renal disease develops within the first 3 years following diagnosis of SLE [2]. Several variables have been associated with the development of SLE nephritis, including male sex, ethnicity (Hispanic American and African American)and disease diagnosis before age 33 years [3-5]. The incidence and prevalence of SLE varies considerably across the countries.

Lupus nephritis (LN) is a common manifestation of SLE. The disease is tightly linked to the production of autoantibodies and circulating immune complexes, i.e. immune complex glomerulonephritis which leads to their deposition and glomerular inflammation [6, 7]. Although LN contributes substantially to the overall mortality in SLE, cardiovascular disease remains the major cause of death in these patients [6-8].

Although not always available, a kidney biopsy is essential in establishing diagnosis and prognosis for this disease. The prognosis of the lesion is predicted by the class, activity and chronicity of the glomerular pathology [8]. Histological evidence of lupus nephritis is present in most patients with SLE, even when they do not yet have clinical manifestations. Current classification of the International Society of Nephrology/Renal Pathology Society (ISN/RPS 2003) of LN provide clearer distinctions between the histological classes, and improve diagnostic. LN prognosis can usually be improved by treatment, but it is potentially toxic, prolonged, and complex [9].

Studies have demonstrated that patient survival has increased significantly to 72% at 10 years when compared to a 5-year survival rates of 17% in the 1950s [10]. In addition the main causes of death have changed and today in addition to infections [11], atherosclerosis [12] and malignancy [13] are the leading causes [9].

Pathophysiology of Lupus Nephritis

In SLE we observe a wide spectrum of morphologic renal lesions, including glomerulonephritis, vasculopaty and tubular-interstitium diseases [9].

The glomerular patterns of injury are related to the site of accumulation of immunoglobulins, their antigen specificity, and their ability to bind and activate complement and evoke a cellular inflammatory response. The pattern of injury can be divided into three groups, according to the main site of injury: mesangium, endothelium, and epithelium and clinical presentation can help to establish diagnosis [9, 14]. The presence of predominant mesangial hypercellularity (at least three mesangial cells per mesangial region in a three micron thick section) and mesangial immune complex and matrix accumulation, is associated with the presence of microscopic hematuria and subnephrotic proteinuria with well-preserved glomerular filtration rate (GFR) [9, 15]. The endothelial pattern, represented by leukocyte accumulation, endothelial cell injury, and endocapillary proliferation, often coexists with capillary wall destruction, varying degrees of mesangial proliferation and crescent formation[9]. The persistent accumulation of immune complexes in the subendothelial space is associated with more severe injury and chronic changes, including cellular interposition and replication of the glomerular basement membrane (mesangiocapillary pattern). The patient often present with varying degree of dysmorphic hematuria and leucocituria, proteinuria and reduced GFR [9, 16]. The epithelial pattern is characterized by autoantibodies and complement cytotoxic injury on the podocytes resulting in non-exudative, nonproliferative capillary wall lesions. This pattern is associated with proteinuria, often in nephrotic range, with preservation or gradual reduction in GFR [9, 17].

The coexistence of different morphologic patterns in LN is common, leading to a more complex clinical expression of disease in many patients.

In addition, renal vascular complications are frequent encountered in SLE and their occurrence can profoundly alter the clinical course and therapeutic options. The renal vasculopathies include vascular immune complex deposition, non-inflammatory necrotizing vasculopathy, thrombotic microangiopathy, renal vasculitis and renal vein thrombosis [9, 18].

The most common renal vascular lesion is immune complex deposition in the walls of arterioles. Small arteries and the vessels usually appear normal at light microscopy. Vascular deposits are commonly found in glomerular proliferative forms, typically associated with tubulointertitial deposits and their presence do not alter the clinical course and prognosis [9, 19].

Non-inflammatory necrotizing vasculopathy, although less frequently observed, represents a more severe form of immune deposition. It is predominantly observed in pre glomerular arteries. The clinical prognosis is generally poor [9, 20].

Thrombotic microangiopathy involves renal vessels in all forms of glomerular injury patterns, especially in patients with antiphospholipid antibody syndrome and it may occur without a recognizable thrombotic systemic process. In the acute phase, a marked narrowing or total occlusion by intraluminal accumulation of fibrin may be observed. The prognosis of this vasculopathy is variable [9, 21].

Among the renal vasculopathy of SLE the renal vasculitis is the least common. It is characterized by marked elevation of serum creatinine. Two thirds of the patients present with severe blood pressure elevation and the clinical prognosis is poor [9, 22].

Renal vein thrombosis occurs in all ages, with higher incidence in patients with nephrotic syndrome and antiphospholipid antibody syndrome. As in other renal diseases, the renal vein thrombosis appears to be a complication rather than a cause of nephrotic syndrome [9, 23].In about 50% of patients with nephritis, less in those with the mesangial pattern of injury, but in up to three quarters of those with the endothelial pattern of injury, immune aggregates are present in the tubular basement membrane [24]. The presence of inflammation in the tubules, characterized by a predominantly by lymphocytes and monocytes, with a few B cells, plasma cells and natural killer cells, is frequently seen in active disease [9]. In a chronic evolution, the interstitium is expanded with a variable amount of collagen. In rare cases, an acute tubulointerstitial nephritis is seen in the absence of glomerular disease and may present clinically as acute renal failure [25].Detection of lupus anticoagulant (LA) in SLE patients identifies a subgroup of patients who have increased risk to develop poorer renal outcomes [26, 27]. Anticardiolipine antibodies are observed in approximately 70% in SLE patients, lupus anticoagulant in 30%, and antiphospholipid syndrome in 20% [28, 29].The nephropathy associated with the presence of antiphispholipid antibodies clinically manifests as vascular nephropathy, associating hypertension, acute and/or chronic renal insufficiency, and low-grade proteinuria [9]. The histological features are characterized by a vaso-occlusive process associating acute thromboses and chronic vascular lesions [27].

Classification of Renal Involvement

Renal involvement can be classified by clinical, laboratory and biopsy findings. Often the patient is asymptomatic and routine urine analysis should be part of the clinical evaluation of SLE patients [9].

The American College of Rheumatology proposed the following criteria to diagnose and classify renal involvement in patients with SLE: (i) presence of persistent proteinuria of >500 mg/day (or greater than 3+ urine dipstick reaction for albumin); and (ii) presence of cellular casts including red blood cells, hemoglobin, renal tubular cell or mixed[30, 31].

Renal biopsy was first introduced in 1950s. With increasing knowledge of pathogenic mechanisms various patterns of renal injury were identified as separate entities like focal segmental glomerulonephritis, diffuse proliferative glemerulonephritis and membranous glomerulonephritis in 1964 followed by identification of mesangial lesions in 1970s [32].

Based on the pathology of glomerular lesions already cited, WHO (1974) proposed the first classification of lupus nephritis. In this classification any qualitative differences between class III and class IV were not describe and tubulointerstitial and vascular lesions were also not included in this classification [32].

This classification was first modified in 1982 by International Study of Kidney Disease in Children group. In this classification class I was subdivided into two subclasses depending on presence or absence of mesangial immune deposits. Class II included only mesangial lesions which, based on the severity of mesangial hypercellularity were sundivided. Class III lupus nephritis included focal segmental glomerulonephritis with necrotizing lesions and class IV denoted diffuse glomerulonephritis without stipulating criteria for percentage of affected glomeruli. In addition class III and IV were subdivided based on the presence of active, chronic or mixed types of glomerular injury. Class V was also subdivided based on the presence of class III or class IV lesions and a newer class VI was added to denote advanced glomerusclerosis without stipulating the percentage of glomeruli. This classification was cumbersome as numerous subcategories and mixed classes had to be handled. Therefore, many pathologists continued to work with 1974 WHO classification [32,33].

These both classifications were revised and a new one was proposed by the International Society of Nephrology and Renal Society in 2003. This classification preserved the simplicity of WHO classification, incorporated refinements including activity and chronicity indices from 1982 and 1995 classifications and added a number of new modifications. The major objective of this classification was to standardized definitions, emphasize clinically relevant lesions and encourage uniform and reproducible reporting between centers [32].

Histologic examination of renal biopsy should contain a minimum of 10 glomeruli in order to reasonably exclude focal lesions. Immunofluorescence is required for complete analysis including staining for IgG, IgA, IgM, Kappa and lambda lights chains, C3 and Clq complement components [34].

Clinical Presentation

LN may present as acute manifestations (acute renal failure) or as a chronic progressive involvement of kidney (chronic renal disease). Although the term acute renal failure has been used in the last decades, no uniform criteria have been established and more than 35 definitions can be found in the literature. The acronym RIFLE (Risk, Injury, Failure, Loss and End-stage Kidney) was formulated by the Acute Dialysis Quality Initiative (ADQI) to establish a uniform definition for acute kidney injury (AKI). The ADQI working group developed the evidence-based RIFLE definition/classification system for acute renal failure [35]. RIFLE defines three grades of increasing severity of AKI—risk (class R), injury (class I) and failure (class F) and two outcome classes (loss and end-stage kidney disease) in patient with less than 90 days of manifestation. This new classification has been used in SLE patients presenting with LN and found that each increase in severityof the RIFLE category was associated with an increase in renal function progression and a decrease in recovery [36]. In addition, analytical data also confirmed the good discriminative power
of the RIFLE classification system for predicting the prognosis of lupus nephritis patients with AKI [36]. Physicians should use the RIFLE classification to assess theshort-term prognosis of LN, and further investigations or clinical trials should focus onthe RIFLE classification as a means of identifying AKI in severe lupus nephritis [36].

The presence of kidney injury (hematuria, leucocituria, proteinuria or decreased GFR) for more than 90 days defines the presence of chronic renal disease and the patient should be treated according to established protocols. We would like to emphasize that the presence of urine sediment abnormalities and/or proteinuria in the presence of normal GFR already defines the presence of chronic renal disease and treatment to avoid progression and loss of kidney functions should be initiated.

Biomarkers

In an effort to optimize treatment of LN, it is important to establish biomarkers that may help in diagnosis renal involvement in SLE [37]. The ability to predict clinical and laboratory flare would be a valuable tool. In order to be useful in clinical practice such a predictive biomarker should be followed serially, and based on biomarker levels, treatment would be initiated before the development of significant inflammatory injury in the kidney [37]. The presence of such a biomarker is likely to improve complete remissions and reduce chronic kidney damage than waiting to treat until the flare is fully developed.

The traditional clinical biomarkers for SLE, including complement components 3 and 4 (C3, C4) and anti-double-stranded DNA antibodies (ADNA) have low sensitivity (49 to 79%) and specificity (51 to 74%) for concurrent renal flare and do not reliably predict impending flare when measured serially, with sensitivities and specificities around 50 and 70%, respectively [37, 38]. However, there are several potential candidate biomarkers.

Table 1. Histological classifications of Lupus Nephritis.

Classification	1974	1982	2003
Class I	Normal glomeruli by LM[1], IF[2], EM[3].	Normal glomeruli Ia – Normal glomerular morphology by LM, IF, EM. Ib – Normal glomerular morphology by LM, but deposits on IF and EM.	Minimal mesangial lupus. Normal glomeruli by LM, but mesangial immune deposits by IF.
Class II	Purely mesangial disease IIa –Normocellular mesagium by LM but mesangial deposits on IF and EM. IIb – Mesangial hypercellularity with mesangial deposits by IF or EM.	Pure mesangial disease IIa – Mesangial widerning and/or mild hipercellularity(+) IIb – Moderate mesangial cellularity (++)	Mesangial proliferative lupus nephritis. Pure mesangial hipercellularity of any degree or mesangial matrix expansion on LM with mesangial immune deposits. A few subendothelial or subepithelial may be visible by IF or EM but not for LM.
Class III	Focal proliferative glomerulonephritis (<50%)	Focal segmental glomerulonephritis (associated with mild or moderate mesangial hipercellularity IIIa – with active necrotizing lesions IIIb – with active and sclerosing lesions IIIc – with sclerozing lesions	Local lupus nephritis IIIa – active or inactive, segmental or global, endo or extracapillary IIIa-c – glomerulonephritis involving <50% of all glomeruli typically with focal IIIc – subendothelial deposits with or without mesangial alterations; Active lesions: focal proliferative lupus nephritis;

Table 1. (Continued)

Classification	1974	1982	2003
			Active and chronic lesions: focal proliferative and sclerosing lupus nephritis; Chronic inactive lesions with glomerular scars: focal sclerosing lupus nephritis.
Class IV	Diffuse Proliferative glomerulonephritis ($\geq 50\%$)	Difuse glomerulonephritis(severe mesangial, endocapillary and mesangiocapillary proliferation and/or extense subendothelial deposits IVa - without segmental lesions IVb – with active necrotizing lesions IVc - with active and sclerosing lesions IVd - with sclerozing lesions	Difuse lupus nephritis; IV-Sa – active lesions: difuse, segmental, proliferative and sclerosing lupus nephritis; IV-Ga - difuse, global, proliferative and sclerosing lupus nephritis; IV-S(a/c) – active and chronical lesions: difuse, segmental, proliferative and sclerosing lupus nephritis; IV-G(a/c) - active and chronical lesions: difuse, global, proliferative and sclerosing lupus nephritis; IV-S(c) – Chronic inactive lesions with scars: difuse, segmental, sclerosing lupus nephritis; IV-G(c) - Chronic inactive lesions with scars: difuse, global, sclerosing lupus nephritis;

Table 1. (Continued)

Classification	1974	1982	2003
Class V	Membranous glomerulonephritis.	Difuse membranous glomerulonephritis Va – pure membranous glomerulonephritis Vb – associeated with lesions of category II (a or b) Vc - associeated with lesions of category III (a-c) Vd - associeated with lesions of category IV (a-d)	Membranous lupus nephritis; Global or subepithelial immune deposits on their morphologica segmental by LM, IF and EM with or without mesangial alterations. Class V lupus nephritis may occur with class III or IV in which case both will be diagnosed. Show advanced scerosis
Class VI		Advanced sclerosing glomerulonephritis	Advanced sclerotic lupus nephritis. ≥90% glomeruli globally sclerosed without residual activity.

[1]: light microscopy
[2]: immunofluorescence
[3]: electron microscopy

Monocyte chemoattractant protein-1 (MCP-1) is a leukocyte chemotactic factor that is involved in the pathogenesis of renal injury in SLE [39]. It has been shown that uMCP-1 was significantly greater in patients developing a renal flare [40]. However it is important to note that MCP-1 has been associated with histologic findings of scarring in kidney biopsies [37, 40-44].

Neutrophil gelatinase-associated lipocalin (NGAL) is a low molecular-weight antibacterial protein that functions by binding bacterial siderophores and sequestering iron[37]. In a pediatric SLE cohort, uNGAL values above a threshold level had a sensitivity of 90% and a specificity of 100% for identifying patients with concurrent, biopsy-proven lupus nephritis. However in an adult population the sensitivity was only of 50%, a specificity of 91% [37, 45, 46]

Mass spectrometry has been used to identify a protein signature for active LN [47]. Four of these were albumin fragments and the other four were transferrin (TF), 1-acid-glycoprotein (AGP), ceruloplasmin (CP), and lipocalin-type prostaglandin d-synthetase (L-PGDS) [37, 48]. These proteins were not increased in non-renal SLE. TF, AGP, CP, and L-PGDS were measured prospectively in children with SLE nephritis, and several were found to significantly increase 3 months before renal flare and TF was most consistent with a forecaster of impending renal flare [37].

Hepcidin is an iron regulatory hormone made mainly in the liver and seems to be involved in the anemia of chronic inflammation [49,50]. In SLE hepcidin is regulated by IL-6 and TNF alfa, cytokines involved in the pathogenesis of LN. Urine hepcidin-20 increased significantly 4 months before flare and within 4 months of treatment returned to baseline [37, 51]. The clinical performance of complement component C1q (anti-C1q) autoantibodies for detecting renal flare was similar to that of C3, C4, and ADNA [43– 47]. However, prospective studies found that anti-C1q levels began to increase 4 to 6 mo before renal flare [52,53] with a positive predictive values of 50 to 71% [37].

Other biomarkers to anticipate the development of chronic kidney disease and predict renal pathology have been studied [37].

Liver-type fatty acid binding protein (L-FABP) is produced by human proximal tubular cells. In SLE it was measured at the time of diagnostic kidney biopsy in 49 patients, who were divided into those who progressed to chronic kidney disease (CKD) and those who did not [54]. Patients with worsening creatinine had a higher uL-FABP than nonprogressors). No patient with an uL-FABP ≤30 ng/mg Cr progressed, suggesting that the uL-FABP level at the time of kidney biopsy may help forecast the development of CKD in patients with LN [37].

Membrane endothelial protein C receptor (mEPCR) is an integral endothelial membrane protein that facilitates the conversion of protein C to activated protein C [37, 55]. Those patients whose biopsies showed that more than 25% of the cortical peritubular capillaries expressed mEPCR responded poorly to therapy at 6 and 12 mo and tended to develop CKD [56]. Interestingly, mEPCR as a biomarker of response to treatment was independent of biopsy class, activity and chronicity indices, GFR, and tubulointerstitial damage [37, 56].

The transcription factor FOXP3 is important in the development of regulatory T cells [57] and seems to be low in T regulatory cells from patients with active lupus, possibly contributing to the functional defect observed in SLE T regulatory cells [37, 58]. FOXP3 mRNA was measured in urine sediment of patients with active lupus nephritis and it was found to be significantly higher than in quiescent lupus nephritis or normal controls [59]. Furthermore, the level of FOXP3 mRNA seemed to stratify patients into treatment responders and non-responders. Higher levels of FOXP3 mRNA were found in urine of the patients who did not respond to therapy compared with patients who had complete response [59].

A noninvasive test that accurately reflects kidney histology would be useful when deciding on therapy because it will provide significantly what is happening within the kidney at flare than proteinuria, urine sediment, and creatinine [37]. Ideally, these histologic biomarkers would differentiate active inflammation, necrosis, and crescents from fibrosis and chronic changes or from an etiology other than lupus, such as nephrotoxic acute tubular necrosis [37].

A proteomic approach was used to identify a urine protein signature that could noninvasively distinguish LN from other types of proteinuric kidney diseases such as diabetic nephropathy [60] and among patients with different classes of LN [61].Using 120 proteins or protein isoforms, lupus nephritis was separated from other pathologies with a sensitivity of 86% and a specificity of 89% [37]. To differentiate between WHO nephritis classes in a cohort of patients with SLE, a panel of 10 proteins provided the most sensitivity for classification, again using an artificial neural network [61]. The proteins in this panel were primarily plasma glycoproteins such as α-1 acid glycoprotein, α-1 microglobulin, and zinc α-2 glycoprotein [37].

CXCL10 is a chemokine that mediates Th-1 cell migration and is upregulated in SLE [62–64]. Urine sediment mRNA for CXCL10 and its receptor CXCR3 was found to be higher 2 wk before renal biopsy in patients with class IV nephritis compared with other classes. After treatment, CXCL10/CXCR3 urine mRNA was measured prospectively. In class IV patients who responded to treatment, chemokine mRNA levels declined, whereas the non-responders showed a tendency for levels to increase. CXCL10 had a sensitivity and specificity of 73 and 94% and CXCR3 of 65 and 83%, respectively [65].

T cell signal transduction molecule β1 integrin (CD29) is an adhesion molecule important for cell– cell and cell–matrix interactions. Using T cells from patients with active SLE, stimulation of CD29 alone was sufficient to mediate these events, apparently through a focal adhesion kinase signaling cascade [66], with significantly increased expression of CD29 on the lupus T cells. Importantly, increased expression of CD29 was mainly seen in patients with active class IV nephritis and not other types of SLE GN [37].

Although several biomarkers have been studied in LN, no ideal candidate has been identified yet. In addition, prospective studies are needed to determine whether they predict the course of lupus nephritis, such as impending flare, or future outcome [37].

Treatment of Lupus Nephritis

Effective immunosuppressive therapies are available for many patients with SLE, some patients do not respond to initial treatment, and others have a relapsing course of disease after remission [8]. The optimal maintenance immunosuppressive treatment and the duration of therapy for patients with lupus nephritis is not entirely clear. Immunosuppressive regimens for severe lupus nephritis can also be associated with a variety of major adverse effects, such as increased risk of infection, infertility and, bone damage [8].

Current treatment options for lupus nephritis have significantly improved both renal prognosis and overall patient survival. High-dose pulse cyclophosphamide therapy (monthly for the first 6 months followed by quarterly infusion) combined with cortico-steroids has been widely used in the treatment of proliferative lupus nephritis [8].

More recently, mycophenolate mofetil (MMF) has been added to the armamentarium of nephrologists for the treatment of lupus nephritis, in the interest of lower toxicity. Controlled data now exist on the use of MMF as both induction therapy and as maintenance therapy in different ethnic and geographical groups, and in both proliferative and membranous lupus nephritis. Such prevention of scarring and fibrosis is a result of the capacity of MMF to inhibit both mesangial cell proliferation and lymphocyte migration into renal tissue. Such inhibition results from impaired glycosylation, which, in turn, leads to alterations in adhesion molecule functioning. MMF might also decrease the expression of nitric oxide synthase in the renal cortex accompanied by a slowing of the progression of atherosclerosis [8, 67].

Other immunossupressive agents are: Ciclosporin (therapy for diffuse proliferative lupus nephritis); Azathioprine (proliferative lupus nephritis); Abetimus (immunomodulatory agent that reduces the anti-double-stranded DNA levels); Rituximab (clinical trial evidence on this agent is lacking) [8, 68].

Maintenance is a period of less intensive therapy following a period of induction therapy that has achieved a partial or complete response, with the aim of keeping the patient free of disease activity. Maintenance therapies are usually administered orally (corticosteroids, MMF or azathioprine) at the lowest possible dose to maintain response [8, 67, 68].

CONCLUSION

Although advances have been made in diagnosis and treatment, improving significantly mortality over the past decades, the treatment of LN is still not optimal. But significant progression has been made and several biomarkers are under consideration that may significantly improve SLE treatment.

REFERENCES

[1] Kulkarni, O; Hans-Joachim, A. Chemokines in lupus nephritis. *Frontiers in Bioscience*, 13 May 1, 2008, 3312-3320.

[2] Korbet, SM; Lewis, EJ; Schwartz, MM; Reichlin, M; Evans, J; Rohde, RD. Factors predictive of outcome in severe lupus nephritis. Lupus Nephritis Collaborative Study Group. *Am J Kidney Dis*, 2000, 35, 904-14.

[3] Seligman, VA; Lum, RF; Olson, JL; Li, H; Criswell, LA. Demographic differences in the development of lupus nephritis: a retrospective analysis. *AmJ Med*, 2002, 112, 726-9.

[4] Hopkinson, ND; Jenkinson, C; Muir, KR; Doherty, M; Powell, RJ. Racial group, socioeconomic status, and the development of persistent proteinuria in systemic lupus erythematosus. *Ann Rheum Dis*, 2000, 59, 116-9.

[5] Houng, DL; Papo, T; Beaufils, H; Wechsler, B; Blétry, O; Baumelou A; et al. Renal involvement in systemic lupus erythematosus. *Medicine*, 1999, 78, 148-66.

[6] Mortensen, ES; Rekvig, OP. *J Am Soc Nephrol*, 2009, 20, 696-704.

[7] Mortensen, ES; Fenton, KA; Rekvig, OP: Lupus nephritis: The central role of nucleosomes revealed. *Am J Pathol*, 2008, 172, 275-283.

[8] Gordon, C; Jayne, D; Pusey, C; et al. European consensus statement on the terminology used in the management of lupus glomerulonephritis. *Lupus*, 2009, 18,, 257-263.

[9] Molino, C; Fabbian, F; Longhini, C. Clinical approach to lupus nephritis: recent advances. *Eur J Intern Med.*, 2009, 20, 447-53

[10] Bono, L; Cameron, JS; Hicks, JA. The very long-term prognosis and complications of lupus nephritis and its treatment. *QJ Med*, 1999, 4, 211-8.

[11] Kang, I; Park, SH. Infectious complications in SLE after immunosuppressive therapies. *Curr Opin Rheumatol*, 2003, 15, 528-34.

[12] Zonana-Nacach, A; Barr, SG; Madger, LA; Petri, M. Damage in systemic lupus erythematosus and its association with corticosteroids. *Arthritis Rheum*, 2000, 43, 1801-8.

[13] Bernatsky, S; Ramsey-Goldman, R; Clarke, A. Exploring the links between systemic lupus erythematosus and cancer. *Rheum Dis Clin North Am*, 2005, 31, 387-402.

[14] Fries, JW; Mendrick, DL; Rennke, HG. Determinants of immune complex-mediated glomerulonephritis. *Kidney Int*, 1988, 34, 333-45.

[15] Berden, JHM. Lupus nephritis. *Kidney Int*, 1997, 52, 538-58.

[16] Schwartz, MM. The pathology of lupus nephritis. *Semin Nephrol*, 2007, 27, 22-34.

[17] Austin, HA; Illei, GG. Membranous lupus nephritis. *Lupus*, 2005, 14, 65-71.

[18] Appel, GB; Pirani, CL; D'Agati, V. Renal vascular complications of systemic lupus erythematosus. *J Am Soc Nephrol*, 1994, 4, 1499-515.

[19] Pirani, CL; Olesnicky, L. Role of electronmicroscopy in the classification in the classification of lupus nephritis. *Am J Kidney Dis*, 1982, 2, 150-63.

[20] Tsumagari, T; Fukmoto, F; Kjnio, M; Tanaka, K. Incidence and significance of intrarenal vasculopathies in patients with systemic lupus erythematosus. *Hum Pathol*, 1985, 16, 43-9.

[21] Banfi, G; Bertani, T; Boeri, V; Faraggiana, T; Mazzucco, G; Monga, G; et al. Renal vascular lesions as a marker of a poor prognosis in patients with lupus nephritis. *Am J Kidney Dis*, 1991, 18, 240-8.

[22] Grishman, E; Gerber, MA; Churg, J. Vascular lesions in lupus nephritis. *Mod Pathol*, 1988, 1, 235-41.

[23] Appel, GB; Williams, GS; Meltzer, JI; Pirani, CL. Renal vein thrombosis, nephritic syndrome, and systemic lupus erythematosus. *Ann Intern Med*, 1976, 85, 310-7.

[24] Stewart Cameron, J. Lupus nephritis. *J Am Soc Nephrol*, 1999, 10, 413-24.

[25] Mori, Y; Kishimoto, N; Yamahara, H; Kijima, Y; Nose, A; Uchiyama-Tanaka, Y; et al. Predominant tubulointerstitial nephritis in a patient with systemic lupus nephritis. *Clin Exp Nephrol*, 2005, 9, 79-84.

[26] Natejumnong, C; Ruangkanchanasetr, P; Aimpun, P; Supaporn, T. Significance of antiphospholipid antibodies in lupus nephritis. *J Med Assoc Thai*, 2006, 89 (Suppl2), S121-8.

[27] Daugas, E; Nochy, D; Huong, DL; Duhaut, P; Beaufils, H; Caudwell, V; et al. Antiphospholipid syndrome nephropathy in systemic lupus erythematosus. *JAmSocNephrol*, 2002, 13, 42-52

[28] Love, PE; Santoro, SA. Antiphospholipid antibodies: anticardiolipin and the lupus anticoagulant in systemic lupus erythematous (SLE) patients and non-SLE disorders. *Ann Intern Med*, 1990, 112, 682-98.

[29] Huong, DL; Papo, T; Beaufils, H; Wechsler, B; Bletry, O; Baumelou, A; et al. Renal involvement in systemic lupus erythematosus. A study of 180 patients from a single center. *Medicine*, 1999, 78, 148-66.

[30] Tan, EM; Cohen, AS; Fries, JF; et al. The 1982 revised criteria for the classification of systemic lupus erythematosus. *Arthritis Rheum*, 1982, 25, 1271-7.

[31] Hochberg Markowitz, GS; D'Agati, VD. The ISN/RPS 2003 classification of lupus nephritis: an assessment at 3 years. *Kidney Int.*, 2007, 71, 491-5.

[32] Markowitz, GS; D'Agati, VD. Classification of lupus nephritis. *Curr Opin Nephrol Hypertens.*, 2009, 18, 220-5.

[33] Schrier, Robert, W. Diseases of the kidney and urinary tract. 8 ed. USA: Philadelphia. *Lippincott Williams & Wilkins*, 2007, 1680.

[34] Bellomo, R; Ronco, C; Kellum, JA; et al. The ADQI workgroup: acute renal failure—definition, outcome measures, animal models, fluid therapy and information technology needs: the Second International Consensus Conference of the Acute Dialysis Quality Initiative (ADQI) Group. *Crit Care,* 2004, 8, R204-R212.

[35] Chen, T; Deng, X; Chen, B. *Nephrol Dial Transplant,* 2009, in press.

[36] Rovin, BH; Zhang, X. Biomarkers for Lupus Nephritis: The Quest Continues. Clin J Am Soc Nephrol., 2009, in press.

[37] Rovin, BH; Birmingham, DJ; Nagaraja, HN; Yu, CY; Hebert, LA. Biomarker discovery in human SLE nephritis. *Bull NYU Hosp Jt Dis,* 2007, 65, 187-193.

[38] Rovin, BH. The chemokine network in systemic lupus erythematosis nephritis. *Frontiers Biosci,* 2007, 13, 904-922.

[39] Rovin, BH; Song, H; Birmingham, DJ; et al. Urine chemokines as biomarkers of human systemic lupus erythematosus activity. *J Am Soc Nephrol,* 2005, 16, 467-473.

[40] Gharaee-Kermani, M; Denholm, EM; Phan, SH. Costimulation of fibroblast collagen and transforming growth factor B1 gene expression by monocyte chemoattractant protein-1 via specific receptors. *J Biol Chem,* 1996, 271, 17779-84.

[41] Sakai, N; Wada, T; Furuichi, K; et al. MCP-1/CCL2-dependent loop for fibrogenesis in human peripheral CD14-positive monocytes. *J Leukocyte Biol,* 2006, 79, 555-563.

[42] Giunti, S; Tesch, GH; Pinach, S; et al. Monocyte chemoattractant protein-1 has prosclerotic effects both in a mouse model of experimental diabetes and in vitro in human mesangial cells. *Diabetologia,* 2008, 51, 198-207.

[43] Wada, T; Furuichi, K; Segawa-Takeada, C; et al. MIP-1a and MCP-1 contribute to crescents and interstitial lesions in human crescentic glomerulonephritis. *Kidney Int,* 56, 1999, 995-1003.

[44] Pitashny, M; Schwartz, N; Qing, X; et al. Urinary lipocalin-2 is associated with renal disease activity in human lupus nephritis. *Arthritis Rheum,* 2007, 56, 1894-1903.

[45] Hinze, CH; Suzuki, M; Klein-Gitelman, M; et al. Neutorphil gelatinase-associated lipocalin (NGAL) anticipates the course of global and renal childhood-onset systemic lupus erythematosus disease activity. *Arthritis Rheum.,* 2009, 60, 2772-81.

[46] Suzuki, M; Ross, GF; Wiers, K; et al. Identification of a urinary proteomic signature for lupus nephritis in children. *Pediatr Nephrol,* 2007, 22, 2047-57.

[47] SuzuKi, M; Wiers, K; Brooks, EB; et al. Initial validation of a novel protein biomarker panel for active pediatric lupus nephritis. *Pediatr Res,* 2009, 65, 530-536.

[48] Nemeth, E; Rivera, S; Gabayan, V; et al. IL-6 mediates hypoferremia of inflammation by inducing the synthesis of the iron regulatory hormone hepcidin. *J Clin Invest,* 2004, 113, 1271-76.

[49] Andrews, NC. Anemia of inflammation: the cytokine-hepcidin link. J Clin Invest 2004, 113, 1251-53.

[50] Zhang, X; Jin, M; Wu, H; et al. Biomarkers of lupus nephritis determined by serial urine proteomics. *Kidney Int,* 2008, 74, 799-807.

[51] Coremans, IEM; Spronk, PE; Bootsma, H; et al. Changes in antibodies to C1q predict renal relapse in system lupus erythematosus. *Am J Kidney Dis,* 1995, 26, 595-601.

[52] Siegert, CEH; Daha, MR; Tseng, CMES; et al. Predictive value of IgG autoantibodies against C1q for nephritis in systemic lupus erythematosus. *Ann Rheum Dis,* 1993, 52, 851-856.

[53] Rovin, BH; McKinley, A; Song, H; Prosek, J. Urine liver-fatty acid binding protein in patients with systemic lupus erythematosus. *J Am Soc Nephrol*, 2008, 19, 776A.

[54] Ye, X; Fukudome, K; Tsuneyoshi, N; et al. The endothelial cell protein C receptor (EPCR) functions as a primary receptor for protein C activation on endothelial cells in arteries, veins, and capillaries. *Biochem Biophys Res Commun*, 1999, 259, 671-677.

[55] Izmirly, PM; Barisoni, L; Buyon, JP; et al. Expression of endothelial protein C receptor in cortical peritubular capillaries associates with a poor clinical response in lupus nephritis. *Rheumatology*, (Oxf), 2009, 48, 513-519.

[56] Banham, AH; Powrie, FM; Suri-Payer, E. FOXP3 + regulatory T cells: Current controversies and future perspectives. *Eur J Immunol*, 2009, 36, 2832-36.

[57] Valencia, X; Yarboro, C; Illei, GG; Lipsky, PE. Deficient CD4+CD25high T regulatory cell function in pateints with active systemic lupus erythematosus. *J Immunol*, 2007,, 178, 2579-2588.

[58] Wang, G; Lai, FM; Tam, LS; et al. Urinary FOXP3 mRNA in patients with lupus nephritis—relation with disease activity and treatment response. *Rheumatology* (Oxf), 2009, 48, 755-760

[59] Varghese, SA; Powell, TB; Budisavljevic, MN; et al. Urine biomarkers predict the cause of glomerular disease. *J Am Soc Nephrol*, 2007, 18, 913-922.

[60] Oates, JC; Varghese, S; Bland, AM; et al. Prediction of urinary protein markers in lupus nephritis. *Kidney Int*, 2005, 68, 2588-92.

[61] Bauer, JW; Baechler, EC; Petri, M; et al. Elevated serum levels of interferon-regulated chemokines are biomarkers for active human systemic lupus erythematosus. *PLoS Med*, 2006, 3, 2274-2284.

[62] Amoura, Z; Combadiere, C; Faure, S; et al. Roles of CCR1 and CXCR3 in the T cell-mediated response occurring during lupus flares. *Arthritis Rheum*, 2003, 48, 3487-3496

[63] Narumi, S; Takeuchi, T; Kobayashi, Y; Konishi, K. Serum levels of ifn-inducible protein-10 relating to the activity of systemic lupus erythematosus. *Cytokine*, 200, 12, 1561-1565.

[64] Avihingsanon, Y; Phumesin, P; Benjachat, T; et al. Measurement of urinary chemokine and growth factor messenger RNAs: A noninvasive monitoring in lupus nephritis. *Kidney Int*, 2006, 69, 747-753.

[65] Nakayamada, S; Saito, K; Nakano, K; Tanaka, Y. Activation signal transduction by beta1 integrin in T cells from patients with systemic lupus erythematosus. *Arthritis Rheum*, 2007, 56, 1559-1568.

[66] Appel, AS; Appel, GB. An update on the use of mycophenolate mofetil in lupus nephritis and other primary glomerular diseases. *Nature Clinical Practice Nephrol*, 2009, 5, 132-42.

[67] Navaneethan, S; Viswanathan, G; Strippoli, GFM. Treatment Options for Proliferative Lupus Nephritis An Update of Clinical Trial Evidence. *Drugs*, 2008, 68, 2095-2104.

Chapter 7

CLINICAL FEATURES OF AXONAL GUILLAIN–BARRÉ SYNDROME

Akiyuki Hiraga[1,2]*, *Masahiro Mori*[1] *and Satoshi Kuwabara*[1]

[1]Department of Neurology, Graduate School of Medicine, Chiba University
[2]Department of Neurology, Chiba Rosai Hospital, Japan

ABSTRACT

Guillain–Barré syndrome is currently classified into 2 major forms based on pathologic and electrophysiologic criteria: (1) acute inflammatory demyelinating polyneuropathy (AIDP), by far the most common form in western countries; and (2) acute motor axonal neuropathy (AMAN), which is more prevalent in East Asia (China and Japan). AMAN is characterized by electrophysiologic and pathologic evidence of axonal degeneration of the motor nerves as well as functional conduction failure or other pathophysiology. It is possibly associated with anti-ganglioside antibodies; in particular, IgG antibodies to the gangliosides GM1, GM1b, GD1a and GalNAc-GD1a, which may be induced by particular infectious agents such as *Campylobacter jejuni* or *Haemophilus influenza*. Although AMAN appears to be similar to AIDP, there are important clinical differences. AMAN is a pure motor syndrome, with infrequent and mild involvement of the autonomic nervous system. When sensory fibres are also affected, this axonal subtype is called acute motor and sensory axonal neuropathy. Patients with AMAN often show hyperreflexia in the recovery phase. AMAN has a rapid progression in its early stage and has an earlier nadir than AIDP. AMAN has 2 patterns of clinical recovery, rapid and prolonged, in contrast to the relatively uniform recovery seen in AIDP. Electrophysiologic evidence of axonal degeneration is thought to be an indicator of poor prognosis. However, the most severely disabled AMAN patients are able to walk independently within a few years, indicating that electrodiagnosis of AMAN is not always a marker of poor recovery. This review provides an update on the clinical features, recovery pattern and long-term prognosis in AMAN patients.

---

* Corresponding author: Department of Neurology, Chiba Rosai Hospital, 2-16 Tatsumidai-Higashi, Ichihara-shi, Chiba 290-0003, Japan., Telephone number: +81-436-74-1111, Fax number: +81-436-74-1151, E-mail: hiragaa@yahoo.co.jp

Based on pathologic and electrophysiologic observations, Guillain-Barré syndrome (GBS) has been regarded as a type of demyelinating neuropathy. In 1986, Feasby et al. identified a severe axonal type of GBS coupled with poor recovery and demonstrated severe wallerian-like degeneration in the peripheral nerves at autopsy [1]. In the 1990s, a pure motor axonal form of GBS, designated acute motor axonal neuropathy (AMAN), was recognized in northern China. This form, which resulted in summer epidemics in children or young adults [2-4], was later reported in other countries [5-13]. GBS is currently divided into 2 major categories based on pathologic and electrophysiologic criteria: (1) acute inflammatory demyelinating polyneuropathy (AIDP, the classical demyelinating form), and (2) AMAN (the pure motor axonal form). AMAN is characterized by electrophysiologic and pathologic evidence of axonal degeneration of the motor nerves as well as functional conduction failure or other pathophysiology. Moreover, it is possibly associated with anti-ganglioside antibodies; in particular, IgG antibodies to the gangliosides GM1, GM1b, GD1a and GalNAc-GD1a [14-22]. *Campylobacter jejuni* infection is the most common antecedent infection in patients with axonal GBS, and this bacterium is likely to share epitopes homologous with gangliosides expressed on human peripheral motor axons (molecular mimicry) [23-26].

The incidence of AMAN varies according to country. AMAN accounted for only 7% of GBS patients reported in England [27] and 3% of such patients in a multicenter study done in 11 western countries [28]. In contrast, it constitutes 65% patients in a study in northern China [4] and 39% in Japan [23]. The low percentages of patients with AMAN in western countries may have affected study results, and most previous studies of the clinical features and prognosis in GBS patients in western countries focused on AIDP. AIDP and AMAN may have different immunopathogeneses and target molecules, which could account for the differences in patterns of clinical features observed between these 2 forms. The present review provides an update of the clinical features of AMAN patients, focusing especially on data from Japan and northern China.

Signs and Symptoms

AMAN is a pure motor syndrome with a rapid onset of muscle weakness and absent reflexes. It usually affects all 4 limbs and can involve the cranial nerves. Although the AMAN form of GBS appears to be similar to the AIDP form, there are some important clinical differences. The following discussion outlines the clinical features of AMAN focusing especially on the differences between AMAN and AIDP, which are summarized in Table 1.

Weakness

Onset of lower limb weakness and an ascending symmetrical paralysis of all 4 extremities are typical in AMAN [2]. Weakness patterns are typically distal dominant [2, 5]. Some anti-ganglioside antibodies, such as GM1b [20], GalNac-GD1a [18, 29] and GM1 [12, 30], which are strongly associated with AMAN, are also reported to be associated with distal-dominant weakness. However, patients whose weakness initially begins in the hand [31], as well as those in whom weakness is completely restricted to the lower limbs, have also been reported [32]. In addition to limb weakness, neck muscle weakness can occur in AMAN patients [2]. Neck weakness is common in patients with anti-GT1a antibodies [33, 34]. Muscle atrophy, reflecting severe axonal damage, has been seen in severely disabled patients with AMAN, but its frequency has not been investigated.

Sensory Symptoms

In contrast to AIDP, which commonly results in the development of sensory nerve dysfunction, AMAN is thought to be a pure motor syndrome. When sensory fibres are also affected, it is called acute motor and sensory axonal neuropathy (AMSAN) [35]. In AMSAN, sensory symptoms can be the sole initial manifestation [35]. Although AMAN is pure motor syndrome, some patients showed mild sensory symptoms such as mild paraesthesia. In fact, 2–19% patients showed paraesthesia of the hands and feet [2, 4].

Pain

Pain occurs frequently in GBS [36]. Severe pain has been reported in a patient with severe AMSAN, and such pain may reflect sensory nerve damage [37]. Because AMAN is a pure motor syndrome without sensory nerve involvement, pain is thought to be minor symptoms in AMAN. However, a recent report showed that 10 of 16 AMAN patients experienced pain [38]. Neuropathic pain is not expected to be relevant in pure motor GBS, because this type of pain results from degeneration or regeneration of sensory fibres. Patients with pure motor GBS who reported pain did not have clinical or electrophysiological evidence of sensory symptoms or involvement; therefore, pain in the acute phase of pure motor GBS is likely to be of nociceptive origin, probably due to activation of the nervi nervorum by inflammation or inflammatory mediators [38]. However, this theory needs further exploration [38]. Moreover, pain can be the initial symptom in AMAN [7].

Deep Tendon Reflexes

Although the presence of "areflexia (loss of tendon jerks)" or "distal areflexia with definite hyporeflexia of the biceps and knee jerks" is required for diagnosis of GBS [39], some AMAN patients manifest hyperreflexia in the recovery phase. Chinese patients with AMAN often develop hyperreflexia during the early phase of recovery [2]. A Japanese study found that hyperreflexia was common in AMAN patients (26%) 3–4 weeks after onset [40], and these patients often had anti-GM1 antibodies and milder disability peak. Increased motor neuron excitability was postulated as a possible mechanism of hyperreflexia. Outside Asia, another case report from Europe showed hyperreflexia 4 weeks after onset [41]. Apart from these, patients with electrophysiologically confirmed AMAN having anti-GM1 antibody who showed preserved tendon reflexes in the acute phase [42] and patients with electrophysiologically confirmed AMAN having anti-GM1b and anti-GalNAc-GD1a antibodies with hyperreflexia in the acute phase also have been reported [43]. These patients did not fulfil the clinical criteria for GBS [39]. However, recognition of the preserved or exaggerated tendon reflexes in AMAN is important in view of the differential diagnosis of myelopathy.

Cranial Nerve Palsy

Cranial nerve palsy is relatively infrequent in AMAN compared with AIDP [4, 7, 44]. However, bulbar palsy, jaw, tongue and pharynx as well as facial palsy are sometimes present [2]. Cranial nerve palsy was reported in 47–57% of patients with AMAN and 75–100% of patients with AIDP in northern China [4, 44], whereas a recent India study showed that cranial nerve involvement was equally frequent in both AIDP (64%) and AMAN (64%) [13]. Extraocular involvements and ptosis are rare. Specific anti-ganglioside antibodies are known to be related to frequent cranial nerve palsy such as, ophthalmoplegia with anti-GQ1b antibody [26, 45, 46] and bulbar palsy with anti-GT1a antibody [33, 34, 45]. Although cranial nerves are affected bilaterally in typical cases, unilateral involvement in a patient with AMAN was also reported [47]. Loss of taste was reported in GBS patients as a rare symptom [48], but no electrodiagnostic information was available for these patients. Thus, the occurrence of loss of taste in AMAN patients is not clear.

Respiratory Failure

AMAN patients often develop respiratory failure and require ventilatory support [49]. In AMSAN patients, respiratory failure commonly occurs, reflecting severe axonal disease [35]. Among Chinese patients, 22–38% of those with AMAN required respiratory assistance compared with 25–44% of those with AIDP [2, 4, 44]. In Japan, 9% of AMAN and 30% of AIDP patients required mechanical ventilation at nadir [50] whereas a Pakistani study showed that mechanical ventilation was required in 16% of AIDP and 29% of AMAN patients [51]. Furthermore, a Taiwanese study showed as many as 32% of AIDP and 17% of AMAN patients required ventilatory assistance [7], and a recent India study showed that 23% of AIDP and 14% of AMAN required mechanical ventilation [13]. One report showed that AIDP patients more often needed mechanical ventilation [52], whereas a recent report indicated that in Fisher/Guillain–Barré overlap syndrome, more often associated with AMAN than with the AIDP pattern, a significant number of patients needed mechanical ventilation [46]. These findings indicate that the incidence of respiratory failure in AMAN appears to be lower than or equal to that in AIDP.

Autonomic Disturbance

In addition to motor and sensory deficits, GBS is often associated with a variety of autonomic findings, including cardiovascular, vasomotor or sudomotor dysfunction affecting both the sympathetic and parasympathetic systems [53, 54]. In the first description of axonal

GBS, by Feasby et al., 3 of 5 patients showed autonomic disturbance [1]. Cardiac arrhythmias and blood pressure alterations also occur in AMAN [2].

AIDP is frequently associated with autonomic disturbance. However, involvement of the autonomic nervous system is infrequent and mild in AMAN [7, 23, 55]. On autonomic function tests, AMAN patients showed normal cardiovascular autonomic function, but some expressed hypoactivity in sudomotor or skin vasomotor function, and patients with severe AMAN may have generalized hypohidrosis [55]. On the other hand, cases with patchy hyperhidrosis are also reported in AMAN [2].

According to the diagnostic criteria for GBS, the presence of bladder or bowel dysfunction raises uncertainty in diagnosis [39]. This is presumably because GBS patients should be clearly differentiated from those with acute myelopathy, in which urinary retention is common. However, urinary symptoms and bowel dysfunction are not rare in GBS. Urinary symptoms (voiding difficulty, retention and urgency) were more common in AIDP (39%) than in AMAN (19%), and urinary retention occurred nearly as often in AMAN (7%) as in AIDP (11%). The most common urinary symptom in AMAN is voiding difficulty. Urinary dysfunction appears to involve both hypoactive and hyperactive lumbosacral nerves [56, 57]. Constipation was present in 18% of AIDP and 8% of AMAN patients [56] and can be severe [58].

Erectile dysfunction [56, 58] and pupillary disturbance [59] were seen in AMAN, but are rare symptoms.

Disease Progression

AMAN shows an earlier nadir than AIDP [5, 60]. In Chinese patients with AMAN (children or young adults), the mean onset to nadir was 5.9 days [2]. The mean periods between onset and nadir were longer in AMAN patients (18.0 days) than in those with AIDP (11.5 days) in Japan [60]. Most AMAN patients had reached the nadir at the time of their first examination. In the subgroup of those with mild disability who were able to walk independently at the first neurologic examination, 88% of AMAN patients versus 65% of AIDP patients had reached the nadir. The remaining 35% of the AIDP patients progressed to nadir over the next 1–2 weeks and were unable to walk at nadir [60].

Disease Severity at Nadir

In northern China, 66% of AMAN patients were bed-bound at nadir compared with 88% of AIDP patients [44]. In Japan, the Hughes functional grading scale at nadir in AMAN and AIDP showed no differences [50, 60]; 50% of AMAN and 45% of AIDP patients were bed-bound at nadir, whereas 41% of AMAN patients were able to walk without assistance at nadir. In a Pakistani study, weakness of both the arms and legs was significantly more severe in AMAN patients than in AIDP patients [51].

Table 1. Comparison between the 2 forms of Guillain–Barré syndrome.

	AMAN	AIDP
Antecedent infection	Campylobacter jejuni	Cytomegalovirus
	Haemophilus influenza	Epstein-Barr virus
Epidemics	Summer in northern china	None
High-frequency region	North China, Japan	Western countries
Respiratory failure	Common	Common
Cranial palsies	Infrequent	Frequent
Tendon reflexes	Usually absent, occasionally preserved or exaggerated	Absent
Sensory symptoms	Rare	Common
Autonomic dysfunction	Infrequent	Frequent
Micturition disturbance	Infrequent	Frequent
Electrophysiology	Axonal degeneration or reversible conduction block/slowing	Demyelination
Anti-ganglioside antibodies	GM1, GM1b, GD1a and GalNAc-GD1a	None
Time to nadir	Earlier	Later
Recovery pattern	Rapid or prolonged	Uniform (good)

AIDP = acute inflammatory demyelinating polyneuropathy; AMAN = acute motor axonal neuropathy

AMAN often produces severe disability. However, considerable numbers of patients manifest only mild disability. Some predictors are associated with disease severity at nadir in AMAN. *Haemophilus influenzae* has been recognized as the second most frequent preceding pathogen in axonal GBS, and *H. influenzae*-related GBS is suggested to be associated with milder disease and faster recovery compared with *Campylobacter jejuni*-related GBS [61].

Recovery Patterns: Rapid and Prolonged

Autopsy studies of AMAN patients have detected extensive wallerian-like degeneration in the ventral roots [3]. Electrophysiologic evidence of axonal degeneration is thought to be an indicator of poor prognosis [8, 62-67]. However, recovery in AMAN patients is often rapid [9, 44, 50, 68, 69].

Among Chinese AMAN patients, recovery was well [2]. In a report of 32 AMAN and 8 AIDP patients in northern China [44], some AMAN patients had rapid clinical recovery and the recovery time in AIDP and AMAN patients were similar. In a Japanese study, the AMAN group had a higher percentage of patients with slow (unable to walk independently at 6 months) and rapid (improvement by 2 Hughes functional grades or more during the first 4 weeks) recovery than the AIDP group [50]. This confirmed that 2 patterns of clinical recovery (rapid and prolonged) were found in AMAN patients, in contrast to the relatively uniform recovery seen in AIDP patients. These 2 recovery patterns were also noted in an earlier study of GBS patients with anti-GM1 antibodies, most of whom had AMAN [9]. The good potential for recovery from AMAN suggests that extensive axonal degeneration is not always the underlying pathophysiology. The rapid recovery of AMAN may be explained by early resolution of physiologic conduction failure at the nodes of Ranvier in the motor fibres [15, 44, 70] or by collateral sprouting of surviving axons [68], and prolonged recovery of AMAN patients is explained by severe axonal degeneration.

Long-Term Prognosis of Severely Disabled Patients with AMAN

In the first description of 5 cases of axonal GBS by Feasby et al., 1 patient died and 3 of 4 survivors showed poor recovery; only 1 in 5 patients could walk without assistance 1 year after onset [1]. Initial indications were that this axonal GBS form had a worse prognosis than demyelinating forms of the disease, and it was suggested that recovery might require axonal regeneration along the entire length of the nerve fibres [71]. In the intervening years, it has become apparent that recovery from axonal GBS is not always poor.

In a multicenter study of 369 GBS patients in 11 western countries [28], axonal GBS accounted for 3% of cases, and 10% of those with the axonal form and 17% with the demyelinating form could not walk or were dead 48 weeks after onset. The numbers of patients unable to walk and those who died did not differ significantly for the axonal and demyelinating forms. Of 32 AMAN and 8 AIDP patients in northern China [44], more than 90% of the AMAN patients and all of those with AIDP could walk 5 metres with a walker or support. The Chinese AMAN patients, however, were markedly younger (median age, 10 years) than the AIDP patients (median age, 42 years). A comparison of the prognosis for AMAN and AIDP patients, therefore, is difficult to make. In a study conducted in Japan, long-term prognosis did not differ between AMAN and AIDP [50]. In that study, 8% of the 97 patients with GBS (6 AMAN and 2 AIDP) could not walk independently 6 months after onset. Four of the 6 AMAN patients could walk independently 1 year after onset, and the other 2 could walk independently 28 or 57 months after onset. It is generally believed that no further recovery can be expected 2–3 years after GBS [72]. However, in a Dutch study, 21% of the GBS patients continued to improve after 2.5–6.5 years [73]. A Japanese study showed that most severely disabled AMAN patients could walk independently within a period of a few years [50]. The mechanism of improvement in severely disabled AMAN patients several years after onset is not clear, but axonal regeneration along the long course of the nerve may account for it. AIDP can be accompanied by secondary axonal degeneration in severe cases, and AMAN could be associated with functional conduction block as well as axonal degeneration [15]. These might explain why the long-term prognoses in AMAN and AIDP are almost equal.

Future Study

Since the 1990s, many studies investigating anti-ganglioside antibodies and their relationship to GBS have revealed some clinical variants or atypical cases of the disease, such as electrodiagnostically confirmed AMAN, presented with preserved or exaggerated tendon reflexes or severe sphincter dysfunction. To reflect these findings, the clinical criteria for GBS [39] should be reconsidered, for example, to include laboratory data about anti-ganglioside antibodies.

As mentioned earlier in this paper, AMAN is common in northern China and Japan but infrequent in western countries. A larger survey comparing AMAN with AIDP should be undertaken by countries in these 2 regions to clarify additional details about the clinical features of AMAN. Most AMAN patients in China are younger (children or young adults) than those in Japan. Because age is one of the most important predictive factors of prognosis in GBS, the difference in clinical features and prognosis between AMAN and AIDP should also be clarified, especially in Japan, using a national survey.

REFERENCES

[1] Feasby, TE; Gilbert, JJ; Brown, WF; Bolton, CF; Hahn, AF; Koopman, WF; Zochodne, DW. An acute axonal form of Guillain-Barré polyneuropathy. *Brain,* 1986, 109, 1115-1126.

[2] McKhann, GM; Cornblath, DR; Griffin, JW; Ho, TW; Li, CY; Jiang, Z; Wu, HS; Zhaori, G; Liu, Y; Jou, LP; Liu, TC; Gao, CY; Mao, JY; Blaser, MJ; Mishu, B; Asbury, AK. Acute motor axonal neuropathy: a frequent cause of acute flaccid paralysis in China. *Ann Neurol,* 1993, 33, 333-342.

[3] Griffin, JW; Li, CY; Ho, TW; Xue, P; Macko, C; Gao, CY; Yang, C; Tian, M; Mishu, B; Cornblath, DR. Guillain-Barré syndrome in northern China: the spectrum of neuropathological changes in clinically defined cases. *Brain,* 1995, 118, 577-595.

[4] Ho, TW; Mishu, B; Li, CY; Gao, CY; Cornblath, DR; Griffin, JW; Asbury, AK; Blaser, MJ; McKhann, GM. Guillain-Barré syndrome in northern China: relationship to *Campylobacter jejuni* infection and anti-glycolipid antibodies. *Brain,* 1995, 118, 597-605.

[5] Visser, LH; van der Meché, FGA; van Doorn, PA; Meulstee, J; Jacobs, BC; Oomes, PG; Kleyweg, RP; Meulstee, J. Guillain-Barré syndrome without sensory loss (acute motor neuropathy): A subgroup with specific clinical, electrodiagnostic and laboratory features. *Brain,* 1995, 118, 841-847.

[6] Rees, JH; Soudain, SE; Gregson, NA; Hughes, RAC. *Campylobacter jejuni* infection and Guillain-Barré syndrome. *N Engl J Med,* 1995, 333, 1374-1379.

[7] Lyu, RK; Tang, LM; Cheng, SY; Hsu, WC; Chen, ST. Guillain-Barré syndrome in Taiwan: a clinical study of 167 patients. *J Neurol Neurosurg Psychiatry,* 1997, 63, 494-500.

[8] Emilia-Romagna Study Group on Clinical and Epidemiological Problems in Neurology. A prospective study on the incidence and prognosis of Guillain-Barré syndrome in Emilia-Romagna region, Italy (1992-1993). *Neurology,* 1997, 48, 214-221.

[9] Kuwabara, S; Asahina, M; Koga, M; Mori, M; Yuki, N; Hattori, T. Two patterns of clinical recovery in Guillain-Barré syndrome with IgG anti-GM1 antibody. *Neurology,* 1998, 51, 1656-1660.

[10] Ogawara, K; Kuwabara, S; Mori, M; Hattori, T; Koga, M; Yuki, N. Axonal Guillain-Barré syndrome: relation to anti-ganglioside antibodies and *Campylobacter jejuni* infection in Japan. *Ann Neurol,* 2000, 48, 624-631.

[11] Chiò, A; Cocito, D; Leone, M; Giordana, MT; Mora, G; Mutani, R; Piemonte Valle d'Aosta Register for Guillain-Barré Syndrome. Guillain-Barré syndrome: a prospective, population-based incidence and outcome survey. *Neurology,* 2003, 60, 1146-1150.

[12] Dourado, ME; Duarte, RC; Ferreira, LC; Queiroz, JW; Illa, I; Perez-Perez, G; Guerrant, RL; Jerônimo, SM. Anti-ganglioside antibodies and clinical outcome of patients with Guillain-Barré syndrome in northeast Brazil. *Acta Neurol Scand,* 2003, 108, 102-108.

[13] Gupta, D; Nair, M; Baheti, NN; Sarma, PS; Kuruvilla, A. Diplomate-American Board. Electrodiagnostic and clinical aspects of Guillain-Barré syndrome: an analysis of 142 cases. *J Clin Neuromuscul Dis,* 2008, 10, 42-51.

[14] Kusunoki, S; Chiba, A; Kon, K; Ando, S; Arisawa, K; Tate, A; Kanazawa, I. N-acetylgalactosaminyl GD1a is a target molecule for serum antibody in Guillain-Barré syndrome. *Ann Neurol,* 1994, 35, 570-576.

[15] Kuwabara, S; Yuki, N; Koga, M; Hattori, T; Matsuura, D; Miyake, M; Noda, M. IgG anti-GM1 antibody is associated with reversible conduction failure and axonal degeneration in Guillain-Barré syndrome. *Ann Neurol,* 1998, 44, 202-208.

[16] Ho, TW; Willison, HJ; Nachamkin, I; Li, CY; Veitch, J; Ung, H; Wang, GR; Liu, RC; Cornblath, DR; Asbury, AK; Griffin, JW; McKhann, GM. Anti-GD1a antibody is associated with axonal but not demyelinating forms of Guillain-Barré syndrome. *Ann Neurol,* 1999, 45, 168-173.

[17] Yuki, N; Ho, TW; Tagawa, Y; Koga, M; Li CY; Hirata, K; Griffin, JW. Autoantibodies to GM1b and GalNAc-GD1a: relationship to *Campylobacter jejuni* infection and acute motor axonal neuropathy in China. *J Neurol Sci,* 1999, 164, 134-138.

[18] Kaida, K; Kusunoki, S; Kamakura, K; Motoyoshi, K; Kanazawa, I. Guillain-Barré syndrome with antibody to a ganglioside, N-acetylgalactosaminyl GD1a. *Brain,* 2000, 123, 116-124.

[19] Kuwabara, S; Ogawara, K; Mizobuchi, K; Koga, M; Mori, M; Hattori, T; Yuki, N. Isolated absence of F waves and proximal axonal dysfunction in Guillain-Barré syndrome with antiganglioside antibodies. *J Neurol Neurosurg Psychiatry,* 2000, 68, 191-195.

[20] Yuki, N; Ang, CW; Koga, M; Jacobs, BC; van Doorn, PA; Hirata, K; van der Meché, FG. Clinical features and response to treatment in Guillain-Barré syndrome associated with antibodies to GM1b ganglioside. *Ann Neurol,* 2000, 47, 314-321.

[21] Ogawara, K; Kuwabara, S; Koga, M; Mori, M; Yuki, N; Hattori, T. Anti-GM1b IgG antibody is associated with acute motor axonal neuropathy and *Campylobacter jejuni* infection. *J Neurol Sci,* 2003, 15, 210, 41-45.

[22] Hiraga, A; Kuwabara, S; Ogawara, K; Misawa, S; Kanesaka, T; Koga, M; Yuki, N; Hattori, T; Mori, M. Patterns and serial changes in electrodiagnostic abnormalities of axonal Guillain-Barré syndrome. *Neurology,* 2005, 64, 856-860.

[23] Kuwabara, S. Guillain-Barré syndrome: epidemiology, pathophysiology and management. *Drugs,* 2004, 64, 597-610.

[24] Yuki, N. Carbohydrate mimicry: a new paradigm of autoimmune diseases. *Curr Opin Immunol,* 2005, 17, 577-582.

[25] Hughes, RAC; Cornblath, DR. Guillain-Barré syndrome. *Lancet,* 2005, 366, 1653-1666.
[26] van Doorn, PA; Ruts, L; Jacobs, BC. Clinical features, pathogenesis, and treatment of Guillain-Barré syndrome. *Lancet Neurol,* 2008, 7, 939-950.
[27] Ree, JH; Gregson, NA; Hughes, RAC. Anti-ganglioside GM_1 antibodies in Guillain-Barré syndrome and their relationship to *Campylobacter jejuni* infection. *Ann Neurol,* 1995, 38, 809-816.
[28] Hadden, RDM; Cornblath, DR; Hughes, RAC; Zielasek, J; Hartung, HP; Toyka, KV; Swan, AV. Electrophysiological classification of Guillain-Barré syndrome: clinical associations and outcome. *Ann Neurol,* 1998, 44, 780-788.
[29] Hao, Q; Saida, T; Yoshino, H; Kuroki, S; Nukina, M; Saida, K. Anti-GalNAc-GD1a antibody-associated Guillain-Barré syndrome with a predominantly distal weakness without cranial nerve impairment and sensory disturbance. *Ann Neurol,* 1999, 45, 758-768.
[30] Jacobs, BC; van Doorn, PA; Schmitz, PI; Tio-Gillen, AP; Herbrink, P; Visser, LH; Hooijkass, H; van der Meché, FG. Campylobacter jejuni infections and anti-GM1 antibodies in Guillain-Barré syndrome. *Ann Neurol,* 1996, 40, 181-187.
[31] Mori, I; Koga, M; Hirata, K; Yuki, N. Hand weakness onset Guillain-Barré syndrome. *J Neurol Neurosurg Psychiatry,* 2004, 75, 169-170.
[32] Hambraeus, J; Eeg-Olofsson, K; Askmark, H. Acute motor axonal neuropathy with selective involvement of the lower limbs. *J Clin Neuromuscul Dis,* 2002, 4, 27-30.
[33] Koga, M; Yoshino, H; Morimatsu, M; Yuki, N. Anti-GT1a IgG in Guillain-Barré syndrome. *J Neurol Neurosurg Psychiatry,* 2002, 72, 767-771.
[34] Nagashima, T; Koga, M; Odaka, M; Hirata, K; Yuki, N. Clinical correlates of serum anti-GT1a IgG antibodies. *J Neurol Sci,* 2004, 219, 139-145.
[35] Griffin, JW; Li, CY; Ho, TW; Tian, M; Gao, CY; Xue, P; Mishu, B; Cornblath, DR; Macko, C; McKhann, GM; Asbury, AK. Pathology of the motor-sensory axonal Guillain-Barré syndrome. *Ann Neurol,* 1996, 39, 17-28.
[36] Moulin, DE; Hagen, N; Feasby, TE; Amireh, R; Hahn, A. Pain in Guillain-Barré syndrome. *Neurology,* 1997, 48, 328-331.
[37] Rostásy, KM; Huppke, P; Beckers, B; Brockmann, K; Degenhardt, V; Wesche, B; König, F; Gärtner, J. Acute motor and sensory axonal neuropathy (AMSAN) in a 15-year-old boy presenting with severe pain and distal muscle weakness. *Neuropediatrics,* 2005, 36, 260-264.
[38] Ruts, L; Rico, R; van Koningsveld, R; Botero, JD; Meulstee, J; Gerstenbluth, I; Merkies, IS; van Doorn PA. Pain accompanies pure motor Guillain-Barré syndrome. *J Peripher Nerv Syst,* 2008, 13, 305-306.
[39] Asbury, AK; Cornblath, DR. Assessment of current diagnostic criteria for Guillain-Barré syndrome. *Ann Neurol,* 1990, 27 (suppl), S21-24.
[40] Kuwabara, S; Ogawara, K; Koga, M; Mori, M; Hattori, T; Yuki, N. Hyperreflexia in Guillain-Barré syndrome: relation with acute motor axonal neuropathy and anti-GM1 antibody. J *Neurol Neurosurg Psychiatry,* 1999, 67, 180-184.
[41] Podnar, S; Vodusek, DB. Hyperreflexia in a patient with motor axonal Guillain-Barré syndrome. *Eur J Neurol.,* 2000, 7, 727-730.
[42] Yuki, N; Hirata, K. Preserved tendon reflexes in Campylobacter neuropathy. *Ann Neurol,* 1998, 43, 546-547.

[43] Kuwabara, S; Nakata, M; Sung, JY; Mori, M; Kato, N; Hattori, T; Koga, M; Yuki, N. Hyperreflexia in axonal Guillain-Barré syndrome subsequent to Campylobacter jejuni enteritis. *J Neurol Sci,* 2002, 199, 89-92.

[44] Ho, TW; Li, CY; Cornblath, DR; Gao, CY; Asbury, AK; Griffin, JW; McKhann, GM. Patterns of recovery in the Guillain-Barré syndromes. *Neurology,* 1997, 48, 695-700.

[45] Yoshino, H; Harukawa, H; Asano, A. IgG antiganglioside antibodies in Guillain-Barré syndrome with bulbar palsy. *J Neuroimmunol,* 2000, 105, 195-201.

[46] Funakoshi, K; Kuwabara, S; Odaka, M; Hirata, K; Yuki, N. Clinical predictors of mechanical ventilation in Fisher/Guillain-Barré overlap syndrome. *J Neurol Neurosurg Psychiatry,* 2009, 80, 60-64.

[47] Sakakibara, Y; Mori, M; Kuwabara, S; Katayama, K; Hattori, T; Koga, M; Yuki, N. Unilateral cranial and phrenic nerve involvement in axonal Guillain-Barré syndrome. *Muscle Nerve,* 2002, 25, 297-299.

[48] Odaka, M; Yuki, N; Nishimoto, Y; Hirata, K. Guillain-Barré syndrome presenting with loss of taste. *Neurology,* 2002, 58, 1437-1438.

[49] Vucic, S; Kiernan, MC; Cornblath, DR. Guillain-Barré syndrome: an update. *J Clin Neurosci,* 2009, 16, 733-741.

[50] Hiraga, A; Mori, M; Ogawara, K; Kojima, S; Kanesaka, T; Misawa, S; Hattori, T; Kuwabara, S. Recovery patterns and long term prognosis for axonal Guillain-Barré syndrome. *J Neurol Neurosurg Psychiatry,* 2005, 76, 719-722.

[51] Shafqat, S; Khealani, BA; Awan, F; Abedin, SE. Guillain-Barré syndrome in Pakistan: similarity of demyelinating and axonal variants. *Eur J Neurol,* 2006, 13, 662-665.

[52] Durand, MC; Porcher, R; Orlikowski, D; Aboab, J; Devaux, C; Clair, B; Annane, D; Gaillard, JL; Lofaso, F; Raphael, JC; Sharshar, T. Clinical and electrophysiological predictors of respiratory failure in Guillain-Barré syndrome: a prospective study. *Lancet Neurol,* 2006, 5, 1021-1028.

[53] Lichtenfeld, P. Autonomic dysfunction in the Guillain-Barré syndrome. *Am J Med,* 1971, 50, 772-780.

[54] Zochodne, DW. Autonomic involvement in Guillain-Barré syndrome: a review. *Muscle Nerve,* 1994, 17, 1145-1155.

[55] Asahina, M; Kuwabara, S; Suzuki, A; Hattori, T. Autonomic function in demyelinating and axonal subtypes of Guillain-Barré syndrome. *Acta Neurol Scand,* 2002, 105, 44-50.

[56] Sakakibara, R; Uchiyama, T; Kuwabara, S; Mori, M; Ito, T; Yamamoto, T; Awa, Y; Yamaguchi, C; Yuki, N; Vernino, S; Kishi, M; Shirai, K. Prevalence and mechanism of bladder dysfunction in Guillain-Barré Syndrome. *Neurourol Urodyn,* 2009, 28, 432-437.

[57] Sakakibara, R; Uchiyama, T; Tamura, N; Kuwabara, S; Asahina, M; Hattori, T. Urinary retention and sympathetic sphincter obstruction in axonal Guillain-Barré syndrome. *Muscle Nerve,* 2007, 35, 111-115.

[58] Sawai, S; Sakakibara, R; Uchiyama, T; Liu, Z; Yamamoto, T; Ito, T; Kuwabara, S; Kanai, K; Asahina, M; Yamanaka, T; Odaka, T; Yamaguchi, T; Hattori, T. Acute motor axonal neuropathy presenting with bowel, bladder, and erectile dysfunction. *J Neurol,* 2007, 254, 250-252.

[59] Sakakibara, R; Hattori, T; Kuwabara, S; Yamanishi, T; Yasuda, K. Micturitional disturbance in patients with Guillain-Barré syndrome. *J Neurol Neurosurg Psychiatry,* 1997, 63, 649-653.

[60] Hiraga, A; Mori, M; Ogawara, K; Hattori, T; Kuwabara, S. Differences in patterns of progression in demyelinating and axonal Guillain-Barré syndromes. *Neurology,* 2003, 61, 471-474.

[61] Mori, M; Kuwabara, S; Miyake, M; Noda, M; Kuroki, H; Kanno, H; Ogawara, K; Hattori, T. Haemophilus influenzae infection and Guillain-Barré syndrome. *Brain,* 2000, 123, 2171-2178.

[62] McKhann, GM; Griffin, JW; Cornblath, DR; Mellits, ED; Fisher, RS; Quaskey, SA. Plasmapheresis and Guillain-Barré syndrome: Analysis of prognostic factors and the effect of plasmapheresis. *Ann Neurol,* 1988, 23, 347-353.

[63] Winer, JB; Hughes, RAC; Osmond, C. A prospective study of acute idiopathic neuropathy. I : Clinical features and their prognostic value. *J Neurol Neurosurg Psychiatry,* 1988, 51, 605-612.

[64] The Italian Guillain-Barré Study Group. The prognosis and main prognostic indicators of Guillain-Barré syndrome. A multicentre prospective study of 297 patients. *Brain,* 1996, 119, 2053-2061.

[65] Visser, LH; Schmitz, PIM; Meulstee, J; van Doorn, PA; van der Meché, FGA. The Dutch Guillain-Barré Study Group. Prognostic factors of Guillain-Barré syndrome after intravenous immunoglobulin or plasma exchange. *Neurology,* 1999, 53, 598-604.

[66] Hadden, RDM; Karch, H; Hartung, HP; Hadden, RD; Karch, H; Hartung, HP; Zielasek, J; Weissbrich, B; Schubert, J; Weishaupt, A; Cornblath, DR; Swan, AV; Hughes, RA; Toyka, KV. Plasma Exchange/Sandoglubulin Guillain-Barré Syndrome Trial Group. Preceding infections, immune factors, and outcome in Guillain-Barré syndrome. *Neurology,* 2001, 56, 758-765.

[67] Cornblath, DR; Mellits, ED; Griffin, JW; Cornblath, DR; Mellits, ED; Griffin, JW; McKhann, GM; Albers, JW; Miller, RG; Feasby TE; Quaskey, SA. Motor conduction studies in Guillain-Barré syndrome: description and prognostic value. *Ann Neurol,* 1988, 23, 354-359.

[68] Kuwabara, S; Ogawara, K; Mizobuchi, K; Mori, M; Hattori, T. Mechanisms of early and late recovery in acute motor axonal neuropathy. *Muscle Nerve,* 2001, 24, 288-291.

[69] Kuwabara, S; Mori, M; Ogawara, K; Hattori, T; Yuki, N. Indicators of rapid clinical recovery in Guillain-Barré syndrome. *J Neurol Neurosurg Psychiatry,* 2001, 70, 560-562.

[70] Ho, TW; Hsieh, ST; Nachamkin, I; Willison, HJ; Sheikh, K; Kiehlbauch, J; Flanigan, K; McArthur, JC; Cornblath, DR; McKhann, GM; Griffin, JW. Motor nerve terminal degeneration provides a potential mechanism for rapid recovery in acute motor axonal neuropathy after *Campylobacter* infection. *Neurology,* 1997, 48, 717-724.

[71] Gabriel, CM. Prognosis in the acute motor axonal form of Guillain-Barré syndrome. *J Neurol Neurosurg Psychiatry,* 2005, 76, 622.

[72] Ropper, AH. Severe acute Guillain-Barré syndrome. *Neurology,* 1986, 36, 429-432.

[73] Bernsen, RAJAM; de Jager, AEJ; Schmitz, PIM; van der Meché, FGA. Long-term impact on work and private life after Guillain-Barré syndrome. *J Neurol Sci,* 2002, 201, 13-17.

In: Autoimmune Diseases: Symptoms, Diagnosis and Treatment   ISBN: 978-1-61668-007-7
Editor: Kyle J. Brenner, pp. 277-288   © 2010 Nova Science Publishers, Inc.

Chapter 8

REMOVAL [BLOCKAGE] OF HYPERPRODUCED CYTOKINES - A NEW APPROACH TO THE TREATMENT OF AUTOIMMUNE CONDITIONS

Simon V. Skurkovich

Plasma Gold Bioceutics, Rockville, Maryland

ABSTRACT

Treatment of many autoimmune conditions was for a long period of time based on different preparations that decrease inflammation. Anticytokine therapy, which is a new chapter in immunotherapy, is one of the first pathogenetic approaches to the treatment of autoimmune conditions. Presently, it is clear that normal production of different cytokines in cells is a marker of normal homeostasis and good health. Any hyperproduction caused by exogenous or endogenous cytokine inducers can lead to significant pathological changes. Disturbances of cytokine synthesis can affect different organ systems including immune, endocrine, neuro-psychiatric and others. My colleagues and I pioneered anticytokinotherapy in 1972 and 1974 (2). The use of anticytokinotherapy with specific modifications for different autoimmune diseases has had positive results in clinics around the world (more than 1 billion people suffer from autoimmune diseases worldwide).

Anticytokine therapy is currently at the very early stages of development. We expect that it will be successful in the treatment of such autoimmune diseases as rejection of organ and tissue transplants, multiple sclerosis, schizophrenia, Parkinson's disease, and others. We do not exclude that disturbance of cytokine synthesis can be very important in pathogenesis of atherosclerosis. Removal of some hyperproductive cytokines and their receptors together with the use of antibodies to LDL will be a crucial factor in the treatment of atherosclerosis. According to the editorial of The New England Journal of Medicine (US) anticytokine therapy is a new era in the treatment of autoimmune diseases especially rheumatoid arthritis (44).

INTRODUCTION

Cytokines are produced by many different kinds of cells. Normal production of cytokines is the major factor of homeostasis both in individual cells and in the whole body as well. Any disturbance of cytokine production, mainly their hyper-production, may cause a number of diseases that can be called a cytokine-related pathology (possibly there is pathology associated with hypo-production of cytokines as well). The main treatment of the diseases associated with hyper-production of cytokines is their removal or blockage. We have pioneered anti-cytokine therapy – in 1972 [1] and 1974 [2] where we explained the mechanism of the development of autoimmune conditions and the methods of their treatment.

In one of the studies [2] we proposed that hyper-production of a cytokine can lead to an autoimmune disease; in other words, a disturbance of interferon (a cytokine) production can cause different autoimmune conditions and removing or blocking of the cytokine can have therapeutic effect. In that article we considered it to be either alpha interferon (IFN-α) or gamma interferon (IFN-γ). One of the basic facts that we discovered in 1975 was the presence of interferon (a cytokine) in the blood of patients with autoimmune diseases [3]. In the same year we successfully used anticytokine therapy for the treatment of patients with acute rheumatoid arthritis with antibodies to IFN-α [3]. Later, in 1989 [4], we proposed to treat different autoimmune diseases and AIDS (which is also an autoimmune condition) with antibodies to tumor necrosis factor - alpha (TNF-α) together with antibodies to IFN-α, which makes anti-TNF-α more efficacious. According to research, IFN-α induces the production of TNF-α [5]. After our publication in 1989 [4], in July of 1993 US Patent Office granted a patent to A. Moeller at al. filed in September of 1987 (Monoclonal Antibodies Against Tumor Necrosis Factor (TNF), and Use Thereof) that described the treatment of autoimmune diseases with antibodies to TNF-α [6]. Later, in July of 1999 US Patent Office issued a patent to J. Le et al. which was filed in February of 1994 that described the use of chimeric antibodies to TNF-α for the treatment of autoimmune diseases [7]. In our articles and patents we have mentioned that functionally, all antibodies to TNF-α - monoclonal, chimeric, polyclonal have the same therapeutic action. Thus, we were first to publish a proposal to treat autoimmune diseases with antibodies to TNF-α in 1989.

After publication of our article in "Nature" in 1974 [2] a lot of experimental and later clinical work began. Thus, in 1974 we opened a new chapter in the treatment of autoimmune diseases with the use of anticytokine therapy. This method continues to be developed in different countries. We were the first to publish an article on the clinical use of blockers (antibodies) to IFN-α and IFN-γ for the treatment of autoimmune diseases [3, 10]; beside that we proposed to treat autoimmune conditions with blockers to different other cytokines [8]. First clinical research on the use of a blocker of TNF-α (a chimeric antibody) to treat rheumatoid arthritis was done in England [9]. Although we were the first to publish the use of antibodies to TNF-α for the treatment of different autoimmune diseases we were the second to use anti-TNF-α antibodies for the treatment of rheumatoid arthritis [10]. For technical reasons we used polyclonal antibodies and F(ab)'$_2$ antibody fragments in our clinical trials; the therapeutic activity of these antibodies was not weaker than that of the monoclonal antibodies and in some cases even stronger. When we first used antibodies to IFN-α for the treatment of acute rheumatoid arthritis [3] we used a very high-titer preparation obtained after a long-term immunization of donkeys with human IFN-α [11]. Later we used another type of anti-IFN-α antibodies with a much lower titer to treat rheumatoid arthritis but the effect was not very remarkable [10]. However, we obtained very positive results when we treated patients with antibodies to IFN-γ and antibodies to TNF-α.

Based on the differentiation of Th cells into Th1, Th2, Th3 and Th0 subsets, autoimmune and allergic diseases are sometimes distinguished as Th1 or Th2 diseases, respectively, depending on whether they are mediated by a polarization of Th cells toward either the Th1 or the Th2 subset [12]. Balanced Th1 cytokine production is maintained by the production of cytokines by Th2 cells, which include IL-4, 5, 10 and others, which can inhibit production of Th1 cytokines.

BACTERIA AND VIRUSES AS CYTOKINE INDUCERS

Reaction of the body to the administration of a cytokine inducer is similar to a response of the organism to the introduction of foreign genetic material. There are plenty of cytokine inducers. Some of the most important types of cytokine inducers [mainly inducers of interferons of different types] are bacteria and viruses. This subject caught our attention.

Bacteria. A number of bacteria induce cytokines that cause autoimmune conditions. For example, a protein of group A β-hemolytic streptococcus has been implicated in psoriasis [13], and a subpopulation of CD_4+T-cells in chronic plaque psoriasis skin lesions have been found to produce significant amounts of IFN-γ in response to streptococcal antigens in comparison with controls [14]. The same phenomenon is revealed in different autoimmune conditions, particularly of the skin, e.g., alopecia areata [15]. T-cell clones from alopecia lesions have been reported to release large amounts of IFN-γ and/or TNF-α that down-regulate epithelial cell proliferation [17].

The role of IFN-γ in the development of alopecia areata was revealed in experiments on a strain of knockout mice with the missing gene responsible for the production of IFN-γ. Alopecia areata could not be induced in those mice [18].

Normal skin commensal bacteria *Propionibacterium acnes*, which are implicated in the pathogenesis of inflammatory acne, appear to stimulate a typical Th1 response. T-cell lines from inflamed acne lesions were shown to proliferate in response to *P. acnes* extract and expressed IFN-γ in response to *P. acnes* stimulation [19]. There are other examples where bacteria and fungi induce cytokines that eventually lead to a number of different diseases, mostly of the skin.

Viruses. Some cytokines are induced by different viruses in different situations. In some cases they activate macrophages a catalyst of nitric oxide [NO], which can have toxic effects on different cells, including neurons [20]. In our opinion, there are two categories of viruses based on their ability to induce interferon and other cytokines [21]. First category consists of viruses that induce interferon which protects the cells from the damage by the viruses. This phenomenon was first discovered by Isaacs and Lindenmann [22]. In our opinion [21] the second category of viruses induces interferon and other cytokines which help the viruses survive. In this latter case the interferon, which acts mostly as a pathological agent, together with viruses and other agents which induce this interferon, exerts pathological effect on the organism. It is possible that slow viruses, e.g., scrapie virus, oncogenic viruses, HIV, chronic virus infection, rubella virus, cytomegalovirus, certain other viruses and bacteria, *Mycobacterium leprae*, avian flu and, possibly, H1N1 swine flu, EBV, and coxsackie virus, some viruses or agents which participate in psychiatric and neurological disorders, and some chemical agents, belong to this latter class. We cannot exclude the possibility that interferon induced by category 2 agents helps these viruses and other agents survive or replicate. We also propose that hyperproduction of interferon induced by category 2 agents disturbs the production of normal interferon, which is induced by category 1 viruses. We believe that the most important step in the treatment of patients with cytokine disturbances is the removal or neutralization of interferon induced by category 2 viruses. Thus, anti-interferon(s) therapy may be considered a delicate instrument in the treatment of a wide range of diseases, and, paradoxically, it may even be possible to treat certain viral infections and other conditions not with interferon but with antibodies or blockers which destroy interferons or other cytokines, i.e., with anticytokinotherapy.

SOME DATA RELATED TO TH1 AND TH1/TH2 AUTOIMMUNE DISEASES

In Th1 autoimmune diseases the levels of cytokines in the blood are not very high [e.g., in rheumatoid arthritis or multiple sclerosis]. To the contrary, in Th1/Th2 autoimmune conditions the levels of cytokines are quite high. We were the first to find extremely high levels of IFN-α in the blood of patients with systemic lupus erythemotosus (SLE) [3]. These data were a stimulus for a broad research into the pathogenesis of SLE. Later, high levels of IFN-α were found in the blood of patients with AIDS [23]. In Th1 autoimmune diseases cytokines were also found at the site of pathology; e.g., in rheumatoid arthritis IFN-γ-producing T-cells were found in the synovial fluid; in multiple sclerosis IFN-γ- producing T-cells were found in cerebrospinal fluid and plaques; in corneal transplant rejection IFN-γ-producing T-cells were found in aqueous humor and corneal infiltrating cells; in type 1 diabetes IFN-γ -producing T-cells were found in the islet β-cells; in uveitis IFN-γ-producing T-cells were found in ocular cells; in psoriasis, alopecia, vitiligo, and acne IFN-γ-producing T-cells were found in skin lesions [13, 14, 15, 16, 17, 18,19]

It would be expedient to treat Th1 autoimmune diseases with the use mainly of mono-anticytokinotherapy.

Poly-anticytokinotherapy can be used in some cases of Th1/Th2 autoimmune diseases.

Anticytokine therapy is mostly used for the treatment of Th1 autoimmune diseases. The main therapeutic preparations are blockers of TNF-α and IFN-γ. There are a lot of publications about therapeutic activity of antibodies (blockers) to TNF-α and a number of publications about therapeutic activity of antibodies (blockers) to IFN-γ. Preparations neutralizing biological activity of TNF-α are produced by different companies and at least four of them are licensed in the United States. We would note, however, that neutralization not only of main cytokines may have therapeutic activity, but also of other cytokines that participate in the cytokine cascade involved in the pathogenesis of Th1 autoimmune diseases.

Cautionary note/Warning

Although, TNF-α blockers have good therapeutic effect on the manifestations of autoimmune diseases, sometimes they can cause a number of complications. For example, anti-TNF-α sometimes leads to the development of SLE, infections, reactivation of latent tuberculosis, malignancies, such as lymphoma, worsening of congestive heart failure, and development of inflammatory demyelinating disease of the central nervous system [24]. Most of these conditions were not observed until after the dugs were used for several years in a broad patient population. Additional adverse effects of these therapies continue to appear in the literature, such as anti-TNF-α triggering alopecia areata [25]. For this reason, a Swiss biotechnology company Serono decided to stop the use of their TNF-α blocker for the treatment of psoriasis [26]. Unfortunately, different companies that invested big money in the production of TNF-α blockers do not pay much attention to the creation of TNF-α blockers that are both effective and safe. There is an impression that most of the companies care about material benefits but not about lives and health of patients. More progressive method for the treatment of autoimmune diseases is the method of blocking IFN-γ because this cytokine is one of most important immune regulators. This method has a better therapeutic effect and fewer complications. Therefore, in the USA and other countries, e.g., Switzerland, there appeared a number of publications on the creation of both humanizes and fully human monoclonal antibodies to IFN-γ. A Swiss company NovImmune has developed a fully human anti-IFN-γ monoclonal antibody that they are planning to use for the treatment of autoimmune conditions [27]. Their program is a copy of our pioneering work started over 30 years ago [2], a number of articles, and more than 41 American and seven international patents and several pending patents. Scientists do sometimes forget about the ethical and legal side of their work.

SOME AUTOIMMUNE DISEASES TREATED BY ANTICYTOKINOTHERAPY.

We would like to present some data on anticytokine therapy of different autoimmune diseases. In many countries anticytokine therapy is mainly used for the treatment of rheumatoid arthritis, psoriasis and some other autoimmune diseases. We want to give a short commentary on this treatment and suggest other autoimmune diseases that have a good chance of responding to this therapy:

1. **Rheumatoid arthritis.** As we have mentioned before the first anticytokinotherapy of rheumatoid arthritis was performed using antibodies to IFN-α and later to IFN-γ. TNF-α blockers are known to have good clinical effect but in some cases to cause severe complications. A lot of companies, mostly in the U.S.A., ignore the serious risks associated with the use of TNF-α blockers because they invested a lot of money in these products. Despite this risk they are being widely used in clinical practice. Both TNF-α and IFN-γ blockers have very similar positive therapeutic effects such as reduction of joint pain, decrease in edema, and other pathological manifestations of joint inflammation. However, therapeutic activity of antibodies to IFN-γ is

stronger than that of antibodies to TNF-α. The number of complications during the use of antibodies to IFN-γ was fewer as well [28 and some abstracts]. We were granted patents by US and International patent offices for the treatment of rheumatoid arthritis with IFN-γ blockers [29]. That is why a number of companies in the US and Europe have started production of antibodies to IFN-γ for the treatment of different autoimmune diseases.

There are also some publications about the treatment of rheumatoid arthritis with antibody to IL-6. Alongside with the good therapeutic effect there were some complications as well [30].

2. **Psoriasis.** Psoriasis is a very common disease and TNF-α blockers are actively promoted for its treatment. However, a lot of physicians are very hesitant to treat these patients with these preparations due to a risk of infection and other serious complications. As we have already mentioned before, Serono, Inc. had terminated the use of their TNF-α blocker for the treatment of psoriasis for this very reason. IFN-γ antibodies (blockers) are much more effective and safer than TNF-α blockers and they can be used both intramuscularly and topically [20 and some abstracts]. We first used anticytokine thereapy for the treatment of psoriasis in 1977.

3. Anti-IFN-γ has been successfully used for the treatment of alopecia areata, seborrheic dermatitis, herpes simples virus type 1 and 2 and a number of other Th1 conditions where IFN-γ plays a central role in their pathogenesis [20 and some abstracts].

4. **Multiple sclerosis (MS).** Administration of IFN-γ to patients with MS causes exacerbation of the disease. The therapeutic agent that is widely used for the treatment of MS is IFN-β which stimulates the synthesis of IL-10 which, in turn, decreases the synthesis of IFN-γ to some extent [31, 32]. This treatment is not very effective, most likely because of a relatively minor suppression of IFN-γ. Probably, a virus induces hyperproduction of IFN-γ and this is the main factor in the development of this disease [33]. A recent study by the researchers at the Mayo Clinic (MN, USA) showed that MS is closely correlated with a genetic variant that leads to production of high levels of IFN-γ [34]. The main goal of MS treatment is to reduce production of INF-γ. We performed a double-blind, placebo-controlled clinical trial in MS patients using cytokine blockers (antibody to TNF-α and antibody to INF-γ). Clinical results showed that antibody to TNF-α had no effect on the course of the disease (similar to placebo). However, the group that received anti-INF-γ had a significant increase in the number of patients free of sustained Expanded Disability Status Scale (EDSS) progression and in the mean time without sustained EDSS progression. A significant increase in the number of patients without gadolinium-enhancing lesions was also recorded using magnetic resonance imagining (MRI).

There also is a publication about positive results of the treatment of MS with antibodies to IFN-γ [33]. We were granted a patent by the US Patent Office for the treatment of multiple sclerosis [29].

5. **Prevention of rejection of organs after transplantation.** The first time anticytokinotherapy was used to stop rejection of skin grafts in mice was in 1972 [1] before we published our main proposal on anticytokine therapy in 1974 [2]. Later, we performed a clinical trial of anticytokine therapy in patients who were rejecting their corneal transplant after penetrating keratoplasty. In this study, 2-3 days after the start of a 6-day treatment course in which anti-IFN-γ eye drops were administered, transplant transparency improved and edema decreased in patients. At the end of the first week the transplant became almost fully transparent, eye inflammation disappeared and visual acuity improved. In the remaining three patients, additional treatment courses with the same preparation were needed for comparable improvement. Improvement was maintained for an average of 7 months. Patients given anti-TNF-α had comparable positive results [36, 37, 38]. According to existing data, a Japanese company produces antibodies for the treatment of immunologic diseases of eyes that were described in our patent and our article. The antibodies are being sold mostly in Russia. We plan to test this approach in transplant rejection of various organs [skin, kidneys, heart, liver etc.] using inhibitors of IFN-γ and TNF-α, and possibly anti-CD20. [35]. We got confirmation from the Dutch scientists who used antibodies to IFN-γ and TNF-α to successfully halt skin graft rejection in the rhesus monkey [39].

6. **AIDS.** We decided to include AIDS in this article because AIDS is one of the diseases with an obvious autoimmune component. Removal of cytokines that participate in the replication of viruses can be a very important step in AIDS therapy. One of the main goals in treating AIDS is to reduce HIV viral load. Some time ago, there was a proposal that HIV may belong to a category of viruses that induce cytokines, possibly changing their properties, which in turn increases virus replication (interferon discovered by Isaacs and Lindenmann normally stops viral replication [21]). Taking into account that in AIDS cytokines (e.g., mostly IFN-α, TNF-α, and possibly IFN-γ), and some other cytokines, may increase viral replication, the main goal of treatment must be to reduce serum levels of these cytokines. The reduction of these cytokines could be a decisive factor in the treatment of AIDS. Cytokine reduction may be achieved through the use of antibodies or soluble receptors to these cytokines or by other methods, such as extracorporeal removal. We obtained positive results in AIDS patients after removal of IFN-α from their blood [40]. In addition, positive results were obtained as well with the removal of TNF-α (personal communication, Dr. J. Bellanti, Georgetown University – Washington).

It should be remembered that AIDS is similar to SLE in a number of features, including high titers of IFN-α. In my view, both diseases are caused by different types of retroviruses. I allow myself to make a proposal for the treatment of AIDS that is not based on a factual material but on analogy, which had some positive clinical results. Since this issue is related to the treatment of AIDS which has no cure, any form of influence even without preliminary substantiation is justified. It is known, that salvarsan proposed by P. Ehrlich in 1909 for the treatment of syphilis was clinically used only by analogy.

HIV that causes AIDS, possibly has many common antigenic determinants with endogenious retrovirus that, in my view, causes development of SLE. In AIDS retrovirus leads to severe and fatal diseases. In SLE endogenic retrovirus causes a complicated chronic disease that can go into temporary with remission. It is appropriate to study the plasma or possibly lymphocytes of patients with SLE to find out the activity against HIV retrovirus in vitro and in vivo.

Thus, I propose to collect plasma (or possibly lymphocytes) from patients with SLE during its remission and to use it for the treatment of AIDS.

7. **Dystrophic epidermolysis bullosa [DEB].**

This condition is included in our article because it has not been well studied and scientists have not come up with any ideas for its rational pathogenetic therapy. This disorder has a genetic genesis and proceeds very painfully. Apparently an autoimmune mechanism is involved in this disease. INF-γ could also be involved by altering gene expression [41]. We treated 2 DEB patients with antibodies to IFN-γ. In one case a 14-year-old male with DEB from birth was given a course of anti-IFN-γ antibodies intramuscularly. Before the treatment the boy suffered from multiple erosive, ulcerative skin lesions up to 15 cm in diameter, his temperature was 39.2 C, and he was in a lot of pain. After the second injection of anti-IFN-γ his temperature normalized; pain, swelling and hyperemia around the lesions disappeared. The child began to eat, his general sense of well-being significantly improved and his sleep normalized. In the second case we obtained very similar results [42]. We are trying to draw scientists' attention to potential therapies for these suffering patients.

We have a number of successful cases, which we have not mentioned in this article yet, of treatment of other autoimmune diseases, especially skin Th1 diseases with the use of anticytokine therapy. The article was published in Annals of New York Academy of Sciences as well as several books by German Publisher "Springer". We will mention just one of them. (43)

CONCLUSION

Anticytokine therapy is a new chapter in immunotherapy. Different clinical syndromes could no be explained for many years although, as it is known now, these syndromes were caused by hyperproduction of different cytokines. Right now it is clear that normal production of different cytokines in cells is a marker of homeostasis and good health. Any hyperproduction caused either by an exogenous or an endogenous inducer of cytokines can have significant pathological consequences, especially if the production of this inducer is related to a genetic anomaly. A lot of diseases are connected to an immune system breakdown caused by the disturbance of cytokine synthesis [2]. In general, treatment of many autoimmune conditions was for a long time based on different preparations that decrease inflammation. Anticytokinotherapy is one of the first pathogenetic approaches to the treatment of autoimmune conditions and it has shown successful therapeutic effect in the treatment of a significant number of patients around the world.

Besides, in some neuropsychiatric diseases such as schizophrenia, Parkinson's disease, depression, etc, the role of the disturbances in the synthesis of cytokines is unquestionable, although not well studied. The goal of the researchers should be to find a way to normalize the synthesis of cytokines in these chronic diseases. On the other hand, there is data that allows us to speculate that the development of high intelligence and genius may involve the heightened sensitivity of certain brain cells to unusually high level of some cytokines or other changes in cytokine production [20].

Hyper-production of cytokines also takes place in different other pathologies, for example, in atherosclerosis and renal disease where hemodialysis is needed. Hyper-produced cytokines (TNF-α, IFN-γ, IL-1, and others) can lead to severe pathological manifestation causing atherosclerosis of coronary vessels and finally death. We have recently proposed to treat renal failure by removal of proinflammatory cytokines with administration of antibodies and other cytokine blockers together with the antibodies to the products of protein metabolism instead of kidney dialysis [43].

Thus, we must say that anticytokinotherapy, first carried out by us, is now widely used around the world. It is clear to us that anticytokinotherapy is one of the most important pathogenetic approaches to the treatment of autoimmune diseases. Nowadays some authors characterize anticytokinotherapy as a new era in the treatment of autoimmune diseases, especially rheumatoid arthritis [44]. There is a lot to research in anticytokine therapy. This therapy can be compared with an iceberg and our knowledge is just the tip of this iceberg. A noble goal for scientists is to find out what is hidden under water in order to help a lot of patients.

REFERENCES

[1] Skurkovich, S. V., Klinova, E. G., Alexandrovskaya, I. M., Levina, N. v., Arkhipova, N. A. & Bulycheva, T. I. (1972). *Proc. Thirteenth I.S.B.T. Cong., Washington.*

[2] Skurkovich, S. V., Klinova, E. G., Eremkina, E. I. & Levina, N. V. (1974). Immunosuppressive Effect of an Anti-interferon Serum. *Nature, 247,* 551-552.

[3] Skurkovich, S. V. & Eremkina, E. I. (1975). The probable role of interferon in allergy. *Ann. Allergy, 35,* 356-360.

[4] Skurkovich, S. V. & Skurkovich, B. (1989). Development of autoimmune diseases is connected with the initial disturbance of IFN synthesis in the cells. *J. Interferon Res., 9 (2),* 305.

[5] Lau, A. S. & Williams, B. R. G. (1990). The role of interferon and tumor necrosis factor in the pathogenesis of AIDS. *J. Exp. Pathology, 5,* 111-122.

[6] Moeller, A. & Emling, F. (1993). Monoclonal antibodies against human tumor necrosis factor (IFN), and use thereof. US patent No. 5, 231,024, filed in 1987.

[7] Le, J., Vilcek, J., Dadonna, P., Ghrayed, J., Knight, D. & Seigal, S. (1999). Methods of treating TNF-alpha-mediated disease using chimeric anti-TNF-antibodies., US patent No. 5, 919, *452,* date of patent, filed 1994.

[8] Skurkovich, S. V., Skurkovich, B. & Kelly, J. A. (2002). Anticytokine therapy – new approach to the treatment of autoimmune and cytokine-disturbance diseases. *Medical Hypotheses, 59(6),* 770-780.

[9] Elliott, M. J., Maini, R. N., Feldmann, M., et al. (1994). Randomized double-blind comparison of chimeric monoclonal antibody to tumor necrosis factor alpha (cA2) versus placebo in rheumatoid arthritis. *Lancet, 344(8930),* 1105-1110.

[10] Skurkovich, S. V., Loukina, G. V., Sigidin, Y. A. & Skurkovich, B. (1998). Successful first-time use of antibodies to interferon-gamma alone and combined with antibodies to tumor necrosis factor-alpha to treat rheumatic diseases (rheumatoid arthritis, systemic lupus erythemotosus, psoriatic arthritis, Behcet's syndrome). *Int. J. Immunotherapy, 14(1),* 23-32.

[11] Skurkovich, S. V., Olshansky, A. Y. A., Klinova, E. G. & Eremkina, E. I. (1978). Preparation of monospecific immunoglobulin against human leukocytic-alpha-INF. *Bulletin of experimental biology and medicine, Bexban, 86(11),* 1415-1562.

[12] Mosmann, T. R. & Sad, S. (1996). The expanding universe of T-cell subsets: Th-1, Th-2 and more. *Immunol. Today, 17,* 138-146.

[13] Prinz, J. C. (1997). Psoriasis vulgaris, streptococci and the immune system: a riddle to be solved soon? *Scand. J. Immunol., 45,* 583-586.

[14] Brown, D. W., Baker, B. S., Ovigne, J. M., Hardman, C., Fowles, A. V. & Fry, I. (2000). Skin CD4+T-cells produce interferon-gamma in vitro in response to streptococcal antigens in chronic plaque psoriasis. *J. Invest. Dermatol., 114,* 576-580.

[15] Thein, C., Strange, P, Hansen, E. R. & Baadsgaard, O. (1997). Lesional Alopecia Areata T-lymphocytes downregulate epithelial cell proliferation. *Arch. Dermatol. Res., 289,* 384-388.

[16] Arca, E., Musabak, U., Akar, A., Erbil, A., H. et al. (2004). Interferon-gamma in alopecia areata. *Eur. J. Dermatol., 14,* 33-36.

[17] Zoller, M., McElwee, K. J., Vitacolonna, M. & Hoffmann, R. (2004). The progressive state, in contrast to the stable or regressive state of alopecia areata, is reflected in peripheral blood mononuclear cells. *Exp. Dermatol., 13,* 435-444.

[18] Freyschmidt-Paul, P., Zoeller, M., McElwee, K. J., Sundberg, J., et al. (2004). The functional relevance of the type 1 cytokines IFN-gamma and IL-2 in alopecia areata of C3H/HeJ mice. Plenary Workshop on Alopecia Areata, The 4th Intercontinental Meeting of Hair Researh Societies, Berlin.

[19] Mouser, P. E., Baker, B. S., Seaton, E. D., et al. (2003). Propionibacterium acnes-reactive T helper-1 cells in the skin of patients with acne vulgaris. *J. Invest. Dermatol., 121,* 1226-1228.

[20] Skurkovich, S., Skurkovich, B. & Kelly, J. (2005). Anticytokine therapy, particularly anti-IFN-gamma, in Th1-mediated autoimmune diseases. *Expert Rev. Clin. Immunol., 1(1),* 11-25.

[21] Skurkovich, S., Skurkovich, B. & Bellanti, J. A. (1987). A Unifying Model of the Immunoregulatory Role of the Interferon System: Can Interferon Produce Disease in Humans? *Clinical immunology and immunopathology, 43,* 362-373.

[22] Isaacs, A. & Lindenmann, J. (1957). Virus interference. I. The interferon. *Proc. Royal Soc., B 147,* 258-267.

[23] DeStefano, E., Friedman, R. M., Friedman-Kien, A. E., et al. (1982). Acid-labile human leukocyte interferon in homosexual men with Kaposi's sarcoma and hymphadenopathy. *J. Infect. Dis., 146,* 451-459.

[24] Scheinfeld, N. (2004). A comprehensive review and evaluation of the side effects of the tumor necrosis factor alpha blockers etanercept, infliximab and adalimumab. *J. Dermatolog. Treat., 15,* 280-294.

[25] Ettefagh, L. et al. (2004). Alopecia areata in a patient using infliximab: new insights into the role of tumor necrosis factor on human hair follicles. *Arch. Dermatol., 140,* 1012.

[26] Discontinuation of Onercept in Moderate-To-severe Psoriasis and Canvaxin(reg) in Stage IV Melanoma. (09 Apr 2005). Medical News Today. http://www.medicalnewstoday.com/printerfriendlynews.php?newsid=22446.

[27] Media, Release, (2005). Serono and NovImmune to collaborate in development of two novel treatments for autoimmune diseases; available from: www.novimmune.com/docman/doc_download-3.html

[28] Sigidin Ya., A., Loukina, G. B., Skurkovich, B. & Skurkovich, S. (2001). Randomized, double-blind trial of anti-interferon-gamma antibodies in rheumatoid arthritis. *Scand. J. Rheumatol., 30,* 203-207.

[29] Skurkovich, B., Skurkovich, S. (1997). Treatment of autoimmune diseases. US patent No. US 6,333,032 B1, date of patent 2001, filed.

[30] Nishimoto, N., Yoshizaki, K., Miyasaka, N., et al. (2004). Treatment of rheumatoid arthritis with humanized anti-interleukin-6 receptor antibody: multicenter, double-blind, placebo-controlled trial. *Arthritis Rheum., 50(6),* 1761-1769.

[31] Ling, L. E., Warren, M. K. & Vogel, S. N. (1985). Antagonistic effect of interferon-beta on the interferon-gamma-induced expression of Ia antigen in murine macrophages. *J. Immunol., 135,* 1857-1863.

[32] Ling, L. E., Zafari, M., Reardon, D. et al. (1995). Human type 1 interferon receptor, IFNAR, is a heavily glycosylated 120-130 kD membrane protein. *J. INF Cytokine Res., 15,* 55-61.

[33] Skurkovich, S., Boiko, A., Beliaeva, I., Buglak, A., et al. (2001). Randomized study of antibodies to IFN-gamma and TNF-alpha in secondary progressive multiple sclerosis. *Multiple Sclerosis, 7,* 277-284.

[34] Kantarei, O. H., Goris, A., Hebrink, D. D., Heggartv, S. et al. (2005). IFNG polymorphisms are associated with gender differences in susceptibility to multiple sclerosis. *Genes. Immun., 6(2),* 153-161.

[35] Skurkovich, B. & Skurkovich, S. (1999). Treatment of autoimmune disease, including AIDS. Patent No. 5,888,511, date of patent, filed 1996.

[36] Skurkovich, B. & Skurkovich, S. (2003). Compositions and methods for treating hyperimmune response in the eye. Patent No. 6,534,059 B1, date of patent, filed 2001.

[37] Skurkovich, S., Kasparov, A., Narbut, N. & Skurkovich, B. (2002). Treatment of Corneal Transplant Rejection in Humans with Anti-interferon-gamma antibodies. *American J. Ophthalmology, 133(6),* 829.

[38] Kasparov, A., Narbut, N., Skurkovich, B. & Skurkovich, S. (2004). Treatment of corneal transplant rejection in patients with antibodies to interferon-gamma and antibodies to TNF-alpha. *New technologies in treatment of corneal diseases,* 200-202.

[39] Stevens, H. P., van der Kwast, T. H., van der Meide, P. H., Vuzevski, V. D., et al. (1990). Synergistic immunosuppressive effects of monoclonal antibodies specific for interferon-gamma and tumor necrosis factor alpha. A skin transplantation study in the rhesus monkey. *Transplantation, 50(5),* 856-861.

[40] Bellanti, J. A., Skurkovich, S. V., Peters, S. M., Johl, S., et al. (1987). Preliminary Clinical Trial of Anti-alpha Interferon (IFN) in Patients with AIDS: A possible Approach for Immune Enhancement. III International Conference on AIDS in Washington, D.C., U.S.A.

[41] Buntix, M., Gielen, E., Van Hummelen, P., et al. (2004), *J. Neurosci. Res., 76,* 846.

[42] Korotky, N. G., Sharova, N. M., Skurkovich, B. & Skurkovich, S. (2004). Striking therapeutic effects in a patient with dysplastic epidermolysis bullosa using anti-IFN-gamma (case report). IX International Congress of Dermatology, Beijing.

[43] Skurkovich, B., Skurkovich, S. (2006). Inhibition of IFN-gamma as a Method of Treatment of Various Autoimmune Diseases, Including Skin Diseases. *Cytokines as Potential therapeutic targets for inflammatory skin diseases, Springer,* 1-27.

[44] Skurkovich, B., Millstein, E. & Skurkovich, S. (2009). Method and composition for treatment of renal failure with antiboides and their equivalents as partial or comlete replacement for dialysis. Patent No. US 7,504,106 B2, date of patent 2009, filed 2006.

[45] Editorials (1999). Anticytokine Therapy – a new era in the treatment of rheumatoid arthritis? *New England Journal of Medicine, 340,* 310-311.

In: Autoimmune Diseases: Symptoms, Diagnosis and Treatment   ISBN: 978-1-61668-007-7
Editor: Kyle J. Brenner, pp. 289-302   © 2010 Nova Science Publishers, Inc.

Chapter 9

REVOLUTIONARY BONE MARROW TRANSPLANTATION METHOD FOR STEM CELL DISORDERS

Susumu Ikehara[*]

First Department of Pathology, Regeneration Research Center for,Intractable Diseases, Center for Cancer Therapy, Kansai Medical University, Moriguchi City, Osaka, Japan

ABSTRACT

We have previously proposed that autoimmune diseases are hemopoietic stem cell (HSC) disorders (Proc. Natl. Acad. Sci. USA 87:8341-8344, 1990).

In this review article, we provide evidence that most age-associated diseases such as osteoporosis are mesenchymal stem cell (MSC) disorders and, based on this evidence, we propose a new concept of "stem cell disorders" (SCDs) that includes HSC and MSC disorders.

To treat SCDs, we have recently developed a new strategy (intra-bone marrow-bone marrow transplantation: IBM-BMT) for replacing the abnormal stem cells of recipients with donor-derived normal stem cells (both HSCs and MSCs).

We believe that this strategy heralds a revolution in the field of transplantation (BMT and organ transplantation) and regeneration therapy.

INTRODUCTION

In 1985, we found that allogeneic (but not syngeneic or autologous) bone marrow transplantation (BMT) could be used to treat autoimmune diseases in autoimmune-prone mice

---

[*] Corresponding author: Department of Pathology, Regeneration Research Center for Intractable Diseases, Center for Cancer Therapy, Kansai Medical University, 10-15 Fumizono-cho, Moriguchi City, Osaka 570-8506, Japan. Phone: 81-6-6993-9429; Fax: 81-6-6994-8283; E-mail: ikehara@takii.kmu.ac.jp

[1,2]. Since then, we have confirmed our findings using a variety of autoimmune-prone mice [3,4,5].

Conversely, we have succeeded in inducing autoimmune diseases in normal mice by transplanting T-cell-depleted bone marrow cells (BMCs) or partially-purified hemopoietic stem cells (HSCs) from autoimmune-prone mice to normal mice [6,7]. Based on these findings, we proposed that autoimmune diseases were "stem cell disorders (SCDs)" [6-8].

Our findings have also been confirmed in humans: patients with autoimmune diseases were cured after allogeneic BMT, while autoimmune diseases were found to be transferred to recipients after BMT from donors who were suffering from autoimmune diseases [9].

In this article, we show that various otherwise intractable diseases (including autoimmune diseases) can be cured by our novel BMT method.

Crucial Role of Donor Stromal Cells in Successful Allogeneic Bmt

We have succeeded in treating various autoimmune diseases by conventional allogeneic (allo) BMT [10]. However, in MRL/lpr mice, which are radiosensitive (< 8.5 Gy), we found that conventional intravenous BMT (IV-BMT) had a transient effect on autoimmune diseases, which were found to recur [11]. Therefore, we concentrated on how we could prevent and treat autoimmune diseases in radiosensitive and chimeric-resistant MRL/lpr mice. We have found that three types of cells are essential for successful allo BMT: i) pluripotent hemopoietic stem cells (P-HSCs) [12], ii) natural suppressor cells [13] and iii) stromal cells (including MSCs) [14]. In particular, we have very recently found that stromal cells play a crucial role in preventing graft failure [15,16], since there is a major histocompatibility complex (MHC) restriction between HSCs and stromal cells [17,18]. To prevent the recurrence of autoimmune diseases in MRL/lpr mice, we have finally found that "IBM-BMT" (injection of whole BMCs [containing P-HSCs and MSCs] into the bone marrow cavity) is the best strategy for allo BMT.

Advantages of Ibm-Bmt in Mice

When donor cells are injected into the bone marrow cavity, the cells can effectively interact with donor-derived stromal cells, which support the proliferation, differentiation and even maintenance of HSCs [17,18], resulting in the earlier engraftment of hematolymphoid cells of donor origin, in contrast to the conventional IV-BMT [19]; in the case of IV-BMT, most BMCs (including HSCs and stromal cells) are trapped in the lung [20-22] and liver [23] where they are killed by radio-resistant host cells. In contrast, IBM-BMT can efficiently recruit donor HSCs and stromal cells into the bone marrow, and can rapidly accelerate the proliferation of donor-derived HSCs while simultaneously retaining HSCs [19,24,25]. Using this new strategy, we have succeeded in treating intractable autoimmune diseases in chimeric-resistant MRL/lpr mice [19].

Moreover, it has also been confirmed that IBM-injection is superior to IV-injection in NOD/SCID mice [26-29].

Ibm-Bmt for Organ Transplantation

Since we have previously found that the combination of organ allografts and conventional IV-BMT from the same donors prevents the rejection of organ allografts [30], we attempted to apply IBM-BMT to organ allografts. IBM-BMT was the most effective strategy, since the the radiation dose could be reduced to 4.0Gy x 2 in mouse skin allografts [31]. In addition, we found that IBM-BMT is applicable to allografts of other organs and tissues, such as pancreas islet [32] and leg transplantion [33], lung [34], and heart [35] in rats.

Ibm-Bmt for Regeneration Therapy

As our experiments showed that donor stromal cells could be effectively recruited by "IBM-BMT", we next attempted to prevent osteoporosis in SAMP6; the SAMP6 (a substrain of senescence-accelerated mice) spontaneously develops osteoporosis early in life and is therefore a useful model for examining the mechanisms underlying osteoporosis. After IBM-BMT, the hematolymphoid system was completely reconstituted with donor-type cells. Thus-treated SAMP6 showed marked increases in trabecular bone even at 12 months of age, and the bone mineral density (BMD) remained similar to that of normal B6 mice. Bone marrow stromal cells in "IBM-BMT"-treated SAMP6 were replaced by donor stromal cells [36]. Thus, we succeeded in preventing osteoporosis in SAMP6 by IBM-BMT, which can recruit not only donor HSCs but also MSCs.

Recently, we have also succeeded in curing osteoporosis in the mice by IBM-BMT (Figure 1) [25].

On the basis of our results, we believe that IBM-BMT could well become a powerful strategy in regeneration therapy.

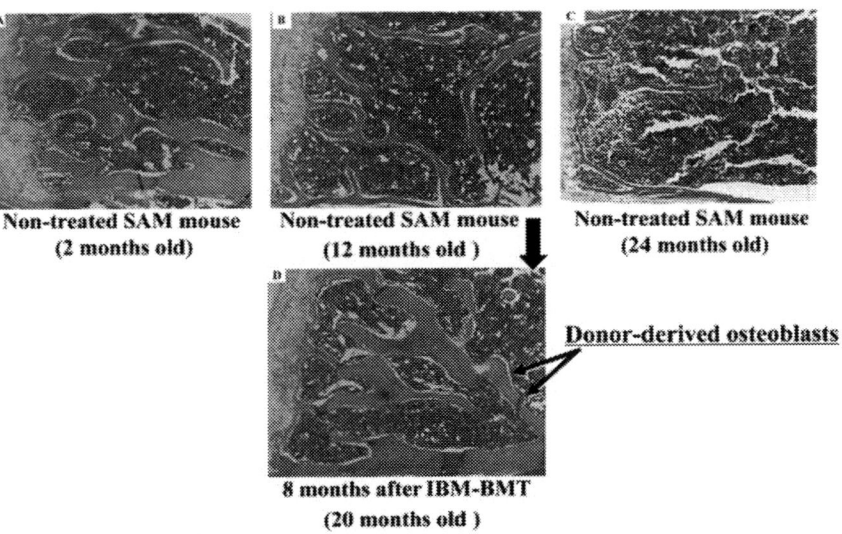

Figure 1. Treatment of osteoporosis in SAMP6 mice by IBM-BMT from normal B6 mice.

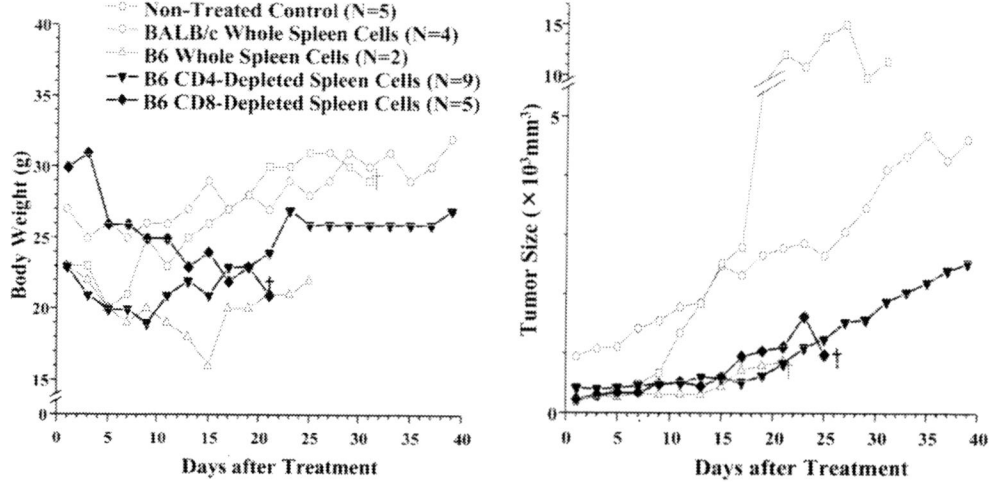

Figure 2. Prevention of GvHD and suppression of tumor growth by IBM-BMT+ DLI (CD4).

We next examined whether senile osteoporosis is attributable to SCDs. By one month after IBM-BMT from SAM to B6 mice [SAM→B6], the hematolymphoid cells had been completely reconstituted by donor-derived cells, and bone marrow stromal cells that could differentiate into osteocytes were also found to be of donor origin. In addition, the recipient C57BL/6 mice showed the features of osteoporosis in the trabecular bone at 12 months of age. Decreases in BMD and increases in urinary deoxypyridinoline (DPD) were also observed [37]. These findings indicate that not only hemopoietic cells but also bone marrow stromal cells in the [SAM→B6] mice are replaced by SAM cells as a result of IBM-BMT, and suggest that the development of senile osteoporosis might be attributable to SCDs, probably MSC disorders, since IV-BMT from SAM to B6 could not induce osteoporosis; the stromal cells of the [SAM→B6] mice treated with IV-BMT were host-derived.

We have also found that IBM-BMT can be used to treat emphysema in Tsk mice, and that the emphysema in these mice can be transferred to normal mice by IBM-BMT, suggesting that emphysema in Tsk mice originates from defects in stem cells in the bone marrow [38]. Thus, IBM-BMT can efficiently reconstitute recipients with both donor-derived normal HSCs and MSCs, which can differentiate into all cells, including hepatocytes [39], epithelial cells [40], nerve cells [41] and retinal cells [42]. Therefore, the use of this method might become a valuable strategy not only for the treatment of intractable diseases such as autoimmune diseases but also in regeneration therapy for injured organs and tissues such as myocardial infarction, cerebral infarction, and Alzheimer's disease.

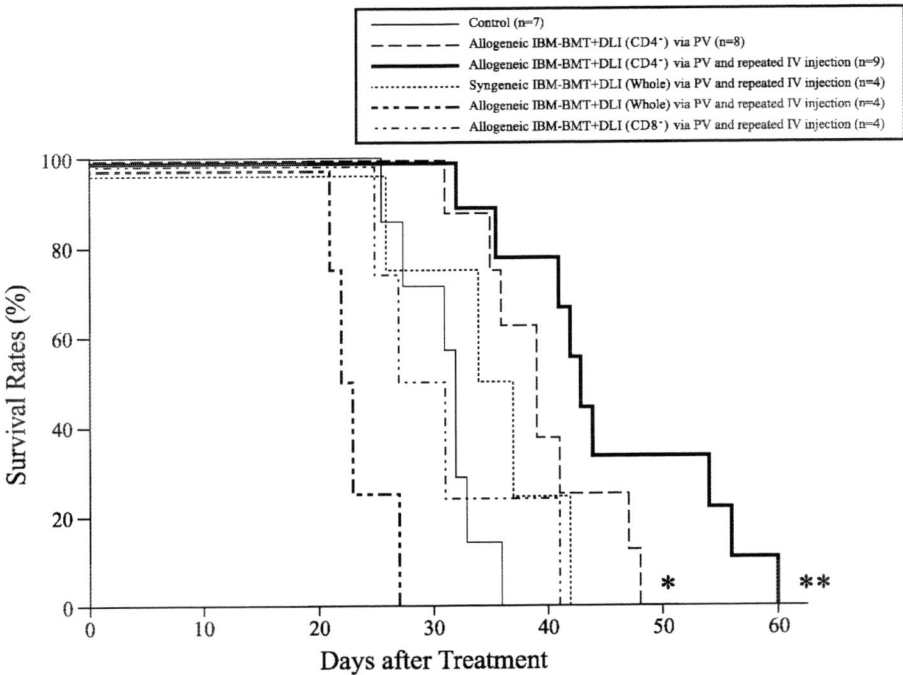

Figure 3. Effects of allogeneic IBM-BMT + DLI using CD4⁻ cells on survival rates of rats implanted with colon cancer cells in the liver. Colon cancer cells (ACL-15) were injected into the liver from the portal vein, and IBM-BMT + single DLI or extensive DLI was carried out, as described in the Materials and Methods and Results. One week after the injection, allogeneic IBM-BMT using T-cell-depleted bone marrow cells and DLI using spleen cells via the portal vain were performed from Brown Norway rats to the F344 rats. In some rats, extensive DLI (once a week) was performed via the tail vein. The rats treated with allogeneic IBM-BMT+ extensive DLI (CD4⁻ cells) (from the PV+ repeated IV) show a better survival rate than those treated with allogeneic IBM-BMT+ single DLI (CD4⁻ cells) (from the PV). The "syngeneic IBM-BMT + extensive DLI (whole)" group showed longevity comparable to the "control" group, but not of the "allogeneic IBM-BMT + extensive DLI (CD4⁻)" group.

IBM-BMT + DONOR LYMPHOCYTE INFUSION (DLI) FOR MALIGNANT TUMORS

It is well known that the graft-versus-leukemia reaction (GvLR) can cure patients of a variety of hematological malignancies [43,44]. Recently, it has been reported that graft-versus-tumor (GvT) effects can induce partial (complete in some) remission of metastatic solid tumors such as breast cancer [45,46,47] and renal cell carcinoma [47,53]. Based on these findings, donor lymphocyte infusion (DLI) has recently been used for the treatment of malignant solid tumors even in humans. However, it is very difficult to completely eradicate the tumors, since extensive DLI induces graft-versus-host disease (GvHD). We therefore attempted to establish a new method for the treatment of malignant tumors, this method consisting of IBM-BMT plus DLI, since we have recently found that IBM-BMT can allow a reduction in radiation doses as a conditioning regimen and prevent GvHD in mice [19,54]. Using the Meth-A cell line (BALB/c-derived fibrosarcoma), we found that IBM-BMT plus the injection of CD4⁺ T-cell-depleted (but not CD8⁺ T-cell-depleted) spleen cells (as DLI) can prevent GvHD while suppressing tumor growth (Figure 2). In addition, we have found that IBM-BMT plus extensive DLI (3 times every 2 weeks) leads to the complete rejection of the tumor, although the success rate (3/50) is not high so far [54].

In addition, we have examined whether this strategy (IBM-BMT plus DLI) is applicable to other tumors in other animals. We have obtained similar results in another system (colon cancer: ACL-15 in rats), as shown in Figure 3 [55]. We are now establishing more efficient strategies to eradicate malignant tumors.

COMPARISON OF NOVEL BMT METHOD WITH CONVENTIONAL BMT METHOD IN HUMANS

In humans, conventional BMT is carried out as shown in Figure 4. Bone marrow needles are inserted into the iliac bones more than 100 times, and the BMCs are collected by the aspiration method (AM). Therefore, contamination with the peripheral blood (particularly T cells) is inevitable. When thus-collected cells are intravenously injected, most cells are trapped in the lung and only a few cells migrate into the bone marrow (Figure 4).

To apply our new BMT methods to humans, we developed (using cynomolgus monkeys) a perfusion method (PM) for collecting BMCs [56]. There is significantly less contamination with T cells when using the PM (<6%) than with the conventional AM (>20%), which consists of multiple bone marrow aspirations from the iliac bones [57,58]. Therefore, T cell-depletion is unnecessary with the PM, and whole BMCs can be used. In contrast, T cell-depletion is necessary in the case of the conventional AM, and the loss of some important cells such as MSCs is inevitable. Furthermore, the number and progenitor activities of the cells harvested using this PM are greater than when using the conventional AM [56,58].

Very recently, we have found that the PM is applicable to the iliac bones as well as the long bones not only in monkeys but also in humans (using autopsy cases) (manuscript in preparation).

The BM fluids obtained from the iliac bones or long bones by the PM are centrifuged, and BMCs are suspended in <10ml of saline (at a high concentration). As shown in Figure 5, the BMC suspension is injected directly into the bone marrow cavity of both tibias of the recipient.

A NEW CONCEPT OF STEM CELL DISORDERS (SCDS)

Finally, I would like to present a new concept of SCDs after a minor modification of my previous proposal [31,59]. As shown in Figure 6, various kinds of stem cells exist. In the bone marrow, HSCs, MSCs, and organ-specific stem cells (OSSCs) should be differentiated from ES-like cells; we have recently found that ES-like cells are present in the bone marrow of even adult humans [60].

HSC disorders are recognized as falling into the following categories: (i) Aplasia of HSCs (aplastic anemia), (ii) Monoclonal or oligoclonal abnormal HSC proliferative syndromes (leukemias and myelodysplastic syndrome), and (iii) Polyclonal abnormal HSC proliferative syndromes (autoimmune diseases) [59,61].

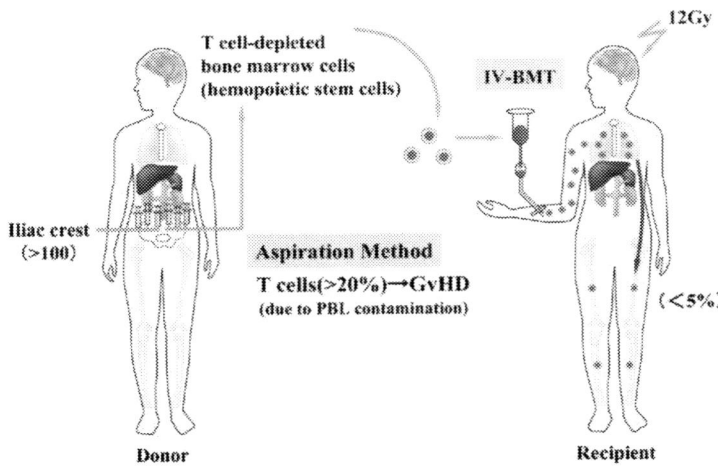

Figure 4. Conventional BMT method for allogeneic BMT. Conventional BMT is carried out using an aspiration method (AM), followed by the intravenous injection of BMCs (IV-BMT).

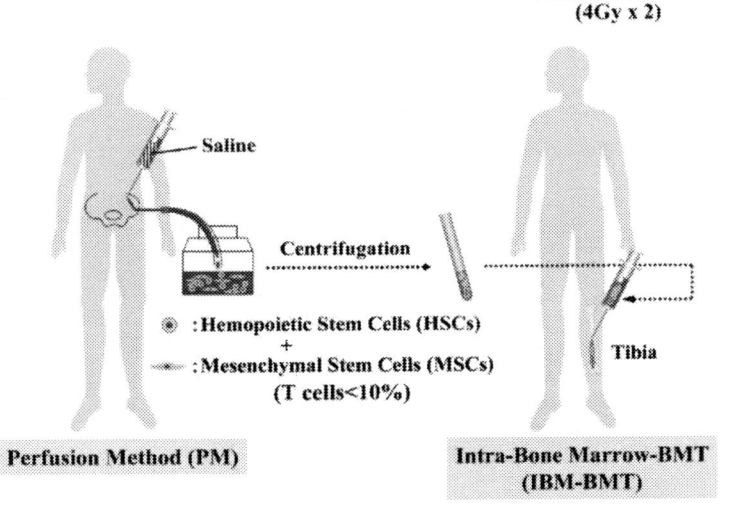

Figure 5. New BMT method for allergenic BMT. The new BMT method is carried out using a perfusion method (PM), followed by IBM-BMT.

On the other hand, there are mesenchymal stem cell disorders, which include age-associated diseases such as osteoporosis [37] and emphysema [39]. It has also been proposed that autoimmune mechanisms are involved in the development of atherosclerosis [59,62-64] and also Alzheimer's disease [65].

Recently, the existence of organ-specific stem cells (OSSCs) or tissue-committed stem cells (TCSCs) has been proposed [59,66], and we would also like to propose that carcinosarcoma (in the liver, lung, and kidney) is due to the malignant transformation of OSSCs. From the findings to date, it is conceivable that all of the body's cells originate in the bone marrow, and that all diseases might therefore originate from defects in the bone marrow. One paper already suggests that gastric cancer originates from bone marrow-derived cells [67].

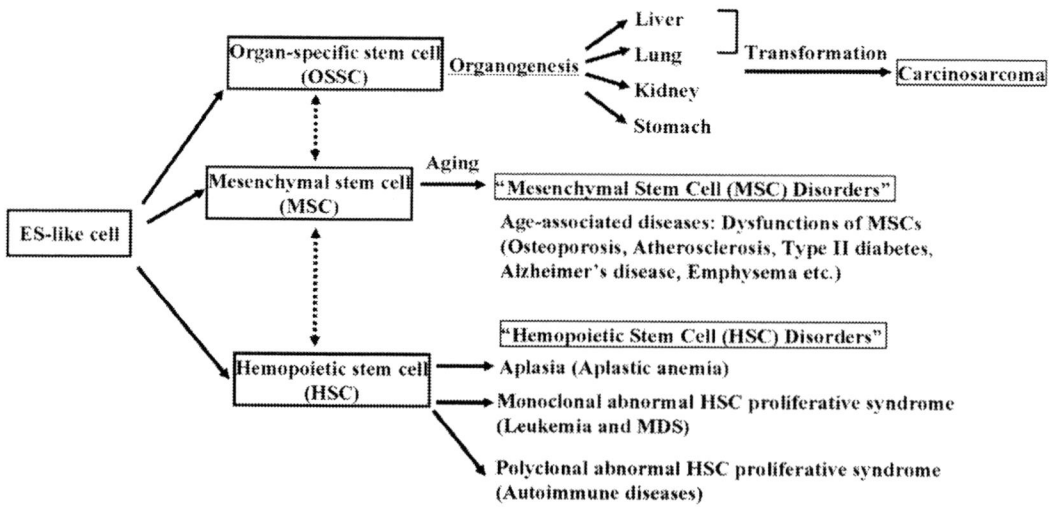

Figure 6. A novel concept of stem cell disorders.

Because most intractable diseases are not only HSC disorders but also MSC disorders, we believe that the use of our new BMT methods (PM + IBM-BMT), which can efficiently collect both HSCs and MSCs and transplant both, will become a valuable strategy for the treatment of various intractable diseases.

In conclusion, this discovery is, in many respects, an "Egg of Columbus"; the combination of "PM + IBM-BMT" is a simple solution that seems obvious in retrospect. It is also a solution that heralds a revolution in the field of transplantation (BMT and organ transplantation) and regeneration therapy.

ACKNOWLEDGMENTS

I thank Mr. Hilary Eastwick-Field and Ms. K. Ando for their help in the preparation of the manuscript. These studies were mainly supported by the 21st Century Center of Excellence (COE) program of the Ministry of Education, Culture, Sports, Science and Technology. Supported also by a grant from Haiteku Research Center of the Ministry of Education, Research on Allergic Disease and Immunology of Health and Labour Sciences Research Grants, a grant from the Science Frontier program of the Ministry of Education, Culture, Sports, Science and Technology, and a grant from the Department of Transplantation for Regeneration Therapy (sponsored by Otsuka Pharmaceutical Company, Ltd.), a grant from Molecular Medical Science Institute, Otsuka Pharmaceutical Co., Ltd. & a grant from Japan Immunoresearch Laboratories Co., Ltd. (JIMRO).

REFERENCES

[1] Ikehara, S., Good, R. A., Nakamura, T., Sekita, K., Inoue, S., Maung Maung, Oo, Muso, E., Ogawa, K. & Hamashima, Y. (1985). Rationale for bone marrow

[1] transplantation in the treatment of autoimmune diseases. *Proc Natl Acad Sci, 82*, 2483-2487.

[2] Ikehara, S., Ohtsuki, H., Good, R. A., Asamoto, H., Nakamura, T., Sekita, K., Muso, E., Tochino, Y., Ida, T., Kuzuya, H., Imura, H. & Hamashima, Y. (1985). Prevention of type I diabetes in nonobese diabetic mice by allogeneic bone marrow transplantation. *Proc Natl Acad Sci, 82*, 7743-7747.

[3] Oyaizu, N., Yasumizu, R., Miyama-Inaba, M., Nomura, S., Yoshida, H., Miyawaki, S., Shibata, Y, Mitsuoka, S., Yasunaga, K., Morii, S., Good, R. A. & Ikehara, S. (1988). (NZW x BXSB)F_1 mouse; A new animal model of idiopathic thrombocytopenic purpura. *J Exp Med, 167*, 2017-2022.

[4] Soe Than, Inaba, M., Inaba, K., Fukuba, Y., Adachi Y. & Ikehara, S. (1992). Bone marrow transplantation as a strategy for treatment of non-insulin-dependent diabetes mellitus in KK-Ay mice. *J Exp Med, 176*, 1233-1238.

[5] Nishimura, M., Toki, J., Sugiura, K., Hashimoto, F., Tomita, T., Fujishima, H., Hiramatsu, Y., Nishioka, N., Nagata, N., Takahashi, Y. & Ikehara, S. (1994). Focal segmental glomerular sclerosis, a type of intractable chronic glomerulonephritis, is a stem cell disorder. *J Exp Med, 179*, 1053-1058.

[6] Ikehara, S., Kawamura, M., Takao, F., Inaba, M., Yasumizu, R., Soe Than, Hisha, H., Sugiura, K., Koide, Y., Yoshida, T. O., Ida, T., Imura, H. & Good, R. A. (1990). Organ-specific and systemic autoimmune diseases originate from defects in hematopoietic stem cells. *Proc Natl Acad Sci, 87*, 8341-8344.

[7] Kawamura, M., Hisha, H., Li, Y., Fukuhara, S. & Ikehara, S. (1997). Distinct qualitative differences between normal and abnormal hemopoietic stem cells in vivo and in vitro. *Stem Cells, 15*, 56-62.

[8] Ikehara, S. (2003). A new concept of stem cell disorders and their new therapy. *J Hematother Stem Cell Res, 12*, 643-653.

[9] Marmont, A. M. (1994). Immune ablation followed by allogeneic or autologous bone marrow transplantation: A new treatment for severe autoimmune diseases? *Stem Cells, 12*, 125-135.

[10] Ikehara, S. (2003). A novel strategy for allogeneic stem cell transplantation: perfusion method plus intra-bone marrow injection of stem cells. *Exp Hematol, 31*, 1142-1146.

[11] Ikehara, S., Yasumizu, R., Inaba, M., Izui, S., Hayakawa, K., Sekita, K., Toki, J., Sugiura, K., Iwai, H., Nakamura, T., Muso, E., Hamashima, Y. & Good, R. A. (1989). Long-term observations of autoimmune-prone mice treated for autoimmune disease by allogeneic bone marrow transplantation. *Proc Natl Acad Sci USA, 86*, 3306-3310.

[12] Doi. H., Inaba, M., Yamamoto, Y., Taketani, S., Mori, S., Sugihata, H., Toki, J., Hisha, H., Inaba, K., Sogo, S., Adachi, M., Matsuda, T., Good, R. A. & Ikehara, S. (1997). Pluripotent hemopoietic stem cells are c-kit$^{<low}$. *Proc Natl Acad Sci USA, 94*, 2513-2517.

[13] Sugiura, K., Inaba, M., Ogata, H., Yasumizu, R., Inaba, K., Good, R. A. & Ikehara, S. (1988). Wheat germ agglutinin-positive cells in a stem cell-enriched fraction of mouse bone marrow have potent natural suppressor activity. *Proc Natl Acad Sci USA, 85*, 4824-4826.

[14] Ikehara, S. (2001). Treatment of autoimmune diseases by hematopoietic stem cell transplantation. *Exp Hematol, 29*, 661-669.

[15] Kushida, T., Inaba, M., Hisha, H., Ichioka, N., Esumi, T., Ogawa, R. & Ikehara, S. (2001). Crucial role of donor-derived stromal cells in successful treatment for intractable autoimmune diseases in MRL/lpr mice by BMT via the portal vein. *Stem Cells, 19*, 226-235.

[16] Fan, T., Hisha, H., Jin, T., Yu, C., Lian, Z., Guo, S., Cui, Y., Feng, B., Yang, G., Li, Q. & Ikehara, S. (2001). Successful allogeneic bone marrow transplantation (BMT) by injection of bone marrow cells via portal vein: Stromal cells as BMT-facilitating cells. *Stem Cells, 19*, 144-150.

[17] Hashimoto, F., Sugiura, K., Inoue, K. & Ikehara, S. (1997). Major histocompatibility complex restriction between hematopoietic stem cells and stromal cells in vivo. *Blood, 89*, 49-54.

[18] Sugiura, K., Hisha, H., Ishikawa, J., Adachi, Y., Taketani, S., Lee, S., Nagahama, T. & Ikehara, S. (2001). Major histocompatibility complex restriction between hematopoietic stem cells and stromal cells in vitro. *Stem Cells, 19*, 46-58.

[19] Kushida, T., Inaba, M., Hisha, H., Ichioka, N., Esumi, T., Ogawa, R. & Ikehara, S. (2001). Intra-bone marrow injection of allogeneic bone marrow cells: A powerful new strategy for treatment of intractable autoimmune diseases in MRL/lpr mice. *Blood, 97*, 3292-3299.

[20] Van Hennik, P. B., De Koning, A. E. & Ploemacher, R. E. (1999). Seeding efficiency of primitive human hematopoietic cells in nonobese diabetic/severe combined immune deficiency mice: implications for stem cell frequency assessment. *Blood, 94*, 3055-306.

[21] Cashman, J. D. & Eaves, C. J. (2000). High marrow seeding efficiency of human lymphomyeloid repopulating cells in irradiated NOD/SCID mice. *Blood, 96*, 3979-3981.

[22] Panoskaltsis-Mortari, A., Price, A., Hermanson, J. R., Taras, E., Lees, C., Serody, J. S. & Blazar, B. R. (2004). In vivo imaging of graft-versus-host-disease in mice. *Blood, 103*, 3590-3598.

[23] Zhang, Y., Yasumizu, R., Sugiura, K., Hashimoto, F., Amoh, Y., Lian, Z., Cherry, Nishio, N. & Ikehara, S. (1994). Fate of allogeneic or syngeneic cells in intravenous or portal vein injection: possible explanation for the mechanism of tolerance induction by portal vein injection. *Eur J Immunol, 24*, 1558-1565.

[24] Ichioka, N., Inaba, M., Kushida, T., Esumi, T., Takahara, K., Inaba, K., Ogawa, R., Iida, H. & Ikehara, S. (2002). Prevention of senile osteoporosis in SAMP6 mice by intra-bone marrow injection of allogeneic bone marrow cells. *Stem Cells, 20*, 542-551.

[25] Takada, K., Inaba, M., Ichioka, N., Ueda, Y., Taira, M., Baba, S., Mizokami, T., Wang, X., Hisha, H., Iida, H. & Ikehara, S. (2006). Treatment of senile osteoporosis in SAMP6 mice by intra-bone marrow injection of allogeneic bone marrow cells. *Stem Cells, 24*, 399-405.

[26] Wang, J., Kimura, T., Asada, R., Harada, S., Yokota, S., Kawamoto, Y., Fujimura, Y., Tsuji, T., Ikehara, S. & Sonoda, Y. (2003). SCID-repopulating cell activity of human cord blood-derived CD34- cells assured by intra-bone marrow injection. *Blood, 101*, 2924-2931.

[27] Yahata, T. & o, K., Sato, T., Miyatake, H., Nakamura, Y., Muguruma, Y., Kato, S. & Hotta, T. (2003). A highly sensitive strategy for scid-repopulating cell assay by direct injection of primitive human hematopoietic cells into NOD/SCID mice bone marrow. *Blood, 101*, 2905-2912.

[28] Mazurier, F., Doedens, M., Gan, O. I. & Dick, J. E. (2003). Rapid myeloerythroid repopulation after intrafemoral transplantation of NOD/SCID mice reveals a new class of human stem cells. *Nat Med, 9*, 959-963.

[29] Castello, S., Podesta, M., Menditto, V. G., Ibatici, A., Pitto, A., Figari, O., Scarpati, D., Magrassi, L., Bacigalupo, A., Piaggio, G. & Frassoni, F. (2004). Intra-bone marrow injection of bone marrow and cord blood cells: An alternative way of transplantation associated with a higher seeding efficiency. *Exp Hematol, 32*, 782-787.

[30] Nakamura, T., Good, R. A., Yasumizu, R., Inoue, S., Maung Maung Oo, Hamashima, Y. & Ikehara, S. (1986). liver allografts in mice by combination with allogeneic bone marrow transplantation. *Proc Natl Acad Sci, 83*, 4529-4532.

[31] Ikehara, S. (2008). A novel method of bone marrow transplantation (BMT) for intractable autoimmune diseases. *J Autoimmun, 30*, 108-115.

[32] Ikebukuro, K., Adachi, Y., Suzuki, Y., Iwasaki, M., Nakano, K., Koike, Y., Mukaide, H., Yamada, Y., Fujimoto, S., Seino, Y., Oyaizu, H., Shigematsu, A., Kiriyama, N., Hamada, Y., Kamiyama, Y. & Ikehara, S. (2006). Synergistic effects of induction in transplantation of allogeneic pancreatic islets. *Bone Marrow Transplantation, 38*, 657-664.

[33] Esumi, T., Inaba, M., Ichioka, N., Kushida, T., Iida, H. & Ikehara, S. (2003). Successful allogeneic leg transplantation in rats by combination of intra-bone marrow (IBM) injection of donor bone marrow cells. *Transplantation, 76*, 1543-1548.

[34] kaneda, H., Adachi, Y., Saito, Y., Ikebukuro, K., Machida, H., Suzuki, Y., Minamino, K., Zhang, Y., Iwasaki, M., Imamura, H. & Ikehara, S. (2005). Long-term observation after simultaneous lung and intra-bone marrow-bone marrow transplantation. *J Heart Lung Transplant, 24*, 1415-1423.

[35] Guo, K., Inaba, M., Li, M., An, J., Cui, W., Song, C., Wang, J., Cui, Y., Sakaguchi, Y., Tsuda, M., Omae, M., Li, Q. Wang, X., Feng, W. & Ikehara, S. (2008). Long-Term Donor-Specific Tolerance in Rat Cardiac Allografts by Intra-Bone Marrow Injection of Donor Bone Marrow Cells. *Transplantation, 85*, 93-101.

[36] Ichioka, N., Inaba, M., Kushida, T., Esumi, T., Takahara, K., Inaba, K., Ogawa, R., Iida, H. & Ikehara, S. (2002). Prevention of senile osteoporosis in SAMP6 mice by intra-bone marrow injection of allogeneic bone marrow cells. *Stem Cells, 20*, 542-551.

[37] Ueda, Y., Inaba, M., Takada, K., Fukui, J., Sakaguchi, Y., Tsuda, M., Kushida, T., Iida, H. & Ikehara, S. (2007). Induction of senile osteoporosis in normal mice by intra-bone marrow-bone marrow transplantation from osteoporosis-prone mice. *Stem Cells, 25*, 1356-1363.

[38] Adachi, Y., Oyaizu, H., Taketani, S., Minamino, K., Yamaguchi, K., Shultz, L. D., Iwasaki, M., Tomita, M., Suzuki, Y., Nakano, K., Koike, Y., Yasumizu, R., Sara, M., Hirama, N., Kubota, I., Fukuhara, S. & Ikehara, S. (2006). Treatment and transfer of emphysema by a new bone marrow transplantation method from normal mice to Tsk mice and vice versa. *Stem Cells, 24*, 2071-2077.

[39] Wang, X., Ge, S., McNamara, G., Hao, Q. L., Crooks, G. M. & Nolta, J. A. (2003). Albumin expressing hepatocyte-like cells develop in the livers of immune-deficient mice transmitted with highly purified human hematopoietic stem cells. *Blood, 101*, 4201-4208.

[40] Spees, J. L., Olson, S. D., J. Ylostalo, J., Lynch, P. S., Smith, J., Perry, A., Peister, A., Wang, M. Y. & Prockop, D. J. (2003). Differentiation, cell fusion, and nuclear fusion

during ex vivo repair of epithelium by human adult stem cells from bone marrow stroma. *Proc Natl Acad Sci, 100*, 2397-2402.

[41] Mezey, E., Key, S., Vogelsang, G., Szalayova, I., Lange, G. D. & Crain, B. (2003). Transplanted bone marrow generates new neurons in human brains. *Proc Natl Acad Sci, 100*, 1364-1369.

[42] Tomita, M., Adachi, Y., Yamada, H., Takahashi, K., Kikuchi, K., Oyaizu, H., Ikebukuro, K., Kaneda, H., Matsumura, M. & Ikehara, S. (2002). Bone marrow-derived stem cells can differentiate into retinal cells in injured rat retina. *Stem Cells, 20*, 279-83.

[43] Thomas, E. D. & Blume, K. G. (1999). Historical markers in the development of allogeneic hematopoietic cell transplantation. *Biol Blood Marrow Transplant, 5*, 341-346.

[44] Weiden, P. L., Flournoy, N., Thomas, E. D., Rentice, R., Fefer, A., Buckner, C. D. & Storb, R. (1979). Antileukemic effect of graft-versus-host diseases in human recipients of allogeneic-marrow grafts. *N Engl J Med*, 300, 1068-1073.

[45] Ben-Yosef, R., Or, R., A. Nagier A. & Slavin, S. (1996). Graft-versus-tumor and graft-versus-leukaemia effect in patient with concurrent breast cancer and acute myelocytic leukaemia. *Lancet, 348*, 1242-1243.

[46] Eibi, B., Schwaigofer, H., Nachbaur, D., Marth, C., Gächter, A., Knapp, R., Böck, G., Gassner, C., Schiller, L., Petersen, F. & Niederwieser, D. (1996). Evidence for a graft-versus-tumor effect in a patient treated with marrow ablative chemotherapy and allogeneic bone marrow transplantation for breast cancer. *Blood, 88*, 1501-1508.

[47] Ueno, N. T., Rondon, G., Mitza, N. Q., Geisler, D. K. &erlini, P., Giralt, S. A. & ersson, B. S., Claxton D. F., Gajewski, J. L., Khouri, I. F., Körbling, M., Mehra, R. C., Przepiorka, D., Rahman, Z., Samuels, B. I., van Besien, K., Hortobagy, G. N. & Champlin, R. E. (1998). Allogeneic peripheral-blood progenitor-cell transplantation for poor-risk patients with metastatic breast cancer. *J Clin Oncol, 16*, 986-993.

[48] Childs, R. W., Clave, E., Tisdale, J., Plante, M., Hensel, N. & Barrett, J. (1999). Successful treatment of metastatic renal cell carcinoma with a nonmyeloablative allogeneic peripheral-blood progenitor-cell transplant: evidence for a graft-versus-tumor effect. *J Clin Oncol, 17*, 2044-2049.

[49] Childs, R., Chernoff, A., Contentin, N., Bahceci, E., Schrum, P. D., Leitman, S., Read, E. J., Tisdale, J., Dunbar, C., Linehan, W. M., Young, N. S. & Barrett, A. J. (2000). Regression of metastatic renal-cell carcinoma after nonmyeloablative allogeneic peripheral-blood stem-cell transplantation. *N Engl J Med, 343*, 750-758.

[50] Appelbaum, F. R. & Sandmaaire, B. (2002). Sensitivity of renal cell cancer to nonmyeloablative allogeneic hematopoietic cell transplantation: unusual or unusually important? *J Clin Oncol, 20*, 1965-1967.

[51] Bregni, M., Dodero, A., Peccatori, J., Pescarollo, A., Bernardi, M., Sassi, I., Yoena, C., Zaniboni, A., Bordignon, C. & Corradini, P. (2002). Nonmyeloablative conditioning followed by hematopoietic cell allografting and donor lymphocyte infusions for patients with metastatic renal and breast cancer. *Blood, 99*, 4234-4236.

[52] Hentschke, P., Barkholt, L., Uzunel, M., Mattsson, S., Weisäll, P., Pisa, P., Martola, S., Albiin, N., Wernerson, A., Söderberg, M, Remberger, M., Thörne, A. & Ringdén, O. (2003). Low-intensity conditioning and hematopoietic stem cell transplantation in patients with renal and colon carcinoma. *Bone Marrow Transplant, 31*, 253-261.

[53] Rini, B. I., Zimmerman, T., Stadler, W. M., Gajewski, T. F. & Uogelzang, N. J. (2002). Allogeneic stem-cell transplantation of renal cell cancer after nonmyeloablative chemotherapy: feasibility, engraftment, and clinical results. *J Clin Oncol, 20*, 2017-2024.

[54] Suzuki, Y., Adachi, Y., Minamino, K., Zhang, Y., Iwasaki, M., Nakano, K., Koike, Y. & Ikehara, S. (2005). A new strategy for treatment of malignant tumor: Intra-bone marrow-bone marrow transplantation plus CD4⁻ donor lymphocyte infusion. *Stem Cells 23*, 365-337.

[55] Koike, Y., Adachi, Y., Suzuki, Y., Iwasaki, M., Koike-Kiriyama, N., Minamino, K., Nakano, K., Mukaide, H., Shigematsu, A, Kiyozuka, Y., Tubura, A., Kamiyama, Y. & Ikehara, S. (2007). Allogeneic intra-bone marrow-bone marrow transplantation plus donor lymphocyte infusion suppresses growth of colon cancer cells implanted in skin and liver of rats. *Stem Cells 25*, 385-391.

[56] Kushida, T., Inaba, M., Ikebukuro, K., Ichioka, N., Esumi, T., Oyaizu, H., Yoshimura, T., Nagahama, T., Nakamura, K., Ito, T., Hisha, H., Sugiura, K., Yasumizu, R., Iida, H. & Ikehara, S. (2002). Comparison of bone marrow cells harvested from various bones of cynomolgus monkeys various ages by perfusion or aspiration methods: A preclinical study for human BMT. *Stem Cells, 20*, 155-162.

[57] Kushida, T., Inaba, M., Ikebukuro, K., Nagahama, T., Oyaizu, H., Lee, S., Ito, T., Ichioka, N., Hisha, H., Sugiura, K., Miyashima, S., Ageyama, N., Ono, F., Iida, H., Ogawa, R. & Ikehara, S. (2000). A new method for bone marrow cell harvesting. *Stem Cells, 18*, 453-456.

[58] Inaba, M., Adachi, Y., Hisha, H., Hosaka, N., Maki, M., Ueda, Y., Koike, Y., Miyake, T., Fukui, J., Cui, Y., Mukaide, H., Koike, N., Omae, M., Mizokami, T., Shigematsu, A., Sakaguchi, Y., Tsuda, M., Okazaki, S., Wang, X., Li, Q., Nishida, A. &o, Y., Guo, K., Song, C., Cui, W., Feng, W., Katou, J., Sado, K., Nakamura, S. & Ikehara, S. (2007). Extensive studies on perfusion method plus intra-bone marrow-bone marrow transplantation using cynomolgus monkeys. *Stem Cells, 25*, 2098-2103.

[59] Ikehara, S. (2003). A new concept of stem cell disorders and their new therapy. *J Hematother Stem Cell Res, 12*, 643-653.

[60] Peterini, M., Pacini, S., Trombi, L., Fazzi, R., Montali, M., Ikehara, S. & Abraham, N. G. (2008). Identification and purification of mesodermal progenitor cells (MPCs) from human adult bone marrow. Stem Cells Dev. In press.

[61] Ikehara, S. (2002). Autoimmune diseases as stem cell disorders: Treatment by allogeneic bone marrow transplantation. In: *Molecular Pathology of Autoimmune Diseases* (eds. Theofilopoulos AN, Bona CA) Taylor & Francis, USA, 566-572.

[62] Ikehara, S. (2005). Intra-bone marrow-bone marrow transplantation. *Ann NY Acad Sci 1051*, 1-9.

[63] Fernandes, G., Alonso, D. R., Tanaka, T., Thaler, H. I., Yunis, E. J. & Good, R. A. (1983). Influence of diet on vascular lesions in autoimmune-prone B/W mice. *Proc Natl Acad Sci* USA, *80*, 874-77.

[64] Rose, N. & Afanasyeva, M. 2003. Autoimmunity: busting the atherosclerotic plaque. *Nature Medicine, 9*, 641-642.

[65] Baron, R., Harpaz, I., Nemirovsky, A., Coheu, H. & Monsonego, A. (2007). Immunity and neuronal repair in the progression of Alzheimer's disease: brief overview. *Exp Gerontol, 42*, 64-69.

[66] Ratajczak., M. Z., Kucia, M., Reca, R., Majka, M., Janowska-Wieczorek, A. & Rayajczak., J. (2004). Stem cell plasticity revisited: CXCR4-positive cells expressing mRNA for early muscle, liver and neural cell "hide out" in the bone marrow. *Leukemia, 18*, 29-40.

[67] Houghton, J., Stoicov, C., Nomura, S., Roger, A. B., Carlson, J., Li, H., Cai, X., Fox, J. G., Goldenring, S. R. & Wang, T. C. (2004). Gastric cancer originating from bone marrow-derived cells. *Science, 306*, 1568-1571.

Chapter 10

IMMUNOLOGICAL CONTROL OF ADULT NEURAL STEM CELLS

Oscar Gonzalez-Perez[1,2*], *Alfredo Quiñones-Hinojosa*[3] *and Jose Manuel Garcia-Verdugo*[4]

[1]Neuroscience Laboratory, Psychology School, University of Colima, Colima, Mexico 28040
[2]Neuroscience Department, Centro Universitario de Ciencias de la Salud, Universidad de Guadalajara. Guadalajara, Jal. Mexico 44340
[3]Department of Neurosurgery, Brain Tumors Surgery Program, the Johns Hopkins. University School of Medicine, Baltimore, MD, USA 21205.
[4]Laboratorio de Morfología Celular. Unidad Mixta CIPF-UVEG, 46013 Valencia, CIBERNED, Spain

ABSTRACT

Adult neurogenesis occurs only in discrete regions of adult central nervous system: the subventricular zone and the subgranular zone. These areas are populated by adult neural stem cells (**aNSC**) that are regulated by a number of molecules and signaling pathways, which control their cell fate choices, survival and proliferation rates. For a long time, it was believed that the immune system did not exert any control on neural proliferative niches. However, it has been observed that many pathological and inflammatory conditions significantly affect NSC niches. Even more, increasing evidence indicates that chemokines and cytokines play an important role in regulating proliferation, cell fate choices, migration and survival of NSCs under physiological conditions. Hence, the immune system is emerging is an important regulator of neurogenic niches in the adult brain, which may have clinical relevance in several brain diseases.

---

[*] Corresponding author: Facultad de Psicologia Universidad de Colima Av. Universidad 333 Colima, COL 28040 Mexico Tel/Fax:. +52 (312) 316-1091 E-mail: osglez@gmail.com

INTRODUCTION

For most of last century, it was believed that cell proliferation in the brain was limited to glial cells, the supportive cells found around neurons. In the 1960s, newborn neurons were first described [1]. In the 1980's and 1990's, neurogenesis was demonstrated in the telencephalon of lizards, adult birds and in several mammalian species: mouse, rat, rabbit, cow, primate and humans [2-9]. In mammals, new neurons are continuously added to restricted brain regions, the olfactory bulb and the hippocampus. In these regions, new neurons are functional and appear to modulate olfaction and memory formation, respectively. New neurons in the adult nervous system derive from adult neural stem cells (aNSC), a group of cells that can self-renew and differentiate into all types of neural cells, including neurons, astrocytes and oligodendrocytes.

The brain is an immune-privileged organ because the selective permeability of the blood-brain barrier only allows certain substances and cells to enter and leave. Under normal physiological conditions, only macrophages, T cells and dendritic cells can access the brain [10-12]. After damage, an inflammatory process is initiated by the activation of astrocytes and microglia. This event is followed by parenchymal infiltration of macrophages and lymphocytes. The recruited immune cells release many anti- and pro-inflammatory mediators, chemokines, neurotransmitters and reactive oxygen species. This process generates the production and releasing of multiple inflammatory factors, which produces a positive feedback loop that results in both detrimental and positive consequences to neurogenesis [11, 13, 14]. Recently, it has been demonstrated that immune system regulates aNSC population through production of chemokines and cytokines [12, 13, 15]. aNSC have been proposed as an alternative for brain repair therapies but the molecular mechanisms that control survival, proliferation and cell fate are to be elucidated. In this chapter, we summarize emergent evidence indicating that immune mediators control aNSC population under physiological and pathological conditions.

1. THE BRAIN NICHES OF ADULT NEURAL STEM CELLS

Active neurogenesis occurs only in discrete regions of the adult central nervous system. There are two regions were adult neurogenesis has been indisputably described: the subventricular zone (**SVZ**) and the subgranular zone within the hippocampus (**SGZ**). Some reports claim that neurogenesis may also occur in other brain areas, including amygdala [16], neocortex [17, 18], substantia nigra [19, 20], and striatum [21, 22]. However, neurogenesis in these areas appears to occur either at substantially lower levels or under non-physiological conditions.

1.1. The Subventricular Zone (SVZ)

The most important germinal region is the SVZ (Figure 1), which contains a subpopulation of astrocytes that function *in vivo* as aNSCs. SVZ astrocyte NSCs are also known as Type-B cells. Currently Type-B cells are divided into two subtypes: B1 and B2.

Type-B1 cells make contact with the ventricular cavity while B2 cells do not. Type-B1 cells show one short primary cilium towards the ventricular cavity (Figure1), which is important to control cell proliferation and posse a long expansion that contact blood vessels [23]. Type-B1 cells give rise to intermediate neural progenitors defined actively proliferating transit amplifying progenitors or Type-C cells. Type-C cells symmetrically divide to produce migrating neuroblasts (Type-A cells) that migrate ventrally through the RMS into the olfactory bulb to become interneurons [24-26], which appear to regulate the olfaction process [27]. Recently, it has been described that Type-B cells *in vivo* generate oligodendrocytes that migrate into the corpus callosum and fimbria fornix [28, 29]. Blood vessels play an important role in the SVZ and there is evidence that the activation of neurogenic niches is regulated by this vascular network [30].

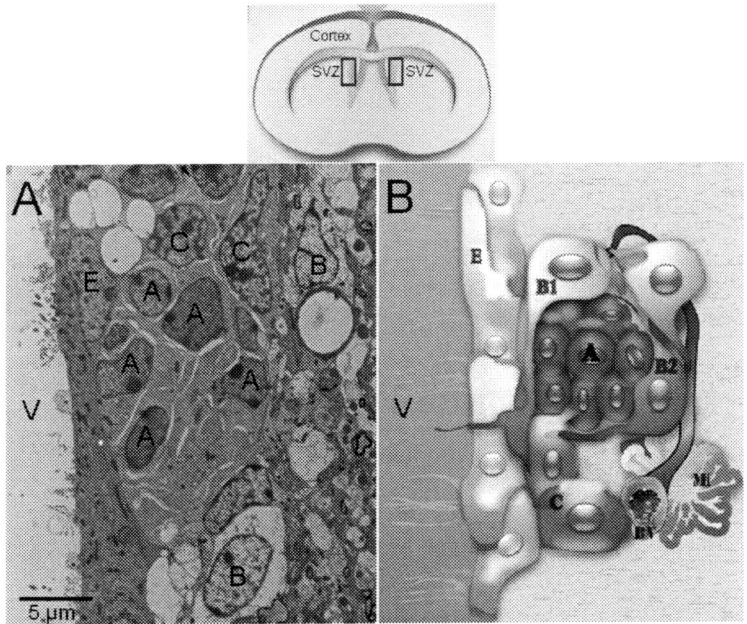

Figure 1. The adult subventricular zone in rodent. This neurogenic niche has been well-characterized by electron microscopy (A). Type-A cells (migrating neuroblasts) have an elongated cell body with one or two processes, profuse lax chromatin with small nucleoli (2 to 4), a scarce dark cytoplasm, abundant free ribosomes, microtubules oriented along the long axis of the cells, and nuclei occasionally invaginated. Their cytoplasmic membrane showed cell junctions intercalated with large intercellular spaces. Type-B cells have a light cytoplasm with a few ribosomes, extensive intermediate filaments and nuclei are typically invaginated. Their cell profiles are irregular that filled intercellular spaces between neighboring cells. Type-C cells are large and semi-spherical; their nuclei contain deep invaginations, lax chromatin occasionally clumped and large reticulated nucleoli. Type-C-cell cytoplasm is more electron-lucent than Type-A cells, but more electron-dense than Type-B cells, because it contains a few ribosomes and no intermediate filaments. Schematic drawing of the adult SVZ shows the cell organization of this region (B). Ependymal cells (Type-E cells) formed an epithelial monolayer that separates the SVZ from the lateral ventricles. These cells have spherical nuclei with lax chromatin, lateral cytoplasmic processes heavily interdigitated with apical junction complexes. The cell membrane contacting the ventricle contains microvilli and cilia, and their cytoplasm is electron-lucent with many mitochondria and basal bodies in the apical pole. A: Type- A cell; B: Type-B cell; C: Type-C cell cell; E: Ependymal cell; BV: Blood vessel; Mi: Microglia cell; V: Ventricle.

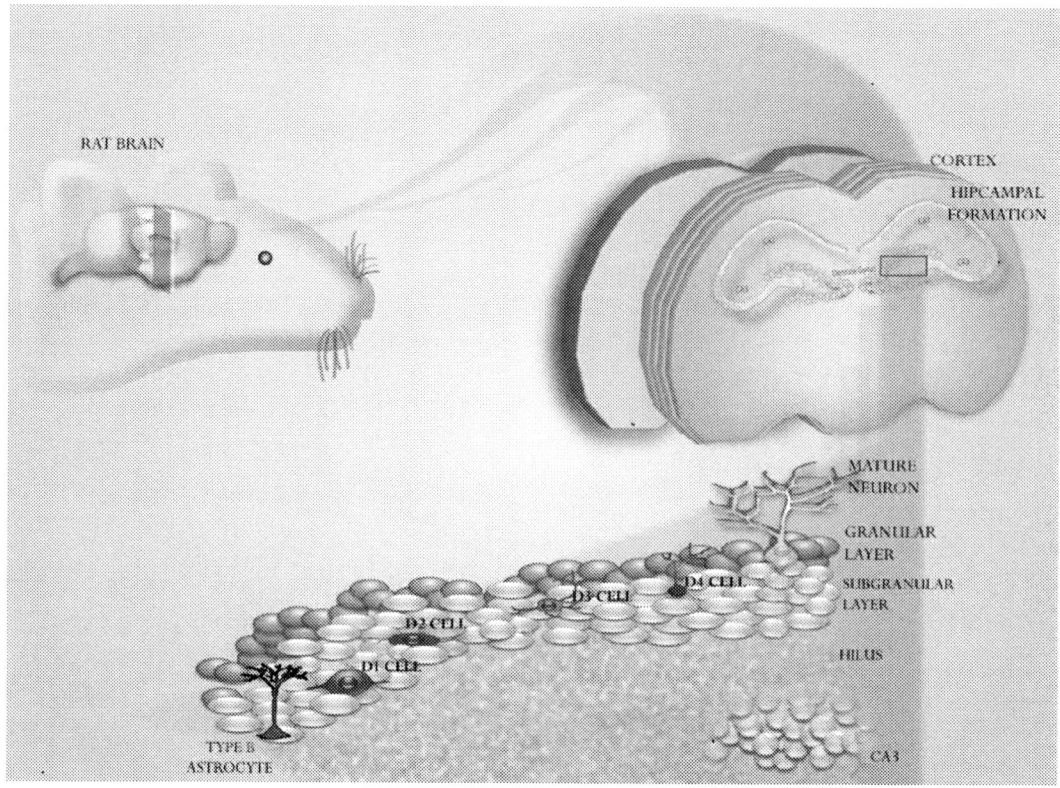

Figure 2. Schematic drawing of adult SGZ in rodent. Dentate gyrus of adult hippocampus continuously produces new neurons throughout life. Type-B cells are the primary progenitors that give rise to intermediate progenitors named Type-D cells, which give rise to granulate neurons.

1.2. The Subgranular Zone (SGZ)

The SGZ of the dentate gyrus in the hippocampus is a proliferative region that contains neuronal progenitors that give rise to granular neurons (Figure 2). The primary progenitors in this region are Type-B astrocytes, which have shown *in vitro,* via neurosphere and adherent monolayer cultures, multipotential properties. *In vivo*, SGZ Type-B cells appear to have limited capacity for differentiation. Therefore, some authors consider SGZ precursors as neuronal progenitors instead of aNSCs. SGZ Type-B cells divide asymmetrically to give rise to type-D cells that differentiate locally into mature granular neurons. The function of these newly generated neurons appears to play a role in memory process, learning and depression [31].

1.3. Microglia in Neurogenic Niches

Microglia is the main immune effector cell in the nervous system, which have a hematopoietic origin [32] and populate the CNS throughout adulthood [33, 34]. Under physiological conditions microglia is a quiescent cell population, which constantly excavates the CNS for damaged neurons, plaques, and infectious agents [34, 35]. In both, the adult SVZ and SGZ, microglia is abundant and, remarkably, is in close contact to aNSC (Type-B cells), which suggest that local interactions are possible between immune cells and multipotential progenitors (figure 3). Attracted by endogenous and exogenous chemotactic factors, microglial cells constitute the "first line of defense" of the CNS against injury or infections [34]. During inflammation or brain injury, microglia is capable of secreting neurotrophic or neuron survival factors upon activation [35], some of these effects are summarized in the figure 4. Recent evidence indicate that microglia instructs aNSC by secreting factors essential for neurogenesis, but not NSC maintenance, self-renewal, or propagation [36]. These effects seem to be mediated a number of factors, such as: interleukin-1 (IL-1) and tumor necrosis factor alpha (TNF-α) that serve as autocrine activators [11, 37, 38]; interferon gamma (IFN-γ), which thrive the immune response toward a cytotoxic response mediated by Th1 cells [39-42]; insulin-like growth factor-1 (IGF-1) that promotes cell proliferation [43]; interleukin-4 (IL-4) that increases phagocytotic properties of microglia [44, 45]; leukemia inhibitory factor (LIF) that is usually related to growth promotion and cell differentiation [15, 46-48]. It has been suggested that microglia modulation of aNSC is mediated by activation of mitogen activated protein kinase and phosphatidylinositol-3-kinase/Akt signaling pathways [49]. However, other inflammatory cells produce chemokines and cytokines, which can also influence implicated proliferation, differentiation, survival, and migration of aNSC [50-55]. Their effects will be described in detail in the next section.

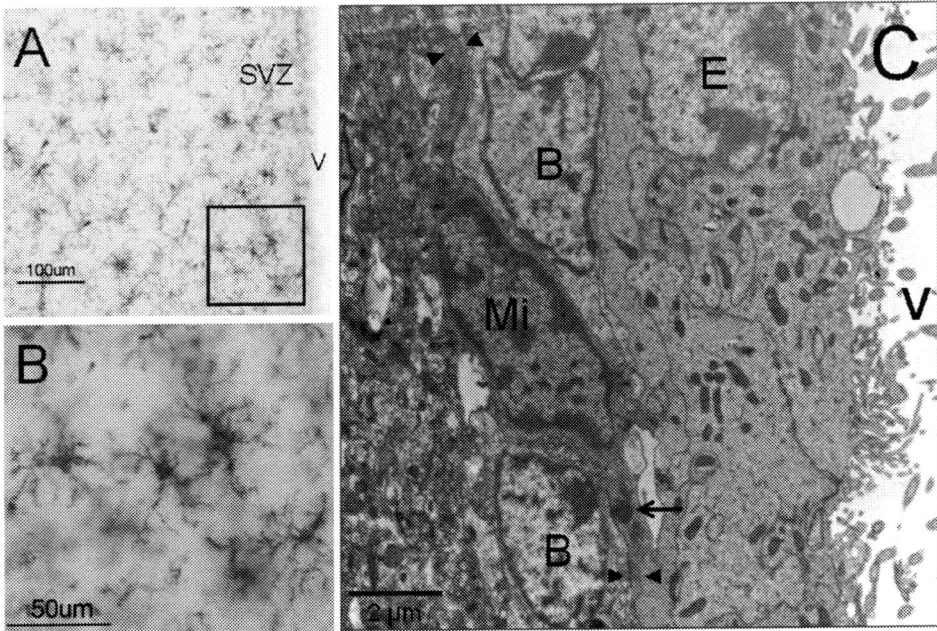

Figure 3. Microglia cells in the rodent SVZ. Iba-1 immunocytochemistry to detect microglia cells by light microscopy (A-B). In their "resting" stage microglia displays multiple thin branches, which confer a 'bushy' morphology to these cells. By electron microscopy (C), microglia (Mi) shows a typical dark nucleus and electrodense corpus in their cytoplasm (arrow). Frequently, microglial cytoplasmic expansions (arrow heads) are in close contact with Type-B cells. B: Type-B cell; E: Ependymal cell; V: Ventricle.

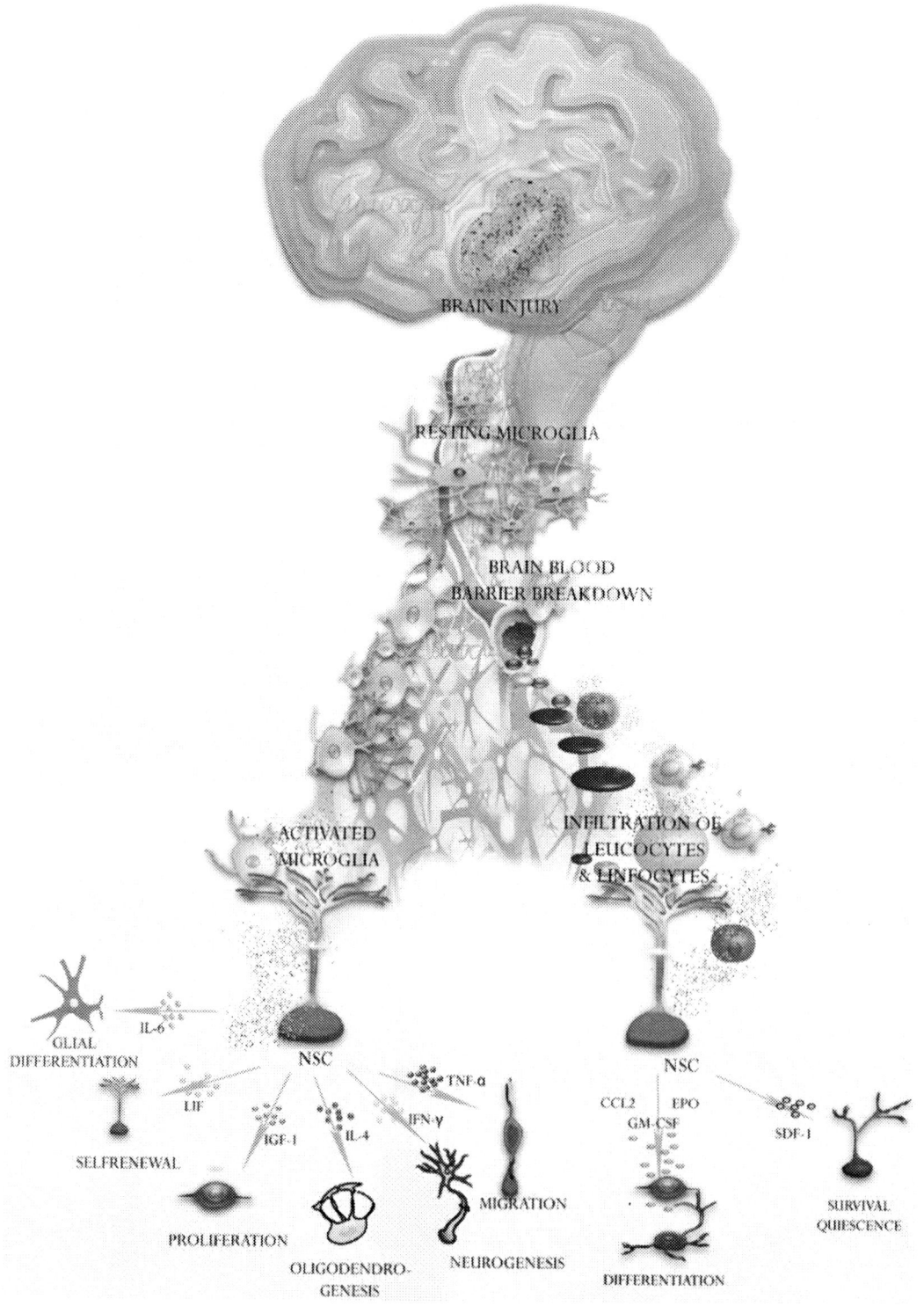

Figure 4. Effects of immune cells on aNSC. Cell effectors such as microglia, lymphocytes and leucocytes can induce a wide variety of effects on aNSC upon brain injury.

2. IMMUNOLOGICAL CONTROL OF ADULT NEURAL STEM CELLS

2.1. Cytokines and Chemokines

There are two types of immunological mediators: cytokines and chemokines. Cytokines are polypeptide regulators that have important roles in cellular communication [13]. Most, if not all, cells are regulated by cytokines. In the central nervous system, neuropoietic cytokines are a group of glycoproteins that control neuronal, glial and immune responses to injury or disease. They regulate neuronal growth, regeneration, survival, and differentiation by binding to high affinity receptors. The neuropoietic cytokine family includes interleukin-6 (IL-6), interleukin-18 (IL-18), IFN-γ, LIF, TNF-α, ciliary neurotrophic factor (CNTF) and others [13, 15]. Chemokines are small cytokines or proteins (8–14 kDa) that, according to the sequence motif of conserved N-terminal cysteine residues, are categorized into four groups: α-chemokines (CXC chemokines), which promote the migration of neutrophils and lymphocytes; β-chemokines (CC chemokines), which induce the migration of monocytes, NK cells and dendritic cells; γ-chemokines (C chemokines) that attract T cell precursors to the thymus; and δ-chemokines (CX3C chemokines), which serve as a chemoattractants and as an adhesion molecules [12]. Neurons express several receptors for immunological mediators, such as: CCR3, CXCR4, CXCR2, and CX3CR1, while astrocytes mainly express CXCR4, which make them responsive to chemokine gradients in the brain. CXCR4 is also highly expressed on the CD133+/nestin+ human neural precursors [56, 57]. Interestingly, CXCR4 expression is upregulated when embryonic precursors differentiate into neuronal precursors, whereas CXCL12 appears to drive astroglial differentiation [58]. Cytokines and chemokines alter self-renewal, progenitor cell division and differentiation of neural progenitors via JAK/STAT pathway and the Janus kinase-signal transducer [13, 15].

2.2. Effects of Cytokines and Chemokines on aNSC

After a brain injury, a number of inflammatory and immunological responses occur that modulate aNSC behavior (Table 1). Activated microglia produces IGF-1, which triggers the extracellular signal-regulated kinase (**ERK**) / mitogen-activated protein kinase (**MAPK**) pathway, increasing neurogenesis in the SGZ [43]. Interestingly, 'resting' microglia can also promote aNSC proliferation via the same signaling pathways [49]. Microglia-derived soluble factors such as IL-6 and LIF-1 induces astrocytic differentiation [59]. However, activated microglia appears to have a dual effect on aNSCs, for instance microglia activated by IL-4 drives the generation of oligodendrocytes (the axon supportive and myelin producer cells), whereas the IFN-γ-activated microglia induces a bias towards neurogenesis [44]. Acute LIF or CNTF exposure differentially affects development, growth, amplification and self-renewal of aNSCs [15, 46-48]. Chronic exposure to LIF or CNTF alters the formation of aNSC progenies and promotes aNSC self-renewal [15]. Phosphorylation of STAT3 induced by LIF is essential for maintaining NSC phenotype [60]. Conversely, leptin, which activates STAT3, inhibits differentiation of multipotent cells [15, 61]. aNSCs do not express a functional receptor for IL-6, thus they do not properly respond to IL-6. However, the stimulation of aNSCs with the active fusion protein of IL-6 and sIL-6R, designated as hyper-IL-6, induces aNSCs to differentiate into glutamate-responsive neurons and oligodendrocytes [62]. IFN-γ is pro-neurogenic, promotes neural differentiation and neurite outgrowth of murine aNSCs [39, 40]. However, IFN-γ has shown a dual effect on neurogenesis, because not only stimulate neuronal differentiation [40, 41] and NPC migration, but also inhibits aNSCs proliferation and reduces aNSCs survival [42]. However, the mechanism of this paradoxical effect is unknown. The IFN-γ-induced neuronal differentiation is probably mediated by c-Jun N-terminal kinase (**JNK**) pathway [63]. JNK pathway has been involved in neural differentiation of carcinoma cells, embryonic stem cells and PC12 cells [64-67]. Decreased neurogenesis has been observed by effect of TNF-α [11]. However, other studies indicates that TNF-α is a positive regulator of neurogenesis and promotes neurosphere grown by reducing aNSC apoptosis [68]. However, TNF-α increases the expression of MCP-1, a chemokine that induces migration of aNSCs thorough the MCP-1 receptor CCR2 [37, 38]. MCP-1 has protective effects on neurons against excitotoxicity mediated by NMDA receptors [69]. SDF-1 chemokyne promotes migration of neural progenitors and increases survival of aNSCs [37, 70, 71], but contrasting reports demonstrated that SDF-1 has a dual effect on neural progenitors producing quiescence [72] or inducing cell proliferation [73]. Other chemokine as CCL2 has no effects on proliferation and cell survival, but promotes neuronal differentiation of SVZ progenitors [74].

Hematopoietic growth factors have also been involved in the regulation of adult NSCs (Figure 4). Granulocyte-macrophage colony stimulating factor (GM-CSF) stimulates neuronal differentiation of aNSCs [75]. Granulocyte-colony stimulating factor (G-CSF) drives neuronal differentiation of aNSCs *in vitro* [76] and enhances neurogenesis and functional recovery. Erythropoietin (EPO) drives neuronal differentiation of aNSCs *in vitro* [77, 78]. Interestingly, EPO-receptor deficient mice display reduced neurogenesis [77, 78]. Yet, as findings in this field are relatively recent, there exist a number of cytokines and chemokines to be investigated as possible regulators of neurogenesis and neuroprotection.

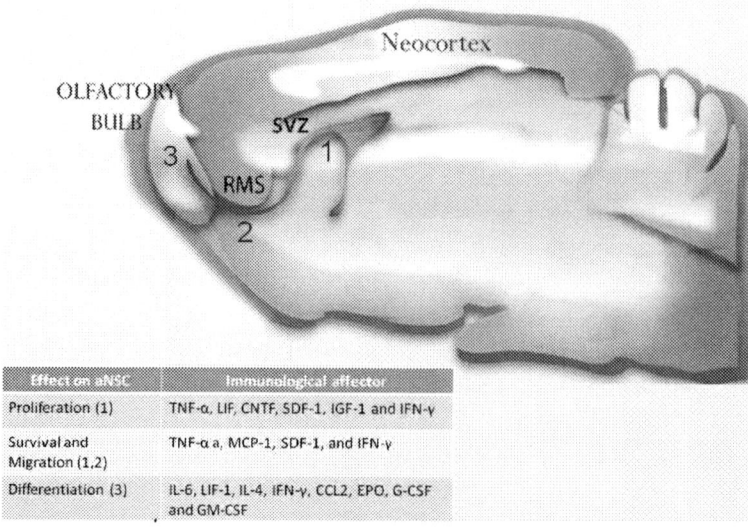

Figure 5. Immunological mediators have multiple effects on aNSC. There are some crucial steps in the neurogenic processs: Proliferation, survival, migration, differentiation. Immune effectors that affect proliferation mainly target the SVZ (1). Effectors that modulate survival and migration aim both SVZ and RMS (2), whereas immunological effects on differentiation are reflected in the olfactory bulb (3).

Table 1. Effects of chemokines and cytokines on adult NSCs

Cytokine / Chemokine	Effect on aNSCs	Reference
IFN-γ	Promotion of differentiation and neurite outgrowth. Reduction of proliferation and survival of multipotent progenitors.	[39, 40, 42]
IGF-1	Increasing of neurogenesis in SGZ	[43]
IL-4	Oligodendrogenesis	[44]
LIF	Neurogenesis promotions and NSC self-renewal (acute exposure)	[15, 46, 47]
CNTF	Neurogenesis promotions and NSC self-renewal (acute exposure)	[15, 79]
Leptin	Inhibition of differentiation of multipotent cells and glial progenitors	[15, 61]
TNF-α	Decreasing of neurogenesis	[11]
H-IL-6	Differentiation into glutamate-responsive neurons and oligodendrocytes	[62]
MCP-1	Migration of NSCs	[37, 38]
SDF-1	Promotion of migration, survival and proliferation of NSCs	[37, 70, 71, 73]
CCL2	Neuronal differentiation of SVZ progenitors	[74]

CONCLUSION

The immunological mediators affect proliferation, survival, migration and differentiation of aNSC (Figure 5). TNF-α, LIF, CNTF, SDF-1 and IGF-1 are considered important regulators of aNSC proliferation. Cell differentiation is driven mainly by IL-6, LIF-1, IL-4, IFN-γ, CCL2, EPO, G-CSF and GM-CSF. Migration of neural progenitors is promoted by MCP-1 and SDF-1, whereas cell survival is positively regulated by TNF-α and SDF-1, but negatively regulated by IFN-γ. In summary, further studies are necessary to elucidate some paradoxical effects on aNSC of immunological factors and signaling pathways involved in these processes.

ACKNOWLEDGMENTS

O.G-P was supported by CONACyT's grant (CB-2008-101476). A.Q-H supported by the National Institute of Health, the Howard Hughes Mediacal Institute, the Robert Wood Johnson Foundation and the Maryland Stem Cell Foundation. J.M.G-V Instituto de Salud Carlos III (Ciberned, Centro de Investigacion Principe Felipe y Red de Terapia Celular, Ministerio de Ciencia e Innovación (SAF2008-01274), Alicia Koplowitz's Foundation. We also thank F. Jáuregui and U. Gómez for assisting with the design and preparation of figures.

REFERENCES

[1] Altman, J. Postnatal neurogenesis and the problem of neural plasticity., in *Developmental neurobiology.*, W.A. Himwich, Editor. 1970, C.C.Thomas: Springfield. 197-237.

[2] Goldman, SA; Nottebohm, F. Neuronal production, migration, and differentiation in a vocal control nucleus of the adult female canary brain. *Proc.Natl.Acad.Sci. USA*, 1983, 80, 2390-2394.

[3] Alvarez-Buylla, A; Nottebohm, F. Seasonal and species differences in the production of long projection neurons in adult birds. *Neuroscience*, 1989, 15, 962.

[4] Galileo, DS; et al., Neurons and glia arise from a common progenitor in chicken optic tectum: Demonstration with two retroviruses and cell type-specific antibodies. *Proc.Natl.Acad.Sci. USA*, 1990, 87, 458-462.

[5] Alvarez-Buylla, A; Garcia-Verdugo, JM; Tramontin, AD. A unified hypothesis on the lineage of neural stem cells. *Nat Rev Neurosci*, 2001, 2, 2(4. 4), 287-93.

[6] Temple, S. The development of neural stem cells. *Nature*, 2001, 414(6859), 112-7.

[7] Gage, FH. Neurogenesis in the adult brain. *J Neurosci*, 2002, 22(3), 612-3.

[8] Sanai, N; et al., Unique astrocyte ribbon in adult human brain contains neural stem cells but lacks chain migration. Nature, 2004, 427(6976), 740-4:

[9] Garcia-Verdugo, JM; et al., The proliferative ventricular zone in adult vertebrates: a comparative study using reptiles, birds, and mammals. *Brain Res Bull*, 2002, 57(6), 765-75.

[10] Hickey, WF. Leukocyte traffic in the central nervous system: the participants and their roles. *Semin Immunol*, 1999, 11(2), 125-37.

[11] Whitney, NP; et al., Inflammation mediates varying effects in neurogenesis: relevance to the pathogenesis of brain injury and neurodegenerative disorders. *J Neurochem,*, 2009, 108(6), 1343-59.

[12] Bonecchi, R; et al., Chemokines and chemokine receptors: an overview. *Front Biosci*, 2009, 14, 540-51.

[13] Miller, RJ; et al., *Chemokine action in the nervous system. J Neurosci*, 2008, 28(46), 11792-5.

[14] Das, S; Basu, A. Inflammation: a new candidate in modulating adult neurogenesis. *J Neurosci Res*, 2008, 86(6), 1199-208.

[15] Bauer, S. Cytokine control of adult neural stem cells. *Ann N Y Acad Sci*, 2009, 1153, 48-56.

[16] Bernier, PJ; et al., Newly generated neurons in the amygdala and adjoining cortex of adult primates. *Proc Natl Acad Sci*, U S A, 2002, 99(17), 11464-9.

[17] Gould, E; et al., Neurogenesis in the neocortex of adult primates. *Science*, 1999, 286(5439), 548-52.

[18] Takemura, NU. Evidence for neurogenesis within the white matter beneath the temporal neocortex of the adult rat brain. *Neuroscience*, 2005, 134(1), 121-32.

[19] Zhao, M; et al., Evidence for neurogenesis in the adult mammalian substantia nigra. *Proc Natl Acad Sci*, U S A, 2003, 100(13), 7925-30.

[20] Yoshimi, K; et al., Possibility for neurogenesis in substantia nigra of parkinsonian brain. *Ann Neurol*, 2005, 58(1), 31-40.

[21] Van Kampen, JM; Robertson, HA. A possible role for dopamine D3 receptor stimulation in the induction of neurogenesis in the adult rat substantia nigra. *Neuroscience,* 2005, 136(2), 381-6.

[22] Bedard, A; Gravel, C; Parent, A. Chemical characterization of newly generated neurons in the striatum of adult primates. *Exp Brain Res,* 2006, 170(4), 501-12.

[23] Han, YG; et al., Hedgehog signaling and primary cilia are required for the formation of adult neural stem cells. *Nat Neurosci,* 2008, 11(3), 277-84.

[24] Lois, C; Alvarez-Buylla, A. Proliferating subventricular zone cells in the adult mammalian forebrain can differentiate into neurons and glia. *Proc.Natl.Acad.Sci.USA,* 1993, 90, 2074-2077.

[25] Lois, C; Alvarez-Buylla, A. Long-distance neuronal migration in the adult mammalian brain. *Science,* 1994, 264, 1145-1148.

[26] Alvarez-Buylla, A; Garcia-Verdugo, JM. Neurogenesis in adult subventricular zone. *J Neurosci,* 2002, 22(3), 629-34.

[27] So, K; et al., The olfactory conditioning in the early postnatal period stimulated neural stem/progenitor cells in the subventricular zone and increased neurogenesis in the olfactory bulb of rats. *Neuroscience,* 2008, 151(1), 120-8.

[28] Menn, B; et al., Origin of oligodendrocytes in the subventricular zone of the adult brain. *J Neurosci,* 2006, 26(30), 7907-18.

[29] Gonzalez-Perez, O; et al., Epidermal Growth Factor Induces the Progeny of Subventricular Zone Type B Cells to Migrate and Differentiate into Oligodendrocytes. *Stem Cells,* 2009, 27(8), 2032-2043.

[30] Shen, Q; et al., Adult SVZ stem cells lie in a vascular niche: a quantitative analysis of niche cell-cell interactions. *Cell Stem Cell,* 2008, 3(3), 289-300.

[31] Aimone, JB; Wiles, J; Gage, FH. Potential role for adult neurogenesis in the encoding of time in new memories. *Nat Neurosci,* 2006, 9(6), 723-7.

[32] Eglitis, MA; Mezey, E. Hematopoietic cells differentiate into both microglia and macroglia in the brains of adult mice. *Proc Natl Acad Sci U S A,* 1997, 94(8), 4080-5.

[33] Cuadros, MA; Navascues, J. Early origin and colonization of the developing central nervous system by microglial precursors. *Prog Brain Res,* 2001, 132, 51-9.

[34] Tambuyzer, BR; Ponsaerts, P; Nouwen, EJ. Microglia: gatekeepers of central nervous system immunology. *J Leukoc Biol,* 2009, 85(3), 352-70.

[35] Pivneva, TA. *Microglia in normal condition and pathology.* Fiziol Zh, 2008, 54(5), 81-9.

[36] Walton, NM; et al., Microglia instruct subventricular zone neurogenesis. *Glia,* 2006, 54(8), 815-25.

[37] Widera, D; et al., MCP-1 induces migration of adult neural stem cells. *Eur J Cell Biol,* 2004, 83(8), 381-7.

[38] Schwamborn, J; et al., Microarray analysis of tumor necrosis factor alpha induced gene expression in U373 human glioblastoma cells. *BMC Genomics,* 2003, 4(1), 46.

[39] Johansson, S; Price, J; Modo, M. Effect of inflammatory cytokines on major histocompatibility complex expression and differentiation of human neural stem/progenitor cells. *Stem Cells,* 2008, 26(9), 2444-54.

[40] Wong, G; Goldshmit, Y; Turnley, AM. Interferon-gamma but not TNF alpha promotes neuronal differentiation and neurite outgrowth of murine adult neural stem cells. *Exp Neurol,* 2004, 187(1), 171-7.

[41] Song, JH; et al., Interferon gamma induces neurite outgrowth by up-regulation of p35 neuron-specific cyclin-dependent kinase 5 activator via activation of ERK1/2 pathway. *J Biol Chem*, 2005, 280(13), 12896-901.

[42] Ben-Hur, T; et al., Effects of proinflammatory cytokines on the growth, fate, and motility of multipotential neural precursor cells. *Mol Cell Neurosci*, 2003, 24(3), 623-31.

[43] Choi, YS; et al., IGF-1 receptor-mediated ERK/MAPK signaling couples status epilepticus to progenitor cell proliferation in the subgranular layer of the dentate gyrus. *Glia*, 2008, 56(7), 791-800.

[44] Butovsky, O; et al., Microglia activated by IL-4 or IFN-gamma differentially induce neurogenesis and oligodendrogenesis from adult stem/progenitor cells. *Mol Cell Neurosci*, 2006, 31(1), 149-60.

[45] von Zahn, J; et al., Microglial phagocytosis is modulated by pro- and anti-inflammatory cytokines. *Neuroreport*, 1997, 8(18), 3851-6.

[46] Bauer, S; Patterson, PH. Leukemia inhibitory factor promotes neural stem cell self-renewal in the adult brain. *J Neurosci*, 2006, 26(46), 12089-99.

[47] Oshima, K; et al., LIF promotes neurogenesis and maintains neural precursors in cell populations derived from spiral ganglion stem cells. *BMC Dev Biol*, 2007, 7, 112.

[48] Covey, MV; Levison, SW. Leukemia inhibitory factor participates in the expansion of neural stem/progenitors after perinatal hypoxia/ischemia. *Neuroscience*, 2007, 148(2), 501-9.

[49] Morgan, SC; Taylor, DL; JM. Pocock, Microglia release activators of neuronal proliferation mediated by activation of mitogen-activated protein kinase, phosphatidylinositol-3-kinase/Akt and delta-Notch signalling cascades. *J Neurochem*, 2004, 90(1), 89-101.

[50] Faiz, M; et al., Substantial migration of SVZ cells to the cortex results in the generation of new neurons in the excitotoxically damaged immature rat brain. *Mol Cell Neurosci*, 2008, 38(2), 170-82.

[51] Liu, XS; et al., Functional response to SDF1 alpha through over-expression of CXCR4 on adult subventricular zone progenitor cells. *Brain Res*, 2008, 1226, 18-26.

[52] Robin, AM; et al., Stromal cell-derived factor 1alpha mediates neural progenitor cell motility after focal cerebral ischemia. *J Cereb Blood Flow Metab*, 2006, 26(1), 125-34.

[53] Tiveron, MC; et al., Molecular interaction between projection neuron precursors and invading interneurons via stromal-derived factor 1 (CXCL12)/CXCR4 signaling in the cortical subventricular zone/intermediate zone. *J Neurosci*, 2006, 26(51), 13273-8.

[54] Yan, YP; et al., Monocyte chemoattractant protein-1 plays a critical role in neuroblast migration after focal cerebral ischemia. *J Cereb Blood Flow Metab*, 2007, 27(6), 1213-24.

[55] Bhattacharyya, BJ; et al., The chemokine stromal cell-derived factor-1 regulates GABAergic inputs to neural progenitors in the postnatal dentate gyrus. *J Neurosci*, 2008, 28(26), 6720-30.

[56] Ni, HT; et al., High-level expression of functional chemokine receptor CXCR4 on human neural precursor cells. *Brain Res Dev Brain Res*, 2004, 152(2), 159-69.

[57] Tran, PB; et al., Chemokine receptors are expressed widely by embryonic and adult neural progenitor cells. *J Neurosci Res*, 2004, 76(1), 20-34.

[58] Peng, H; et al., Differential expression of CXCL12 and CXCR4 during human fetal neural progenitor cell differentiation. *J Neuroimmune Pharmacol*, 2007, 2(3), 251-8.

[59] Nakanishi, M; et al., Microglia-derived interleukin-6 and leukaemia inhibitory factor promote astrocytic differentiation of neural stem/progenitor cells. *Eur J Neurosci*, 2007, 25(3), 649-58.

[60] Burdon, T; Smith, A; Savatier, P. Signalling, cell cycle and pluripotency in embryonic stem cells. *Trends Cell Biol*, 2002, 12(9), 432-8.

[61] Udagawa, J; Nimura, M; Otani, H. Leptin affects oligodendroglial development in the mouse embryonic cerebral cortex. *Neuro Endocrinol Lett*, 2006, 27(1-2), 177-82.

[62] Islam, O; et al., Interleukin-6 and neural stem cells: more than gliogenesis. *Mol Biol Cell*, 2009, 20(1), 188-99.

[63] Kim, SJ; et al., Interferon-gamma promotes differentiation of neural progenitor cells via the JNK pathway. *Neurochem Res*, 2007, 32(8), 1399-406.

[64] Zentrich, E; et al., Collaboration of JNKs and ERKs in nerve growth factor regulation of the neurofilament light chain promoter in PC12 cells. *J Biol Chem*, 2002, 277(6), 4110-8.

[65] Akiyama, S; et al., Activation mechanism of c-Jun amino-terminal kinase in the course of neural differentiation of P19 embryonic carcinoma cells. *J Biol Chem*, 2004, 279(35), 36616-20.

[66] Wang, H; et al., Activation of c-Jun amino-terminal kinase is required for retinoic acid-induced neural differentiation of P19 embryonal carcinoma cells. *FEBS Lett*, 2001, 503(1), 91-6.

[67] Amura, CR; et al., Inhibited neurogenesis in JNK1-deficient embryonic stem cells. *Mol Cell Biol*, 2005, 25(24), 10791-802.

[68] Widera, D; et al., Tumor necrosis factor alpha triggers proliferation of adult neural stem cells via IKK/NF-kappaB signaling. *BMC Neurosci*, 2006, 7, 64.

[69] Eugenin, EA; et al., MCP-1 (CCL2) protects human neurons and astrocytes from NMDA or HIV-tat-induced apoptosis. *J Neurochem*, 2003, 85(5), 1299-311.

[70] Peng, H; et al., Stromal cell-derived factor 1-mediated CXCR4 signaling in rat and human cortical neural progenitor cells. *J Neurosci Res*, 2004, 76(1), 35-50.

[71] Molyneaux, KA; et al., The chemokine SDF1/CXCL12 and its receptor CXCR4 regulate mouse germ cell migration and survival. *Development*, 2003, 130(18), 4279-86.

[72] Krathwohl, MD; Kaiser, JL. HIV-1 promotes quiescence in human neural progenitor cells. *J Infect Dis*, 2004, 190(2), 216-26.

[73] Gong, X; et al., Stromal cell derived factor-1 acutely promotes neural progenitor cell proliferation in vitro by a mechanism involving the ERK1/2 and PI-3K signal pathways. *Cell Biol Int*, 2006, 30(5), 466-71.

[74] Liu, XS; et al., Chemokine ligand 2 (CCL2) induces migration and differentiation of subventricular zone cells after stroke. *J Neurosci Res*, 2007, 85(10), 2120-5.

[75] Kruger, C; et al., The hematopoietic factor GM-CSF (granulocyte-macrophage colony-stimulating factor) promotes neuronal differentiation of adult neural stem cells in vitro. *BMC Neurosci*, 2007, 8, 88.

[76] Schneider, A; et al., The hematopoietic factor G-CSF is a neuronal ligand that counteracts programmed cell death and drives neurogenesis. *J Clin Invest*, 2005, 115(8), 2083-98.

[77] Chen, ZY; et al., Endogenous erythropoietin signaling is required for normal neural progenitor cell proliferation. *J Biol Chem*, 2007, 282(35), 25875-83.

[78] Shingo, T; et al., Erythropoietin regulates the in vitro and in vivo production of neuronal progenitors by mammalian forebrain neural stem cells. *J Neurosci*, 2001, 21(24), 9733-43.

[79] Shimazaki, T; Shingo, T; Weiss, S. The ciliary neurotrophic factor/leukemia inhibitory factor/gp130 receptor complex operates in the maintenance of mammalian forebrain neural stem cells. *J Neurosci,* 2001, 21(19), 7642-53.

In: Autoimmune Diseases: Symptoms, Diagnosis and Treatment   ISBN: 978-1-61668-007-7
Editor: Kyle J. Brenner, pp. 317-327   © 2010 Nova Science Publishers, Inc.

Chapter 11

TEMPOROMANDIBULAR JOINT DISORDERS AND SYSTEMIC LUPUS ERYTHEMATOSUS

*L F Andre Costa[1] and Simone Appenzeller[2]**

[1] Rheumatology Unit, Department of Internal Medicine Faculty of Medical Sciences-
State University of Campinas, Campinas, Brazil
[2] Neuroimaging Lab, Faculty of Medical Sciences, State University of Campinas,
Campinas, Brazil

ABSTRACT

Temporomandibular joint disorder (TMD) is the most common cause of orofacial pain and has multifactorial etiologies. Commonly, temporomandibular joint (TMJ) is often a forgotten joint in rheumatologic evaluation, but well known affected in several diseases, including systemic lupus erythematosus (SLE). It is important for clinicians and rheumatologists to be able to recognize symptoms of TMD. TMD involvement may be secondary to systemic inflammation and arthritis or a clinical manifestation of an independent pathology, such as infections, degeneration and osteonecrosis. Since there are overlapping signs and symptoms, the diagnosis can be confusing. It is therefore important for clinicians and rheumatologists to be able to recognize symptoms of TMD. Imaging may help to establish diagnosis. Several imaging modalities are available, including X-rays, tomography and magnetic resonance imaging. Since TMD may lead to severe disabilities, early diagnosis, as well as timely and appropriate management is warranted.
In this chapter, we describe the most frequent TMD associated with SLE and provide an overview of the evaluation of the common TMJ in a simplified version that will help to identify the clinical findings and imaging patterns.

---

[*] Corresponding author: Disciplina de Reumatologia, Departamento de Clínica Médica Faculdade de Ciências Médicas, Universidade Estadual de Campinas (UNICAMP) Distrito de Barão Geraldo, Campinas-SP, Brazil. - CEP 13081-970, E-mail: appenzellersimone@yahoo.com

INTRODUCTION

Temporomandibular disorders (TMD) are a collective term that refers to a number of clinical problems that involve the masticatory musculature and/or the temporomandibular joint (TMJ). It has been identified as a major cause of nondental pain in the orofacial region and is considered to be a subclassification of musculoskeletal disorders [1]. The most important symptom, and the reason most patients seek medical attention is pain, usually localized in the muscles of mastication, the preauricular area, and/or the TMJ. Common complaints include jaw ache, earache, headache, and facial pain. In addition to pain, limited or asymmetric jaw moment and joint sounds have been frequently observed [1].

Systemic lupus erythematosus (SLE) is a chronic inflammatory disease of unknown etiology. Joint disease is common in SLE and often one of the earliest manifestations. It may occur in up to 90% of the patients during the disease course. Joint involvement varies from inflammatory arthralgias requiring minimal therapy up to deforming arthritis with erosions [2-4]. Frequently, arthritis is polyarticular and involves small to medium joints in a symmetrical distribution [2]. The small joints of the hand, the wrist and the knees are commonly involved. Most of the time arthritis of SLE is non-erosive and rarely deforming, as opposed to rheumatoid arthritis. Early morning stiffness is a commonly observed symptom and often disabling. Involvement of the elbows, shoulder, or ankles is less frequently [5].

SLE patients frequently present TMJ pathology [6-8] and its symptoms mimic characteristics of the more common TMDs. Pain, clicking and functional limitation predominate in the clinical picture of TMJ in SLE. On the other hand, these signs and symptoms are non-specific and may be found in several non-dysfunctional conditions [9].

We intend to help the reader with a thorough understanding of the potentially complications associated with SLE in TMJ, identify patients at risk and preventative treatment initiated when appropriate.

Anatomy, Epidemiology and Etiopathogenesis of TMD

The TMJ is composed of the temporal bone and the mandible, as well as the articular disk, a specialized dense fibrous structure, several ligaments, and numerous associated muscles. The TMJ is a compound joint that can be classified by anatomic type as well as by function [10].

Anatomically the TMJ is a diarthrodial joint, which is a discontinuous articulation of two bones permitting freedom of movement, which is limited by muscles and ligaments. Its fibrous connective tissue capsule is well innervated and well vascularized. It is also a synovial joint, lined on its inner aspect by a synovial membrane, which secretes synovial fluid. The fluid acts as a joint lubricant and supplies the metabolic and nutritional needs of the nonvascularized internal joint structures [10].

Functionally the TMJ is a compound joint, composed of four articulating surfaces: the articular facets of the temporal bone and of the mandibular condyle and the superior and inferior surfaces of the articular disk. The articular disk divides the joint into two compartments. The lower compartment permits hinge motion or rotation. The superior compartment permits sliding (or translatory) movements [10].

TMD is a common condition in clinical practice. Cross-sectional epidemiological studies have shown that about 75% of included subjects have at least one sign of TMD and about 33% have at least one symptom [1]. Signs and symptoms of TMD generally increase in frequency and severity from the second through the fourth decade of life. Although it may affect both males and females, it is 1.5 to 2 times more prevalent in women than in men [11]. However, the reason for a female predominance is still not well understood. Hormonal, constitutional factors, and psychosocial gender differences, have been considered possible etiologic factors [12]. Although most individuals present with mild and transient symptoms and may not require treatment, approximately 10% of patients suffering from TMD develop severe disorders associated with chronic pain [12]. It is estimated that only 5–6% of affected patients are currently in treatment [1, 3, 6, 7].

TMD has a multifactorial etiology [1]. Predisposing factors include pathophysiological, structural, and/or psychological conditions that adversely affect the masticatory system and increase the risk of developing TMD. Skeletal malformations, past injuries, inappropriate dental treatment and inadequate occlusion are common predisposing factors [1]. Psychologic predisposing factors include emotional, personality, and attitude features [1].

In patients without inflammatory joint disease, TMD is characterized by intra-articular positional and/or structural abnormalities [19], presenting therefore a non-inflammatory starting point. The pathological process is characterized by deterioration and abrasion of articular cartilage, local thickening and remodeling of the bone. The changes are associated with the superimposition of secondary inflammatory changes [19]. Non-inflammatory arthropathies can progress to the inflammatory types through increasing concentrations of degradation products within the joint [18] such pro-inflammatory cytokines, proteinases and free radicals that damage the articular tissues of the TMJ [19]. Inflammatory joint diseases, on the other hand, are associated with synovial thickening and pannus formation. Degenerative changes occur later during the course of the disease and have been confirmed to aggravate the degree of tissue destruction and dysfunction within the TMJ [18, 19].

Classification of Temporomandibular Disorders

A classification of TMDs should be in agreement with the classification of synovial joint disorders, as generally used by rheumatologists and orthopedic surgeons (Table 1) [17].

Gold standard for diagnosing TMD is based on assessment of the patient's history and findings from clinical examination.

Clinical investigation should include the following questions [1]:

1. Are you having difficulties or pain, when opening your mouth?
2. Does your jaw get stuck, locked, or go out?
3. Are you having difficulties or pain chewing, talking, or using your jaws?
4. Are you aware of noises in the jaw joint?
5. Do you have pain in or about ears, temples, or cheeks?
6. Does your bite feel uncomfortable or unusual?
7. Do you have frequent headaches?
8. Have you had a recent injury to your head, neck, or jaw?

9. Have you previously been treated for a jaw joint problem?

Physical evaluation should include [1]:

(a) Measuring range of motion of the mandible on opening and right and left laterotrusion;
(b) Palpation for preauricular TMJ tenderness;
(c) Palpation for TMJ crepitus;
(d) Palpation for TMJ clicking;
(e) Palpation for tenderness in the masseter and temporalis muscles;
(f) Assessment of excessive occlusal wear, excessive tooth mobility, or migration, in the absence of periodontal disease, and soft tissue alterations, for example, buccal mucosal ridging, lateral tongue scalloping;
(g) Examine symmetry and alignment of the face, mandible and dental arches.

Table I. General classification of Joint disorders

Articular disorders	Nonarticular disorders
Noninflammatory Arthropathies: • *Primary osteoarthrosis;* • *Secondary osteoarthrosis (trauma, previous surgery, avascular necrosis)* • *Mechanical derangements (articular disc displacement)*	Muscle disorders: • *Muscle pain;* • *Myofacial pain and dysfunction;* • *Fibromyalgia;* • *Myotonic dystrophies;* • *Myositis ossificans progressiva*
Inflammatory arthropathies: • *Synovitis;* • *Capsulitis;* • *Rheumathoid arthritis;* • *Seronegative polyarthritis;* • *Ankylosing spondilytis;* • *Psoriatic arthritis.*	Growth disorders: • *Structural deformity of the craniofacial bones*
Growth disorders: • *Non-neoplastic: developmental (hypoplasia, hyperplasia, dysplasia;* • *Non-neoplastic: acquired (condylolysis, (post) juvenile osteoarthrosis or rheumatoid arthritis;* • *Neoplasm: pseudotumors, benign, malignant.*	Miscellaneous nonarticular disorders: • *Heterotopic bone formation*
Diffuse connective tissue disorders: • *scleroderma, Sjogren syndrome, rheumatic fever, polymyalgia rheumatic, arteritis temporalis*	
Miscellaneous articular disorders: • *Traumatic arthritis, neurogenic arthropathy, congenital abnormalities*	

Adapted from de Bont L.G. *et al.* and Miloro *et al.* (16, 17).

TMD Diagnosis with imaging

Studies have shown that physical examination alone is inaccurate in determining the status of the joint [20]. Accuracy of the clinical diagnosis for the specific status of the joint is obtained in only 50 to 60% of the patients [20]. The primary aim for imaging the TMJ is that internal derangement disease and its concomitant pathology is treated differently according to the underlying disease. There are diverse techniques for imaging the TMJ: plain radiography, computerized tomography, arthrography, ultrasound and magnetic resonance imaging (MRI).

Plain film depicts only the mineralized part of the joint, not the cartilage and soft tissues. It is therefore valuable for determining the presence of osseous changes and traumatic injury to the osseous components of the joint [20]. Negative findings on plain film are frequently observed, but cannot exclude abnormalities affecting the soft-tissue. In addition, superimposition of adjacent anatomic structures can make interpretation difficult. Panoramic radiography cannot be used to evaluate the condyle and glenoid fossa due to superimposition of other structures [20]. Unfortunately, the articular disc cannot be seen by conventional radiography or computed tomography (CT).

Ultrasound (US) has been evaluated as a screening technique in recent years to evaluate disk displacement in TMJ [20]. High-frequency transducers allow a fast and accurate assessment of the small joints and the periarticular soft tissues in experienced hands. US of the TMJ is easy to perform and comfortable to the patient, with low cost and high availability. US can be used for diagnosing TMJ disc position abnormalities in a similar way as MRI at closed mouth position and also at opened-mouth position. However, because of the ability to be performed in real-time, (the articular disk can be evaluated during the mouth-opening movement), US has a great advantage with respect to other imaging modalities. Recent studies have evaluated the usefulness of US in the diagnosis of internal derangement when compared with the gold-standard imaging technique (MRI) or pathology [1]. Recent studies have found that a retrospective interpretation of US studies had an accuracy of 88% at the closed-mouth position and 86% at the maximum mouth opening. US can assess the presence of effusion, cartilage thickness and distension synovial proliferation, and capsular distention, with more difficulties in detecting osseous pathology [1]. However, US should be considered as an imaging technique modality when therapeutic injection guided into the superior and inferior joint spaces are considered for treatment.

CT has been used and applied in the past to study the complex anatomic structures of the TMJ and the pathology such as ankylosis, condyle fracture, and osseous changes. CT allows noninvasive imaging of both osseous and soft-tissue abnormalities related to disk damage. However, the accuracy of the disk displacement was only 40 to 67% in CT in studies of autopsy specimen materials [20]. Moreover, some reports pointed out that radiographic signs of arthrosis may not be associated with clinical symptoms of pain dysfunction [20]. Advantages of CT over MRI include the specialized imaging capabilities for assessing bone detail, and 3D assessment, usefull in evaluating congenital, traumatic, and postsurgical conditions involving the TMJ. Arthrography is an imaging method by which radiopaque contrast dye is injected into the lower TMJ spaces under fluoroscopic guidance to image the soft tissue structures [21].

MRI has gradually replaced arthrography and arthrotomography, to image soft tissue structures. MRI allows excellent depiction of the TMJ anatomy and abnormalities because of its inherent tissue contrast and high resolution [20]. MRI has become the examination of choice in evaluating the TMJ, because of its noninvasive nature and its ability to differentiate the cortex, marrow, hyaline cartilage, muscle, fluid, and fibrous tissue. MR imaging plays a main role in establishing a definitive diagnosis of TMJ disorders, thereby facilitating correct management [22]. Information about disk position, joint fluid, bone marrow changes, and bone structure at multiple levels of the joint can be obtained from MRI. The technique, however, is expensive compared with plain radiography and conventional tomography. MRI is also contraindicated in patients who have pacemakers, intracranial vascular clips, and metal particles in their eyes or other vital structures. Relative contraindications include obesity, claustrophobia, and the inability to remain motionless during the examination [21, 22].

Systemic Lupus Erythematosus and TMJ Involvement

TMJ arthritis is a common finding in rheuatic diseases. TMJ arthritis may be caused by systemic conditions, such as SLE, or more localized conditions related to trauma, infection, or degenerative changes. In Table II, it is showed the principal arthritic disorders.

Arthritis

Usually, in SLE arthritis is polyarticular and involves small to medium joints in a symmetric distribution. TMJ involvement generally occurs simultaneously to other joint involvement. Isolated TMJ arthritis is rarely observed. It is commonly nonerosive, although, several authors have described the occurrence of erosions [23, 24].

More typical symptoms of TMJ arthritis are morning stiffness, swelling over the TMJ area, and problems to obtain a good dental occlusion [25] and signs of inflammation. Pain is normally exacerbated with join motion.

In conventional radiograph, it is possible to see subchondral sclerosis, condylar flattening, marginal lipping, erosion, osteophyte formation, bone cysts, and narrowing of the joint space [26]. MRI findings are bone destruction or deformation and soft-tissue abnormalities: normal disc position and abnormal disc structure (fragmentation, poor delineation, severe flattening) or severely destroyed disc [25].

Table II. Classification of Arthritic Conditions Affecting the Joint

Low-inflammatory Arthritic Disorders	Degenerative joint disease (Osteoarthritis) Post-traumatic arthritis
High-inflammatory Arthritic Disorders	Infectious arthritis Rheumatoid arthritic conditions • *adult and juvenile* Metabolic arthritic conditions • *gouty arthritis* • *psoriatic arthritis* • **lupus erythematosus** • *ankylosing spondylitis* • *Reiter's Syndrome* • *arthritis associated with ulcerative colitis*

Adapted from Mercuri LG (24).

Infectious arthritis

Infection is a frequent problem in the course and management of SLE [35-37]. However, infectious arthritis affecting the TMJ is uncommon [1, 21]. Patients who have a compromised immune condition are more prone to infectious arthritis [21]. Even though the source of the bacteria is usually at a distant site, spread from dental infections of maxillary teeth has been reported in which the bacteria are thought to spread through the pterygoid plexus of veins to the joint [38]. Rapid diagnostic and therapeutic intervention is necessary when an infection of the TMJ is suspected because joint distention is frequently painful and permanent changes in joint function can happen [17].

Symptoms of infectious arthritis are unilateral pain, tenderness, swelling, redness of TMJ region, and systemic findings of the infection such as fever and chills [1]. Patients usually exhibit inability to occlude the teeth and a posterior open bite on the ipsilateral side as a result of the increased joint fluid [1, 17]. Prompt diagnostic and therapeutic intervention is required when an infection of the TMJ is suspected because joint distention is usually painful and permanent changes in joint function can occur [17].

X-rays are normal in the early stages, although widening of the joint space due to accumulation of inflammatory exudates may be seen. Later during the course of the diseasebony destruction may be seen [1]. Magnetic resonance imaging is an excellent modality for identifying the place of the exudates [39].

Osteonecrosis

Osteonecrosis is a clinic-radiological pathology characterized by death of bone marrow and trabecular bone as a consequence of disruption of vascular supply to the bone. It is a final common pathway of a number of conditions that include both traumatic and non-traumatic etiologies, such as trauma, and inflamation [40-43].

Osteonecrosis occurs in 5% to 10% of patients with SLE and often involves multiple joints [44]. The prevalence of symptomatic osteonecrosis in SLE has been described to be close to 12% and often involves multiple joints. Glucocorticoid therapy, presence of arthritis and the use of cytotoxic drugs are independent risk factors for the development of osteonecrosis
in SLE [44]. The role of anti-phospholipid antibodies in the development of this condition is controversial. The time of onset of osteonecrosis in SLE is usually within the first month of high dose corticosteroid treatment [44]. High risk patients should be closely monitored so that early osteonecrosis can be diagnosed by sensitive techniques such as magnetic resonance imaging and radioisotope bone scanning. The long term prognosis of early stage necrosis is favorable in SLE patients when the necrotic area is less than 25% [44].Whenever moderate or high dose corticosteroid therapy is undertaken, the risk of bone necrosis must be recognized.

SLE patients receiving corticosteroids and complaining of joint pains should be promptly evaluated for osteonecrosis. A normal radiograph would not exclude osteonecrosis and when required, other more sensitive modalities such as magnetic resonance or radionucleide bone scanning should be used.

The clinical course of patients with osteonecrosis is unpredictable, but frequently they will lead to painful, arthritic joints often requiring major surgical procedures as treatment.

The incidence of osteonecrosis of the mandibular condyle is unknown because various reports describing this phenomenon have presented biased populations [45].

Clinically, pain is the most common symptom, with limitation of movement when the joint is affected [46]. Magnetic resonance imaging is the best imaging modality for these conditions, although its results may be false-negative when lesions are small [46, 47]. CT and three dimensional–CT scanning also may disclose bone necrosis and defects in the condyle [46] Treatment includes unloading the condyle to relieve condylar stress, treating underlying systemic diseases and surgical intervention as necessary [46].

Temporomandibular Joint Disorders, Systemic Lupus Erythematosus and Psychological Conditions

It has been suggested that chronic pain conditions and depressive disorders share common pathophysiologic characteristics [27], and possibly, there are a similar risk of a major life stressor precipitating a chronic pain condition such as TMD [28].

Neuropsychiatric manifestations are present in 14–75% of the patients with lupus [29, 30] and various works showed a link between this disease and stress/anxiety [31-33]. Stress maintained in a chronic way may not only produce a worsening of the lupus symptomatology, but it can also produce negative complex consequences at various levels [22].

We can hypothesize that TMD in lupus patients would be also triggered by emotional conditions found in SLE.

Treatment of TMJ in SLE

Conservative treatments are endorsed for the initial care of nearly all TMD patients because the majority of patients with TMD achieve good relief of symptoms with conservative treatment [1]. Patient education is important and should emphasize rest of the masticatory system through voluntary limitation of mandibular function. Home physiotherapeutic program of moist heat and/or ice to the affected areas, massage of the affected muscles and gentle range of motion exercises is also indicated [1].

The changing maladaptive habits and behavior is an important part of the overall treatment program for TMD patients. Use of dental therapies such as stabilization or repositioning appliance appears to enhance the effect of behavioral treatment [1].

Pharmacological management of TMD is strictly associated with the correct diagnosis. Treatment of degenerative and inflammatory etiologies include analgesics, anti-inflammatory agents, muscle relaxants, corticosteroids, anti-anxiety agents, and low-dose antidepressants [1]. Infectious etiology should be treated with antibiotics according to the most probable organism. However obtaining cultures from blood and from synovial fluid is important for adequate treatment. Treatment of ON of TMJ is still controversial. Core decompression has been described in hip involvement, but further studies are necessary to determine the best treatment for ON in SLE.

CONCLUSIONS

In this chapter, we summarized some of the more frequent TMD associated with SLE. Application of this finding by physicians in their daily practice may lead to earlier identification and quick management of TMD. It is important signs to referral for additional consultations or examinations because of the possible overlapping symptomatology between SLE/TMD and other medical disorders.

REFERENCES

[1] Atsü, SS; Ayhan-Ardic, F. Temporomandibular disorders seen in rheumatology practices: a review. *Rheumatol Int.*, 2006, 26, 781-7.
[2] Lahita, R. Systemic lupus erythematosus. 3rd ed. New York, NY: *Churchill Livingstone*, 1999.
[3] Alarcon-Segovia, D; Abud-Mendoza, C; Díaz-Jouanen, E; Iglesias, A; De Los Reyes, V; Hernández-Ortiz, J. Deforming arthropathy of the hands in systemic lupus erythematosus. *J Rheumatol*, 1988, 15, 65-69.
[4] Richter-Cohen, M; Steiner, G; Smolen, JS; Isenber, DA. Erosive arthritis in systemic lupus erythematosus: analysis of a distinct clinical and serologic subset. *Br J Rheumatol*, 1998, 37, 421-424.
[5] Ostendorf, B; Scherer, A; Specker, C; Modder, U; Schneider, M. Jaccoud's arthropathy in systemic lupus erythematosus: differentiation of deforming and erosive patterns by magnetic resonance imaging. *Arthritis Rheum*, 2003, 48, 157-65.
[6] Liebling, MR; Gold, RH. Erosions of the temporomandibular joint in systemic lupus erythematosus. *Arthritis Rheum*, 1981, 24, 948-50.
[7] Gerbracht, D; Shapiro, L. Temporomandibular joint erosions in systemic lupus erythematosus. *Arthritis Rheum*, 1982, 25, 597.
[8] Jonsson, R; Lindval, A; Nyberg, G. Temporomandibular joint involvement in systemic lupus erythematosus. *Arthritis Rheum*, 1983, 26, 1506-10.
[9] Costa, AL; D'Abreu, A; Cendes, F. Temporomandibular joint internal derangement: association with headache, joint effusion, bruxism, and joint pain *J Contemp Dent Pract.*, 2008, 9, 9-16.
[10] DuBrul, EL. *Sicher's oral anatomy*. 7th ed. St.Louis (MO): C.V. Mosby; 1980, 146-61, 174-209.
[11] Dworkin, SF; Huggins, KH; LeResche, L; Von Korff, M; Howard, J; Truelove, E; Sommers, E. Epidemiology of signs and symptoms in temporomandibular disorders: clinical signs in cases and controls. *J Am Dent Assoc.*, 1990, 120, 273-81.
[12] Vignolo, V; Vedolin, GM; de Araujo Cdos, R; Rodrigues Conti, PC. Influence of the menstrual cycle on the pressure pain threshold of masticatory muscles in patients with masticatory myofascial pain. *Oral Surg Oral Med Oral Pathol Oral Radiol Endod.*, 2008, 105, 308-15.
[13] Fricton, JR; Olsen, T. Predictors of outcome for treatment of temporomandibular disorders. *J Orofac Pain*, 1996, 10, 54-65.

[14] de Bont, LG; Stegenga, B. Pathology of temporomandibular joint internal derangement and osteoarthrosis. *Int J Oral Maxillofac Surg.*, 1993, 2, 71-4

[15] Stegenga, B; De Bont, LG; Van Der, KB; Boering, G. Classification of temporomandibular joint osteoarthrosis and internal derangement. I. Diagnostic significance of clinical and radiographic symptoms and signs. *J Craniomandibular Pract*, 1992, 10, 96 106.

[16] Stegenga, B; De Bont, LG. Classification of temporomandibular joint osteoarthrosis and internal derangement. II. Specific diagnostic criteria. *J Craniomandibular Pract*, 1992, 10, 107-17.

[17] de Bont, LG; Dijkgraaf, LC; Stegenga, B. Epidemiology and natural progression of articular temporomandibular disorders. *Oral Surg Oral Med Oral Pathol Oral Radiol Endod.*, 1997, 83, 72-6

[18] Miloro, PE; Ghali, GE; Larsen, PE. Peterson's principles of oral and maxillofacial surgery. 2nd ed. Hamilton, *Ont; London: B C Decker*, 2004.

[19] Tanaka, E; Detamore, MS; Mercuri, LG. Degenerative disorders of the temporomandibular joint: etiology, diagnosis, and treatment. *J Dent Res.*, 2008, 87, 296-307.

[20] Vilanova, JC; Barceló, J; Puig, J; Remollo, S; Nicolau, C; Bru, C. Diagnostic imaging: magnetic resonance imaging, computed tomography, and ultrasound. *Semin Ultrasound CT MR.*, 2007, 28 184-91.

[21] Lewis, EL; Dolwick, MF; Abramowicz, S; Reeder, SL. Contemporary imaging of the temporomandibular jointDent *Clin North Am.*, 2008, 52(4), 875-90.

[22] Rao, VM. Bacelar, MT. MR imaging of the temporomandibular joint. *Neuroimaging Clin N Am.*, 2004, Nov, 14, 761-75.

[23] van Vugt, RM; Derksen, RH; Kater, L; Bijlsma, JW. Deforming arthropathy or lupus and rupus hands in sustemic lupus erythematosus. *Ann Rheum Dis.*, 1998, 57, 540-4.

[24] Fernandez, A; Quintana, G; Rondon, F; Restrepo, JF; Sa´nchez, A; Matteson, EL. Lupus arthropathy: a case series of patients with rhupus. *Clin Rheumatol.*, 2006, 25, 164-7.

[25] Larheim, TA. Role of Magnetic Resonance Imaging in the Clinical Diagnosis of the Temporomandibular *Joint. Cell Tissue Organs.*, 2005, 180, 6–21.

[26] Laskin, DM. Temporomandibular joint pain. In: ED; Harris, RC; Budd, GS; Firestein, MC; Genovese, JS; Sergent, S; Ruddy, CB; Sledge, (Eds). Kelley's Textbook of Rheumatology. Philadelphia: *Elsevier Saunders*, 2005, 637-648.

[27] Magni, G. On the relationship between chronic pain and depression when there is no organic lesion. *Pain*, 1987, 31, 1-21.

[28] Korszun, A; Hinderstein, B; Wong, M. Comorbidity of depression with chronic facial pain and temporomandibular disorders. *Oral Surg Oral Med Oral Pathol Oral Radiol Endod.*, 1996, 82, 496-500.

[29] Haupt, M. Psychiatric disorders in rheumatic diseases, as exemplified by systemic lupus erythematosus. *Z Rheumatol*, 2004, 63, 122-130.

[30] Appenzeller, S; Carnevalle, AD; Li, LM; Costallat, LT; Cendes, F. Hippocampal atrophy in systemic lupus erythematosus. *Ann Rheum Dis.*, 2006, 65, 1585-9

[31] Adams, SG; Dammers, PM; Saia, TL; Brantley, PJ; Gaydos, GR. Stress, depression and anxiety predict average symptom severity and daily symptom fluctuation in systemic lupus erythematosus. *J Behav Med*, 1994, 17, 459-477.

[32] Schubert, C; Lampe, A; Rumpold, G; et al. Daily psychosocial stressors interfere with the dynamics of urine neopterin in a patient with systemic lupus erythematosus: An integrative single-case study. *Pychosom Med*, 1999, 6, 876-882.

[33] Schubert, C; Geser, W; Noisternig, B; Konig, P; Rumpold, G; Lampe, A. Stressful life events and skin diseases: An additional perspective from research on psychosomatic dynamics in systemic lupus erythematosus. *Psychother Psychosom*, 2002, 71, 123-126.

[34] Peralta-Ramírez, MI; Coín-Mejías, MA; Jiménez-Alonso, J; Ortego-Centeno, N; Callejas-Rubio, JL; Caracuel-Romero, A; Pérez-García, M. Stress as a predictor of cognitive functioning in lupus. *Lupus.*, 2006, 15, 858-64.

[35] Picillo, U; Italian, G; Marcialis, MR; Ginolfi, F; Abbate, G; Tufano, MA. Bilateral femoral osteomyelitis with knee arthritis due to Salmonella enteritidis in a patient with systemic lupus erythematosus. *Clin Rheumatol.*, 2001, 20, 53-6.

[36] Huang, JL; Hung, JJ; Wu, KC; Lee, WI; Chan, CK; Ou, LS. Septic Arthritis in Patients with Systemic Lupus Erythematosus: Salmonella and Nonsalmonella Infections Compared Semin *Arthritis Rheum.*, 2006, 36, 61-7.

[37] Van de Laar, MA; Meenhorst, PL; Van Soesbergen, RM; Olsthoorn, PG; Van der Korst, JK. Polyarticular Salmonella bacterial arthritis in a patient with systemic lupus erythematosus. *J Rheumatol*, 1989, 16, 231-4.

[38] Murakami, K; Matsumoto, K; Iizuka, T. Suppurativ arthritis of the temporomandibular joint: report of a case with special reference to arthroscopic observations. *J Maxillofac Surg*, 1984, 12, 41-5.

[39] Heffez, LB; Mafee, MF; Rosenberg, HM. Imaging atlas of the temporomandibular joint. 1st ed. Philadelphia, PA: *Williams & Wilkins*, 1995.

[40] Schellhas, KP; Wilkes, CH; Fritts, HM; Omlie, MR; Lagrotteria, LB. MR of osteochondritis dissecans and avascular necrosis of the mandibular condyle. *AJR Am J Roentgenol*, 1989, 152, 551-560.

[41] Lanigan, DT; Hey, JH; West, RA. Aseptic necrosis following maxillary osteotomies: report of 36 cases. *J Oral Maxillofac Surg*, 1990, 48, 142-156.

[42] lida, K; Kurita, K; Tange, K; Yoshida, K. Necrosis of the articular tubercle after repeated injections of sodium hyaluronate in the temporomandibular joint: a case report. *Int J Oral Maxillofac Surg*, 1998, 27, 278-279.

[43] Glimcher, MJ; Kenzora, JE. The biology of osteonecrosis of the femoral head and its clinical implications: An abridged communication. *Clin Ortho*, 1978, 130, 47-50.

[44] Gladman, DD; Chaudhry-Ahluwalia, V; Ibanez, D; Bogoch, E; Urowitz, MB. Outcomes of symptomatic osteonecrosis in 95 patients with systemic lupus Erythematosus. *J Rheumatol*, 2001, 28, 2226-9.

[45] Chuong, R; Piper, MA; Boland, TJ. Osteonecrosis of the mandibular condyle. Pathophysiology and core decompression. *Oral Surg Oral Med Oral Pathol Oral Radiol Endod.*, 1995, 79, 539-45

[46] Soulafa, A. Almazrooa and Sook-Bin Woo Bisphosphonate and Nonbisphosphonate-Associated Osteonecrosis of the Jaw: *A Review J Am Dent Assoc*, 2009, 140, 864-875.

[47] Gebhard, KL; Maibach, HI. Relationship between systemic corticosteroids and osteonecrosis. *Am J Clin Dermatol*, 2001, 2, 377-388.

In: Autoimmune Diseases: Symptoms, Diagnosis and Treatment   ISBN: 978-1-61668-007-7
Editor: Kyle J. Brenner, pp. 329-339   © 2010 Nova Science Publishers, Inc.

Chapter 12

FATIGUE IN GUILLAIN-BARRÉ SYNDROME: ACTIVITY-DEPENDENT CONDUCTION BLOCK

Hiroyuki Nodera[1] and Atsuko Nodera[2]*

[1]Department of Neurology and Neuroscience, Weill Cornell Medical College, New York, NY USA,
[2]Department of Neurology, Tokushima University, Tokushima Japan

ABSTRACT

Fatigue is commonly reported by patients with Guillain-Barré syndrome (GBS), even long after the patients "recover" from the weakness and when no apparent weakness by brief muscle strength testing is present. Fatigue may be a major limiting factor for GBS survivors in social life. The causes for the fatigue are multifactorial, including dysfunction of central and peripheral nervous systems, including depression and other mental conditions. However, the objective analysis of fatigue in GBS may not be straightforward, since many patients with such condition show unremarkable results of conventional nerve conduction studies. The authors discuss little known concept of activity-dependent conduction block (ADCB), a conduction characterized by nerve conduction failure induced by high frequency nerve transmission as occurring in prolonged muscle contraction. The mechanism behind this is transient hyperpolarization of axon membrane by activation of Na^+-K^+-ATP pump, which is triggered by axonal depolarization when impulse transmission and influx of Na^+ occur. Neurophysiologic techniques to identify ADCB include recording of compound muscle action potentials (CMAP) serially before and after supramaximal voluntary muscle contraction. In ADCB there is temporary conduction block after muscle contraction, demonstrated as lower CMAP amplitudes, prolongation of CMAP durations, and lower conduction velocities. Better recognition of fatigue in GBS by appropriate tests and potential therapeutic intervention based on the pathophysiology is important.

---

* Corresponding author: Department of Neurology and Neuroscience, Weill Cornell Medical College, 1305 York Avenue, Rm 217, New York, NY 10021 USA, E-mail: hin2003@med.cornell.edu, phone: 646-962-3202

INTRODUCTION

The long-term prognosis of Guillain-Barré syndrome (GBS) is considered to be favorable in majority of the patients. However, many of such patients with "full recovery by physicians" do complain of fatigue and may limit the quality of life after returning to the social life. The possible mechanisms for fatigue in GBS will be discussed, focusing on a concept called "activity-dependent conduction block".

Fatigue in GBS

The long-term prognosis of GBS is highly variable and its prediction depends on many factors. Van Koningsveld and colleagues studied the prognostic factors of the 388 participants from randomised clinical trials and found three variables that were predictive of poor outcome at 6 months: age, preceding diarrhea, and GBS disability score at 2 weeks after entry (van Koningsveld et al., 2007). However, even though there is no or little neurological deficit by standard neurological examinations, residual dysfunction is common in GBS. The residual signs in a group of seriously paralyzed GBS patients are reported (follow-up 2-24 years). Thirty-five percent of the patients had recovered completely at the time of the follow-up examination, 35% had minimal residual motor signs and 30% had a moderate or severe residual paresis. The most serious residua were found distally in the legs. More than half of the patients considered themselves to be cured. The others were more or less handicapped by their sequelae. Of the adults, 60% resumed work, 25% found a less demanding job and 15% did not return to work (de Jager and Minderhoud, 1991). Many patients with GBS suffer from severe residual fatigue that has an uncertain basis. Garssen determined the relative contribution of peripheral and central factors during a 2-min fatiguing sustained maximal voluntary contraction (MVC) in 10 neurologically well-recovered GBS patients and 12 age- and sex-matched healthy controls. Physiological fatigue was defined as the decline of voluntary force during an MVC of the biceps brachii. Relative amounts of peripheral fatigue and central activation failure were determined combining voluntary force and force responses to electrical stimulation. Surface electromyography was used to determine muscle-fiber conduction velocity. During the first minute of sustained MVC, peripheral fatigue developed more slowly in patients than in controls. Central fatigue only occurred in patients. The muscle-fiber conduction velocity was higher in patients. The initial MVC, decrease of MVC, initial force response, and initial central activation failure did not significantly differ between the groups. Although peripheral mechanisms cannot be excluded in the pathogenesis of residual fatigue after GBS, these results suggest that central changes are involved (Garssen et al., 2007).

Various neurological diseases demonstrate fatigue (Tables 1 and 2). Since the perception of fatigue is subjective, no exact definition exists because of overlap between the lay notion of tiredness and the clinically relevant symptom of fatigue. It is not the same as muscle weakness, depression, or muscle fatigability, and it is not a non-specific outcome of chronic illness. For clinical use, fatigue is best defined as difficulty in initiation of or sustaining voluntary activities (Chaudhuri and Behan, 2004), but also defined as a reduction of the maximal force-generating capacity of a muscle induced by exercise. Experienced fatigue has both psychological and physiological dimensions and relates to personal experience; it can best be quantified with questionnaires such as Fatigue Severity Scale (Krupp et al., 1989).

Mechanism of fatigue in GBS

Central causes

Figure 1 shows the responsible lesions for central fatigue associated with central neurological diseases. Post-stroke fatigue is considered to be due to interruption of the connection between the prefrontal cortex and thalamus as well as disturbance of the limbic integration for cortically-driven voluntary activities (Chaudhuri and Behan, 2004). Fatigue is caused in patients with posterior fossa lesions including Chiari malformations likely due to changes in ascending serotonergic tone and amounts of substance P. In hypothalamic, pituitary, and diencephalic lesions, fatigue is associated with endocrine disturbance and changes in bodyweight and sleep pattern, further explained by reduced concentrations of cytokines, substance P, leptons, and prostagrandins. Although fatigue is one of the most disabling residual symptoms and seriously affects quality of life in GBS patients, its pathophysiological mechanisms remain unknown, but the role of afferent sensory input in the perceived sensation of central fatigue is proposed. Since GBS most affects large myelinated fibers which conduct proprioceptive afferent sensation, whereas pain transmission through unmyelinated C fibers are relatively intact. This sensory mismatch generates a high perception of effort probably because unpleasant or painful sensations associated with motor activities are registered earlier than normal (Chaudhuri and Behan, 2004). Also, fatigue in GBS is explained by peripheral mechanisms. Garssen and colleagues performed standardized nerve conduction (NC) studies in 13 fatigued patients who were relatively well recovered GBS (6 men, 7 women; aged 26-66 (mean age of 52.1 years)), mean 5.7 years after diagnosis (range 3.1-12.1 years). Most NC values in GBS patients were remarkably restored and within normal values. No correlations were found between the electrophysiological findings and the fatigue scores, muscle strength, or functional scores. They concluded that fatigue in GBS is not explained by residual nerve dysfunction, using conventional NC measurements (Garssen et al., 2006b). However, it has been understood that the degree of conduction failure by demyelination is not constant, and influenced by multiple factors such as temperature and exercise. Thus, the absence of demyelination in the baseline tests does not necessarily exclude the possibility of transient conduction failure in certain conditions, such as transient conduction block induced by exercise (activity-dependent conduction block) (ADCB).

Peripheral Cause: Activity-Dependent Conduction Block

Saltatory transmission of the myelinated peripheral nerve is influenced by number of factors. The most notable example is clinically called Uhthoff's phenomenon in multiple scletrosis, that is transient worsening of symptoms on elevation of body temperature (e.g. during a hot bath), originally described by Uhthoff in 1889. This phenomenon was electrophysiologically confirmed that demyelinating axons demonstrated conduction slowing at higher temperature (Rasminsky, 1973). If excessive, demyelinating axon eventually causes transient conduction block. Despite of the long recognition, the pathomechanism of Uhthoff's phenomenon has not been fully elucidated. The potential etiology of Uhthoff's phenomenon may be multifactorial, including heat itself, effects of serum calcium level, blockade of ion channels, circulatory changes, heat shock proteins, and unidentified humoral substances (Guthrie and Nelson, 1995).

Less recognized phenomenon of transient worsening of axonal conduction is called ADCB or frequency-dependent conduction block, defined as transient conduction block (CB) induced by brief exercise. ADCB has been clinically and electrophysiologically observed in various demyelinating peripheral nerve diseases such as chronic inflammatory demyelinating polyneuropathy (CIDP), diabetic neuropathy, and multifocal motor neuropathy (MMN) (Kuwabara et al., 1999; Cappelen-Smith et al., 2000; Nodera et al., 2006; Krishnan et al., 2008).

Cappelen–Smith et al. studied patients with CIDP (Cappelen-Smith et al., 2000). By using the conventional technique of nerve conduction studies, they stimulated the median nerve at the wrist and recorded over the abductor pollicis brevis, comparing the compound muscle action potential (CMAP) parameters at baseline and serially recording after 1 minute of maximal voluntary contraction (MVC). Transient conduction block, manifested as decreased CMAP amplitude, was identified.

Neurophysiologic Tests to Identify ADCB

There have been several techniques to assess ADCB, which will be discussed in this section.

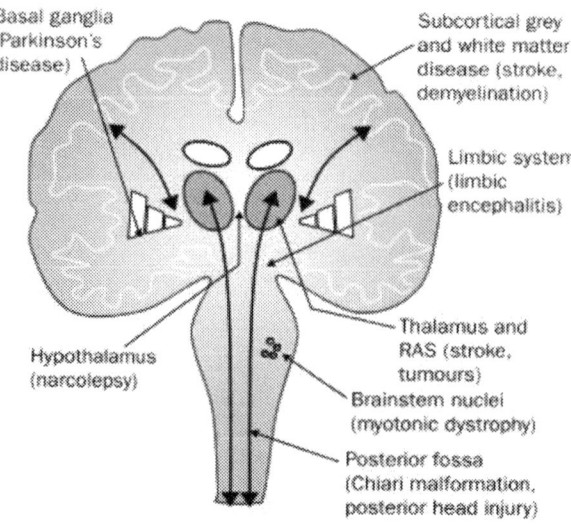

Figure 1. Responsible lesions for central fatigue in neurological diseases (Chaudhuri and Behan, 2004). RAS = reticular activating system

Table 1. Neurological disorders associated with central fatigue (Chaudhuri and Behan, 2004)

Symptomatic
Cerebral vasculitis and cerebrovascular diseases
Channelopathies
Developmental disorders (cerebral palsy, Chiari malformations)
Dysautonomic states
Encephalitis lethargica
Granulomatous disorders (neurosarcoid, Wegener's granulomatosis)
Hypothalamic and pituitary diseases
Intracranial infections (meningitis and encephalitis)
Metabolic encephalopathy and mitochondrial diseases
Migraine
Motor neuron disease
Multiple sclerosis
Multiple system atrophy
Myotonic dystrophy
Narcolepsy and related sleep disorders
Paraneoplastic (limbic encephalitis, opsoclonus-myoclonus)
Parkinson's disease and other parkinsonian disorders
Posterior head injury
Post-Guillain Barré syndrome fatigue
Postinfective fatigue states (poliomyelitis, Lyme disease, Qfever, and viral fatigue)
Postoperative (posterior fossa and cardiopulmonary bypass surgery)
Idiopathic
Chronic fatigue syndrome/myalgic encephalomyelitis

Table 2. Neurological disorders associated with peripheral fatigue revised from Chaudhuri and Behan (Chaudhuri and Behan, 2004).

Muscle disorders
Polymyositis and dermatomyositis
Muscular dystrophies
Metabolic myopathies
Mitochondrial disorders
Neuromuscular junction disorders
Autoimmune myasthenia gravis (generalised)
Lambert-Eaton myasthenic syndrome
Peripheral nerve disorders
Guillain-Barré syndrome (GBS)
Chronic Inflammatory Demyelinating Polyneuropathy (CIDP)

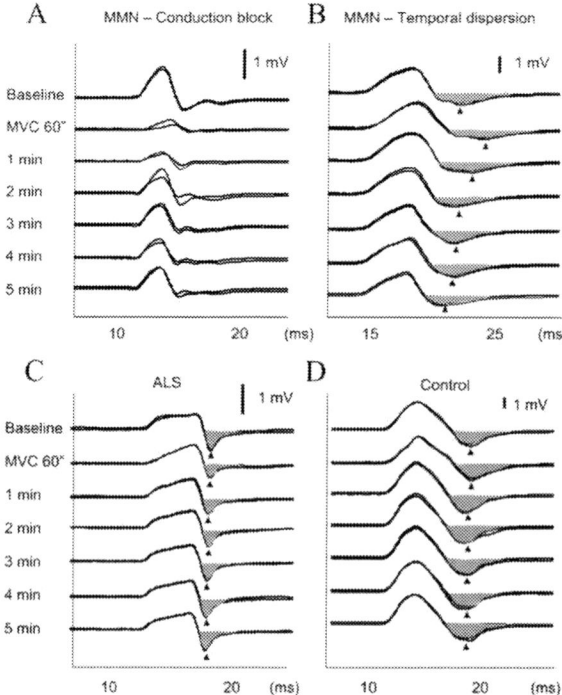

Figure 2. Activity-dependent conduction block in multifocal motor neuropathy (MMN) stimulated by magnetic stimulation of the cervical nerve root (Nodera et al., 2006). Note: (1) In MMN, two patterns of abnormality are identified. In conduction block (Panel A), the response amplitudes are transiently smaller, maximum immediately after 60 second maximum voluntary contraction (MVC) of the abductor pollicis brevis with slow recovery over the next few minutes. In temporal dispersion (Panel B), the response amplitudes are stable, but the response duration transiently increases. The positive segment (downward deflection) shown in gray demonstrates greater prolongation than the negative phase (upward deflection), because phase cancellation of the multiple motor units with different degrees of demyelination inhibits the prolongation of the negative phase

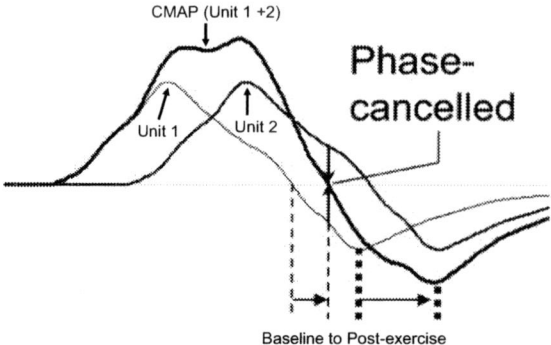

Figure 3. The explanation for Figure 2 showing greater prolongation of the positive phase in activity-dependent conduction block in multifocal motor neuropathy. The figure assumes that only two motor units comprise the compound muscle action potential (CMAP). Demyelination is to be present only in Unit 2 and CMAP to be the sum of Units 1 and 2, as shown in the thick line. Because there is phase cancellation between the negative phase (upward deflection) of the Unit 2 and the positive phase (downward deflection) of the Unit 1, the sum CMAP does not show significant prolongation of the negative phase. On the other hand, since no phase cancellation affects the positive phase, the positive phase shows greater degree of prolongation in the positive phase (Nodera et al., 2006)

Second, Kaji, Nodera, and Hitomi demonstrated ADCB in multifocal motor neuropathy (MMN) and CIDP by stimulating cervical nerve roots by magnetic stimulation over cervical spine (Kaji et al., 2000; Nodera et al., 2006; Hitomi et al., 2007). In detail, recording electrode is placed over abductor pollicis brevis (APB) or abductor digiti minimi, same placement as used in the routine nerve conduction study. As shown in Figure 2, normal controls showed almost identical morphology of the CMAPs (Figure 2D). However, detailed analysis demonstrates mild prolongation of CMAP duration, most notable in the positive phase (gray area) and positive peak (arrowhead), maximum immediately post exercise. ALS patients showed similar changes (Figure 2C). On the other hand, the patients with MMN showed two patterns of abnormality, CB and temporal dispersion. Figure 2A depicts the example of CB, which shows transient increase of distal latency (onset latency) and response amplitude maximum at immediate postexercise and slowly recovers few minutes after exercise. Figure 2B shows an example of temporal dispersion. As seen in normal controls (Figure 2D), there is transient prolongation of CMAP durations, more noticeable in the positive phase. In comparison to the normal control, the degree of prolongation in MMN is much greater, lasting 1-2 minutes after exercise. The reason for greater change of CMAP duration in the positive phase is unknown. One of the explanations is shown in Figure 3. Let's assume that there are only two motor units comprising the CMAP. A motor unit is a group of muscle fibers innervated by a single motoneuron, thus behaving similarly with transient conduction failure such as CB and temporal dispersion. Provided that demyelination s present only in Unit 2, CMAP as the sum of Units 1 and 2 changes its morphology as shown in the thick line. Because there is phase cancellation between the negative phase (upward deflection) of the Unit 2 and the positive phase (downward deflection) of the Unit 1, the sum CMAP does not show significant prolongation of the negative phase. On the other hand, since no phase cancellation affects the positive phase, the positive phase shows greater degree of prolongation in the positive phase.

Third, carpal tunnel syndrome (CTS), one of the most common entrapment neuropathy, has been reported to demonstrate ADCB (Kiernan et al., 1996; Miller et al., 1996; Cappelen-Smith et al., 2003; Burke, 2006; Watson et al., 2006). As ADCB is able to be demonstrated by the same technique as reported in CIDP (Cappelen-Smith et al., 2000), Watson reported the clinical usefulness of repetitive stimulation in CTS (Watson et al., 2006). Repetitive stimulation testing is useful in detecting impairment of neuromuscular junctions, such as myasthenia gravis, Lambert-Eaton myasthenic syndrome, botulism, and so forth. Decrement of the amplitudes and areas of the CMAP by low-frequency repetitive stimulation (typically 10 stimulations at 2-3 Hz) is observed in these conditions and increment of the amplitudes and areas is suggestive of pre-synaptic neuromuscular junction disorders such as Lambert-Eaton myasthenic syndrome and botulism. Watson and colleagues performed repetitive nerve stimulation test by stimulating median nerve at the wrist and recording over APB, 20 stimulations ranging from 1 Hz to 30 Hz (Watson et al., 2006). In normal controls, a phenomenon called "pseudofacilitation" occurs, that is mild increase in CMAP amplitude (usually up to 30%). The explanation of pseudofacilitation includes (1) shortening of muscle fibers, (2) increase of muscle conduction velocity, and (3) transient muscle membrane hyperpolarization due to activation of Na^+-K^+-ATPase (McComas et al., 1994; Rutkove, 2000; van Dijk et al., 2000). In CTS, however, repetitive stimulation rather shows decrement of the CMAP amplitudes (Figure 4), notable in patients with severe CTS and at high stimulation frequency (Figure 5)(Watson et al., 2006). Since repetitive stimulation is painful, especially in patients with demyelinating neuropathy who have much higher stimulation threshold than normal nerves, it is advisable to limit the number of stimulation and stimulation frequency at minimum. To the author's knowledge, there has not been any report of the usefulness of repetitive stimulation testing in GBS.

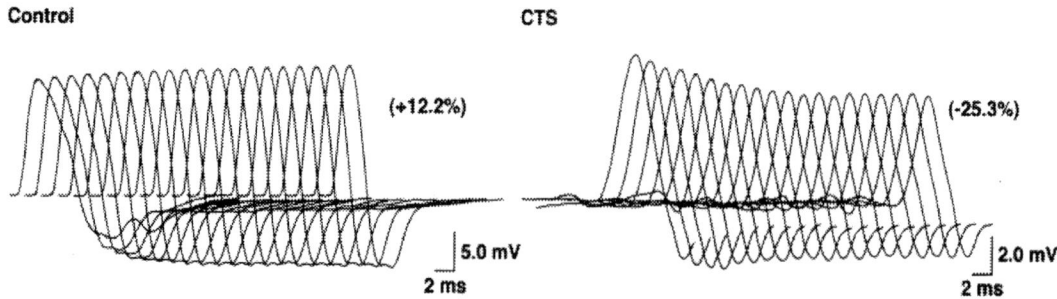

Figure 4. Typical thenar motor recordings (compound muscle action potentials: CMAP) from a control subject and a patient with carpal tunnel syndrome (CTS) in response to 20 stimuli delivered at 30 HZ. Note the characteristic increase in CMAP amplitudes between the 1st and 20th response in the control subject and the decrease in CMA amplitudes in the CTS subject (Watson et al., 2006)

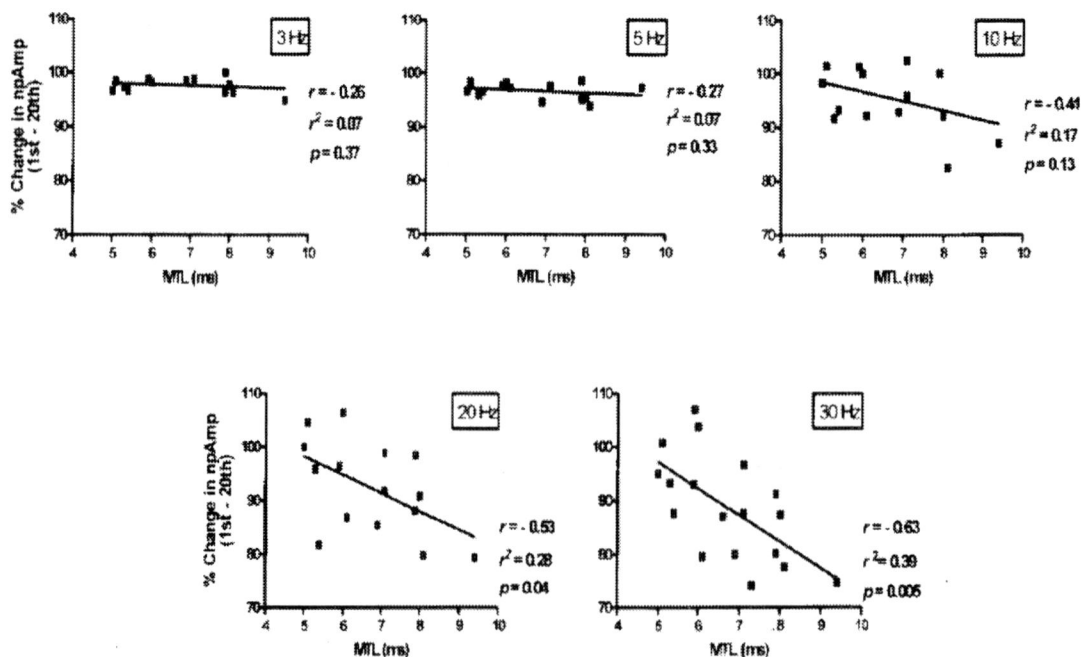

Figure 5. The association of the percent change in compound muscle action potentials (CMAPs) with distal motor terminal latency (MTL) in CTS subjects while stimulating the median nerve and recording over the thenar eminence at increasing frequencies (3, 5, 10, 20, and 30 HZ) (Watson et al., 2006). Note that (1) decrement of the CMAP amplitude is greater in severe CTS (longer distal motor terminal latency) and (2) CMAP decrement is greater at higher frezuencies

Therapy for Fatigue in GBS

Only a handful clinical trials has been conducted for fatigue in patients with GBS. Garssen and colleagues performed a randomised, double blind, placebo controlled, crossover trial of amantadine (Garssen et al., 2006a). Amantadine is a NMDA receptor antagonist which blocks presynaptic dopamine reuptake and stimulates postsynaptic receptors, thus is theoretically effective for fatigue. Seventy-four patients with GBS with severe fatigue, defined as a mean fatigue score ≥ 5 on the Fatigue Severity Scale (FSS), were randomized. The primary outcome measure was improvement of FSS (≥ 1), while the secondary outcome measures were impact of fatigue, anxiety, and depression, handicap, and quality of life. Up to 200 mg daily dose of amantadine was given to the patients. There was no significant difference in any of the primary and secondary measures.

Another potential therapeutic intervention for fatigue in GBS, although no clinical data is available, would be to block Na^+-K^+-ATPase by digitalis and other agents, especially if ADCB is confirmed. In central nervous system demyelination such as multiple sclerosis and Pelizaeus-Merzbacher disease, promising effect of digitalis has been reported (Kaji and Sumner, 1989a; Kaji and Sumner, 1989b; Nezu et al., 1996). Still, since Na^+-K^+-ATPase is integral for normal central and peripheral nervous system, careful therapeutic intervention is essential.

Recently, the sustained release form of 4-animopyridine (3,4 DAP) was approved by Food and Drug Administration for the treatment of fatigue in multiple sclerosis, another demyelinating disease. Its pharmaceutical mechanism of action is to block axonal fast K^+ channel, thus extending the depolarizing phase of the axon membrane. Whether the same therapeutic strategy is beneficial also in GBS is an open question.

CONCLUSION

Fatigue in GBS is underappreciated by physicians, but it limits the long-term quality of life in GBS sufferers who superficially appear to be "cured". Various mechanisms affecting both central and peripheral nervous systems are proposed, including activity-dependent conduction block. New medication for fatigue based on its pathophysiology is awaited.

REFERENCES

Burke, D. Frequency-dependent conduction block in carpal tunnel syndrome. *Muscle Nerve*, 2006, 33, 587-8.

Cappelen-Smith, C; Kuwabara, S; Lin, CS; Mogyoros, I; Burke, D. Activity-dependent hyperpolarization and conduction block in chronic inflammatory demyelinating polyneuropathy. *Ann Neurol*, 2000, 48, 826-32.

Cappelen-Smith, C; Lin, CS; Burke, D. Activity-dependent hyperpolarization and impulse conduction in motor axons in patients with carpal tunnel syndrome. *Brain*, 2003, 126, 1001-8.

Chaudhuri, A; Behan, PO. Fatigue in neurological disorders. *Lancet* 2004; 363: 978-88.

de Jager AE, Minderhoud JM. Residual signs in severe Guillain-Barre syndrome: analysis of 57 patients. *J Neurol Sci*, 1991, 104, 151-6.

Garssen, MP; Schillings, ML; Van Doorn, PA; Van Engelen, BG; Zwarts, MJ. Contribution of central and peripheral factors to residual fatigue in Guillain-Barre syndrome. *Muscle Nerve*, 2007, 36, 93-9.

Garssen, MP; Schmitz, PI; Merkies, IS; Jacobs, BC; van der Meche, FG; van Doorn, PA. Amantadine for treatment of fatigue in Guillain-Barre syndrome: a randomised, double blind, placebo controlled, crossover trial. *J Neurol Neurosurg Psychiatry*, 2006a, 77, 61-5.

Garssen, MP; van Doorn, PA; Visser, GH. Nerve conduction studies in relation to residual fatigue in Guillain-Barre syndrome. *J Neurol*, 2006b, 253, 851-6.

Guthrie, TC; Nelson, DA. Influence of temperature changes on multiple sclerosis: critical review of mechanisms and research potential. *J Neurol Sci*, 1995, 129, 1-8.

Hitomi, T; Kaji, R; Murase, N; Kohara, N; Mezaki, T; Nodera, H; et al. Dynamic change of proximal conduction in demyelinating neuropathies: a cervical magnetic stimulation combined with maximum voluntary contraction. *Clin Neurophysiol*, 2007, 118, 741-50.

Kaji, R; Bostock, H; Kohara, N; Murase, N; Kimura, J; Shibasaki, H. Activity-dependent conduction block in multifocal motor neuropathy. *Brain*, 2000, 123 (Pt 8), 1602-11.

Kaji, R; Sumner, AJ. Effect of digitalis on central demyelinative conduction block in vivo. *Ann Neurol*, 1989a, 25, 159-65.

Kaji, R; Sumner, AJ. Ouabain reverses conduction disturbances in single demyelinated nerve fibers. *Neurology*, 1989b, 39, 1364-8.

Kiernan, M; Mogyoros, I; Burke, D. Changes in excitability and impulse transmission following prolonged repetitive activity in normal subjects and patients with a focal nerve lesion. *Brain*, 1996, 119 (Pt 6), 2029-37.

Krishnan, A; Lin, C; Kiernan, M. Activity-dependent excitability changes suggest Na+/K+ pump dysfunction in diabetic neuropathy. *Brain*, 2008, 131, 1209-16.

Krupp, LB; LaRocca, NG; Muir-Nash, J; Steinberg, AD. The fatigue severity scale. Application to patients with multiple sclerosis and systemic lupus erythematosus. *Arch Neurol*, 1989, 46, 1121-3.

Kuwabara, S; Nakajima, Y; Hattori, T; Toma, S; Mizobuchi, K; Ogawara, K. Activity-dependent excitability changes in chronic inflammatory demyelinating polyneuropathy: A microneurographic study. *Muscle Nerve*, 1999, 22, 899-904.

McComas, AJ; Galea, V; Einhorn, RW. Pseudofacilitation: a misleading term. *Muscle Nerve*, 1994, 17, 599-607.

Miller, T; Kiernan, M; Mogyoros, I; Burke, D. Activity-dependent changes in impulse conduction in a focal nerve lesion. *Brain*, 1996, 119 (Pt 2), 429-37.

Nezu, A; Kimura, S; Osaka, H; Kobayashi, T; Ohtsuki, N. Effect of digitalis on conduction dysfunction in Pelizaeus-Merzbacher disease. *J Neurol Sci*, 1996, 141, 49-53.

Nodera, H; Bostock, H; Izumi, Y; Nakamura, K; Urushihara, R; Sakamoto, T; et al. Activity-dependent conduction block in multifocal motor neuropathy: magnetic fatigue test. *Neurology*, 2006, 67, 280-7.

Rasminsky, M. The effects of temperature on conduction in demyelinated single nerve fibers. *Arch Neurol*, 1973, 28, 287-92.

Rutkove, SB. Pseudofacilitation: A temperature-sensitive phenomenon. *Muscle Nerve*, 2000, 23, 115-8.

van Dijk JG; van der Hoeven BJ; van der Hoeven H. Repetitive nerve stimulation: effects of recording site and the nature of 'pseudofacilitation'. *Clin Neurophysiol* 2000, 111, 1411-9.

van Koningsveld R; Steyerberg EW; Hughes RA; Swan AV; van Doorn PA; Jacobs BC. A clinical prognostic scoring system for Guillain-Barre syndrome. *Lancet Neurol* 2007, 6, 589-94.

Watson BV; Brown WF; Doherty TJ. Frequency-dependent conduction block in carpal tunnel syndrome. *Muscle Nerve* 2006, 33, 619-26.

Chapter 13

COULD COMPUTERIZED DEVICES FOR OPTIC NERVE HEAD ANALYSIS FIND OUT LOSS OF GANGLION CELLS IN NOT-GLAUCOMATOUS DAMAGE?

Michele Iester[*], *Marina Papadia and Alessandro Bagnis*

Laboratorio clinico anatomo-funzionale per la diagnosi e il trattamento del glaucoma e delle malattie neuro-oftalmologiche, Clinica Oculistica, Department of Neurological Sciences, Ophthalmology, Genetic, University of Genoa, Italy

Multiple sclerosis (MS) is a chronic neurological autoimmune disease that can affect vision. Visual complaints might be one of the first signs of MS and the ophthalmologist can be the first physician consulted, therefore familiarity with the pathology and appropriate diagnosis are of great importance. This pathology typically occurs in young people (mean age between 20 and 40 years) and the incidence is higher in women. The aetiopathology is still unknown, but seems to be multifactorial. The environment seems to play an important role and migration studies showed that people moving before age 15 have the same risk level as the native population of the nation they move in. Genetics has an important role too: the association with HLA-DR2 antigen is proved, and the association of MS susceptibility with two or more genes is suspected. First degree family members of MS patients have approximately 10 times greater chance to develop the pathology compared to controls. Another etiological theory is that the infection of a virus in childhood might cause in genetically predisposed patients the activation of the immune system after years of latency. Demyelination of the optic nerve caused by the autoimmune attack leads to ganglion cell loss and subsequent nerve atrophy [1]. The tissue damage often involves the prechiasmatic visual pathways. With the progession of the disease, demyelination is associated with mononuclear cell infiltration and removal of myelin by macrophages. At the end stage of the pathology common findings are gliotic lesions ("plaques") that derive from astrocytic proliferation with production of glial fibrils.

---

[*] Corresponding author: Associate Professor, Clinica Oculistica, Università di Genova, Viale benedetto XV, 5, 16132 Genoa, Italy, Phone: 010 353 8455, Fax: 010 353 8494, e-mail: iester@unige.it

A descriptive postmortem study of patients with multiple sclerosis and in vivo magnetic resonance imaging studies found the presence of RNFL atrophy in association with optic nerve atrophy, although neither was measured quantitatively [2-5].

Clinically, in 1974 Frisen and Hoyt noted that in multiple sclerosis RNFL was different from healthy subjects [6], in particular, in patients with multiple sclerosis, RNFL abnormalities have been found in up to 80% by inspection of red-free retinal photographs [2,3]. Also optic disc pallor detected by direct ophthalmoscopy or by slides has been described in up to 71% of eyes previously affected by optic neuritis [3,4].

Because clinical assessment is somewhat subjective, prone to interobserver variability, and does not produce quantitative data, in the last decades new computerized techniques have been developed to quantify retinal ganglion cells objectively [7]. On the marketing there are many different systems, those with more capacity to detect a morphometric changes are the Nerve Fiber Analyzer (GDx VCC), the Heidelberg Retina Tomograph 3 (HRT 3) and the Optical Coherence Tomograph 3 (OCT 3). The other systems, such as the Optical Coherence Tomograph Scanning Laser Ophthalmoscopy (OCT SLO), are at the moment good to evaluate the posterior pole morphologically, but they are not provided with an algorithm able to quantify any loss of ganglion cells.

The clinical application of HRT, GDx VCC and OCT has been clearly demonstrated in glaucoma, where reduction of the RNFL outside the optic nerve head (ONH) and the enlargement of the optic cup [8-11] can be hereby quantified. Furthermore the correlation between retinal nerve fiber layer thickness (RNFLt) and visual field loss and could potentially be used as an indicator of early glaucomatous changes [12-15].

Nowadays new applications of these instruments are evaluated. They could be helpful in the diagnosis of pathologies characterized by ganglion cell loss.

RETINAL NERVE ANALYZER - GDX VCC

This instrument analyzes RNFL of each eye using a confocal scanning laser polarimeter with a 780 nm polarized light source. The image analyzer allows ignoring retinal vessels when assessing RNFL [13,14]. Such technique is highly reproducible and has already been fully described by many authors [14-22].

Briefly, a complete scan consists of 128 X 256 pixels. The field of view used by the system is 40° X 20°. Upon data acquisition, a computer algorithm calculates the amount of retardation at each measured retinal position. A retardation map describes the change in the state of polarization (retardation) at each location within the field of view. Each pixel represents the amount of retardation at a particular location. The GDx VCC compensates for corneal birefringence using a variable cornea compensator that allows compensation for each specific cornea individually.

For the analysis of each image, four points are positioned: one on the extreme superior, nasal, inferior and temporal outer margin of optic nerve head to create an ellipse approximately placed around the inner margin of the peripapillary scleral ring. Retardation information is than obtained for a 10 pixel width ellipse concentric with the disc margin. Using the standard ellipse which appears as a 10 pixel green ellipse on the GDx display, the system assesses the RNFLT at 1.75 disc diameter (DD) from the outer edge of the optic nerve head. To evaluate in a better way the possible RNFL loss the 360° circumference is divided into 36 segments measuring 10° each and the RNFLT is calculated for each segment.

HEIDELBERG RETINA TOMOGRAPH (HRT)

The HRT is a confocal scanning diode laser with a wavelength of 670 nm. A series of confocal images based on the depth of the ONH (8 images for 1 mm) is obtained at consecutive focal planes, each 386 x 386 pixels in size that the computer converts into a single tridimensional topographic image. The depth of each topographic image series ranges between 0.5 mm and 4.0 mm depending on individual differences in the optic disc morphology. For each eye, three 15° confocal scanning laser tomographic images are obtained and a mean three-dimensional image is created and the mean standard deviation of the height of each pixel is calculated. The optic disc margin defined as the inner edge of Elshnig's ring is outlined by an experienced observer. The technique including its reproducibility and reliability have already been described in detail elsewhere [23-28]. The HRT variables are measured for the optic disc both as a whole and in four separate disc sectors. This disc sectioning is different from previous studies in which the optic nerve head is divided into six sectors: superotemporal, superonasal, nasal, inferonasal, inferotemporal and temporal [29].

Disc Area or Global Area, Cup Shape Measure (CSM), Rim Volume or Volume Above Reference (RV), Height Variation Contour (HVC), Retinal Nerve Fiber Layer Thickness (RNFLT), Rim Area (RA), Inferior Area Below Reference (ABRI), Inferior Effective Area (EAI), Nasal Mean Height Contour (MHCN), Temporal Mean Height Contour (MHCT), Superior Peak Height Contour (PHCS), Cup Area or Area Below Reference (CA), and Cup Volume or Volume Below Reference (CV) are some of the HRT parameters.

Based on the confocal laser scanning measurements of the optic nerve head, different classification methods have been introduced such as the Moorfields regression analysis, the discriminant formulas and the Glaucoma Probability score [30].

OPTICAL COHERENCE TOMOGRAPHY (OCT)

Cross-sectional imaging of peripapillary RNFL was performed with the Stratus OCT (model 3000, software version 4.04, Carl Zeiss Meditec, Dublin, CA). While seated, the subject's chin was steadied on a chin rest. The OCT lens was adjusted for the patient's refractive error. After the other eye was covered, the machine was aligned to register an image of the fundus through the pupil. The subject was then instructed to fixate on a target the eye examined, to bring the optic nerve head within view of the examiner in real time. The Z-offset was adjusted to bring the OCT image into view. Polarization was adjusted to obtain the strongest signal. The aiming circle was adjusted by the operator to match the optic nerve head so that the nerve head scan would acquire a circular B-scan OCT image at a radius of 1.73 mm around the center of the optic nerve head. The scan circle around the disc thus had a diameter of 3.46 mm. If the amount of peripapillary atrophy exceeded the scan circle, which was visible and controlled by the operator, the patient was excluded [7].

The fast RNFL scans were used to calculate the overall and quadrantic RNFL thickness. The following criteria were used to assess scan quality: the fundus image should be clear enough to see the optic disc and the scan circle, color saturation should be even and dense across the entire scan, signal strength should be 6 or more, and there should be red color visible in the retinal pigment epithelium layer and RNFL, with no missing or blank area within the scan pattern. The scans were assessed to ascertain proper detection of RNFL boundaries by the software.

The RNFL analysis uses an automated computer algorithm to identify the anterior and posterior margins of the RNFL. This delineation is carried out by the computer calculating the boundary where the red reflectivity exceeds a set threshold. The data points between the 2 white lines delineating the RNFL then make up the RNFL thickness. The analysis algorithm averages the measurements around the circular scan to obtain 17 parameters per scan. These include the single mean RNFL thickness, the average thickness within each of 4 quadrants (temporal, superior, nasal, and inferior), and average thickness within each of 12 sectors corresponding to clock hours [7].

In literature some authors are trying to use these new imaging devices to detect loss of ganglion cells in MS. Parisi et al. tried to measure the ONH changes in ON by using OCT and they assessed axonal loss after a single clinical episode of unilateral optic neuritis. In particular, 14 multiple sclerosis patients previously affected by optic neuritis has demonstrated to have a reduction in RNFL thickness [31]. A 46% reduction of total RNFL thickness in affected eyes compared with control eyes was found, as well as a 28% reduction compared with unaffected fellow eyes. Furthermore the unaffected fellow eye RNFL thickness was reduced by 26% relative to control eyes.

It has been shown that the reductions in RNFL thickness in affected patient eyes compared with control and unaffected patient eyes were highly significant by using OCT [32-34]. These results were obtained using the most recent- and higher resolution-model of OCT (Stratus OCT Model 3000) and they found less reduction compared with control eyes but a similar reduction compared with unaffected fellow eyes. The lower reduction compared to control subjects in this study could be due to greater accuracy of the Stratus OCT and also because of differences in RNFL thickness in the control groups studied. A nonsignificant reduction in unaffected eyes compared to control eyes was found in this study [32], which again was of lower magnitude to the findings of Parisi and colleagues [31].

Fellow eye abnormalities do occur in unilateral optic neuritis [33], and a possible explanation for the difference between the two study findings (as well as technical differences relating to the OCT model used) is that the unaffected eyes in this study had a lesser degree of subclinical involvement than those in the study by Parisi and colleagues all of whom had clinically definite multiple sclerosis [31].

Some authors tried to study the ONH changes in ON and the reduction of the RNFLt by means of Optical Coherence Tomography (OCT) [33,34] and they confirmed the findings. Using HRT, Trip et al. detected relevant changes in the amount of ganglion cells. In particular they found a significant difference between the ON eyes and the unaffected fellow eyes for RV and mRNFLt [34]. In a recent study, Iester et al also showed a similar degree of RNFL loss by HRT and GDx VCC in patients with isolated optic neuritis and in those with multiple sclerosis [35]. The HRT Cup shape measure, which is the most sensitive parameter in distinguish normal from glaucomatous ONHs, does not show any difference between controls and both ON and unaffected eyes of MS patients. Also the Nerve Fiber Indicator did not have a good diagnostic capacity as in glaucoma clinics and they found a poor agreement between HRT and GDX VCC. However few GDx parameters show a good capacity to distinguish ON eyes and those without history of ON.

HRT, OCT and GDx VCC are to different confocal scanning techniques able to distinguish normal from glaucomatous eyes. Although the systems have been introduced to detect the ganglion cell loss in glaucomatous disease, the published data showed that some parameters of the GDx VCC and OCT have the capacity to distinguish eyes with old optic neuritis from the fellow ones. However, at this moment, only the HRT RNFLt seems to be able to detect MS changes. However HRT has been introduced to detect change of cup shape and change of volume due to loss of tissue such as in glaucoma and therefore might be not accurate in detecting MS neuritis. In MS disease patients can have loss of ganglion cells but without creating a deep cup, because astroglia cells can occupied the space. The only parameter able to detect a loss of ganglion cells was the mean RNFL thickness, which quantifies the ganglion cells on the outer edge of the rim, by using a reference plane as for software [35]. Indeed, the HRT Cup Shape Measure which is the most sensitive parameter in distinguish normal from glaucomatous ONHs, did not show any difference between normal patients and the two groups (post optic neuritis and without history). CSM indicated that the measurement was normal both in glaucoma and in normal control group. MS patients can suffer from loss of ganglion cells without creating a deep cup as astroglia cells can indeed occupy the damaged space. It seems likely that similar pathophysiological mechanisms of axonal damage occur in acute optic neuritis lesions as in other inflammatory multiple sclerosis lesions, regardless of whether it is clinically isolated or part of multiple sclerosis.

In a different way the GDx VCC is able to detect ganglion cell loss, it uses the difference in the retardation time that polarized light needs to cross the microtubule of the ganglion cell. A less diagnostic capacity has been showed by the GDx Nerve Fiber Indicator which was able to distinguish the two MS subgroups, and when the results were compared to normal database no significant difference was found, but the NFI values in the subgroup with the optic neuritis was higher than in the other subgroup and borderline in the normal confidence interval [35]. However GDx VCC could be able to detect also small differences between the two eyes: one with a large amount of ganglion cell loss post-ON and the other one with some subclinical involvement of the optic disc, but with a smaller loss of ganglion cells.

The OCT is able to assess in RNFL thickness based on the algorithm inside the system. It is able to quantify what Frisen and Hoyt found ophthalmoscopically [6].

The published data could suggest that after an optic neuritis, the optic disc decreases the number of ganglion cells. This loss is not like a glaucomatous damage where an increase of the cupping occurs. In MS optic neuritis the ganglion cell loose their own microtubule, but the space seems to be filled by astroglia. Imaging technologies could detect a different degree of RNFL loss between the eyes with ON and the unaffected fellow eyes, although they can not distinguish ON eyes from healthy control eyes yet. These new methods to assess the loss of RNFL could be very useful in clinics, but further studies needs to be done towards this direction.

REFERENCES

[1] Gartner, S. Optic neuropathy in multiple sclerosis. *Arch Ophthalmol*, 1953, 50, 718-726.

[2] MacFadyen, DJ; Drance, SM; Douglas GR; et al. The retinal nerve fiber layer, neuroretinal rim area, and visual evoked potentials in MS. *Neurology*, 1988, 38, 1353-1358.

[3] Elbol, P; Work, K. Retinal nerve fiber layer in multiple sclerosis. *Acta Ophthalmol*, (Copenh) 1990, 68, 481- 486.

[4] Trobe, JD; Glaser, JS; Cassady, JC. Optic atrophy. Differential diagnosis by fundus observation alone. *Arch Ophthalmol*, 1980, 98, 1040-1045.

[5] Kerrison, JB; Flynn, T; Green, WR. Retinal pathologic changes in multiple sclerosis. *Retina*, 1994, 14, 445- 451.

[6] Frisen, L; Hoyt, WF. Insidious atrophy of retinal nerve fibers in multiple sclerosis. Funduscopic identification in patients with and without visual complaints. *Arch Ophthalmol*, 1974, 92, 91-97.

[7] Iester, M; Garway-Heath, DF; Lemij, H. Optic nerve head and retinal nerve fiber analysis. *Dogma, Savona*, 2005.

[8] Airaksinen, PJ; Drance, SM; Douglas, GR; Mawson DK. Diffuse and localized nerve fiber loss in glaucoma. *Am J Ophthalmol*, 1984, 98, 566-571.

[9] Airaksinen, PJ; Drance, SM; Douglas, GR; Schulzcr, M; Wijsman, K. Visual field and retinal nerve fiber layer comparisons in glaucoma. *Arch Ophthalmol*, 1985, 103, 205-207.

[10] Caprioli, J; Miller, JM. Measurements of retinal nerve fiber layer surface height in glaucoma. *Ophthalmology*, 1989, 96, 633-641.

[11] Iester, M; Courtright, P; Mikelberg, FS. Retinal nerve fiber layer height in high-tension glaucoma and healthy eyes. *J Glaucoma*, 1998, 7, 1-7.

[12] Kamal, DS; Viswanthan, AC; Garway-Heath, DF; et al. Detection of optic disc change with the HRT before confirmed visual field change in ocular hypertensives converting to early glaucoma. *Br J Ophthalmol*, 1999, 83, 290-294.

[13] Chauhan, BC; McCormick, TA; Nicolela, MT; LeBlanc, RP. Optic disc and visual field changes in a prospective longitudinal study of patients with glaucoma. *Arch Ophthalmol*, 2001, 119, 1492-1499.

[14] Weinreb, RN; Shakiba, S; Zangwill, L. Scanning laser polarimetry to measure the nerve fiber layer of normal and glaucomatous eyes. *Am J Ophthalmol*, 1995, 119, 627-636.

[15] Tjon-Fo-Sang, MJ; Lemij, HG. The sensitivity and specificity of nerve fiber layer measurements in glaucoma as determined with scanning laser polarimetry. *Am J Ophthalmol*, 1997, 123, 62-9.

[16] Waldock, A; Potts, MJ; Sparrow, JM; Karwatowski, WSS. Clinical evaluation of scanning laser polarimetry: I Intraoperator reproducibility and design of a blood vessel removal algorithm. *Br J Ophthalmol*, 1998, 82, 252-259.

[17] Waldock, A; Potts, MJ; Sparrow, JM; Karwatowski, WSS. Clinical evaluation of scanning laser polarimetry: II Polar profile shape analysis. *Br J Ophthalmol*, 1998, 82, 260-266.

[18] Weinreb, RN; Dreher, AW; Coleman, A; Quigley, H; Shaw, B; Reiter, K. Histopathologic validation of four-ellipsometry measurements of retinal nerve fiber layer thickness. *Arch Ophthalmol*, 1990, 108, 557-560.

[19] Zhou, Q; Weinreb, RN. Individualized compansation for anterior segment birefringence during scanning laser polarimetry. *Invest Ophthalmol Vis Sci*, 2002, 43, 2221-2228.

[20] Zangwill, L; Berry, CA; Garden, VS; Weinreb, RN. Reproducibility of retardation measurements with the Nerve Fiber Analyzer II. *J Glaucoma*, 1997, 384-389.

[21] Hoh, ST; Ishikawa, H; Greenfield, DS; Liebmann, JM; Chew, SJ; Ritch, R. Peripapillary nerve fiber layer thickness measurement reproducibility using scanning laser polarimetry. *J Glaucoma*, 1998, 7, 12-15.

[22] Weinreb, RN; Shakiba, S; Sample, PA; et al. Association between quantitative nerve fiber layer of normal and glaucomatous eyes. *Am J Ophthalmol*, 1995, 120, 732-738.

[23] Dreher, AW; Tso, PC; Weinreb, RN. Reproducibility of topographic measurements of the normal and glaucomatous nerve head with the laser tomographic scanner. *Am J Ophthalmol*, 1991, 111, 221-229.

[24] Kruse, FE; Burk, ROW; Völcker, HE; et al. Reproducibility of topographic measurements of the optic nerve head with laser tomographic scanning. *Ophthalmology*, 1989, 96, 1320-1324.

[25] Cioffi, GA; Robin, AL; Eastman, RD; et al. Confocal laser scanning ophthalmoscope: reproducibility of optic nerve head topographic measurements with the confocal scanning laser ophthalmoscope. *Ophthalmology*, 1993, 100, 57-62.

[26] Weinreb, RN; Lusky, M; Bartsch, DU; Morsman, D. Effect of repetitive imaging on topographic measurements of the optic nerve head. *Arch Ophthalmol*, 1993, 111, 636-638.

[27] Mikelberg, FS; Wijsman, K; Schulzer, M. Reproducibility of topographic parameters obtained with the Heidelberg Retina Tomograph. *J Glaucoma*, 1993, 2, 101-103.

[28] Chauhan, BC; LeBlanc, RP; McCormick, TA; Rogers, JB. Test-retest variability of topographic measurements with confocal scanning laser tomography in patients with glaucoma and control subjects. *Am J Ophthalmol*, 1994, 118, 9-15.

[29] Iester, M; Swindale, NV; Mikelberg, FS. Sector based analysis of optic nerve head shape parameters and visual field indices in healthy and glaucomatous eyes. *J Glaucoma*, 1997, 6, 370-6.

[30] Iester, M; Perdicchi, A; Capris, E; Siniscalco, A; Calabria, GA; Recupero, SM. Comparison between discriminant analysis models and 'glaucoma probability score' for the detection of glaucomatous optic nerve head changes. *J Glaucoma*, (in press).

[31] Parisi, V; Manni, G; Spadaro, M; et al. Correlation between morphological and functional retinal impairment in multiple sclerosis patients. *Invest Ophthalmol Vis Sci*, 1999, 40, 2520-2527.

[32] Kerrison, JB; Flynn, T; Green, WR. Retinal pathologic changes in multiple sclerosis. *Retina*, 1994, 14, 445-451.

[33] Trip, SA; Schlottmann, PG; Jones, SJ; Garway-Heath, DF; Thompson, AJ; Plant, GT; Miller, DH. Quantification of optic nerve head topography in optic neuritis: a pilot study. *Br J Ophthalmol*, 2006, 90, 1128-1131.

[34] Trip, SA; Schlottmann, PG; Jones, SJ; Altmann, DR; Garway-Heath, DF; Thompson, AJ; Plant, GT; Miller, DH. Retinal nerve fiber layer axonal loss and visual dysfunction in optic neuritis. *Ann Neurol*, 2005, 58, 383-391.

[35] Iester, M; Cioli, F; Uccelli, A; Bandini, F; Papadia, M; Mancardi, GL; Calabria, GA. Retinal nerve fiber layer measurements and optic nerve head analysis in multiple sclerosis patients. *Eye* 2009, 23, 407-12.

None of the authors has proprietary interest in development or marketing of any product or instrument mentioned in this article

Part of these data has been published in: "Iester M, Cioli F, Uccelli A, Bandini F, Papadia M, Mancardi GL, Calabria GA. Retinal nerve fiber layer measurements and optic nerve head analysis in multiple sclerosis patients. Eye 2009, 23, 407-12".

Chapter 14

STRUCTURAL BIOLOGY INSIGHTS INTO THE AUTOANTIGENS OF THE MYELIN SHEATH

Petri Kursula
Department of Biochemistry, University of Oulu, Oulu, Finland and
CSSB-HZI, DESY, Hamburg, Germany

ABSTRACT

The fast 'saltatory' conduction of nerve impulses is mandatory for vertebrates, and the normal functioning of the nervous system requires a coordinated interplay between neurons and glia. One specific region of intercellular interactions is the myelin sheath, a tightly packed multilayered membrane structure, which is formed around myelinated axons in both the central (CNS) and peripheral nervous systems (PNS). Defective myelin in inherited or autoimmune disease causes severe neurological disorders, affecting both CNS and PNS. In addition, axonal regeneration in the adult CNS after neuronal injury is limited by myelin proteins interacting with the axonal surface. Myelin contains a specific set of proteins, which have unique properties and interact closely with membranes; several of them are also implicated as autoantigens. When structural and functional data on these molecules are obtained, we will be able to better understand the functions of myelin and the ways, in which its deficiencies may lead to disease. In this chapter, the current knowledge about myelin protein 3-dimensional structure and the interactions of myelin proteins with their ligands will be discussed, with specific emphasis on the implications for understanding autoimmune diseases of the nervous system, such as multiple sclerosis and Guillain-Barré syndrome.

THE MYELIN SHEATH

The rapid conduction of nerve impulses is mandatory for the normal functioning of the nervous system of vertebrates, which requires the coordinated interplay between neurons and glia. Cell proliferation, neuronal sprouting, and myelination are crucial processes involved in nervous system development and regeneration after injury. An important location of intercellular interaction is the myelin sheath, which is formed around myelinated axons by myelinating glial cells, *i.e.* Schwann cells in the PNS and oligodendrocytes in the CNS. De- or dysmyelination in hereditary or autoimmune diseases leads to severe, chronic neurological disorders, affecting both CNS and PNS. Axonal regeneration in the adult CNS after neuronal trauma is limited by myelin-specific components.

AUTOIMMUNE DISEASES RELATED TO MYELIN

Neuropathic diseases of the CNS and PNS create a serious medical and social problem. They often affect young people, leading to a chronic disability, the inability to work, and a dependence on social support for decades. One of the most common and best-characterized myelin-related diseases is multiple sclerosis (MS), with a prevalence of approximately 100 per 100 000 citizens in Europe; and even higher in Northern Europe, including Scandinavian countries and Scotland. MS is characterized by the presence of plaques in the CNS, in which myelin is destroyed. Most commonly, the disease starts to develop between the ages of 20 and 40 years, and females are more prone to get MS. The first phase of the disease is characterized most often by a relapsing-remitting cycle, and a secondary progressive MS develops during later years in life. The primary cause of MS is unknown, although both genetic and environmental factors have been highlighted, including molecular mimicry related to certain virus infections. At the molecular level, MS is characterized by autoimmunity towards the specific components of myelin, such as MBP and MOBP (Kaushansky *et al.* 2009b; Meinl & Hohlfeld 2002).

Guillain-Barré syndrome (GBS) is a group of autoimmune conditions, in which the immune response is directed against myelinated nerves (Hughes & Cornblath 2005). For the axonal forms, recent evidence suggests that microbial infections, especially of certain forms of *C. jejuni*, are involved in disease onset, *via* molecular mimicry against axonal gangliosides (Komagamine & Yuki 2006; Vucic *et al.* 2009; Yuki & Kuwabara 2007). On the other hand, antibodies against myelin proteins are likely to be involved in the AIDP (acute inflammatory demyelinating polyradiculoneuropathy) subtype of GBS (Hughes & Cornblath 2005). AIDP is reminiscent of the animal model EAN, which can be induced by different myelin proteins.

MAJOR AUTOANTIGENS OF MYELIN AND THEIR STRUCTURE

Myelin, the insulating, multi-layered membrane structure surrounding an axon, provides an increase in the speed of nerve impulses; thus, it is essential for proper functioning of the vertebrate nervous system. Myelin is mainly composed of lipid and protein, the latter constituting 20% of its dry weight. The two most abundant proteins in CNS myelin are the proteolipid protein and the myelin basic protein (MBP); they represent 50% and 30%, respectively, of the total myelin protein (Benjamins & Morell 1978).

The proteins present in myelin present one of the systematically largest gaps in our current structural knowledge of the protein universe (Xie & Bourne 2005). Several questions related to the structure of myelin proteins remain unanswered at the moment. What do their folded structures look like, both alone and in complex with other molecules? How do some of these molecules interact with the surface molecules of the neuronal membrane, and how do they contribute to the overall compact structure of the myelin sheath? And last but not least, what can we learn about the myelin-related handicapping diseases that affect both the central and peripheral nervous systems by studying the structures of the myelin proteins and their ligands?

The myelin proteins, in general, have unique biochemical and biophysical properties; this is related to the specific environment found in the tightly packed membrane environment. Such common properties of myelin-specific proteins include: 1) myelin-specific proteins interact intimately with the membrane; most of them are either peripheral or integral membrane proteins; 2) the cytoplasmic myelin proteins, and the cytoplasmic domains of transmembrane myelin proteins, often carry a high positive charge, with pI values often exceeding 10; 3) many myelin proteins are intrinsically disordered, or carry disordered cytoplasmic domains; 4) at the sequence level, the myelin-specific proteins share very little homology with other known protein sequences, making structure prediction difficult; 5) many of the myelin proteins are present at very high local concentrations *in vivo*. The following paragraphs of this chapter will give brief structural insights into the myelin-specific proteins that have received the most attention with respect to autoimmunity.

MYELIN BASIC PROTEIN (MBP)

MBP is essential for the formation of CNS myelin, and it is able to interact with a wide range of ligands, often polyanionic in nature (Boggs 2006), and including, for example, cytoskeletal proteins (Barylko & Dobrowolski 1984; Boggs & Rangaraj 2000; Boggs 2006; Dobrowolski *et al.* 1986; Hill & Harauz 2005). Due to the large number of charged residues and a low overall hydrophobicity, there is significant intramolecular electrostatic repulsion in MBP; thus, MBP is an extended, intrinsically unstructured protein in aqueous solution (Harauz *et al.* 2004). The MBP family comprises numerous developmentally regulated isoforms, of which the 18.5-kDa species is the most abundant in adult human myelin, and has been studied the most. This isoform further undergoes complex posttranslational modifications (PTM), giving rise to charge isomers designated as components C1 to C8 (Zand *et al.* 1998), of which C1 is the least modified, *i.e.* the 'wild-type' form, and C8 mimics the form seen, for example, in the aggressive Marburg variant of multiple sclerosis (Beniac *et al.* 1999).

The structural data currently available for MBP is, while extensive, usually not high-resolution, owing to the fact that MBP is an intrinsically disordered molecule. Firstly, several crystal structures are available on short MBP peptides bound to immune system molecules (He *et al.* 2002; Li *et al.* 2000; Li *et al.* 2001; Li *et al.* 2005; Smith *et al.* 1998). Also NMR studies have been carried out on such peptides in solution (Fares *et al.* 2006; Mantzourani *et al.* 2006; Mantzourani *et al.* 2008; Spyranti *et al.* 2009). Secondly, low-resolution methods, such as SAXS (Haas *et al.* 2004; Krigbaum & Hsu 1975; Majava *et al.* 2008; Majava *et al.* 2010; Mendz *et al.* 1992) and electron microscopy (Beniac *et al.* 1997; Ridsdale *et al.* 1997), have been used to obtain shapes and molecular dimensions of MBP at different environments.

Recently, several in-depth reviews have been published on the structural properties of MBP (Harauz & Musse 2007; Harauz *et al.* 2004; Harauz *et al.* 2009; Musse & Harauz 2007;

Boggs 2006; Tzakos *et al.* 2005; Katsara *et al.* 2008). Thus, with regard to MBP, in this chapter, mainly the latest results from our own laboratory are discussed. MBP has been characterized to have two CaM binding sites, one of which is the main immunodominant epitope in the middle region of the protein, and the other binding site lies close to the C-terminus of MBP (Libich & Harauz 2008; Libich *et al.* 2003). Our initial structural analyses provided a model (Figure 1) for the interaction between CaM and the C-terminal binding site from MBP (Majava *et al.* 2008). This work was then extended to cover also full-length MBP (Majava *et al.* 2010). We determined the 3D structure of a complex between full-length MBP and its ligand calmodulin, at different stoichiometric ratios (Figure 2). The results indicate that upon complex formation, MBP remains extended while two CaM molecules successively bind to it. The C-terminal binding site is saturated first, while the central binding site is only occupied at higher CaM concentrations. It is likely that CaM is able to regulate the membrane interactions of MBP. Interestingly, a variety of post-translational modifications have also been shown to occur at or near the main epitope in the central region of MBP (Kim *et al.* 2003; Majava *et al.* 2009; Persaud *et al.* 1988), and it is likely that such modifications may modulate the involvement of MBP in disease. Notably, the conformation of MBP in aqueous solution and bound to membrane surfaces is significantly different (Figure 3).

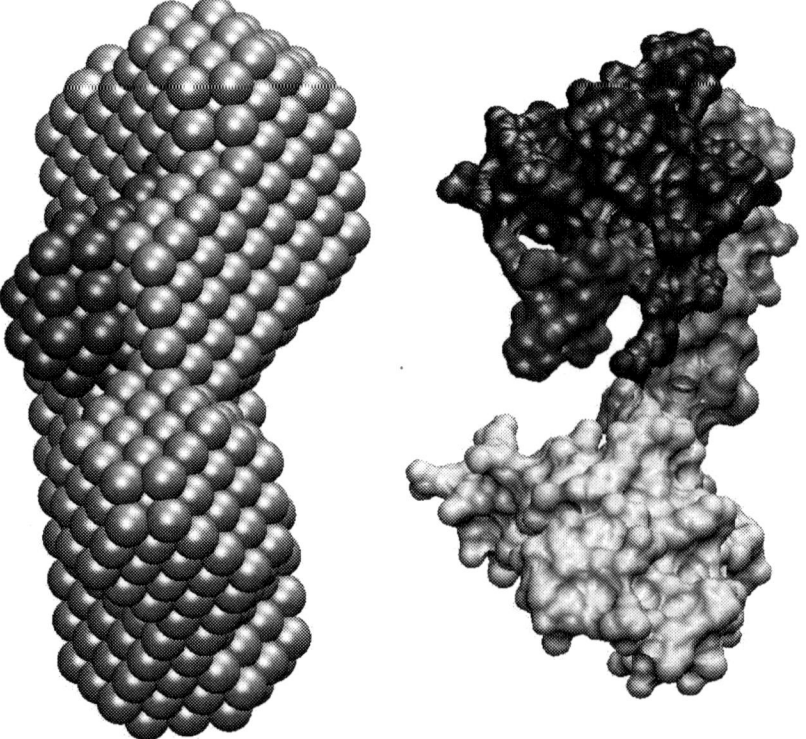

Figure 1. Solution structure of the complex between CaM and a peptide from the C-terminus of MBP. Left panel: a two-component shape of the complex; Right panel: a rigid body model. The peptide parts are shown in red. The central helix and the N- and C-terminal lobes of CaM in the rigid body model are shown in green, yellow, and blue, respectively. Reprinted from (Majava et al. 2008).

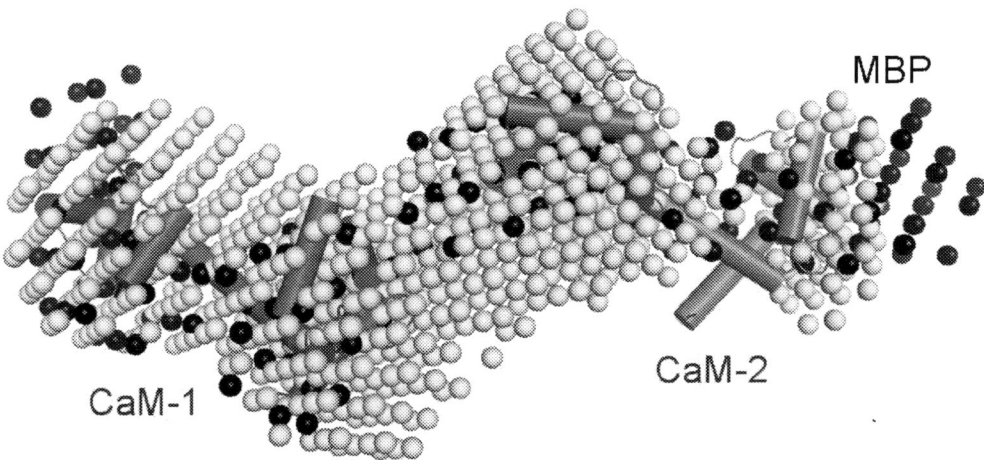

Figure 2. The solution structure of full-length 18.5-kDa MBP bound to two molecules of CaM. The result was obtained by synchrotron small-angle X-ray scattering (Majava et al. 2010). Black, MBP alone is an elongated disordered molecule; Yellow, the structure of a complex between one MBP molecule and two CaM molecules; Magenta, the observed locations of the two bound CaM molecules, CaM-1 is bound first (high-affinity site close to C terminus of MBP) and CaM-2 at high CaM concentrations.

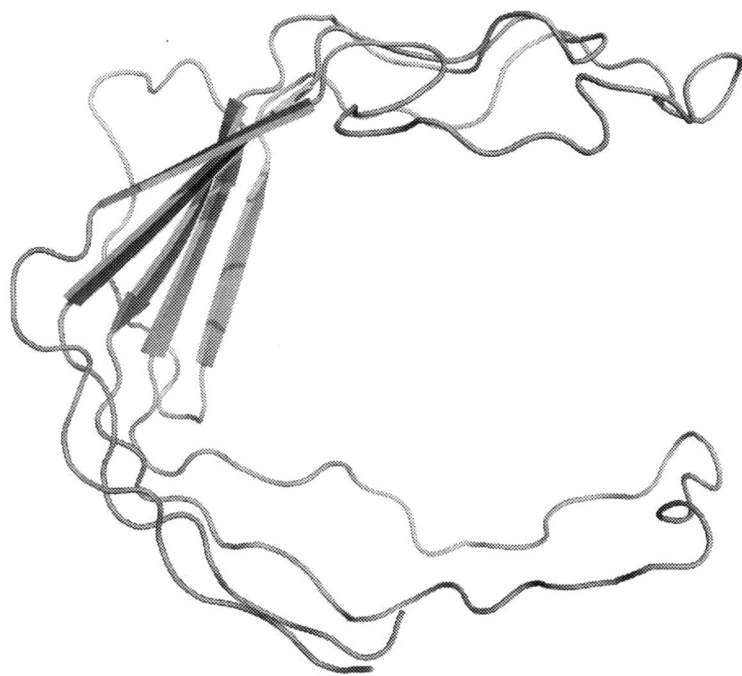

Figure 3. A 3D model of MBP bound to a lipid monolayer, obtained from electron microscopy experiments with single particle reconstruction and molecular modeling (Beniac et al. 1997; Ridsdale et al. 1997). In contrast to aqueous solution, MBP is a folded molecule, although not globular.

MYELIN/OLIGODENDROCYTE BASIC PROTEIN (MOBP)

The myelin/oligodendrocyte associated basic protein (MOBP) is an abundant protein of the CNS myelin (Yamamoto *et al.* 1994). It is a basic protein, for which no structural information has been available, and which for long has been though to be intrinsically disordered, *via* analogy to MBP. MOBP has been implicated in autoimmune CNS disease (de Rosbo *et al.* 2004; Holz *et al.* 2000; Kaushansky *et al.* 2007; Kaushansky *et al.* 2009a; Kaushansky *et al.* 2009b; Kaye *et al.* 2000; Maatta *et al.* 1998). A major encephalitogenic epitope in multiple sclerosis is found near the N-terminus of MOBP (de Rosbo *et al.* 2004), and this region, in fact, is predicted to fold into a FYVE domain (Kursula 2008), while the C-terminal region of MOBP is likely to be disordered. FYVE domains are small folded entities binding zinc and membranes. The MS epitope is in the area of a loop structure, which is likely to be the part of MOBP inserting into the surface of the inner leaflet of the myelin membrane. While MOBP has been implicated as one of the major targets of autoimmune attack in MS (Kaushansky *et al.* 2009b; Kaye *et al.* 2000; Montague *et al.* 2006), not much is known about its structure, function, or interactions with other molecules and membranes (Kursula 2008).

MYELIN/OLIGODENDROCYTE GLYCOPROTEIN (MOG)

MOG is one of the major myelin autoantigens in the CNS, and it has been originally characterized as the main antigen of an animal model of MS, experimental autoimmune encephalomyelitis (EAE) (Lebar *et al.* 1979; Lebar *et al.* 1986). MOG is also one of the major antigens involved in the autoimmune response in MS (de Rosbo & Ben-Nun 1998). MOG is a transmembrane protein harboring a single extracellular Ig domain, a transmembrane domain, and another membrane-associated domain in the middle of its cytoplasmic region.

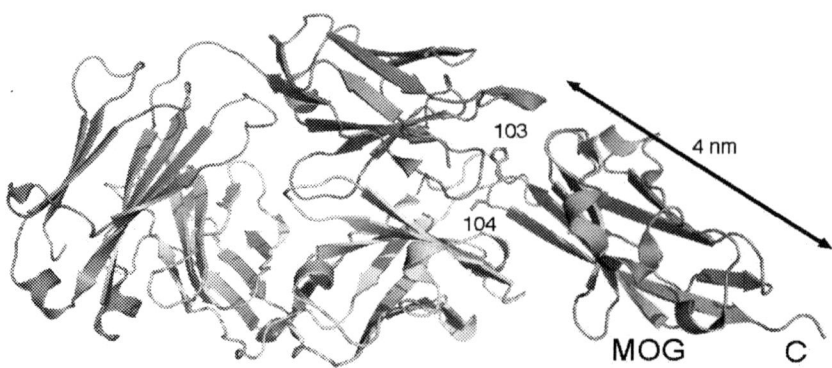

Figure 4. The crystal structure of the MOG extracellular domain (green) bound to its specific antibody Fab fragment (yellow/orange) (Breithaupt et al. 2003). To give an idea of the relevant dimensions, the extracellular space in normal compact myelin is 2 nm, which corresponds to the short dimension of a single Ig domain fitting between the apposing membrane surfaces. The long dimension of the MOG Ig domain is around 4 nm (arrow). The C terminus and the loop (103-104) recognized by the antibody are labeled.

Interestingly, the crystal structure of the MOG extracellular Ig domain has been determined in the presence (Figure 4) and absence (Figure 5) of a specific antibody fragment (Breithaupt *et al.* 2003; Clements *et al.* 2003). The antibody used was the Fab fragment of the demyelinating 8-18C5 monoclonal antibody. Thus, the atomic details of antibody-antigen interactions can be revealed in this case (Breithaupt *et al.* 2008). Antibody binding to the MOG extracellular domain is highly likely to compromise its cell adhesion function, within the tightly packed membrane multilayer, and to lead to myelin abnormalities. A number of studies have also been carried out to identify peptide epitopes within MOG that would be relevant for the autoimmune response; these studies have been reviewed before (de Rosbo & Ben-Nun 1998), and the results relevant to human disease are summarized in Figure 5.

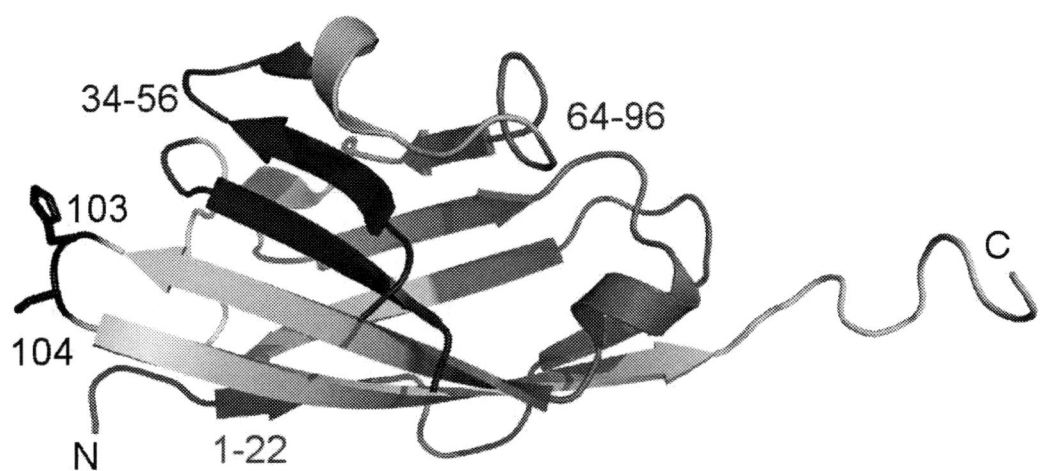

Figure 5. Some experimentally determined epitopes mapped onto the MOG extracellular domain crystal structure. The N and C termini are also labeled, the C terminus enters into the extracellular face of the myelin membrane (to the right).

PERIPHERAL MYELIN PROTEIN 2 (P2)

P2 is a small folded protein, and a member of the fatty acid binding protein family (Chmurzynska 2006). It is expressed in the cytoplasmic face of compact myelin formed by Schwann cells in the PNS (Eylar *et al.* 1980; Hahn *et al.* 1987; Trapp *et al.* 1984), and its lipid-binding activity suggests it may serve important functions in generating and maintaining the unique lipid composition of the myelin membrane (Uyemura *et al.* 1984). P2 can be used to induce an animal model of autoimmune peripheral neuropathy (Nomura *et al.* 1987; Suzuki *et al.* 1980; Uyemura *et al.* 1982), and thus, P2 is possibly one of the autoantigens in the human disorder Guillain-Barre syndrome (Hughes & Cornblath 2005; Hughes *et al.* 1999; Rostami 1997), which is an autoimmune disease of the peripheral nervous system. The fact that P2 has during recent years been largely neglected, despite its obvious importance in PNS myelin, is highlighted by the observation that a recent encyclopedic work on myelin, its components, and disorders, includes chapters on all other major, and several minor, myelin proteins, except for P2 (Lazzarini *et al.* 2004).

The crystal structure of P2 has been determined from both bovine (Jones *et al.* 1988) and equine (Hunter *et al.* 2005) sources. In addition, we have recently determined a high-resolution crystal structure of the human P2 protein, as well as its solution structure using SAXS and SRCD methods (unpublished data). Visualization of the surface charge distribution of P2, which is unique among the FABP family, suggests possible mechanisms of membrane interaction and lipid transfer. In fact, our recent results indicate that P2 is able to affect significantly the properties of artificial membranes when bound to their surface (Knoll *et al.* 2010).

The main autoimmune epitope of P2 locates at residues 58-73 (Rostami & Gregorian 1991), and a peptide corresponding to this region has been been used extensively to induce and study the animal model of GBS, experimental autoimmune neuritis (EAN). The minimal T cell epitope of P2 includes a subset of this region, residues 61-70 (Olee *et al.* 1990). In EAN, a 16-mer of the P2(58-73) peptide has also been used for treatment and vaccination (Stienekemeier *et al.* 2001). At the structural level (Figure 6), the epitope localizes to a beta-strand-loop-beta-strand unit, on the side opposite to the helical domain suggested to be important in lipid transfer to the membrane surface.

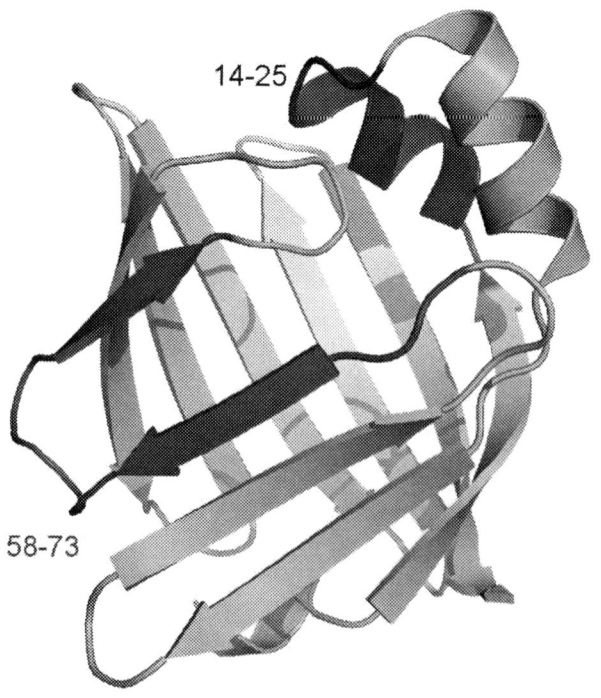

Figure 6. The crystal structure of equine P2 (Hunter et al. 2005), and the localization of the EAN epitope (residues 58-73, in red) within the structure. In addition, the epitope recognized by GB syndrome patients in a recent study (Inglis et al. 2007) is shown in blue. Note the small domain formed by the two helices on the top right; this domain forms a 'lid' on top of the lipid-binding cavity in the centre of the 10-stranded beta barrel structure.

MYELIN-ASSOCIATED GLYCOPROTEIN (MAG)

The myelin-associated glycoprotein (MAG) is a cell adhesion molecule having 5 extracellular Ig domains and one of two cytoplasmic tails generated by alternative splicing (Tropak *et al.* 1988). The transmembrane domain of MAG is a hydrophobic stretch of 20 amino acid residues. A cysteine residue within the MAG transmembrane domain is a target for palmitoylation, occurring posttranslationally *via* a thioester linkage (Pedraza *et al.* 1990). Sites of special interest from the structural point of view include the cytoplasmic tails and the first 2 Ig domains. Ig domain 1 binds sialic acid, and is connected to Ig domain 2 *via* an unususal disulfide bridge (Pedraza *et al.* 1990). No experimentally determined 3D structures for any domains of MAG exist.

Of special interest is the homology between the first two Ig domains of MAG and the corresponding domains in members of the sialoadhesin family (Kelm *et al.* 1996), including, among others, sialoadhesin and the avian Schwann cell myelin protein (SMP). The first extracellular domain of all the family members is a V-type Ig domain, containing the sialic acid binding site. The two distinctive properties of this domain are the presence of an intrasheet disulfide bridge, and the linkage of the first and second Ig domains *via* another disulfide bridge (Kursula 2001; Pedraza *et al.* 1990). The structure of this domain from sialoadhesin has been determined by X-ray crystallography (May *et al.* 1998; Zaccai *et al.* 2007), and comparison of the family members has highlighted residues involved in direct sialic acid binding, that are almost completely conserved throughout the family. An important residue for sialic acid binding by MAG is Arg118 within the first Ig-like domain (Tang *et al.* 1997). A theoretical model for the structure of the first two Ig domains of MAG has been presented before (Kursula 2000; Kursula 2001; Kursula 2008).

As the result of alternative mRNA splicing of exon 12, two isoforms of MAG are produced, differing only by the carboxy-terminal portion of their cytoplasmic domain (Tropak *et al.* 1988). The length of the cytoplasmic tail of S-MAG is 46 residues, and that of L-MAG 90 amino acids. The MAG isoforms share a common cytoplasmic domain of 36 amino acids, which is followed by the isoform-specific carboxy-terminal domains of 10 or 54 amino acids for S- and L-MAG, respectively (Salzer *et al.* 1987). At the primary sequence level, neither of the MAG cytoplasmic domains shares a significant degree of homology with other proteins. However, there are a few short sequence motifs, such as phosphorylation consensus sequences, that have been used to predict the functional properties of the MAG cytoplasmic domains (Arquint *et al.* 1987; Salzer *et al.* 1987). Experimental data from CD spectroscopy indicates that while the S-MAGct is devoid of secondary stucture in solution, the L-MAGct most likely comprises a folded domain (Kursula 2000). Similar results have been obtained with secondary structure prediction algorithms (Kursula 2000). Of the MAG cytoplasmic domains, that of S-MAG is known to bind zinc and tubulin (Kursula *et al.* 1999a; Kursula *et al.* 2001). The L-MAG cytoplasmic domain interacts with S100 proteins (Kursula *et al.* 1999b), is phosphorylated by Fyn kinase, protein kinase C, and protein kinase A (Kursula *et al.* 2000; Umemori *et al.* 1994), and has a tendency to dimerize (Kursula 2000).

MAG has been implicated as a major antigen in autoimmune peripheral neuropathies (Andersson *et al.* 2002; Gabriel *et al.* 1996; Jaskowski *et al.* 2004; Kuijf *et al.* 2009; Lunn *et al.* 2002; Steck *et al.* 2006), and the involved epitopes are located to a large extent in the carbohydrate moieties of the extracellular domain (Frail *et al.* 1984). The structural basis of MAG-related autoimmunity remains to be elucidated.

2',3'-CYCLIC NUCLEOTIDE 3'-PHOSPHODIESTERASE (CNPASE)

CNPase is a myelin-specific enzyme whose *in vitro* catalytic activity has been well-characterized (Drummond *et al.* 1962); however, its *in vivo* function remains a mystery. The reaction catalyzed by CNPase, the cleavage of 2',3'-cyclic ribonucleotide phosphates to yield 2'-OH ribonucleotides, seems to have no clear counterpart *in vivo*. CNPase is one of the most abundant myelin proteins, and in fact, the most abundant protein of the non-compact regions of myelin. CNPase is isoprenylated and attached to the plasma membrane (Braun *et al.* 1991). While structural information on the CNPase catalytic domain has become available (Kozlov *et al.* 2003; Sakamoto *et al.* 2004), it is still lacking concerning the full-length protein, and the interactions of the enzyme with substrates and other ligands (Myllykoski & Kursula 2010).

The enzymatic activity of CNPase is known to be reduced in and around MS plaques (Riekkinen *et al.* 1972; Trotter *et al.* 1984), and CNPase has been identified as a putative autoantigen (Morris-Downes *et al.* 2002; Walsh & Murray 1998). Immunodominant epitope clusters have been characterized at residues 343-373 and 356-388 (Muraro *et al.* 2002). Both of the latter epitopes reside within the catalytic domain, close to the C-terminus of CNPase. Figure 7 indicates the mapping of these epitopes onto the crystal structure of human CNPase catalytic domain. The epitope principally occupies the 'backside' of CNPase, away from the catalytically active pocket. It includes 4 beta strands and two surface loops.

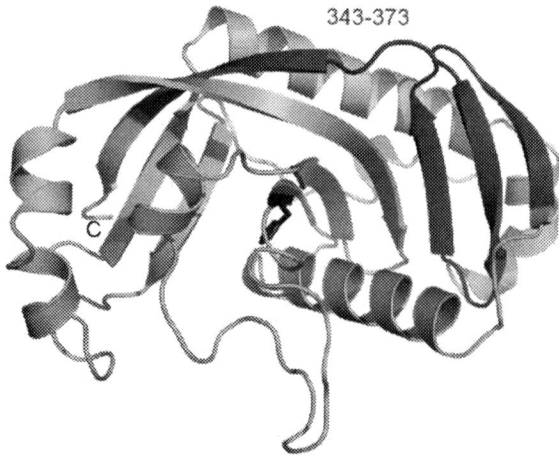

Figure 7. Mapping of a putative disease-linked autoimmune epitope, residues 343-373, onto the crystal structure of the C-terminal catalytic phosphodiesterase domain of CNPase. The side chain of the active-site residue His310 is also shown in blue to localize the catalytic center, and the C terminus is labelled.

MYELIN PROTEIN ZERO (P0)

P0 is a quantitatively major protein of PNS compact myelin, comprising up to 50% of total myelin protein (Adelmann & Linington 1992; Everly *et al.* 1973; Kitamura *et al.* 1976). The extracellular domain of P0 is glycosylated, and the protein also contains a single transmembrane domain and a highly basic cytoplasmic domain. P0 is one of the putative PNS autoantigens (Favereaux *et al.* 2003), and can be used to induce EAN in animal models (Suzuki *et al.* 1980; Zhu *et al.* 2001; Zou *et al.* 2000). Functionally, P0 most likely acts as molecular glue between successive turns of the myelin membrane.

The crystal structure of the extracellular domain of P0 has been determined (Shapiro *et al.* 1996), in the absence of glycan moieties. The structure comprises a single Ig domain (Figure 8), and has been used to map inherited P0 mutations in 3D space. Autoimmune peptide epitopes detected in experimental studies on neuropathy include, for example, residue ranges 56-71, 106-125, and 180-199 (Adelmann & Linington 1992; Miletic *et al.* 2005; Zhu *et al.* 2001). These are mapped onto the P0 structure in Figure 8, with the exception of 180-199, which lies interestingly in the cytoplasmic domain of P0. In addition, a major epitope in P0 lies within the HNK-1 carbohydrate epitope (Voshol *et al.* 1996).

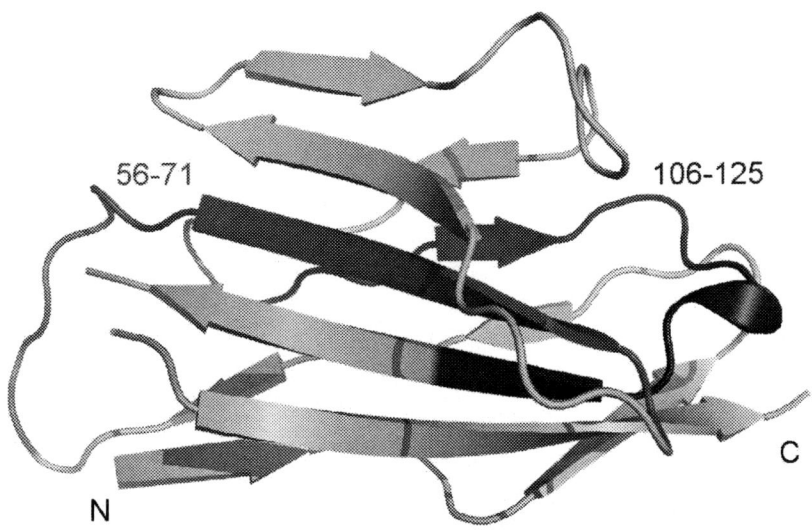

Figure 8. The crystal structure of the extracellular domain of myelin protein P0. Two extracellular peptide epitopes, which have been suggested to be neuritogenic, are mapped onto the structure. The N and C termini are also indicated; the C terminus is close to the outer leaflet of the myelin membrane, leading to the transmembrane domain (to the right).

HOW CAN STRUCTURAL INFORMATION AID IN UNDERSTANDING AUTOIMMUNE DISEASE?

The importance of accurate biochemical and biophysical data in the overall understanding of nervous system structure and function, as well as the etiology of neurological myelin-related diseases, must not be underestimated. Obtaining 3D information on myelin proteins, both alone and in complex with other molecules, is crucial to the understanding of their function in the myelin sheath.

It should be remembered that for full-length myelin proteins, little structural information is available (Kursula 2008). For example, the extracellular domains of both MOG and P0 were solved in the absence of their respective other domains or glycan moieties, which could play roles in the protein structure and its involvement in autoimmunity. It should also be borne in mind that crystal structures, although providing very high-resolution data, often do not necessarily represent the conformation or even the oligomeric status observed in solution. A simple example of this was recently provided by our work on the complex between calmodulin and calcineurin A (Majava & Kursula 2009). Thus, if possible, crystal structure data should always be validated by independent methods, which mostly are carried out in near-physiological conditions.

CONCLUSION

Knowledge of the 3-dimensional structures of myelin proteins will help us understand their function and involvement in disease; this knowledge will also give us a higher-resolution view of the intimate interactions between the axonal membrane and the plasma membrane of the myelin-forming cell, *i.e.* Schwann cell in the PNS and oligodendrocyte in the CNS. The results will also illuminate the mechanisms by which myelin causes inhibition of axonal regeneration following neuronal trauma.

ACKNOWLEDGMENTS

The author wishes to thank all past and present collaborators for their hard work and fruitful discussions. This work has been supported by the Academy of Finland and the Sigrid Juselius Foundation (Finland).

REFERENCES

Adelmann, M. & Linington, C. (1992). Molecular mimicry and the autoimmune response to the peripheral nerve myelin P0 glycoprotein. *Neurochem Res 17*, 887-891.

Andersson, M., Yu, M., Soderstrom, M., Weerth, S., Baig, S., Solders, G. & Link, H. (2002). Multiple MAG peptides are recognized by circulating T and B lymphocytes in polyneuropathy and multiple sclerosis. *Eur J Neurol 9*, 243-251.

Arquint, M., Roder, J., Chia, L.S., Down, J., Wilkinson, D., Bayley, H., Braun, P. & Dunn, R. (1987). Molecular cloning and primary structure of myelin-associated glycoprotein. *Proc Natl Acad Sci U S A 84*, 600-604.

Barylko, B. & Dobrowolski, Z. (1984). Ca^{2+}-calmodulin-dependent regulation of F-actin-myelin basic protein interaction. *Eur J Cell Biol 35*, 327-335.

Beniac, D.R., Luckevich, M.D., Czarnota, G.J., Tompkins, T.A., Ridsdale, R.A., Ottensmeyer, F.P., Moscarello, M.A. & Harauz, G. (1997). Three-dimensional structure of myelin basic protein. I. Reconstruction via angular reconstitution of randomly oriented single particles. *J Biol Chem 272*, 4261-4268.

Beniac, D.R., Wood, D.D., Palaniyar, N., Ottensmeyer, F.P., Moscarello, M.A. & Harauz, G. (1999). Marburg's variant of multiple sclerosis correlates with a less compact structure of myelin basic protein. *Mol Cell Biol Res Commun 1*, 48-51.

Benjamins, J.A. & Morell, P. (1978). Proteins of myelin and their metabolism. *Neurochem Res 3*, 137-174.

Boggs, J.M. (2006). Myelin basic protein: a multifunctional protein. *Cell Mol Life Sci 63*, 1945-1961.

Boggs, J.M. & Rangaraj, G. (2000). Interaction of lipid-bound myelin basic protein with actin filaments and calmodulin. *Biochemistry 39*, 7799-7806.

Braun, P.E., De Angelis, D., Shtybel, W.W. & Bernier, L. (1991). Isoprenoid modification permits 2',3'-cyclic nucleotide 3'-phosphodiesterase to bind to membranes. *J Neurosci Res 30*, 540-544.

Breithaupt, C., Schafer, B., Pellkofer, H., Huber, R., Linington, C. & Jacob, U. (2008). Demyelinating myelin oligodendrocyte glycoprotein-specific autoantibody response is focused on one dominant conformational epitope region in rodents. *J Immunol 181*, 1255-1263.

Breithaupt, C., Schubart, A., Zander, H., Skerra, A., Huber, R., Linington, C. & Jacob, U. (2003). Structural insights into the antigenicity of myelin oligodendrocyte glycoprotein. *Proc Natl Acad Sci U S A 100*, 9446-9451.

Chmurzynska, A. (2006). The multigene family of fatty acid-binding proteins (FABPs): function, structure and polymorphism. *J Appl Genet 47*, 39-48.

Clements, C.S., Reid, H.H., Beddoe, T., Tynan, F.E., Perugini, M.A., Johns, T.G., Bernard, C.C. & Rossjohn, J. (2003). The crystal structure of myelin oligodendrocyte glycoprotein, a key autoantigen in multiple sclerosis. *Proc Natl Acad Sci U S A 100*, 11059-11064.

de Rosbo, N.K. & Ben-Nun, A. (1998). T-cell responses to myelin antigens in multiple sclerosis; relevance of the predominant autoimmune reactivity to myelin oligodendrocyte glycoprotein. *J Autoimmun 11*, 287-299.

de Rosbo, N.K., Kaye, J.F., Eisenstein, M., Mendel, I., Hoeftberger, R., Lassmann, H., Milo, R. & Ben-Nun, A. (2004). The myelin-associated oligodendrocytic basic protein region MOBP15-36 encompasses the immunodominant major encephalitogenic epitope(s) for SJL/J mice and predicted epitope(s) for multiple sclerosis-associated HLA-DRB1*1501. *J Immunol 173*, 1426-1435.

Dobrowolski, Z., Osinska, H., Mossakowska, M. & Barylko, B. (1986). Ca^{2+}-calmodulin-dependent polymerization of actin by myelin basic protein. *Eur J Cell Biol 42*, 17-26.

Drummond, G.I., Iyer, N.T. & Keith, J. (1962). Hydrolysis of ribonucleoside 2',3'-cyclic phosphates by a diesterase from brain. *J Biol Chem 237*, 3535-3539.

Everly, J.L., Brady, R.O. & Quarles, R.H. (1973). Evidence that the major protein in rat sciatic nerve myelin is a glycoprotein. *J Neurochem 21*, 329-334.

Eylar, E.H., Szymanska, I., Ishaque, A., Ramwani, J. & Dubiski, S. (1980). Localization of the P2 protein in peripheral nerve myelin. *J Immunol 124*, 1086-1092.

Fares, C., Libich, D.S. & Harauz, G. (2006). Solution NMR structure of an immunodominant epitope of myelin basic protein. Conformational dependence on environment of an intrinsically unstructured protein. *FEBS J 273*, 601-614.

Favereaux, A., Lagueny, A., Vital, A., Schmitter, J.M., Chaignepain, S., Ferrer, X., Labatut-Cazabat, I., Vital, C. & Petry, K.G. (2003). Serum IgG antibodies to P0 dimer and 35 kDa P0 related protein in neuropathy associated with monoclonal gammopathy. *J Neurol Neurosurg Psychiatry 74*, 1262-1266.

Frail, D.E., Edwards, A.M. & Braun, P.E. (1984). Molecular characteristics of the epitope in myelin-associated glycoprotein that is recognized by a monoclonal IgM in human neuropathy patients. *Mol Immunol 21*, 721-725.

Gabriel, J.M., Erne, B., Miescher, G.C., Miller, S.L., Vital, A., Vital, C. & Steck, A.J. (1996). Selective loss of myelin-associated glycoprotein from myelin correlates with anti-MAG antibody titre in demyelinating paraproteinaemic polyneuropathy. *Brain 119*, 775-787.

Haas, H., Oliveira, C.L., Torriani, I.L., Polverini, E., Fasano, A., Carlone, G., Cavatorta, P. & Riccio, P. (2004). Small angle x-ray scattering from lipid-bound myelin basic protein in solution. *Biophys J 86*, 455-460.

Hahn, A.F., Whitaker, J.N., Kachar, B. & Webster, H.D. (1987). P2, P1, and P0 myelin protein expression in developing rat sixth nerve: a quantitative immunocytochemical study. *J Comp Neurol 260*, 501-512.

Harauz, G., Ishiyama, N., Hill, C.M., Bates, I.R., Libich, D.S. & Fares, C. (2004). Myelin basic protein-diverse conformational states of an intrinsically unstructured protein and its roles in myelin assembly and multiple sclerosis. *Micron 35*, 503-542.

Harauz, G., Ladizhansky, V. & Boggs, J.M. (2009). Structural polymorphism and multifunctionality of myelin basic protein. *Biochemistry 48*, 8094-8104.

Harauz, G. & Musse, A.A. (2007). A tale of two citrullines--structural and functional aspects of myelin basic protein deimination in health and disease. *Neurochem Res 32*, 137-158.

He, X.L., Radu, C., Sidney, J., Sette, A., Ward, E.S. & Garcia, K.C. (2002). Structural snapshot of aberrant antigen presentation linked to autoimmunity: the immunodominant epitope of MBP complexed with I-Au. *Immunity 17*, 83-94.

Hill, C.M. & Harauz, G. (2005). Charge effects modulate actin assembly by classic myelin basic protein isoforms. *Biochem Biophys Res Commun 329*, 362-369.

Holz, A., Bielekova, B., Martin, R. & Oldstone, M.B. (2000). Myelin-associated oligodendrocytic basic protein: identification of an encephalitogenic epitope and association with multiple sclerosis. *J Immunol 164*, 1103-1109.

Hughes, R.A. & Cornblath, D.R. (2005). Guillain-Barre syndrome. *Lancet 366*, 1653-1666.

Hughes, R.A., Hadden, R.D., Gregson, N.A. & Smith, K.J. (1999). Pathogenesis of Guillain-Barre syndrome. *J Neuroimmunol 100*, 74-97.

Hunter, D.J., Macmaster, R., Roszak, A.W., Riboldi-Tunnicliffe, A., Griffiths, I.R. & Freer, A.A. (2005). Structure of myelin P2 protein from equine spinal cord. *Acta Crystallogr D Biol Crystallogr 61*, 1067-1071.

Inglis, H.R., Csurhes, P.A. & McCombe, P.A. (2007). Antibody responses to peptides of peripheral nerve myelin proteins P0 and P2 in patients with inflammatory demyelinating neuropathy. *J Neurol Neurosurg Psychiatry 78*, 419-422.

Jaskowski, T.D., Martins, T.B., Litwin, C.M. & Hill, H.R. (2004). Immunoglobulin (Ig) M antibody against myelin associated glycoprotein (MAG): A comparison of methods. *J Clin Lab Anal 18*, 247-250.

Katsara, M., Ramsland, P.A., Tselios, T., Matsoukas, J. & Apostolopoulos, V. (2008). A structural perspective of peptides from myelin basic protein. In Boggs, J.M. (Ed.), *Myelin Basic Protein* (pp. 87-103) New York: Nova Science Publishers, Inc.

Kaushansky, N., Altmann, D.M., Ascough, S., David, C.S., Lassmann, H. & Ben-Nun, A. (2009a). HLA-DQB1*0602 determines disease susceptibility in a new "humanized" multiple sclerosis model in HLA-DR15 (DRB1*1501;DQB1*0602) transgenic mice. *J Immunol 183*, 3531-3541.

Kaushansky, N., Eisenstein, M., Zilkha-Falb, R. & Ben-Nun, A. (2009b). The myelin-associated oligodendrocytic basic protein (MOBP) as a relevant primary target autoantigen in multiple sclerosis. *Autoimmun Rev*

Kaushansky, N., Zilkha-Falb, R., Hemo, R., Lassman, H., Eisenstein, M., Sas, A. & Ben-Nun, A. (2007). Pathogenic T cells in MOBP-induced murine EAE are predominantly focused to recognition of MOBP21F and MOBP27P epitopic residues. *Eur J Immunol 37*, 3281-3292.

Kaye, J.F., Kerlero de Rosbo, N., Mendel, I., Flechter, S., Hoffman, M., Yust, I. & Ben-Nun, A. (2000). The central nervous system-specific myelin oligodendrocytic basic protein (MOBP) is encephalitogenic and a potential target antigen in multiple sclerosis (MS). *J Neuroimmunol 102*, 189-198.

Kelm, S., Schauer, R. & Crocker, P.R. (1996). The Sialoadhesins--a family of sialic acid-dependent cellular recognition molecules within the immunoglobulin superfamily. *Glycoconj J 13*, 913-926.

Kim, J.K., Mastronardi, F.G., Wood, D.D., Lubman, D.M., Zand, R. & Moscarello, M.A. (2003). Multiple sclerosis: an important role for post-translational modifications of myelin basic protein in pathogenesis. *Mol Cell Proteomics 2*, 453-462.

Kitamura, K., Suzuki, M. & Uyemura, K. (1976). Purification and partial characterization of two glycoproteins in bovine peripheral nerve myelin membrane. *Biochim Biophys Acta 455*, 806-816.

Knoll, W., Natali, F., Peters, J., Nanekar, R., Wang, C. & Kursula, P. (2010). Dynamic properties of a reconstituted myelin sheath. *Spectroscopy*, in press.

Komagamine, T. & Yuki, N. (2006). Ganglioside mimicry as a cause of Guillain-Barre syndrome. *CNS Neurol Disord Drug Targets 5*, 391-400.

Kozlov, G., Lee, J., Elias, D., Gravel, M., Gutierrez, P., Ekiel, I., Braun, P.E. & Gehring, K. (2003). Structural evidence that brain cyclic nucleotide phosphodiesterase is a member of the 2H phosphodiesterase superfamily. *J Biol Chem 278*, 46021-46028.

Krigbaum, W.R. & Hsu, T.S. (1975). Molecular conformation of bovine A1 basic protein, a coiling macromolecule in aqueous solution. *Biochemistry 14*, 2542-2546.

Kuijf, M.L., Eurelings, M., Tio-Gillen, A.P., van Doorn, P.A., van den Berg, L.H., Hooijkaas, H., Stork, J., Notermans, N.C. & Jacobs, B.C. (2009). Detection of anti-MAG antibodies in polyneuropathy associated with IgM monoclonal gammopathy. *Neurology 73*, 688-695.

Kursula, P. (2001). The current status of structural studies on proteins of the myelin sheath (Review). *Int J Mol Med 8*, 475-479.

Kursula, P. (2008). Structural properties of proteins specific to the myelin sheath. *Amino Acids 34*, 175-185.

Kursula, P. (2000). *Acta Univ Oul D*. Oulu, Finland: Oulu University Press.

Kursula, P., Lehto, V.P. & Heape, A.M. (2000). S100beta inhibits the phosphorylation of the L-MAG cytoplasmic domain by PKA. *Brain Res Mol Brain Res 76*, 407-410.

Kursula, P., Lehto, V.P. & Heape, A.M. (2001). The small myelin-associated glycoprotein binds to tubulin and microtubules. *Brain Res Mol Brain Res 87*, 22-30.

Kursula, P., Merilainen, G., Lehto, V.P. & Heape, A.M. (1999a). The small myelin-associated glycoprotein is a zinc-binding protein. *J Neurochem 73*, 2110-2118.

Kursula, P., Tikkanen, G., Lehto, V.P., Nishikimi, M. & Heape, A.M. (1999b). Calcium-dependent interaction between the large myelin-associated glycoprotein and S100beta. *J Neurochem 73*, 1724-1732.

Lazzarini, R.A., Griffin, J.W., Lassman, H., Nave, K.A., Miller, R.H. & Trapp, B.D. (2004). *Myelin biology and disorders*. San Diego, CA: Elsevier Academic Press.

Lebar, R., Lubetzki, C., Vincent, C., Lombrail, P. & Boutry, J.M. (1986). The M2 autoantigen of central nervous system myelin, a glycoprotein present in oligodendrocyte membrane. *Clin Exp Immunol 66*, 423-434.

Lebar, R., Vincent, C. & Fischer-le Boubennec, E. (1979). Studies on autoimmune encephalomyelitis in the guinea pig--III. A comparative study of two autoantigens of central nervous system myelin. *J Neurochem 32*, 1451-1460.

Li, Y., Huang, Y., Lue, J., Quandt, J.A., Martin, R. & Mariuzza, R.A. (2005). Structure of a human autoimmune TCR bound to a myelin basic protein self-peptide and a multiple sclerosis-associated MHC class II molecule. *EMBO J 24*, 2968-2979.

Li, Y., Li, H., Dimasi, N., McCormick, J.K., Martin, R., Schuck, P., Schlievert, P.M. & Mariuzza, R.A. (2001). Crystal structure of a superantigen bound to the high-affinity, zinc-dependent site on MHC class II. *Immunity 14*, 93-104.

Li, Y., Li, H., Martin, R. & Mariuzza, R.A. (2000). Structural basis for the binding of an immunodominant peptide from myelin basic protein in different registers by two HLA-DR2 proteins. *J Mol Biol 304*, 177-188.

Libich, D.S. & Harauz, G. (2008). Backbone dynamics of the 18.5 kDa isoform of myelin basic protein reveals transient alpha-helices and a calmodulin-binding site. *Biophys J 94*, 4847-4866.

Libich, D.S., Hill, C.M., Haines, J.D. & Harauz, G. (2003). Myelin basic protein has multiple calmodulin-binding sites. *Biochem Biophys Res Commun 308*, 313-319.

Lunn, M.P., Crawford, T.O., Hughes, R.A., Griffin, J.W. & Sheikh, K.A. (2002). Anti-myelin-associated glycoprotein antibodies alter neurofilament spacing. *Brain 125*, 904-911.

Maatta, J.A., Kaldman, M.S., Sakoda, S., Salmi, A.A. & Hinkkanen, A.E. (1998). Encephalitogenicity of myelin-associated oligodendrocytic basic protein and 2',3'-cyclic nucleotide 3'-phosphodiesterase for BALB/c and SJL mice. *Immunology 95*, 383-388.

Majava, V. & Kursula, P. (2009). Domain swapping and different oligomeric states for the complex between calmodulin and the calmodulin-binding domain of calcineurin a. *PLoS One 4*, e5402.

Majava, V., Petoukhov, M.V., Hayashi, N., Pirila, P., Svergun, D.I. & Kursula, P. (2008). Interaction between the C-terminal region of human myelin basic protein and calmodulin: analysis of complex formation and solution structure. *BMC Struct Biol 8*, 10.

Majava, V., Wang, C., Myllykoski, M., Kangas, S.M., Kang, S.U., Hayashi, N., Baumgärtel, P., Heape, A.M., Lubec, G. & Kursula, P. (2010). Structural analysis of the complex between calmodulin and full-length myelin basic protein, an intrinsically disordered molecule. *Amino Acids*, in press.

Mantzourani, E.D., Blokar, K., Tselios, T.V., Matsoukas, J.M., Platts, J.A., Mavromoustakos, T.M. & Grdadolnik, S.G. (2008). A combined NMR and molecular dynamics simulation study to determine the conformational properties of agonists and antagonists against experimental autoimmune encephalomyelitis. *Bioorg Med Chem 16*, 2171-2182.

Mantzourani, E.D., Tselios, T.V., Grdadolnik, S.G., Brancale, A., Platts, J.A., Matsoukas, J.M. & Mavromoustakos, T.M. (2006). A putative bioactive conformation for the altered peptide ligand of myelin basic protein and inhibitor of experimental autoimmune encephalomyelitis [Arg91, Ala96] MBP87-99. *J Mol Graph Model 25*, 17-29.

May, A.P., Robinson, R.C., Vinson, M., Crocker, P.R. & Jones, E.Y. (1998). Crystal structure of the N-terminal domain of sialoadhesin in complex with 3' sialyllactose at 1.85 A resolution. *Mol Cell 1*, 719-728.

Meinl, E. & Hohlfeld, R. (2002). Immunopathogenesis of multiple sclerosis: MBP and beyond. *Clin Exp Immunol 128*, 395-397.

Mendz, G.L., Jamie, I.M. & White, J.W. (1992). Effects of acyl chain length on the conformation of myelin basic protein bound to lysolipid micelles. *Biophys Chem 45*, 61-77.

Miletic, H., Utermohlen, O., Wedekind, C., Hermann, M., Stenzel, W., Lassmann, H., Schluter, D. & Deckert, M. (2005). P0(106-125) is a neuritogenic epitope of the peripheral myelin protein P0 and induces autoimmune neuritis in C57BL/6 mice. *J Neuropathol Exp Neurol 64*, 66-73.

Montague, P., McCallion, A.S., Davies, R.W. & Griffiths, I.R. (2006). Myelin-associated oligodendrocytic basic protein: a family of abundant CNS myelin proteins in search of a function. *Dev Neurosci 28*, 479-487.

Morris-Downes, M.M., McCormack, K., Baker, D., Sivaprasad, D., Natkunarajah, J. & Amor, S. (2002). Encephalitogenic and immunogenic potential of myelin-associated glycoprotein (MAG), oligodendrocyte-specific glycoprotein (OSP) and 2',3'-cyclic nucleotide 3'-phosphodiesterase (CNPase) in ABH and SJL mice. *J Neuroimmunol 122*, 20-33.

Muraro, P.A., Kalbus, M., Afshar, G., McFarland, H.F. & Martin, R. (2002). T cell response to 2',3'-cyclic nucleotide 3'-phosphodiesterase (CNPase) in multiple sclerosis patients. *J Neuroimmunol 130*, 233-242.

Musse, A.A. & Harauz, G. (2007). Molecular "negativity" may underlie multiple sclerosis: role of the myelin basic protein family in the pathogenesis of MS. *Int Rev Neurobiol 79*, 149-172.

Myllykoski, M. & Kursula, P. (2010) Expression, purification, and initial characterization of different domains of recombinant mouse 2',3',-cyclic nucleotide 3'-phosphodiesterase, an enigmatic enzyme from the myelin sheath. *BMC Res Notes 3*, 12.

Nomura, K., Hamaguchi, K., Ohno, R., Hosokawa, T., Negishi, T., Yamashita, T., Suzuki, M. & Uyemura, K. (1987). Cell-mediated immunity to bovine P2 protein and neuritogenic synthetic peptide in experimental allergic neuritis. *J Neuroimmunol 15*, 25-35.

Olee, T., Powell, H.C. & Brostoff, S.W. (1990). New minimum length requirement for a T cell epitope for experimental allergic neuritis. *J Neuroimmunol 27*, 187-190.

Pedraza, L., Owens, G.C., Green, L.A. & Salzer, J.L. (1990). The myelin-associated glycoproteins: membrane disposition, evidence of a novel disulfide linkage between immunoglobulin-like domains, and posttranslational palmitylation. *J Cell Biol 111*, 2651-2661.

Persaud, R., Fraser, P., Wood, D.D. & Moscarello, M.A. (1988). The glycosylation of human myelin basic protein at threonines 95 and 98 occurs sequentially. *Biochim Biophys Acta 966*, 357-361.

Ridsdale, R.A., Beniac, D.R., Tompkins, T.A., Moscarello, M.A. & Harauz, G. (1997). Three-dimensional structure of myelin basic protein. II. Molecular modeling and considerations of predicted structures in multiple sclerosis. *J Biol Chem 272*, 4269-4275.

Riekkinen, P.J., Rinne, U.K., Arstila, A.U., Kurihara, T. & Pelliniemi, T.T. (1972). Studies on the pathogenesis of multiple sclerosis. 2',3'-Cyclic nucleotide 3-phosphohydrolase as marker of demyelination and correlation of findings with lysosomal changes. *J Neurol Sci 15*, 113-120.

Rostami, A. & Gregorian, S.K. (1991). Peptide 53-78 of myelin P2 protein is a T cell epitope for the induction of experimental autoimmune neuritis. *Cell Immunol 132*, 433-441.

Rostami, A.M. (1997). P2-reactive T cells in inflammatory demyelination of the peripheral nerve. *J Infect Dis 176 Suppl 2*, S160-3.

Sakamoto, Y., Tanaka, N., Ichimiya, T., Kurihara, T. & Nakamura, K.T. (2004). Three-dimensional structure of a cyclic-nucleotide phosphodiesterase from human brain. *Nucleic Acids Symp Ser (Oxf)* 157-158.

Salzer, J.L., Holmes, W.P. & Colman, D.R. (1987). The amino acid sequences of the myelin-associated glycoproteins: homology to the immunoglobulin gene superfamily. *J Cell Biol 104*, 957-965.

Shapiro, L., Doyle, J.P., Hensley, P., Colman, D.R. & Hendrickson, W.A. (1996). Crystal structure of the extracellular domain from P0, the major structural protein of peripheral nerve myelin. *Neuron 17*, 435-449.

Smith, K.J., Pyrdol, J., Gauthier, L., Wiley, D.C. & Wucherpfennig, K.W. (1998). Crystal structure of HLA-DR2 (DRA*0101, DRB1*1501) complexed with a peptide from human myelin basic protein. *J Exp Med 188*, 1511-1520.

Spyranti, Z., Tselios, T., Deraos, G., Matsoukas, J. & Spyroulias, G.A. (2009). NMR structural elucidation of myelin basic protein epitope 83-99 implicated in multiple sclerosis. *Amino Acids*

Steck, A.J., Stalder, A.K. & Renaud, S. (2006). Anti-myelin-associated glycoprotein neuropathy. *Curr Opin Neurol 19*, 458-463.

Stienekemeier, M., Falk, K., Rotzschke, O., Weishaupt, A., Schneider, C., Toyka, K.V., Gold, R. & Strominger, J.L. (2001). Vaccination, prevention, and treatment of experimental autoimmune neuritis (EAN) by an oligomerized T cell epitope. *Proc Natl Acad Sci U S A 98*, 13872-13877.

Suzuki, M., Kitamura, K., Uyemura, K., Ogawa, Y., Ishihara, Y. & Matsuyama, H. (1980). Neuritogenic activity of peripheral nerve myelin proteins in Lewis rats. *Neurosci Lett 19*, 353-358.

Tang, S., Shen, Y.J., DeBellard, M.E., Mukhopadhyay, G., Salzer, J.L., Crocker, P.R. & Filbin, M.T. (1997). Myelin-associated glycoprotein interacts with neurons via a sialic acid binding site at ARG118 and a distinct neurite inhibition site. *J Cell Biol 138*, 1355-1366.

Trapp, B.D., Dubois-Dalcq, M. & Quarles, R.H. (1984). Ultrastructural localization of P2 protein in actively myelinating rat Schwann cells. *J Neurochem 43*, 944-948.

Tropak, M.B., Johnson, P.W., Dunn, R.J. & Roder, J.C. (1988). Differential splicing of MAG transcripts during CNS and PNS development. *Brain Res 464*, 143-155.

Trotter, J.L., Wegescheide, C.L. & Garvey, W.F. (1984). Regional studies of myelin proteins in human brain and spinal cord. *Neurochem Res 9*, 133-146.

Tzakos, A.G., Kursula, P., Troganis, A., Theodorou, V., Tselios, T., Svarnas, C., Matsoukas, J., Apostolopoulos, V. & Gerothanassis, I.P. (2005). Structure and function of the myelin proteins: current status and perspectives in relation to multiple sclerosis. *Curr Med Chem 12*, 1569-1587.

Umemori, H., Sato, S., Yagi, T., Aizawa, S. & Yamamoto, T. (1994). Initial events of myelination involve Fyn tyrosine kinase signalling. *Nature 367*, 572-576.

Uyemura, K., Suzuki, M., Kitamura, K., Horie, K., Ogawa, Y., Matsuyama, H., Nozaki, S. & Muramatsu, I. (1982). Neuritogenic determinant of bovine P2 protein in peripheral nerve myelin. *J Neurochem 39*, 895-898.

Uyemura, K., Yoshimura, K., Suzuki, M. & Kitamura, K. (1984). Lipid binding activities of the P2 protein in peripheral nerve myelin. *Neurochem Res 9*, 1509-1514.

Voshol, H., van Zuylen, C.W., Orberger, G., Vliegenthart, J.F. & Schachner, M. (1996). Structure of the HNK-1 carbohydrate epitope on bovine peripheral myelin glycoprotein P0. *J Biol Chem 271*, 22957-22960.

Vucic, S., Kiernan, M.C. & Cornblath, D.R. (2009). Guillain-Barre syndrome: an update. *J Clin Neurosci 16*, 733-741.

Walsh, M.J. & Murray, J.M. (1998). Dual implication of 2',3'-cyclic nucleotide 3' phosphodiesterase as major autoantigen and C3 complement-binding protein in the pathogenesis of multiple sclerosis. *J Clin Invest 101*, 1923-1931.

Xie, L. & Bourne, P.E. (2005). Functional coverage of the human genome by existing structures, structural genomics targets, and homology models. *PLoS Comput Biol 1*, e31.

Yamamoto, Y., Mizuno, R., Nishimura, T., Ogawa, Y., Yoshikawa, H., Fujimura, H., Adachi, E., Kishimoto, T., Yanagihara, T. & Sakoda, S. (1994). Cloning and expression of myelin-associated oligodendrocytic basic protein. A novel basic protein constituting the central nervous system myelin. *J Biol Chem 269*, 31725-31730.

Yuki, N. & Kuwabara, S. (2007). Axonal Guillain-Barre syndrome: carbohydrate mimicry and pathophysiology. *J Peripher Nerv Syst 12*, 238-249.

Zaccai, N.R., May, A.P., Robinson, R.C., Burtnick, L.D., Crocker, P.R., Brossmer, R., Kelm, S. & Jones, E.Y. (2007). Crystallographic and in silico analysis of the sialoside-binding characteristics of the Siglec sialoadhesin. *J Mol Biol 365*, 1469-1479.

Zand, R., Li, M.X., Jin, X. & Lubman, D. (1998). Determination of the sites of posttranslational modifications in the charge isomers of bovine myelin basic protein by capillary electrophoresis-mass spectroscopy. *Biochemistry 37*, 2441-2449.

Zhu, J., Pelidou, S.H., Deretzi, G., Levi, M., Mix, E., van der Meide, P., Winblad, B. & Zou, L.P. (2001). P0 glycoprotein peptides 56-71 and 180-199 dose-dependently induce acute and chronic experimental autoimmune neuritis in Lewis rats associated with epitope spreading. *J Neuroimmunol 114*, 99-106.

Zou, L.P., Ljunggren, H.G., Levi, M., Nennesmo, I., Wahren, B., Mix, E., Winblad, B., Schalling, M. & Zhu, J. (2000). P0 protein peptide 180-199 together with pertussis toxin induces experimental autoimmune neuritis in resistant C57BL/6 mice. *J Neurosci Res 62*, 717-721.

Chapter 15

AUTOIMMUNE INITIATION OF MULTIPLE SCLEROSIS: MOLECULAR ASPECTS

C. Fred Westall[*]
Institute for Disease Research, Temecula, California, USA

ABSTRACT

Multiple sclerosis (MS) is considered to be initiated by an autoimmune attack on myelin proteins by a mimic within a protein from some unidentified microorganism. Experimental allergic encephalomyelitis (EAE) is the model for MS. Different peptides from four myelin proteins are potent known EAE immunogens. The contribution of particular amino acids to encephalitogenicity within several immunogens and the minimum adjuvant requirements have been ascertained. Thus, the EAE initiation process at a molecular level is known. Using this EAE molecular information with known aspects of clinical MS, e.g. patient's age, variable histology, clinical immunological data, epidemiology, etc., the molecular initiation process of the autoimmune aspects of MS is defined. This definition includes: a.) type of organism providing the mimic, b.) estimation of single versus multiple immunogens, c.) location of the mimic, d.) involvement of adjuvant molecules and other inflammatory agents, e.) elucidation of magnetic resonance imaging (MRI) data, f.) dissection of confusing cellular immunology data, and g.) explanation of variable histological lesion locations. With this information various therapeutic options are discussed.

INTRODUCTION

Multiple sclerosis (MS) is a slowly progressive disease of the central nervous system (CNS) distinguished by areas of demyelination. It is characterized by unpredictable relapses, remissions and stationary phases, which can last for weeks, months or even years. In latter life a more progressive form without the defined relapses usually develops (McAlpine, Lumsden

---
[*] Corresponding author: E-mail: fcwestallidr@roadrunner.com

and Acheson, 1972). The onset of multiple sclerosis is extremely variable. The average age of onset for women is 28 years and men 32 years. Symptoms may develop rapidly in the course of minutes, hours or days. Also the frequency of the initial symptoms of MS vary considerably: motor weakness in one or more limbs, 40%; optic neuritis, 22%; paresthesia, 21%; double vision, 12%; vertigo/vomiting, 5% and disturbance of micturation, 5%.

ALLERGIC ENCEPHALOMYELITIS

Experimental allergic encephalomyelitis (EAE), considered a model for MS, is an autoimmune attack on the central nervous system myelin. Clinical signs include paralysis, loss of balance, an incontinence of urine and feces. Lesions consist characteristically of dense infiltration of mononuclear leukocytic cells surrounding blood vessels (Kies, 1965).

Various central nervous system (CNS) myelin proteins---myelin basic protein, proteolipid protein, myelin-associated oligodendrocyte glycoproteins, and myelin-associated oligodendrocyte basic protein---are capable of inducing acute EAE in a variety of mammals when they are injected with the appropriate adjuvant (Kies and Alvord, Jr., 1959; Roboz-Einstein et al. 1962; Sakai et al., 1988; Tuohy et al., 1988; Amor et al., 1994). Linear encephalitogenic sequences within these proteins have been described (Table 1) (Westall, et al., 1971; Shapira, et al., 1971; Karkhanis et al., 1975; Westall, Thompson, and Lennon, 1977; Tuohy et al., 1988, 1989; Endoh et al., 1990; Greer et al., 1992; Amor et al., 1994; Mendel, Kerelero de Rosbo and Ben-Nun, 1995). In some cases the contribution to encephalitogenicity by the individual amino acids within a site has been elucidated. This work has centered with the encephalitogenic tryptophan peptide from myelin basic protein---phe-ser-trp-gly-ala-glu-gly-gln-arg (Eylar et al., 1970; Westall et al., 1971; Westall, 1972; Sasaki, 1974; Suzuki and Sasaki 1974; Westall and Thompson, 1977b; Khanarian et al., 1979) (Table 2). Whole brain injections also produce only EAE. Therefore, the myelin of the central nervous system appears to be unique in possessing a plethora of disease-producing immunogens.

A. Types of EAE

There are several forms of EAE, hyperacute, acute, and chronic/relapsing. Hyperacute is induced in Lewis rats by injection of guinea pig myelin basic protein (MBP) with *B. pertussis* (Levine, 1974; Lennon et al., 1976). Clinical signs initially appear within a week. A specific peptide derived from guinea pig MBP with *B. pertussis* also induces hyperacute EAE (Westall, Thompson and Lennon, 1977) (Table 3). Acute EAE, which develops within 2 weeks, can be initiated in different mammalian species with any one of four myelin proteins as described above.

Chronic relapsing EAE imitates MS more closely, both clinically and histologically (Lassmann and Wisniewski, 1979). It has been induced in monkeys, rabbits and guinea pigs by sensitization with CNS tissue and complete Freund's adjuvant. True relapsing EAE was initially observed in juvenile Hartley and strain 13 guinea pigs (Raine and Stone, 1977) and later in rats (Panitech and Ciccone, 1981) and mice. In juvenile guinea pigs, the relapsing

EAE was produced with whole CNS material, but only acute disease resulted when MBP was used. MBP is the prime protein encephalitogenic for guinea pigs. Furthermore, the tryptophan peptide from MBP, phe-ser-trp-gly-ala-glu-gly-gln-arg, is by far the most significant encephalitogenic region within MBP for guinea pigs (Westall et al, 1971). If the tryptophan residue in MBP is destroyed, MBP's encephalitogenicity vanishes (Chao and Einstein, 1970). Since MBP presents only one encephalitogen to guinea pigs, it was suggested that multiple antigens, were necessary for chronic EAE and maybe MS (Raine and Traugott, 1982). However, it was shown in rats (Panitech and Ciccone, 1981) and mice (Fritz, Chou and Mc Farlin, 1983) that MBP could produce chronic/relapsing EAE. Also MOG produces relapsing EAE in mice (Kerleo de Rosbo, Mendel and Ben-Nun, 1995) and rats (Johns et al., 1995).

What is the difference between guinea pigs and the other species with respect to chronic/relapsing EAE? In these other species a variety of myelin proteins are encephalitogenic---MBP, lipoprotein, MOG and myelin oligodendrocyte basic protein. Furthermore, there are multiple regions (immunogens) within these proteins which are themselves encephalitogenic in these species (see Table 1).These species, unlike the guinea pig, "see" multiple immunogenic regions even when only whole protein is injected. Therefore the rule that chronic relapsing EAE requires multiple immunogens is upheld. The guinea pig work suggests that a combination of strong (from MBP) and weak (from other CNS tissue) immunogens are also necessary. Since the individual peptide encephalitogens are of varying potency, non-guinea pig test animals would also see simultaneous strong and weak immunogens, when whole protein is injected.

Are their exceptions to these "rules" for chronic relapsing EAE induction? In the case of the Lewis rat, MOG peptide 35-55 is able to induce relapsing EAE (Johns et al., 1995). However, it is known that this long sequence contains at least both T cell and B cell epitopes (Bernard et al., 1997). Therefore, this example is not an exception. Furthermore 200 ug, an enormous amount for induction, per animal were used. It is interesting that Linington et al. at lower doses (1993) were unable to detect any neurological symptoms in Lewis rats using this peptide.

The mouse, however, presents an interesting story. In recent years there has been considerable work on mouse encephalitogens. In fact not only whole protein produces relapsing EAE, but synthetic peptides from these proteins are also claimed to be active (Amor et al., 1994; Kerlero de Rosbo, Mendel, Ben-Nun, 1995). This would seem to argue against the necessity of multiple immunogens for relapsing EAE induction. However, it is very difficult to compare this work with the studies involving other species. In the mouse a) usually multiple sites of injection, b) multiple adjuvants, c) large amounts of adjuvants, considering the size of the mouse, and d) large amounts of encephalitogenic peptide are employed. This last difference is particularly disturbing. Encephalitogenic peptide dose response curves are quite sharp (Young et al., 1974) (Table 4).

A few extra microorganisms can reduce the encephalitogenicity greatly. In some mice experiments the molar ratio of peptide to whole protein used for comparison is as much as 100 fold. When 1 ug is sufficient to induce potent EAE in guinea pigs (Young et al., 1974; Westall, 1978) or rats (Westall, Thompson and Lennon, 1977), why are 150-200 ug (Amor et al., 1994) used for induction in mice or the 200 ug of peptide 35-55 in Lewis rats as mentioned above. (Johns et al.,1995)? Table 3 and 4 compare acute EAE production in guinea pigs and Lewis rats using synthetic encephalitogens. It would appear at best to this author with over 40 years of encephalitogenic peptide experience, that the mouse work is employing immunological procedures and mechanisms which are totally different from those in other test species. These results also bring into question the contribution of impurities, even with synthetic peptides. An impurity of ½ % of a 200 ug preparation is still 1 ug!

Because of the large amounts of immunogen and the use of multiple adjuvants for induction, one could easily question whether the mouse is a very good model for MS. Furthermore, it has been shown in mice that MBP inducing relapsing EAE produces not only activated lymphocytes to MBP, but also to lipoprotein (Perry, Barzaga-Gilbert and Trotter, 1991). In the mouse weak encephalitogens might "allow other encephalitogenic structures" to be processed. To ascertain the differences between mouse relapsing EAE and the relapsing EAE seen in other species, encephalitogenic dose response curves and the effects of different adjuvant combinations, need to be performed. In any event, for best results in producing relapsing EAE relevant to MS, a series of immunogens must be present and that these immunogens are of varying potency. This last point probably is crucial. For each species except guinea pig, MBP for example, presents a very potent encephalitogen and one or more weaker ones. In the case of the guinea pig, other CNS material must provide the secondary immunogen(s).

Table 1. Major Defined Encephalitogenic Sequences[1]

Encephalitogen	Active EAE species	References
Myelin Basic Protein		
fswgaegqr-tryptophan pep.	Guinea pig, rabbit, monkey	Westall et al. 1971; Eylar, Westall and Brostoff, 1971
tthygslpqk-mid-peptide	Rabbit, DR rat	Shapira et al., 1971; Smeltz, Wolf and Swanborg, 1998
pqksqrtqdenpv-hyperacute	Lewis rat, monkey	Westall, Thompson and Lennon, 1977; Levine, 1974
fklggrdsr	Rabbit, monkey	Westall and Thompson, 1978; Eylar et al., 1972; Karkhanis et al., 1975
c-terminal	rat	Westall and Thompson, 1977
sequence 89-101	mouse	Jansson et al. 1991
sequence 1-9	mouse	Zamvil et al. 1986
Lipoprotein		
hslgkwlghpdkf	Mice	Tuohy et al, 1989
ntwttcqsiafpsk	Mice	Greer et al. 1992
yktticgkglsatv	Mice	Tuohy et al., 1988
dyeylinvihafqyv	Mice	Amor et al., 1993
Oligodendrocytic glycoprotein		
mevgwyrppfsrvvhlyrngk Also 1-22; 43-57;92-106	mice	Kerlero de Rosbo and Ben-Nun, 1996; Amor et al, 1994
Oigodendrocyte basic protein		
Residues 15-36	mice	Kerlero de Rosbo et al, 2004

[1] The decision of what should be included as a "major" encephalitogenic sequence is quite arbitrary. The result depends upon the laboratories testing the sequence and the animal being tested. The purpose of the table is primarily to show that there are several proteins which are encephalitogenic and within these proteins are numerous encephalitogenic regions.

Table 2 Encephalitogenicity in Guinea Pigs of Synthetic Variants of the Tryptophan Region Of Myelin Basic Protein (Phe Ser Trp Gly Ala Glu Gly Gln Arg)A

Sequence	References	Clinical Activity
PheSerTrpGlyAlaGlnGlyGlnLys	Westall et al., 1971	++
SerArgPheSerTrpGlyAlaGluGlyGlnLys	Eylar et al., 1970	++
SerArgPheSerTrpGlyAlaGluGlyGln ---	Eylar et al., 1970	-
SerArgPheSerTrpGlyAlaGluGlyGlnArg	Westall et al., 1971	++
SerArgPheSerTrpGlyAlaGluGlyGlnIle	Westall et al., 1971	-
SerArgPheSerTrpGlyAlaGluGlyIleLys	Westall et al., 1971	-
SerArgPheSerTrpGlyAlaIleGlyGlnLys	Westall et al., 1971	++
SerArgPheSerPheGlyAlaGluGlyGlnLys	Westall et al, 1971	-
SerArgPheSerValGlyAlaGluGlyGlnLys	Westall et al., 1971	-
SerArgPheAlaTrpGlyAlaGluGlyGlnLys	Westall et al., 1971	++
SerArgValSerTrpGlyAlaGluGlyGlnLys	Westall et al., 1971	+
PheSerTrpAlaAlaGluGlyGlnLys	Westall, 1972	-
GlySerTrpGlyAlaGluGlyGlnArg	Westall, 1972	+
PheSerTrpGlyAlaGluGlyGluArg	Westall, 1972	-
PheSerTrpGlyAlaGluGlySerArg	Westall and Thompson, 1977b	+
PheSerTrpGlydAlaGluGly Ser Arg	Khanarain et al, 1979	-
PheSerTrpGlyGlyGluGlyGlnArg	Suzuki and Sasaki, 1974	-
PheSerTrpGlyAlaGluGlyAsnArg	Sasaki, 1974	+
PheGlyTrpGlyAlaGluGlyGlnArg	Suzuki and Sasaki, 1974	++
PheSerTrpGlyAlaGlyGlyGlnArg	Suzuki and Sasaki, 1974	++
PheSerTrpGlyAlaGluGlyGlnGlyArg	Westall, 1972	+
PheSerTrpGlyAlaGluGlyGlyGlnArg	Westall, 1972	+

All peptides containing smaller segments of the tryptophan region were inactive (Eylar et al., 1970; Westall, 1972). However, using large amounts of synthetic adjuvant Nagai (1978a) was able to induce EAE in guinea pigs with the sequence trp-gly-glu-gly-gln-arg.

[a]The antigens were dissolved just prior to injection in normal saline and emulsified with Freund's complete adjuvant.

Table 3. The Effect of *B. Pertussis* on the Encephalitogen-Icity of Myelin Basic Proteins in Lewis Rats[1]

Encephalitogen	Dose	Clinical	Day of Onset	Number of Deaths
Guinea pig MBP	316	5/5	9,9,10,10,10	5/5
	100	5/5	9,10,10,10,11	5/5
	31.6	5/5	9,9,9,9,10	5/5
	10	5/5	9,10,10,10,11	5/5
	3.2	5/5	10,10,11,11,11	5/5
	1.0	5/5	11,12,12,13,14	5/5
Lewis rat MBP	316	5/5	10,11,11,11,11	4/5
	100	5/5	10,10,11,11,11	5/5
	31.6	4/4	11,12,12,12,14	0/5
	10.0	5/5	12,13,13,15,15	0/5
	3.2	4/5	14,15,17,17	0/5
	1.0	0/5	-----------------	

Table 3. (Continued)

Encephalitogen	Dose	Clinical	Day of Onset	Number of Deaths
Human MBP	316	5/5	8,8,8,9,9	2/5
	100	5/5	8,9,10,10,10	1/5
	31.6	5/5	9,10,11,11,11	1/5
	10.0	5/5	11,12,12,12,15	0/5
	3.2	0/5	------------------	
Monkey MBP	316	5/5	11,11,11,11,12	4/5
	100	5/5	11,11,12,13,13	3/5
	31.6	5/5	12,12,13,13,15	2/5
	10.0	5/5	12,13,15,15,19	0/5
	3.2	0/5	------------------	
Pig MBP	316	5/5	7,7,10,10,10	1/5
	100	5/5	8,9,11,11,11	2/5
	31.6	5/5	10,11,11,12,13	0/5
	10.0	3/5	12,12,13	0/5
	3.2	0/5	------------------	
Cow MBP	316	5/5	10,11,12,12,12	5/5
	100	5/5	10,12,12,12,12	5/5
	31.6	5/5	12,12,12,13,13	3/5
	10.0	2/5	12,12	0/5
	1.0	0/4	------------------	
Rabbit MBP	316	5/5	10,10,10,11,12	
	100	5/5	11,11,12,12,12	
	31.6	5/5	12,13,13,13,13	
	10.0	0/5	------------------	
Sheep MBP	316	5/5	10,11,11,12,14	1/5
	100	5/5	12,12, 13, 14,14	1/5
	31.6	1/5	14	0/5
Guinea Pig				
Peptide 70-88	0.3-4.9	33/33	Mean day 9	27/33
	0.01-0.08	13/14	Mean day 13	7/14
Peptide 73-86	1.9	12/12	Mean day 10	8/12
	0.3	8/8	Mean day 13	3/8
Rat Peptide 68-86	4.9	4/5	Mean day 13	0/5

[1] HEAE was distinguished from ordinary EAE clinically by a combination of early onset (usually 9-10 days), rapid and severe course and high incidence of mortality and cerebral signs (irritability, seizures, coma and spasticity). Histologic lesions characteristic of HEAE were found in all recipients of GPMBP. Histologic lesions in recipients of large doses (31.6-316 ug) of MBP other than guinea pig also had features of HEAE when examined on days 11-15.

Table 4. Induction of EAE in Guinea Pigs Using the Tryptophan Peptide from Myelin Basic Protein

Dose ug	Clinical	% Clinical	Histological	% Hist
10.00	11/42	26.1	25/42	59.5
3.30	17/51	34.0	29/51	56.8
1.00	30/51	58.8	34/51	66.7
0.33	6/26	23.1	18/26	69.2

It should also be noted that many of the peptide encephalitogens described for the mouse are substantially longer, 15-20 residues, than those described for other species, 9-11 residues (see Table 1). The probability of a mimic occurring in a microbial system which would trigger an autoimmune response against human myelin is directly related to the number of residues of the immunogen, the longer the immunogen the lower the probability. While some of these peptides might serve as multi-antigens, it is highly unlikely that a single mimic could imitate these long peptides.

B. Adjuvants

In order to improve immune responses to potential immunogens, a large number of substances, mostly bacterial, were studied to find general immunostimulants. These were collectively termed "adjuvants" (Freund, Stern and Pisani, 1947; Kabat, Wolf, and Bezer, 1947; Morgan, 1947). The most popular of these is Freund's complete adjuvant, which is an oil emulsion of *Mycobacteria*. With respect to autoimmune induction, the oil emulsion may or may not be required. With EAE, it appears essential. However, artificial castration (LHRH, immunogen, Carelli et al., 1982) and experimental autoimmune orchitis (aspermatogenous protein, immunogen, Toullet et al, 1977; Hagopian et al, 1977) are induced in aqueous solution.

Freund's adjuvant has been chemically defined further. Ellouz et al (1974) reported that the minimum molecular requirement for use as an adjuvant was n-acetyl-muramyl-L-ala-D-isogln (MDP or muramyl dipeptide). This molecule is found in a wide variety of bacterial cell walls. Other studies have shown that it can act as an adjuvant, a general, immunostimulant and anti-neoplastic drug. It also has been found to be pyrogenic (Kotani et al., 1977), a naturally found sleep factor (Martin et al., 1984) and a mimic of serotonin (Root-Bernstein and Westall, 1983, 1990). The single term "adjuvant" has been used whether one is discussing antibody stimulation, delayed hypersensitivity enhancement, pyrogenicity, anti-infectious effects, mitogenic responses, or autoimmune disease induction. Actually a given adjuvant may augment one or more of these actions (for review see Chedid, Audibert and Johnson, 1978). With the chemical definition of adjuvants (Ellouz et al., 1974) and the use of synthetic modifications, the different potential actions have been chemically distinguished (Adam et al., 1981).

Much work has been performed on muramyl dipeptide's ability to assist in the production of antibody against a large number of antigens. In these cases MDP appears to be functioning as a general immunostimulant (Chedid, Audibert, Johnson, 1978; Adam et al., 1981). It also does not have to be injected with the antigen or even at the same time as the antigen (Chedid et al., 1976). Since the immunogen-adjuvant complex is required (see below) for autoimmune disease initiation, MDPs function in autoimmune disease seems to be much more than just a general immunostimulant. This is further supported by the activity of synthetic modifications of muramyl dipeptide. As can be seen in Table 5, the specificity of adjuvanticity and autoimmune disease induction are similar, but decidedly different.

EAE induction by a myelin protein or its encephalitogenic peptides is dependent upon concomitant injection of Freund's complete adjuvant (FCA) or one of a number of other adjuvants or inducer types. While the encephalitogen and the inducer may be injected separately, they must be injected at the same site and within a very limited period of time to be active in EAE induction (Waksman, Adams and Mansmann, 1957). Depending upon the particular protein or peptide used and the species of the host animal, the adjuvant may be *Mycobacterium tuberculosis* or a close relative (Freund, Stern and Pisani, 1947; Kabat, Wolf, Bezer, 1947; Morgan, 1947), an active bacterial subunit, e.g. n-acetyl muramyl dipeptide (Ellouz et al., 1974; Nagai et al, 1978a; Nagai et al., 1978b), *B. pertussis* (Levine and Wenk, 1965; Lennon et al., 1976; Westall, Thompson and Lennon, 1977) or homogenates of whole spinal cord with and without synthetic adjuvants (Levine and Wenk, 1965), usually in an oil emulsion.

Nagai et al. (1978a, b) showed that n-acetyl-muramyl dipeptide (MDP) in the oil emulsion with the whole myelin basic protein, or the encephalitogenic tryptophan peptide of myelin basic protein, would induce EAE in guinea pigs. Maeda et al (1980) produced EAE in various strains of rats using MDP and whole myelin basic protein. Carilli et al., (1982) found that n-acetyl muramyl dipeptide with LHRH in an aqueous solution could induce artificial autoimmune castration. Lee and Schneider (1962) and Shaw et al. (1962), using whole proteins, have demonstrated that the ability of the encephalitogen-adjuvant combination to induce acute EAE is dependent upon the proportion of the constituents. Encephalitogenicity disappears if the proportion of adjuvant is too great or too small (Shaw et al., 1962; Simon and Anzil, 1974).

Westall (1978) noted the interesting dose response curve for both the tryptophan peptide and n-acetyl muramyl dipeptide---the minimum dose of each required for disease induction was equal on the molar basis. This led Root-Bernstein and Westall (1990) to show with nuclear magnetic resonance that the two physically formed a complex. The tryptophan peptide alone has only a slight interaction with the emulsion, whereas both muramyl dipeptide alone or in combination with the tryptophan peptide interacts considerably with the emulsion. They also found that LHRH and n-acetyl muramyl dipeptide formed a complex. In this case the complex formed in aqueous solution. More importantly they found that those combinations, whether involving tryptophan peptide, LHRH or adjuvant modifications, which did not produce disease, also did not physically form a complex. However, with respect to artificial castration, the adjuvant could be chemically attached and still disease would ensue. This association is not required for the adjuvant to act solely as a general immunostimulant (Hosmalin et al, 1987).Thus it appeared that for the induction of autoimmune disease added restrictions are placed upon the adjuvant. The immunogen and the adjuvant work as a unit.

Table 5. Comparison between the Specificity for Adjuvanicity and EAE Induction for MDP[1]

	Clinical EAE	Adjuvanticit
Nac-Mur-L-Ala-D-Glu-Gly	3/5	poor
Nac-Mur-Gly-D-isoGln	10/10	weak
Nac-Mur-D-Ala-D-isoGln	2/5	weak
Nac-Mur-L-Ala-D-isoGln	10/10	strong
Nac-Mur-L-Ser-D-isoGln	10/10	strong
Nac-Mur-L-Ala-D-isoGln-L-Lys-D-Ala	5/5	strong
Nac-Mur-LAla-D-isoGln-L-Lys	5/5	strong

[1] EAE data from Nagai et al., 1978b. Adjuvant activity data Chedid, Audibert, and Johnson, 1978.

Walter Moore and his associates investigated the tertiary structure of myelin basic protein and the encephalitogenic peptides derived from this protein. (Mendz, Moore and Carnegie, 1982; Chapman, Littlemore and Moore, 1978; Chapman and Moore, 1976). The tryptophan peptide---phe-ser-trp-gly-ala-glu-gly-gln-arg---has a distinct bent structure in aqueous solution. The oil emulsion would aid in maintaining this structure. In fact a sequence change which alters this bent form, eliminates the molecule's EAE activity. This was seen spectacularly with two sequence changes: a.) the change of an L-alanine for glycine and b.) the D-alanine for L-alanine. These are the most minimal sequence changes that can be made in the structure. However, the glycine permits a bend at the glycine-tryptophan bond. Alanine hinders it. The D-alanine change causes the molecule to twist away from the bent form. Obviously the tertiary structure of this small peptide is crucial for its activity. (Khanarian et al, 1979; Moore et al., 1981).

The conformation of the heptadecapeptide, phe-lys-leu-gly-gly-arg-asp-ser-arg-ser-gly-ser-pro-met-ala-arg-arg, comprising the encephalitogenic sequence in Rhesus monkey and rabbit has also been studied (Price, Mendz and Martenson 1988). Mendz and Moore (1983) also studied another rabbit encephalitogenic sequence. In both cases a bent form is found. Likewise, Fermandjian et al (1987), using 1H-NMR, found evidence for a MDP structure involving two successive beta turns. As mentioned above, using nuclear magnetic resonance, Root-Bernstein and Westall (1990) extensively studied the tryptophan/n-acetyl muramyl dipeptide and LHRH/n-acetyl muramyl dipeptide interactions. They found that the combinations indeed interacted and that immunologically-inactive modifications did not form a complex. (Tables 2, 6 and 7)

Table 6. Minimum Structural Requirements for Adjuvant Activity Induction of EAE in Guinea PIGs[1]

	Encephalitogenicity
Nac-Mur-L-Ala-D-isoGln	++
Nac-Mur-L-Ala	-
Nac-Mur-L-Ala-D-isoGln-L-Lys	++
L-Ala-D-isoGln-L-Lys-D-Ala	-
Nac-Mur-L-Ala-D-isoGln-L-Lys-D-Ala –L-Lys-D-Ala	++
Nac-Mur-L-Ala-D-Glu-NH2	++
Nac-Mur-L-Ala-D-Glu-Gly	+
Nac-Mur-L-Ser-D-Glu-NH2	++
Nac-Mur-Gly-D-Glu-NH2	++
Nac-Mur-D-Ala-D-Glu-NH2	+
Nac-Mur-D-Ala	-
Nac-Mur-D-Glu-NH2	-
Nac-Mur-L-Ala-D-Glu	+
Nac-Mur-L-Ala-L-Glu	-
Nac-Mur-L-Ala-D-Asp-NH2	-
alpha-Methyl-NAc-Mur-L-Ala-D-Glu-NH2	++
beta-Methyl-NAc-Mur-L-Ala-D-Glu-NH2	+
D-Lactyl-Ala-D-Glu-NH2	+
6-o-Stearoyl-NAc-Mur-L-Ala-D-Glu-NH2	-

[1-2] Nagai et al., 1978b; Chedid, Audibert and Johnson, 1978.

Table 7. Summary of NMR Results of Binding Muramyl Dipeptide and its Derivatives to Immunogens

	Active Adj	EAE Induc	Trp Pep	MSH 4-10	LHRH	LHRH 4-10	LHRH 1-3
Muramyl dipeptide	+	+	+	+	+	+,-	-
N-acetyl-nor-muramyl-L-alanyl-D-isoglutamine	+	unk	+	nd	+	nd	nd
N-acetyl-nor-muramyl-D-alanyl-D-isoglutamine	-	unk	-	nd	-	nd	nd
N-acetyl-muramyl-L-alpha-aminobutyryl-DisogIn	+,-	unk	-	nd	+,-	nd	nd
N-acetyl-muramyul-L-threonyl-D-isoglutamine	+	unk	+,-	nd	+	nd	nd
N-acetyl-muramyl-D-Ala-D-isoglutamine	-	-	-	-	-	-	-
N-acetyl-muramyl-L-Ala-L-isoglutamine	-	-	-	-	-	-	-
Muramic acid	-	-	-	-	-	-	-

Table 8. The Effect of *B. Pertussis* on the Encephalitogeni- City of Myelin Basic Proteins in Guinea PIGs

Encephalitogen	Dose	Numbers of *B. pertussis* Organisms	Clinical	Day of Onset	Day of Death
GPmbp	33ug	0	5/5	17,13,13,14,11	18,14,14,15,14
		10^{10}	5/5	14,17,13,14,19	15,18,14,15,27
		20×10^{10}	4/5	26,25,14,19	20,15
Lew Rat MBP	33ug	0	4/5	--,13,17,13,13	15,20,14,14
		10^{10}	5/5	17,14,18,21,13	18,27,14,20,27
		20×10^{10}	2/5	18,15	
Human MBP	33ug	0	5/5	11,14,11,13,13	12,15,13,14,14
		10^{10}	5/5	13,12,14,13,14	18,12,16,14,18
		20×10^{10}	3/5	26,19,19	20,19
Bovine MBP	33ug	0	4/5	13,13,13,13	15,14,15,15
		10^{10}	¾	10,17,17	12,18,17
		20×10^{10}	4/5	19, 19,18,18	20,19,19
Porcine MBP	33ug	0	5/5	11,13,12,13,13	19,20,19
		20×10^{10}	4/5	27,15,19,19	19,20,19
Monkey MBP	33ug	O	5/5	11,12,14,12,11	15,14,15,14,14
		20×10^{10}		19,25,18,19	19,25,18,20
Rabbit MBP	33ug	0	5/5	12,12,11,12,15	15,14,16,17
		20×10^{10}	4/5	13,13,14,20	14,14,15,20

Table 9. The Effect of *B. Pertussis* on the Encephalitogen-Icity of Myelin Basic Proteins in Rabbits

Encephalitogen	Dose, ug	Number of *B. pertussis* Organisms	Clinical	Day of Onset
Guinea Pig MBP	1000	4 x 10^{10}	1/4	20
	1000	0	3/4	20,20,22
Human MBP	1000	4 x 10^{10}	2/4	22,23
	1000	0	1/4	20
Encephalitogen	Dose, ug	Organisms	Clinical	Day of Onset
Rabbit MBP	1000	4 x 10^{10}	3/4	19,20,23
	1000	0	1/4	23
Bovine MBP	1000	4 x 10^{10}	1/4	18
	1000	0	1/4	20
GP Peptide 70-88	100	4 x 10^{10}	0/4	--

Is the apparent required association between adjuvant and antigen, seen between MDP and tryptophan peptide or LHRH, an apparent requirement for adjuvanticity with other adjuvants and immunogens? While most gram-positive bacteria have an acetylated muramyl structure in their cell-walls, *Mycobacteria*, *Norcardiea*, and *Micromonospora* have an acylated muramyl structure, involving a glycolyl group (Adam et al., 1976). Westall et al. (1975), using a hydrosoluble mycobacterial fraction (Migliore-Samour and Jolles, 1973) prepared by Migliore-Samour and Jolles, induced EAE in guinea pigs using whole myelin basic protein. However, when they attempted to produce EAE using the encephalitogenic tryptophan peptide eight times the adjuvant was required for induction (Westall et al., 1974).

Since the hydrosoluble mycobaterial adjuvant was effective using whole MBP and the tryptophan peptide is the only major encephalitogenic region in guinea pig, two possible explanations can be offered. First, the normal structure of the encephalitogenic peptide compared to its structure within the whole protein is different. Second, the hydrosoluble adjuvant was responding to a much weaker determinant in the whole protein, e.g. the n-terminal region (Barton et al., 1972). In either case the hydrosoluble adjuvant is specifically interacting with a particular immunogen in a different way than is seen with MDP. As stated above the n-acetyl muramyl dipepitde combined with the tryptophan peptide to form an active complex. It is very likely that the multiple carbohydrate units comprising the Mycobacterial fraction could disrupt the complex formation. In any event, the Jolles' hydrosoluble adjuvant is not just acting as a general stimulant, responding with any encephalitogen presented to it.

The whole *Mycobacterium* adjuvant appears to be effective in those mammalian species tested. However, the *B. pertussis* adjuvant shows tremendous variability in species potency. In Lewis rat, but not the Brown Norway (BN) rat, guinea pig myelin basic protein and *B. pertussis*, without the necessity of *Mycobacteria*, will produce a hyperacute form of EAE in Lewis rats (Lennon et al., 1976). This also appears in the monkey (Levine and Wenk, 1965; Levine and Wenk 1964; Levine, 1974). However, *B. pertussis* is rather ineffectual in rabbits and guinea pigs (Westall, 1977) (Tables 8-9). Within the guinea pig myelin basic protein is an encephalitogenic seqeuence, pro-gln-lys-ser-gln-arg-ser-gln-asp-glu-asn-pro-val-val, (Westall, Thompson and Lennon, 1977) which when it is injected with *B. pertussis* produces hyperacute EAE. Modified versions of this sequence, which mimic Lewis rat, rabbit, human cow and pig sequences, only produce regular EAE at normal doses. The *Mycobacterium* adjuvant will only produce ordinary EAE with any of these sequences in Lewis rat. The hyperacute site is only active in those species which are also active to *B. pertussis* (Westall, 1977). It is not active in rabbits or guinea pigs even if the *Mycobacterium* adjuvant is used. Also the tryptophan region, which is active with n-acetyl muramyl dipeptide and *Mycobacteria*, is not active in the species which are responsive to *B. pertussis*. These data are interpreted as showing that *B. pertussis* adjuvant has a "special association" with the hyperacute site, and the MDP has a "special association" with the tryptophan peptide.

C. Simultaneous Immune Processing of the Adjuvant and Immunogen

The complex requires that both the immunogen and the adjuvant are processed by the same immune cell. Only an activated system directed against the immunogen can result. There is no chance that excess immunogen or adjuvant can "turn on" suppressor systems. There is no chance that immunogen or adjuvant will be degraded prior to immune processing. There is no chance the adjuvant activated cells will "waste" their efforts on other molecules they encounter before they encounter the immunogen. Is there any other evidence which supports these conclusions? Yes LHRH has been chemically attached to the n-acetylmuramyl dipeptide. This modification should prevent the formation of the complex by complimentary interaction, but it still maintains a 1:1 association. What affect does this have on artificial castration? It still produces disease (Hosmalin et al., 1987; Bernard et al., 1987). The crucial step is the simultaneous processing by the same immune cell of both the adjuvant and immunogen. The linked complex, however, puts both immunogen and adjuvant at risk of premature digestion. However, since both the LHRH and n-acetyl muramyl dipeptide are themselves bent structures, their linked conformation might incorporate much of the complex form, and thus be protected.

MULTIPLE SCLEROSIS

While the cause is unknown, it is generally believed that MS is initiated by an autoimmune attack on the CNS myelin. A microorganism which contains a region on its surface which mimics an antigenic region on one of the myelin proteins instigates the autoimmune process (Jahnke, Fisher and Alvord, 1985; Fujinami and Oldstone, 1985)

A. Immunological Restrictions on Molecular Mimicry

With the availability of information concerning peptide encephalitogens, various investigators have searched the sequences of particularly viral coat proteins for similar structures. In some cases sequences have been synthesized and tested, with little success. While some sequences have initiated T cell activation (Ufret-Vicenty et al., 1998; Wucherpfennig and Stromenger, 1995; Katz-Levy et al., 1999) only one sequence initiates clinical encephalitogencity (Lenz et al, 2001). This sequence was located "in the C-terminus of a protein specified by a gene designated Cpn0483". The protein's location within the organism (*Chlamydia*) is not known. Could the immune system even access the region of the protein during human infection? Furthermore Freund's adjuvant was required to induce disease experimentally. Recently, the validity of molecular mimicry has been questioned (Bar-Or et al., 1999).

Many believe that small peptides do not possess tertiary structures. This is not true. As stated above, the structural work on encephalitogens have shown that slight changes, i.e. a D-alanine for L-alanine, or alanine for glycine, can easily alter the encephalitogencity of a peptide. Therefore, if one is looking for a molecular mimic one should be searching for "structural mimics" and not "sequential mimics". The immune system, like hormonal systems, recognizes three dimensional shapes, and not sequences. This is, however, not enough. The contributions of the individual amino acids must be ascertained. For example, not all nine residues of encephalitogenic peptide from myelin basic protein---phe-ser-trp-gly-ala-glu-gly-gln-arg--- are equally important. The phenylalanine can be replaced by other hydrophobics, especially ring structures. The arginine can be replaced by other positive structures. The glutamine can be substituted by serine but not glutamate, etc. This presents a major problem for molecular mimicry. There are very few immunologically-active peptides which have been analyzed to this degree (See Table 2).

B. Multiple Sclerosis Initiation

The author examined (2006a) the known sequences from bacteria and viruses which infect or are normally present in humans. No distinction was made between pathogens and non-pathogens or with the location of the protein within the microorganism. Sequences within these proteins were compared to the three best chemically defined encephalitogenic regions: the tryptophan peptide (phe-ser-trp-gly-ala-glu-gly-gln-arg), hyperacute site (pro-gln-lys-ser-his-qln-arg-thr-qln-asp-glu-asn-pro-val) and the mid-region (thr-thr-his-tyr-gly-ser-leu-pro-qln-lys) from myelin basic protein. The procedure outlined in the previous section was followed and was far more rigid than any previous process to identify mimics. The bacteria contained 111 encephalitogenic mimics: 39 corresponding to the midregion, 23 to the tryptophan peptide and 49 to the hyperacute site (Table 10). Very few viruses contained mimics. Almost all the mimics were found in bacteria, rather than viruses. No one immunogen dominated the group. In fact the differences in numbers of mimics seem to reflect more how extensive the immunogen had been defined, rather than any sequential preference. Sites were found in most of the bacteria examined. Gram stain characteristics of a bacterium seem to be irrelevant. The number of mimics found in a particular species seemed to reflect more on the amount of sequence data accumulated about that species. The mimics were located in all parts of the cell and within all parts of the proteins. The majority of the mimics were located in non-pathogenic gut bacteria. Since there are from 20 to 30 potential encephalitogenic regions in four myelin proteins, one must assume that structural mimics are not rare.

Table 10. Human Microorganism Proteins which Contain Potential Mimics of Defined Encephalitogens

Organism	Mid-Region Peptide	Tryptophan Peptide	Hyperacute Peptide
Bacterium			
Burkhoderia	1	1	0
Enteroccus	1	3	8
Bacteroides	6	6	3
Esherichia	7	2	8
Streptococcus	4	3	3
Lactobacillus	6	2	8
Clostridium	3	2	6
Bifidobacteria	1	2	3
Klebsiella	1	0	0
Fusobacteria	1	0	3
Salmonella	1	0	0
Chlamydophia	1	0	1
Haemophilus	1	1	0
Bacillus	1	0	0
Pseudomonas	1	0	0
Actinobacillus	1	0	0
Helicobacter	0	1	0
Serratia	0	0	5
Virus			
Hepatitis B	4	0	0
Hepatitis C	0	1	0
Papillomona	1	0	0
Influenza C	1	0	0
Blue Tongue	0	0	1
Ecovirus	0	0	1
Herpes	0	0	1

Previous to this study it was assumed that mimics were rare, which explained why MS was rare. However, they are not rare. To make matters worse the majority of the mimics are located in normal gut bacteria. If molecular mimicry is important in MS why is MS rare? Can EAE give an explanation? EAE induction first requires two molecules, the immunogen, in the MS case the mimic, and the adjuvant. However, the gut has large concentrations of gram-positive bacteria, which contain either n-acetyl muramyl dipeptide or n-acyl muramyl dipeptide. Therefore that is not a limitation. However, a second requirement is that the adjuvant and, in this case, mimic act together. The bacteria, itself is not being processed by the immune system, but the adjuvant and mimic are. For this to happen in the gut the hydrolytic processes must be activated in such a fashion to produce high concentrations of both adjuvant and mimic, which can then be immunologically processed. Aberrations in the hydrolytic processing of the gut could account for the rarity of MS. Is there any other evidence of gut involvement in MS? Yes. Serotonin metabolism is greatly altered during MS relapses. This was observed (Westall, 200a) by longitudinal measurements of (5-HIAA)/ tryptophan ratios from MS urine. This ratio drops noticeably during relapse. The urinary serotonin reflects gut metabolism and not central nervous system metabolism. As mentioned above n-acetyl muramyl dipeptide is a potent serotonin mimic. If it is elevated one could hypothesize that it would act like serotonin and feedback inhibit serotonin production by inhibition of tryptophan hydrolase production. This would lower serotonin concentrations. However the MDP could also act in place of serotonin at other receptors. This could explain why one sees a reduction of serotonin without any clinical effects.

C. Adjuvants

The importance of adjuvants in induction of experimental autoimmune disease has been known for decades. However, their possible importance in human autoimmune diseases has been essentially ignored. The fact that post viral and vaccinal neuropathies are associated with secondary infections is suggestive (Root-Bernstein and Westall, 1986). Furthermore it appears possible that the immunogens important in MS are mimicked by gut bacterial protein fragments. Some of these same bacteria contain peptidoglycans which have been linked to adjuvanticity. Thus both immunogen mimics and adjuvant molecules are readily available from the same sources. Has there been any association between adjuvants and MS. Yes. Elevated concentrations of peptidoglycans in MS neurological cells, immunological cells and in antigen-presenting cells have been reported (Schrijver el al., 2001). They also found peptidoglycan antibodies in MS CSF. Since the brains examined for this study were from patients who had had MS for over 14 years, the significance is somewhat cloudy. One could argue that the peptidoglycan concentrations in MS cells are secondary events of a chronic process.

Several studies suggest that infections correlate with MS attacks (Sibley, Bamford and Clark, 1985; Buljevac et al., 2002). However, over 80% of the infections are identified as of viral sources and certainly not all of the bacterial infections are from gram-positive (peptidoglycan-containing) bacteria. Furthermore, MS patients have fewer infections than non-sick individuals (Buljevac et al., 2002). Therefore it would seem unlikely that the increased MS peptidoglycan concentrations are from these infections. Most likely they are from the gut. Lehonten (Lehtonen, Eerola and Toivanen, 1997; Lehtonen et al., 1995) (Table 11) found that the concentration of peptidoglycans in normal immunological cells was dependent on age. At birth there were none. This increased until after puberty and then slowly declined in latter life. Therefore, negligible concentrations of peptidoglycans were expected to be found in the MS cells discussed above. Lehonten also concluded that the peptidoglycans were from gut. In any event it would seem that there is an abnormal, i.e. hydrolytic, production of peptidoglycans in MS.

Lipopolysaccharides are the gram-negative bacterial counterpart to peptidoglycans. Lipopolysaccharides have the ability to pass the gut barrier without assistance, a property which has been used by the pharmaceutical industry for some time. These compounds have been shown to grossly affect the blood-brain barrier (Xaio et al, 2001) and cause acute inflammatory responses in CNS parenchyma (Andersson, Perryand Gordon, 1992). One of the enzyme responsible for the breakdown of lipopolysaccharides, arylesterase, has been shown to be deficient in MS myelin (Back, Broch-Moeller and Boeg-Hansen, 1976). Therefore, another bacterial component has been associated with the MS pathology.

Table 11. Age Distribution of Subjects with Muramic Acid in Peripheral Blood Leucocytes

Mean Age	% Positive Subjects	Number in Group
0	0	41
14	60	20
25	23	83
35	17	41
45	0	34
55	5	61
65	7	46
75	0	38

The muamic acid was detected by gas chromatography/ mass spectrometry by the procedure in references, Lehtonen, et al., 1995; Lehtonen, Errola and Toivanen, 1997.

D. Simultaneous Activation of the Immune System by Multiple Immunogens

There is a major difference between chronic relapsing EAE and MS. In chronic EAE, the immunogens are injected in a fixed ratio as determined by the composition of the whole tissue or protein. In the case of MS, if multiple mimics are involved, the mimics encounter the immune system in variable concentrations depending on the microorganisms and hydrolytic enzymes present. This would suggest that MS clinically would present a much more varied disease than the EAE model. Of course this is what is seen.

If chronic relapsing EAE is initiated by the action of multiple immunogens, are there any data supporting simultaneous multi-immunogenic initiation of MS? As was mentioned above mimics of encephalitogenic regions appear rather plentiful. MS' rarity appears to be the result of problems in the processing of the mimic: a) either the presentation of the mimic, through digestive processes involving hydrolytic enzymes, to the immune system or b) the activation of the immune system by the mimic. Both of these processes are under strict hormonal control. This is particularly interesting since it has been suggested (see below) that the histo-clinical variance characteristic of MS is the result of proteolytic processing of myelin antigens in the CNS (Westall, 2006b). The same hormones which control CNS proteolysis also control the gut processes. In any event, MS appears as a hormonal disease which is manifested clinically as an autoimmune attack on CNS myelin (Westall, 2000a, 2007). If the processing, and not the presence of the mimic, is determining disease initiation, why would the immune system only process as single mimic at a time? It would seem more likely that multiple mimics would simultaneously be processed. In other words, MS, like chronic relapsing EAE, its model, is an autoimmune attack on the CNS myelin by the simultaneous activation of the immune system by multiple mimics of myelin antigens. Is there any other data which would support this explanation? Yes.

Various test results on the responses of different myelin proteins to MS activated immune cells have been confusing. Different groups have found myelin basic protein (MBP) (Tejada-Simon et al., 2000), lipoprotein (Trotter et al., 1998; Correale et al., 1995) and oligodendrocyte glycoprotein (MOG) (Kerlero de Rosbo et al., 1997) responsive to the activated MS system. The MOG data is the most impressive. However, when all three immunogens were tested in the same patients, better response was seen with MOG, but the other two showed positives, which certainly presents a complicated multi-antigen activation (Kerlero de Rosbo et al., 1993). Finally, the MOG data shows positive response to multiple regions within the MOG protein. This also supports a complicated multi-antigen activation.

E. Longitudinal Appearance of Cytokines and Other Inflammatory Compounds

The work discussed in this section involves only relapsing-remitting MS. The progressive form of MS usually develops late and therefore has years of chronic overlay.

MS was generally thought to be initiated by an autoimmune attack on myelin, i.e. a form of EAE. However, recent magnetic resonance imaging (MRI) work has suggested that MS is far more complicated (Lassmann, Bruck and Lachinetti, 2007; Filippi and Rocca, 2005; Griffen et al., 2002; Silver et al., 2001, Goodwin et al., 1998). Initially a rather diffuse lesion appears. These lesions develop prior to any external immunological cell invasion. In some cases the lesions develop into the classically described MS lesions. Since the initial lesions lack the presence of bacterial and viral agents or externally-produced immunological cell infiltrates, what triggers these initial lesions?

If bacteria are involved in MS by providing immunological mimics and adjuvants molecules, they should also provide other cell wall components, such as lipo-polysaccharides, which have known inflammatory properties. These agents can pass easily through the gut barrier and tight junction cells, as they are used by the pharmaceutical industry to transport drugs (Wong and Toth, 2001). Mimics and their associated adjuvant molecules initiate an autoimmune process which requires weeks to develop. The lipopolysaccharides and other inflammatory agents can activate inflammation and other degradative processes within hours (Felts et al., 2005) This process could explain the histological picture that has emerged.

Is there evidence for non-CNS MS –related activity? Gut serotonin metabolism, as reflected by the urinary tryptophan/5-hydroxyindole acetic acid ratio, drops during MS relapses (Westall, 2006a). As already mentioned peptidoglycans, which are presumably from the gut appear in abnormal concentrations in MS immunological and neurological cells. Numerous other inflammatory and immunological agents appear in the spinal fluid, serum and urine significantly earlier than the development of the classical MS immune lesions. In fact the concentrations of these agents maximizes in some cases a month or two months prior to the MS relapse (Tables 12 and 13). To the contrary in EAE the concentrations of these compounds rise quickly within days as the clinical disabilities develop and decline rapidly. Therefore the clinical expression of these compounds is quite different in MS.

The principal physiological pathways for metabolic degradation of the extracellular matrix in mammals consist of a family of matrix metalloproteinases (MMP's). MMP activities are controlled by gene transcription, proenzyme activation and activity of tissue inhibitors of MMPs (TIMPS). In MS MMP-9 was increased over controls in 100% of relapsing remitting cases. However, similar levels of MMP-9 were detected during relapses and clinically stable phases of disease (Leppert et al., 1998).

In a small longitudinal study of MS patients in acute relapse, high expression of MMP-9 in CSF coincided with gadolinium-enhancing lesions on MRI (Rosenberg et al., 1996).

However in a cross-sectional study of 40 patients no correlation between the number of active MS lesions and MMP-9 could be established (K. Gijbels, personal communication). Similarly the number of hyperintense MS lesions as found in T2- and proton weighted MRI scans, does not correlate with MMP-9 in CSF (Paemen et al., 1994). Kouwehoven et al. (2002) showed differences in MMPs and TIMPs expression, production, secretion and activity between immature dendritic cells and mature dendritic cells from MS patients and healthy controls, but they were unable to find correlations with clinical variables. In MS TIMP is not upgraded. CSF MMP to TIMP ratios did not differ between MS subtypes, suggesting systemic rather than CNS-restricted changes.

Table 12. Time-Line for the Appearance of Inflammatory and Immunological Compounds Associated with Ms Relaspse

A. Abnormal mRNA Levels in Peripheral Blood Mononuclear Cells from MS Patients[1,2]

Compound	-12	-11	-10	-9	-8	-7	-6	-5	-4	-3	-2	-1	0	+1	+2	+3	+4	+5	+6	+7	+8
Elevated Values																					
Caspase-1								o	o	o	x		o	o							
IL-12p35						o			o		x			o							
IL-12p40						o			x		o			o							
IL-10						o			o		x			o							
CXCR3	o			+				+			x					-				o	
TNF-alpha	o			o				x			-					-				o	
Lymphotoxin	o			o				x			-					-				o	
Reduced Values																					
TGF-b	o			o				x			-						o			o	
IL-10	o			o				x			-						o			o	

1 X refers to maximum value. + and – means that the values are increasing or decreasing to and from the maximum. O indicates essentially baseline values.

2References:
Caspase-1: Furlan et al., 1999a,b
TNF-a, Il-12p35, IL-12p40, and IL-10: van Boxel-Dezaire et al. 1999
CXCR3: Mahad et al., 2003
Tumor necrosis factor-alpha, Transforming growth factor-beta, lymphotoxin, and interleukin-10: Rieckmann et al, 1995

B. Abnormal Serum Levels in MS Patients[1,2].

Compounds	-12			-8			-4			0			-4			-8		
Elevated																		
MMP/TIMP-1	+			+			x			-			-			-		
MMP-3	o			o			o			+			x			o		
Glutamate	o			+			+			x			-			o		

1 X refers to maximum value. + and – means that the values are increasing or decreasing to and from the maximum. O indicates essentially baseline values.

2References:
MMP/TIMP-1 Waubert et al., 1999.
MMP-3 Kanesaka et al., 2006.
Glutamate: Westall, Myers & Ellison, 1980.

Table 13. Inflammatory and Immunological Compounds Related to MS Relapses

Compound	Source	Correlation with MS Relapse	Reference
Kinin B1 receptor	Rna-leucocytic cells	Up-regulated	Prat et al., 2005
Gelainase B	serum	elevated	Lee et al., 1999
PAI-1	plasma	elevated	Onodera et al., 1999
Interleukin-15	Rna-mononuclear cells	No change	Kivisakk et al., 1998
ICAM-1	Serum	Slightly elevated	Alves-Leon et al., 2001
CXCL10	CSF	Increased	Moreira et al., 2006
CCL2	CSF	Lower	Moreira et al., 2006
TNF receptor	serum	Correlates	Khoury et al., 1999
Neopterin	Serum	No correlation	Bagnato et al., 2003
Beta-2 Microglobulin	Serum	No correlation	Bagnato et al., 2003
Uric acid	Serum	Lower	Mostert et al., 2005
TNF-a converting	RNA-leucocytic cells	Up regulated	Seifert et al., 2002
sVCAM-1	Serum/ CSF	Elevated	Matsuda et al., 1995
CCL2	CSF	Decreased	Malmestrom et al., 2006

The Leppert study also found MMP-2 was not upgraded and did not detect MMP-7. Table 12 presents data showing MMP-3 levels were elevated transiently within 1 month after relapse. MMP-3 with its broad specificity can degrade major components of the blood-brain barrier.

Caspase -1 cleaves IL-beta and IL-18 precursor proteins into their secretory forms and it is therefore essential in the early steps of the inflammatory process. It appears to be involved in the blood-derived CNS confined inflammatory process underlying lesion formation in MS. Furlan et al. (1999a,b) found that caspase-1 mRNA levels peak significantly only in the week preceding an acute attack, subside immediately after the beginning of an acute attack, and correlate with the number of new but not persisting enhancing lesions.

Plasminogen activators (PA) convert plasminogen into the serine protease plasmin, which degrades several components of the ECM and activates MMPs. It is significant that one of the earliest detectable signs of inflammation in MS white matter is increased expression of PAs on mononuclear cells in perivascular cuffs (Cuzner et al., 1996). The CSF plasminogen activator, tPA, activity in MS patients was significantly raised, but did not correlate with disease activity (Akenami et al., 1996). Onodera et al. (1999) found the plasma plasminogen activator inhibitor-1 level in patients with active MS 6 times higher than the controls.

Cytokines are a family of polypeptides that regulate immune responses and inflammatory reactions. Three of them, interleukin-1 beta, tumor necrosis factor alpha, and interleulin-6 are secreted mainly by monocytes, but all three can also be synthesized by other immune and non-immune cells including CNS microglia and astrocytes. Interleukin-1 beta and tumor necrosis factor alpha promote the establishment of perivascular infiltrates by increasing adhesiveness between endothelium and leukocytes (Bevilacqua et al., 1995) Interkeukin-6 induces immunoglobulin production of activated B cells. All three cytokines enhance T- and

B-cell immune responses (Dinarello, 1989). Both interleukin-1 beta and tumor necrosis factor alpha stimulate the proliferation of astrocytes and promote gliosis in vivo (Giulian and Lachman, 1985). Maimone et al. (1991) found CSF interleukin-6 in 10 of 34 MS patients. There were no statistical differences between active and stable MS. Frei et al. (1991) found IL-6 concentrations in MS plasma were about 17 times higher than MS CSF. This report supports the hypothesis of a systemic B cell response in MS. The results for tumor necrosis factor were similar. Beck et al. (1988) found that tumor necrosis factor and interferon peaked approximately 2 weeks before exacerbation and then declined. As early as 4 weeks prior to a relapse, tumor necrosis factor alpha and lymphotoxin mRNA expression significantly increased whereas interleukin 10 and transforming growth factor beta mRNA decreased compared to mRNA values of these cytokines at 8 or 12 weeks prior to a relapse (Rieckmann et al., 1995). Serum concentrations decreased significantly before clinical relapse and the appearance of active lesions (Galboiz and Miller, 2002).

Increased levels of soluble intercellular adhesion molecules, sVCAM-1 and sL-selectin and tumor necrosis receptor were found in the blood of clinically active MS patients experiencing a clinical relapse (Hartung et al. 1995).

Elevated CSF glutamic acid concentrations, as much as three times normal, have been reported in active MS lesions (Stover et al., 1997). This aberration can lead to neurologic cell death (Goldsmith, 2000; Werner, Pitt and Raine, 2001). Westall et al., (1980) in a longitudinal study found that the serum glutamate concentrations are elevated in active MS as much as two times normal. The increase in glutamic acid did not occur sharply during the onset of relapse. Instead it appeared to rise gradually within a month or two prior to the onset of the clinical relapse to reach a peak during the relapse and then slowly decline. Since the absolute serum concentration observed were much higher than the CSF levels, the source of the glutamate in the serum was not the CSF. Elevated levels of endogenous glutamate and/or excessive activation of glutamate receptors can stimulate MMP-9 production through a NO synthase pathway (Manabe, Gu and Lipton, 2005). It can also interfere with cystine cellular transfers via competing with the carrier molecule on the cell (Bannai, 1986).

One problem with MS research is that there are limited numbers of longitudinal studies. Clinical researchers tend to compare active MS with inactive MS to controls. Only a few studies watch individual patients as they develop a relapse and as the relapse subsides. This is unfortunate since it tends to give an all or nothing result. This is quite misleading since many of the compounds of interest peak considerably before or after the relapse (Tables 12 and 13). This adds to the confusing nature of the results reported.

Another problem in studying individual compounds and their variance in MS is that different investigators use different techniques with varying sensitivities.

F. Histological Location

Any hypothesis of the pathology of MS must include an explanation of its peculiar variability in symptoms, which of course is reflected in its histology. The most common explanation of the histo-clinical variability is that MS is a collection of diseases, which produce essentially the same clinical result. However when one examines individual patients one sees a continuum of symptoms rather than finite groups of diseases.

For the immune system to attack the myelin or areas in the vicinity of the myelin, the immune cells have to be activated. I already have suggested that this process for MS involves the exposure to the immune system of mimics by abnormal hydrolytic digestion of microorganisms, probably gut bacteria. Once the immune cells are activated they look for the appropriate antigen. Encephalitogenic regions are short peptides. In fact they were originally isolated from proteolytic digestion. These peptides tend to be rather stable. For example the 43-88 MBP region is found in the CSF of active MS patients, even though a variety of proteases inundate the MS lesion (Whitaker, 1997). Extensive digestion of myelin proteins does not necessarily destroy its encephalitogenic and antigenic regions. In fact variable processing of myelin proteins is known to hide known regions and expose newer antigens (Matsuo, 1997). The characteristic histological feature of EAE is called perivascular cuffing. This shows the activated immune cells surrounding the blood vessel, not the myelin. This strongly suggests that the activated cells are encountering initially peptides released from the myelin, presumably due to normal protein turnover. Calculations (Westall, 1974) based on the normal turnover of myelin proteins support the release of a constant gradient of peptides from its structure. The turnover is the result of the action of both intracellular and extracellular proteases. Table 14 lists the proteases associated with oligodendrocytes including their location and specificity.

While the composition of myelin within the CNS is consistent, the concentrations of the individual proteases vary greatly within different locations of the brain. (Table 14) Furthermore, most are under strict control. Therefore the proteases' concentrations are further altered in response to these controls. An individual protein will be processed differently by altering the concentrations and availability of the CNS proteases. Therefore the availability and concentration of myelin antigens will vary with the alterations in proteases. At a specific *time* and *place*, the activated immune cells will be presented with none, one or more antigens. Therefore active immune attack will vary depending on this dynamic character of the proteolytic populations. In MS histology will vary with time in an individual and among patients. This variance in histology is mirrored in variance in clinical signs---all tied to a dynamic hydrolytic process which is constantly altering. This process does not only affect histology, clinical observations, and progression of disease, but also its initiation. Everything is tied to the abnormal function of the hydrolytic controls.

G. Clinical Ramifications

Because hyperacute, acute and relapsing EAE overlap histopathologically and immunologically they provide experimental evidence supporting the concept that certain human demyelinating diseases represent a spectrum of autoimmunity ranging from chronic multiple sclerosis to acute hemorrahagic necrotizing leukoencephalopathy, for which hyperacute EAE is a model (Levine and Wenk, 1964; Levine, 1974). It is generally presumed that adjuvants are only necessary for experimental autoimmune induction. However, this doesn't seem to be the case. Viral neuropathies, quite rare diseases, involve autoimmune attack of the nervous system. The viral attacks are very prevalent events even though the induction of autoimmune disease is very rare. These viral neuropathies have a significant association with secondary infections (see discussion in (Westall and Root-Bernstein, 1986). The secondary infection would provide an adjuvant molecule, not provided by the virus.

Table 14. Proteases Which Have Known Association with Oligodendrocytes

PROTEASE	CHARACTERISTICS	LOCATION
Myelencephron-Specific [A-E]	Increaed by kainic acid—regulated by protease secreted	Highest in medulla oblongata, spinal cord; lowest in corpus callosum, anterior commussure
Caspase-1 (iL-1beta convert [F-H]	Involved in inflammation	Located in oligodendrocytes
Calpain [J-L]	Membrane bound, increased by calpastatin, lipids, activator protein	Located in myelin
Cathepsin [M-N]	Acid protease, increased in MS Seen in MS lesions, degrades myelin basic protein	
MMP-9 [O-Q]	Cysteine protease Induced by liposaccharides	Up in corpus callosum
Cathepsin L [R]	Extracellular-regulated by cistatin C	Located in myelin
Neuropsin [S-T]	Serine protsese, kainite induced, injury induced secreted	Neurons---Oligodendrocytes
Plasminogen Activator [U]	Serine protease	Similar distribution to myelencephalon specific protein Except lower in medulla oblonga, temporal and frontal lobes and cerebral cortex
Cathepsin A [V]	Carbxypeptidase ---increased in MS	
Dipeptidyl peptidase II [W]		Oligodendrocytes
Carboxypeptidase M [X]	Membrane bound	Rich in corpus callosum, pyramidyl and optic tracts; low in ganglia and cortex

[A-E] Scarisbrick et al., 2000
Scarisbrick et al., 2001
Yamanaka et al., 1999
Blaber, et al., 2002
Bernett, et al., 2002
[F-H] Shibata et al., 2000
Furlan et al., 1999b
Hisahara, Okano & Miura, 2003
[J-L] Li and Banik, 1995
Shields and Banik, 1998.
Chakrabarti et al., 1993.
[M-N] Schaecher, Shield and Banik, 2001.
Snyder, et al., 1985.
[O-Q] Berlet, 1986.

Chantry & Glynn 1990
Penkowa et al., 2003
[R] Oh, et al., 1999
[S-T] Stebbins, Jaffe & Moeller, 1998
Tomizawa, et al., 1999
[U] He, et al., 2001
[V] Grynbaum & Marks, 1976
[W] Gorenstein & Sweet, 1985
[X] Nagae, et al., 1992

Chlamydia pneumoniae has been linked to multiple sclerosis (Swanborg, Whittum-Hudson and Hudson, 2003; Stratton and Sriram, 2003). In fact a *Chlamydia pneumoniae*-specific peptide induces EAE in rats (Lenz et al., 2001). N-acetyl muramyl dipeptide is a component of the cell walls of many bacteria especially gram positive organisms. However,

Chlamydia is an exception. It contains no muramic acid. Therefore even though *Chlamyida* contains an encephalitogenic immunogen, its infection of an animal results in no EAE. The investigators who are looking for MS immunogens should also search for MS adjuvants.

Table 15. Suppression of Hyperacute EAE with Myelin Basic Protein in Lewis Rats

Challenge MBP [1]	Suppressor MBP in Saline[2]	Dose (ug) daily	Clinical6 Animals/Group
Rat (35mg)	Rat	1500	0
		750	0
		500	1
		250	1
		125	5
	Guinea Pig	1500	0
		750	0
		375	1
		187	2
		94	4
	Bovine	2000	6
		1000	6
		500	6
		250	4
		125	6
	Rabbit	1000	6
		500	5
		250	6
		125	6
Bovine	Bovine	2000	0
		1000	0
		500	0
		250	0
		125	3
		0	6
Guinea Pig	Guinea Pig	2000	0
	Bovine	2000	6

[1] The basic proteins were prepared in saline, emulsified with CFA and injected intradermally into 10 week-old female Lewis rats as described in reference Lennon et al., 1977. *B. pertussis* vaccine (2 x10^{10} organisms) was injected subcutaneously.

[2] The suppressive dose was given daily IP from day 4-12 after challenge.

One area of therapeutic work has involved specific antigen suppression (Mozes, Sela and Tausig, 1974). This is accomplished by either injecting multiple large doses of a suspected immunogen, for example myelin basic protein, or knocking out specific cell lines which recognize a specific immunogen. Because of the mounting data supporting multiple immunogen involvement in MS this type of therapy appears ill advised. There is an added problem with attempting antigen suppression. MBP is a very effective therapeutic agent against EAE in guinea pigs, but it did not work in a MS trial. Is this because MBP is not the immunogen in MS? Or is it because the correct immunogen within MBP was not tested? Porcine MBP was used in the Salk/ Lilly MS trial (Salk et al, 1980). In guinea pigs the major encephalitogenic region is the tryptophan peptide. With the exception of an arginine for lysine, the sequence of this peptide does not vary among mammalian species. However the MBP encephalitogenic region in Lewis rat varies greatly among mammalian species. In fact porcine is only weakly active in Lewis rats. The Lewis rat encephalitogen is also active in monkeys. If the Lewis rat encephalitogen (the HEAE site) is the region active in humans, the Salk/Lilly experiment never tested the effectiveness of MBP as a therapeutic agent in MS (Table 15).One then would suggest that human MBP should be used, at least in a small initial trial. However, here again one could have a problem. In Lewis rats, Lewis rat MBP is a potent encephalitogen. However guinea pig MBP is much more powerful. It will not only suppress acute EAE but also hyperacute EAE. Rather than looking at specific immunogens or general immunosupressant, one should examine how these immunogens are produced. This work centers on the hormonal control systems involved in hydrolytic processes in the brain, gut and other sites in the human anatomy. Compounds could be produced to specifically alter the action of these hormonal controls systems. This virgin area would certainly have an excellent potential as a MS therapeutic tool.

REFERENCES

Adam, A., Deyys, M., Souvannavong, V., Lefrancier, P., Choay, J. & Lederer, E. (1976). Correlation of structure and adjuvant activity o fn-acetyl-muramyl-l-alanine-d-iosglutamine, its derivatives and analogues. *Biochem. Biophys. Res. Comm., 72*, 339-346.

Adam, A., Petit, J. F., Lefrancier, P. & Lederer, E. (1981). Muramyl dipeptides. *Mol. Cell. Biol., 41*, 27-47.

Akenami, F. O. T., Siren, V., Koshiniemi, M. Simes, M. A.,Teravainen, H., Vaheri, A. (1996). Cerebrospinal fluid activity of tissue plasminogne activator in patients with neurological diseases. *J. Clin. Pathol., 49*, 577-580.

Alves-Leon, S. V., Batista, E., Papais-Alvarenga, R. & Quirico-Santos, T. (2001). Determination of soluble ICAM-1 and TNFalphaR in the cerebrospinal fluid and serum levels in a population of Brazilian patients with relapsing-remitting MS. *Arg. Neuro-Psiquiatr, 59*, 1-7.

Amor, S., Baker, D., Groome, N. & Turk, J. L. (1993). Identification of a major encephalitogenic epitope of proteolipid protein for the induction of EAE in Biozzi AB/H and non-obese diabetic mice. *J. Immunol., 150*, 5666-5672.

Amor, S., Groome, N., Linington, C., et al. (1994). Identification of epitopes of myelin oligodendrocyte glycoprotein for the induction of EAE in SJL and Biozzi AB/H mice. *J. Immunol., 153*, 4339-56.

Andersson, P. B., Perry, V. H. & Gordon, S. (1992). The acute inflammatory response to liposaccharide in CNS parenchyma differs form that in other body tissues. *Neurosci., 48*, 169-186.

Back, U., Boch-Moeller, B. & Boeg-Hansen, T. C. (1976). Host resistance to liposaccharides in the pathogenesis of MS and Membranoproliferative glomerulonephritis. *Lancet II*, 188-191.

Bagnato, F., Durstandi, V., Finamore, L., Volante, G. & Millefiorini, E. (2003). Beta-2 microglobulin and neopterin as markers of disease activity in MS. *Neurol. Sci., 24*, S301-304.

Bannai, S., (1986). Exchange of cystine and glutamate across plasma membrane of human fibroblasts. *J.Biol.Chem., 261*, 2256-2263.

Bar-Or, A. Oiveira, E. M. L., Anderson, D. E. & Hafler, D. (1999). Molecular pathogenesis in MS. *J. Neuroimmunol., 100*, 252-259.

Barton, M. A., McPherson, T. A., Lemieuex, R.U.and Bain, G.O. (1972). Allergic encephalomyelitis. *Can. J. Biochem., 50*, 689-96.

Beck, J., Rondot, P., Catinot. L., Falcoff, E., Kirchner, H. & Wietzerbin, J. (1988). Increased production of interferon gamma and tumor necrosis factor precedes clinical manifestation in MS: Do cytokines trigger off exacerbations? *Acta Neurol. Scand., 78*, 318-323.

Berlet, H. (1986). Acid endopeptidase activty of human myelin elicited by using exogenous MBP as enzyme substrate. *FEBS, 194*, 297-300.

Bernard, J. M., Gras-Masse, H., Drobeacq, H., Tartar, A., et al. (1987). Synthesis of conjugates between luteinizing hormone releasing hormone (LHRH) and MDP models of totally synthetic vaccines. *Int. Pept. Protein Res., 29*, 455-463.

Bernett, M. J., Blaber, S. I., Scarisbrick, I. A., Dhanarajan, P., Thompson, S. M. & Blaber, M. (2002). Crystal structure and biochemical characterization of human kallikrein 6 reveals a trypsin-like kallikrein is expressed in the CNS. *J. Biol. Chem, 277*, 24562-70.

Bevilacqua, M. P., Pobver, J. S., Wheeler, M. E., et al., (1995). Interleukin 1 acts on cultured human vascular endothelium to increase the adhesion of polymorphonuclear leukocytes, monocytes and related leukocyte cell lines. *J. Clin. Invest, 76*, 2003-2011.

Blaber, S. I., Scarisbrick, I. A., Bernett, M. J. et al. (2002). Enzymatic properties of rat myelencephalon-specific protease. *Biochem., 41*, 1165-73.

Buljevac, D., Flach, H. Z., Hop, W. C. J., Hijdra, D., Laman, J. D., et al. (2002). Prospective study on the relationship between infections and MS exacerbations. *Brain, 125*, 952-960.

Carelli, C., Audibert, F., Gailard, J. & Chedid, L. (1982). Immunological castration of female mice by a totally synthetic vaccine administered in saline. *Proc.Natl.Acad. Sci, USA, 79*, 5392-5395.

Chakrabarti, A. K., Banik, N. L., Lobo, D. C.,Terry, E. C. & Hogan E. L. (1993). Calcium-activated neutral proteinase (calpain) in rat brain during development compartmentation and role in myelination. *Brain Res. Dev., 71*, 107-13.

Chantry, A. & Glynn, P. (1990). A novel metalloproteinase originally isolated from brain myelin membranes is present in many tissues.*Biochem. J., 268*, 245-8.

Chao, L. P., Einstein, E. R. (1970). Localization of the active site through chemical modification of the encephalitogenic protein. *J.Biol. Chem., 245*, 6397-6403.

Chapman, B. E., Littlemore, L. T. & Moore, W. J. (1978). Conformation of myelin basic protein and its role in myelin formation. *Adv. Exp. Med. Biol., 100*, 207-220.

Chapman, B. E. & Moore, W. J. (1976). Conformation of myelin basic protein in aqueous solution from NMR spectroscopy. *Biochem. Biophys. Res. Comm., 73*, 758-766.

Chedid, L., Audibert, F. & Johnson, A. G. (1978). Biological activities of muramyl dipeptide, a synthetic glycopeptide analogous to bacterial immunoregulating agents. *Prog. Allergy, 1978*, 63-105.

Chedid, l., Audibert, F, Lefrancier, P., Choay, J. & Lederer, E. (1976). Modulation of the immune response by a synthetic adjuvant and analogs. *Proc. Natl. Acad. Sci., USA, 73*, 2472-2475.

Correale, J., McMillan, M., Carthy, K. M. C., Le, T. & Weiner, L. P. (1995). Isolation and characterization of autoreactive proteolipid protein-peptide specific T cell-clones from MS patients. *Neurology, 45*, 1370-8.

Cuzner, M. L., Gveric, D., Strand, C., Loughlin, A. J., Paemen, L., Opdenakker, G. & Newcombe, J. (1996). The expression of tissue type plasminogen activator, matrix metalloproteinases and endogenous inhibitors in the CNS in MS: comparison of stages in lesion evolution. *J. Neuropath. Exp. Neurol., 55*, 1194-204.

Dinarello, C. A. (1989). Interleukin-1 and its biologically related cytokines. In: *Advances in Immunology, Vol 44*, (153-205) New York, Academic Press.

Ellouz, F., Adam, A., Ciobaru, R. & Lederer, E. (1974). Minimal structural requirements for adjuvant activity of bacterial peptidoglycan derivatives. *Biochem. Biophys. Res Comm. 59*, 1317-1325.

Endoh, M., Kunishita, T., Neihei, J., Nishizawa, M. & Tabira, T. (1990). Susceptibility to proteolipidaproprotein and its encephalitogenic determinants in mice. *Int. Arch. Allergy Appl. Immunol., 92*, 433-439.

Eylar, E. H., Brostoff, S., Jackson, J. & Carter, H. (1972). Allergic encephalomyelitis in monkeys induced by a peptide from the A1 protein. *Proc. Nat. Acad. Sci., USA, 69*, 617-619.

Eylar, E. H., Caccam, J., Jackson, J. J., Westall, F. C. & Robinson, A. B. (1970). EAE: synthesis of disease-inducing site of basic protein. *Science, 168*, 1220-1223.

Eylar, E. H., Westall, F . C. & Brostoff, S. (1971). Allergic encephalomyelitis. *J. Biol. Chem, 256*, 34318-3424.

Felts, P. A., Woolston, A. M., Fernando, H. B., Asquith, S., Gregson, N. A., Mizzi, O. J. & Smith, K. J. (2005). Inflammation and primary demyelination induced by the intraspinal injection of lipopolysaccharide. *Brain, 128*, 1649-1666.

Fermandjian, S., Perly, B., Level, M. & Lefrancier, P. (1987). A comparative 1H-NMR study of MDP and its analogue, muabutide: evidence for a structure involving two successive beta turns. *Carbohydrate Res., 162*, 23-32.

Filippi, M. & Rocca, M. A. (2005). MRI evidence for MS as a diffuse disease of the centralnervous system. *J. Neurol., 252*, Suppl, 5, 16-24.

Frei, K., Fredrikson, S., Fontana, A. & Link, H. (1991). Interleukin-6 is elevated in plasma in MS. *J. Neuroimmunol., 31*, 147-153.

Freund, M., Stern, E. R. & Pisani, T. M. (1947). Isoallergic encephalomyelitis and radiculitis in guinea pigs after one injection of brain and *Mycobacteria* in water –in –oil emulsion. *J. Immunol., 57*, 179-194.

Furlan R., Filippi, M., Bergami, A., Rocca, M. A., et al. (1999a). Peripheral levels of caspase-1 mRNA correlate with disease activity in patients with MS; a preliminary study. *J. Neruol. Neruosrug. Psychiatry, 67*, 785-788.

Furlan, R., Martino, G., Galbiati, F., et al. (1999b). Caspase-1 regulates the inflammatory process leading to autoimmune demyelination. *J. Immunol., 163*, 2403-9.

Fujinami, R. S. & Oldstone, M. B. (1985). Amino acid homology between the encephalitogenic site of MBP and virus: mechanism for autoimmunity. *Science, 230* 1043-1045.

Galboiz, Y. & Miller, A. (2002). Immunological indicators of disease activity and prognosis in MS. *Curr.Opin. Neurol., 15*, 233-237.

Giuliain, D., Lachman, L. B. (1985). Interleukin-1 stimulation of astroglial proliferation after brain injury. *Science, 228*, 497-499.

Goldsmith, P. C. (2000). Neurological responses to elevated glutamate in the medial basal hypothalamus of the infant mouse. *J. Nutr., 130*, 1033S-1038S.

Goodwin, D. E., Rooney, W. D., Sloan, R., Bacchetti, P., et al. (1998). A serial study of new MS lesions and the white matter from which they arise. *Neurology, 51*, 1689-97.

Gorenstein, C. & Sweet, J. E. (1985). Distribution of dipeptidyl peptidase. II In rat spinal cord. *Am J. Anat., 173*, 29-35.

Greer, J. M., Kuchroo, V. K., Sobel, R. A. & Lees, M. J. (1992). Identification and characterization of a second encephalitogenic determinant of myelin proteolipid protein. *J. Immunol., 149*, 783-8.

Griffen, C. M., Chard, D. T., Parker, G. J., Barker, G. J., Thompson, A. J. & Miller, D. H. (2002). The relationship between lesion and normal appearing brain tissue abnormalties in early relapsing remitting MS. *J .Neurol., 249*, 193-9.

Grynbaum, A. & Marks, N. (1976). Characterization of a rat brain catheptic carboxypeptidase inactivating angiotensin. II. *J. Neurochem, 26*, 313-8.

Hagopian, A, Jackson, J. J., Carlo, D. J., Limjuco, G. A. & Eylar, E. H. (1975). Experimental allergic aspermatogenic orchitis. III. Isolation of spermatozoal glycoproteins and their role in allergic aspermatogenic orchitis. *J. Immunol., 115*, 1731-43.

Hartung, H. P., Reiners, K., Archelos, J. J., Michels, M. et al. (1995). Circulating adhesion molecules and tumor necrosis factor receptor in MS: correlation with magnetic resonance imaging. *Ann. Neurol., 38*, 186-193.

He, X. P, Shosaka, S. & Yoshida, S. (2001). Expression of neuropsin in oligodendrocytes after injury to the CNS. *Neurosci. Res., 39*, 455-62.

Hisahara, S., Okano, H. & Miura, M. (2003). Caspase-mediated oligodendrocyte cell death in the pathogenesis of autoimmune demyelination. *Neuro Sci., 46*, 387-97.

Hosmalin, A., Carelli, C., Gaillard, J., Lefrancier, P., Drobecq, H., Leclerc, C., Amar, O., Audibert, F. & Chedid, L. (1987). Structural requirements for the induction of "immunological castration" by linear monomeric LHRH-LYS-MDP administered in saline. *Clin. Immunol. Immunopath., 45*, 447-460.

Jahnke, U., Fisher, E. D. & Alvord, E. C., Jr. (1985). Sequence homology between certain viral proteins and proteins related to encephalomyelitis and neuritis. *Science, 229*, 282-284.

Jansson, L., Olsson,T., Hojeberg, B. & Holdahl, R. (1991). Chronic EAE induced by the 89-101 MBP peptide in BIORIII(H-2r) mice. *Eur. J. Immunol., 21*, 693-9.

Johns, T. G., Kerlero de Rosbo, N., Menon, K., Abo, S., Gonzales, F. & Bernard, C. C. (1995). Demyelinating encephalomyelitis resembling MS after immunization with a peptide from myelin oligodendrocyte glycoprotein. *J. Immunol., 154*, 5536-5541.

Kabat, E. A., Wolf, A. & Bezer, A. F. (1947). The rapid production of acute disseminated encephalomyelitis in Rhesus monkeys by injection of heterologous and homologous brain tissue with adjuvants. *J. Exp. Med., 85*, 11-7.

Kanesaka, T., Mori, M., Hattori, T, Oki, T. & Kuwabara, S. (2006). Serum matrix metalloproteinase-3 levels correlate with disease activity in relapsing-remitting MS. *J. Neurol. Neurosurg. Psychiatry, 77*, 185-188.

Karkhanis, Y. D., Carlo, D. J., Brostoff, S. W. & Eylar, E. H. (1975). Allergic encephalomyelitis. Isolation of an encephalitogenic peptide active in the monkey. *J. Biol.Chem., 250*,1718-1722.

Katz-Levy, Y., Neville, K. L., Girvin, A. M., Vanderlugt, C. L., Pope, J. G., Tan, L. J. & Miller, S. D. (1999). Endogenous presentation of self myelin epitopes by CNS-resistant APCs in Theiler's virus-infected mice. *J.Clin. Invest., 104*, 599-607.

Kerlero,de Rosbo, N. & Ben-Nun, A. (1996). Delineation of a minimal encephalitogenic epitope within the immunodominant region of myelin oligodendrocyte glycoprotein. *Eur. J. Immunol., 26*, 2470-9.

Kerero de Rosbo, N., Hoffman, M., Mendel, I., Yust, I., Kaye, J., Bakimer, R., Fletcher, S., et al. (1997). Predominance of the autoimmune response to myelin oligodendrocyte glycoprotein in MS: reactivity to the extracellular domain of MOG is directed against three main regions. *Eur. Immunol., 27*, 3059-3069.

Kerero de Rosbo, N., Kaye, J. F., Eisentein, M., Mendel, I., Hoeftberger, R., Lassmann , H., Milo, R. & Ben-Nun, A. (2004). The myelin-associated oligodendrocyte basic proein region MOBP 15-36: Encompasses the immunodominant major enephalitogenic epitope for SJL/J mice and predicted epitope for MS-associated HLA-DRB1. *J. Immunol., 173*, 1426-1435.

Kerero de Rosbo, N, Mendel, I. & Ben-Nun, A. (1995). Chronic relapsing EAE with a delayed and an atypical clinical course, induced in PL/J mice by MOG-derived peptide: preliminary analysis of MOG T cell epitopes. *Eur. J. Immunol., 25*, 985-93.

Kerero de Rosbo, N., Milo, R., Lees, M. B., Burger, D., Bernard, C. C. A. & Ben-Nun, A. (1993). Reactivity to myelin antigens in MS. *J. Clin Invest., 92*, 2602-2608.

Khanarian, G., Margeson, S. A., Moore, W. S., Pasaribu, S. J. & Westall, F. C. (1979). Effects of substitution of D-alanine for L-alanine on activity and conformation of an encephalitogenic peptide. *Bbrc, 87*, 236-243.

Khoury, S. J., Orav, E. J., Guttermann, C., Kikinis, R., Jolesz, F. A. & Weiner, H. L. (1999). Changes in serum levels of ICAM and TNF-R correlate with disease activity in MS. *Neurology, 53*, 758-764.

Kies, M. W. (1965). Allergic encephalomyelitis. *Ann. N.Y. Acad. Sci., 122*, 161-169.

Kies, M. W. &Alvord, E. C., Jr. (1959). In: *Allergic encephalomyelitis.*(pp239-299) Springfield, Ill., Thomas.

Kivisakk, P., Matusevicius, D., He, B., Soderstrom, M., Fredrikson, S. & Link, H. (1998). IL-15 mRNA expression is up-regulated in blood and cerebrospinal fluid mononuclear cells in MS. *Clin. Exp. Immunol., 111*, 193-197.

Kotani, S., Watanabe, Y., Shimono, T., Harada, K., et al. (1976). Correlation between the immunoadjuvant activities and pyrogenicities of synthetic N-acetyl muramyl peptides or -amino acids. *Biken J., 19*, 9-13.

Kouwenhoven, M., Ozenci, V., Tjernlund, A., Pashenhov, M., Homman, M., Press, R. & Link, H. (2002). Monocyte-derived dendritic cells express and secrete matrix-degrading metalloproteinases and their inhibitors and are imbalanced in MS. *J. Neuroimmunol., 126*, 161-171.

Lassmann, H., Bruck, W. & Lucchinetti, C. F. (2007). The immunopathology of MS: an overview. *Brain Pathol., 17*, 210-8.

Lassmann, H. & Wisniewski, H. M. (1979). Chronic relapsing EAE. *Arch. Neurol., 36*, 490-497.

Lee, J. M. & Schneider, H. A. (1962). Critical relationships between constituents of the antigen-adjuvant emulsion affecting EAE in a completely susceptible mouse genotype. *J. Exp. Med., 15*, 159-168.

Lee, M. A., Palace, J., Stabler, G., Ford, J., Gearing, A. & Miller, K. (1999). Serum gelatinase B, TIMP-1 and TIMP-2 levels in MS. A longitudinal clinical and MRI study. *Brain, 122*, 191-197.

Lehtonen, l., Eerola, E., Oksman, P. & Toivanen P. (1995). Muramic acid in peripheral blood leukocytes of healthy human subjects. *J. Infect. Dis., 171*, 1060-4.

Lehtonen, L., Eerola, E. & Toivanen, P. (1997). Muramic acid in human peripheral blood leucocytes in different age groups. *Eur. J. Clin. Invest., 27*, 791-92.

Lennon, V. A., Westall, F. C., Thompson, M. & Ward, E. (1976). Antigen, host and adjvant requirements for induction of hyperacute EAE. *Eur. J. Immunol., 6*, 805-810.

Lenz, D. C., Lu, L., Conant, S. B., et al. (2001). A *Chlamydia pneumoniae*-specific peptide induces EAE in rats. *J. Immunol., 167*, 1803-1808.

Leppert, D., Ford, J., Stabler, G., Grygar, C., et al. (1998). Matrix metalloproteinase-9 is selectively elevated in CSF during relapses and stable phases of MS. *Brain, 121*, 2327-2334.

Levine, S. & Wenk, E. J. (1964). Allergic encephalomyelitis: a hyperacute form. *Science, 146*, 1681-1682.

Levine, S. & Wenk, E. J. (1965). A hyperacute form of allergic encephalomyelitis. *Amer. J. Path., 47*, 61-88.

Levine, S. (1974). Hyperacute, neurophilic and localized forms of EAE: a review. *Acta Neuropath., 28*, 174-189.

Li, Z. & Banik, N. L. (1995). The localization of m-calpain in myelin immuno-cykotchemical evidence in different areas of rat brain and nerves. *Brain Res., 697*, 112-21.

Linington, C., Berger, T., Perry, L., Weerth, S., Hinze-Selch, D., Zwang, Y., Lu, H. C. Lassmann, H. & Wekerke, H. (1993). T cells specific for the myelin oligodendrocyte glycoprotein mediate an unusual autoimmune inflammatory response in the CNS. *Eur. J. Immunol., 23*, 1364-72.

McAlpine, D., Lumsden, C. E. & Acheson, E. D. (1972). In: *Multiple Sclerosis. A reappraisal.* (8-32) Edinburgh Churchill, Livingstone.

Maeda, K., Koga, T., Sakamoto, S., Onoue, K., Kotani, S., Kusumoto, S., Shiba, T. & Sumiyoshi, A. (1980). Structural requirements of synthetic n-acetylmuramyl dipeptides for induction of EAE in the rat. *Microbiol. Immunol., 24*, 771-776.

Mahad, D, Lawry, J., Howell, S. J. L. & Woodroofe, M. N. (2003). Longitudinal study of chemokine receptor expression on peripheral lymphocytes in MS: CXCR3 upregulation is associated with relapse. *Mult. Scler., 9*, 189-198.

Maimone, D., Gregory, S., Arnason, B. G. & Reder, A. T. (1991). Cytokine levels in the cerebrospinal fluid and serum of patients with MS. *J. Neuroimmunol., 32*, 67-74.

Malmestrom, C., Andersson, B. A., Haghighi, S. & Lycke, J. (2006). IL-6 and CCL2 levels in CSF are associated with the clinical course of MS: Implications for their possible immunopathogenic roles. *J. Neurommunol., 175*, 176-182.

Manabe, S., Gu, Z. & Lipton, S. A. (2005). Activation of matrix metalloproteinase-9: Neuronal nitric oxide synthase contributes to NMDA-induced retinal ganglion cell death. *Invest. Opthal. Vis. Sci., 46*, 4747-4753.

Martin, S. A., Karnovsky, M. L., Kruger, J. M., Pappenheimer, J. R. & Nieman, K. (1984). Peptiodoglycan as promoters of slow wave sleep. I. Structure of the sleep-promoting factor isolated from human urine. *J. Biol. Chem., 259*, 12652-8.

Matsuda, M., Tsukada, N., Miyagi, K. & Yanagisawa, N. (1995). Increased levels of soluble vascular cell adhesion molecule-1 (VCAM-1) in the cerebrospinal fluid and serum of patients with MS and human T lymphotrophic virus type-1-associated myelopathy. *J. Neuroimmunol, 59*, 35-40.

Matsuo, A., Lee, G. C., Terai, K, Takami, K., Hickey, W. F., McGeer, E. G. & Geer, P. L. (1997). Unmasking of an unusual myelin basic protein epitope during the process of myelin degeneration in humans. *Am. J. Path., 150*, 1253-1266.

Mendel, I., Kerero de Rosbo, N. & Ben-Nun, A. (1995). A myelin oligodendrocyte glycoprotein peptide induces typical chronic EAE in H2b mice: fine specificity and T-cell receptor V beta expression of encephalitogenic cells. *J. Eur. Immunol., 25*, 1951-1959.

Mendz, G. L. & Moore, W. J. (1983). NMR studies of MBP. X. Conformation of a determinant encephalitogenic in the rabbit. *Biochim. Biophys. Acta, 748*, 176-83.

Mendz, G. L., Moore, W. J. & Carnegie, P. R. (1982). Proton NMR evidence for secondary and tertiary structure in myelin basic protein. *Biochem. Biophys. Res. Comm., 105*, 1333-40.

Migliore-Samour, D. & Jolles, P. (1973). Hydrosoluble adjuvant active mycobacterial fractions of low molecular weight. *FEBS Lett., 36*, 317-21.

Moore, W. J., Chapman, B. E., James, G. E., Khanarian, G., Margetson, S. A., Pasaaribu, S. J. & Westall, F. C. (1981). Conformation of encephalitogenic proteins and peptides. *Excerta Medica No., 546*, 198-211.

Moreira, M. A., Souza, A. L. S., Lana-Peixoto, M. A., Teixeira, M. M. & Teixeira, A. L. (2006). Chemokines in he cerebrospinal fluid of patients with active and stable relapsing-remitting MS. *Braz. J. Med. Biol. Res., 39*, 441-445.

Morgan, I. M. (1947). Allergic encephalomyelitis in monkeys in response to injection of normal monkey nervous tissue. *J.Exp. Med., 85*, 131-35.

Mostert, J. P., Ramsaransing, S. M., Heersema, D. J., Heerings, M., Wilczak, N. & De Keyer, J. (2005). *J. Neurol. Sci., 231*, 41-44.

Mozes, E., Sela, M. & Tausig, M. J. (1974). Tolerance to thymus-independent antigens. *Immunology, 27*, 641-646.

Nagae, A., Deddish, P. A., Becker, R. P., et al. (1992). Carboxypeptidase M in brain and peripheral nerves. *J. Neurochem., 59*, 2201-12.

Nagai, Y., Akiyama, K., Suzuki, K., Kotani, S., Watanabe, Y., Shimono, T., Shiba, T., Kusumota, S., Ikuta, F. & Takeda, S. (1978a). Minimum structural requirements for encephalitogen and for adjuvant in the induction of EAE. *Cell. Immunol., 35*, 158-167.

Nagai, Y., Akiyam, K., Kotani, S., Watanabe, Y., Shimono, T., Shiba, T. & Kusmoto, S. (1978b). Structural specificity of synthetic peptide adjuvant for induction of EAE. *Cell Immunol., 35*, 168-172.

Oh, L. Y. S., Larsen, P. H., Krekoski, C. A., Edwards, D. R., Donovan, F., Werb, Z., et al. (1999). Matrix metalloproteinase-9/gelatinase B is required for process outgrowth by oligodendrocytes. *J. Neurosci., 1*, 8464-75.

Onodera, H., Nakashima, I., Fujihara, K., Nagata, T. & Itoyama, Y. (1999). Elevated plasma level of plasminogen activator inhibitor-1 (PAI-1) in patients with relapsing-remitting MS. *Tohoko J. Exp. Med., 189*, 259-265.

Paeman, L., Olsson, T., Soderstrom, M., Van Damme, J. & Opdenakker, G. (1993). Evaluation of gelatinases and IL-6 in the cerebrospinal fluid of patients with optic neuritis, multiple sclerosis and other inflammatory neurological diseases. *Eur. J. Neurol., 1*, 55-63.

Panitech, H. & Ciccone, C. (1981). Induction of recurrent EAE with myelin basic protein. *Ann. Neurol., 9*, 433-438.

Penkowa, M., Espejo, C., Ortega-Aznar, A., Hidalgo, J., Montalban, X. & Martinez-Caceres, E. M. (2003). Metallothionen expression in the CNS of MS patients. *CMLS Cell Mol Life Sci, 60*, 1258-66.

Perry, L. L., Barzaga-Gilbert, E. & Trotter, J. L. (1991). T cell sensitization to proteolipid protein in myelin basic protein-induced relapsing EAE. *J. Neuroimmunol., 33*, 7-15.

Prat, A., Biernacki, K., Saroli, T., Orav, J. E., et al., (2005). Kinin B1 receptor expression on MS mononuclear cells. *Arch. Neurol., 62*, 795-800.

Price, W. S., Mendz, G. L. & Martenson, R. E. (1988). Conformation of a heptadecapeptide comprising the segment encephalitogenic in Rheus monkey. *Biochemistry, 27*, 8990-8999.

Raine, C. S. & Stone, S. H. (1977). Animal model for MS: chronic EAE in inbred guinea pigs. *N.Y. State J. Med., 77*, 1693-1697.

Raine, C. S. & Traugott, U. (1982). The pathogenesis and therapy of MS is based upon the requirement of a combination of myelin antigens for autoimmune demyelination. *J. Neuroimmunol., 2*, 83-91.

Rieckmann, P., Albrecht, M., Kitze, B., Weber, T., et al., (1995). Tumor necrosis factor alpha messenger RNA expression in patients with relapsing-remitting MS is associated with disease activity. *Ann Neurol., 37*, 82-88.

Roboz-Einstein, E., Robertson, D. M., DiCaprio, J. & Moore W. (1962). The isolation from bovine spinal cord of a homologous protein with encephalitogenic activity. *J. Neurochem., 9*, 353-361.

Root-Bernstein, R. S. & Westall, F. C. (1990). Serotonin binding sites II. *Brain Res. Bull., 25*, 826-41.

Root-Bernstein, R. S. & Westall, F. C. (1986). Clinical suppression of EAE by muramyl dipeptide "adjuvant". *Brain Res. Bull., 17*, 473-476.

Root-Bernstein, R. S. & Westall, F. C. (1983). Do muramyl peptides activate serotonin binding sites? *Lancet I*, 653.

Rosenberg, G. A., Dencoff, J. E., Correa, N. Jr., Beiners, M. & Ford, C. C. (1996). Effect of steroids on CSF matrix metalloproteinases in MS: relation to blood-brain barrier injury. *Neurology, 46*, 1626-32.

Sakai, K., Zamvil, S. S., Mitchell, D. J., Lim, M., Rothbard, J. B. & Steinman, L. (1988). Characterization of a major encephalitogenic T cell epitope in SJL/J mice with synthetic oligopeptides of myelin basic protein. *J. Neuroimmunol., 19*, 21-32.

Salk, J., Romine, J. S., Westall, F. C. & Wiederholt, W. C. (1980). Myelin basic protein studies in EAE and MS. A summary with theoretical considerations of multiple sclerosis etiology. Davison, A.N. & Cuzner, M.C. eds. In: *Proceedings of the Liversedge MS*

Society Symposium on the Suppression of *MS and EAE*. (pp 141-153) London, Academic Press. London.

Sasaki, Y. (1974). Studies on encephalitogenic fragments of myelin basic protein. III. Synthesis of H-Arg-Phe-Trp-Gly-Ala-Glu-Gly-Asn-Arg-OH as an analog of encephalitogenic decapeptide. *Chem Pharm. Bull., 22*, 2199-2191.

Scarisbrick, I. A., Asakura, K., Blader, S., et al. (2000). Preferred expression of myelencephalon-specific protease by oligodendrocytes of the adult rat spinal cord white matter. *Glia, 30*, 219-30.

Scarisbrick, I. A.,Isackson, P. J., Ciric, B., Windebank, A. J. & Rodriquez, M. (2001). MSP—a trypsin-like serine protease is abundantly expressed in the human nervous system. *J.Comp. Neurol., 431*, 347-61.

Schaecher, K. E., Shield, D. C. & Banik, N. L. (2001). Mechanism of myelin breakdown in experimental demyelination: a putative role for calpain. *Neurochem. Res., 26*, 731-7.

Schrijver, I. A., van Meurs, M., Melief, M. J., Ang, C. W., et al. (2001). Bacterial peptidoglycan and immune reactivity in the central nervous system in MS. *Brain, 124*, 1544-1554.

Seifert T., Kieseier, B. C., Ropele, S., Strasser-Fuchs, S., Ouehenberger, F., Fazekas, F. & Hartung, H. P. (2002). TACE mRNA expression in peripheral mononuclear cells precedes new lesions on MRI in MS. *Mult. Scler., 8*, 447-451.

Shapira, R., Chou, F. C. H., McKneally, S., Uraban, E. & Kibler, R. F. (1971). Biological activity and synthesis of an enephalitogenic determinant. *Science, 172*, 736-738.

Shaw, C. M., Alvord, E. C., Jr., Fahlberg, W. J., Jr. & Kies W. W. (1962). Adjuvant-antigen relationships in the production of EAE in the guinea pig. *J. Exp. Med., 115*, 169-179.

Shibata, M., Hisahara, S., Hara, H., et al. (2000). Caspases determine the vulnerability fo oligodendrocytes in the ischemic brain. *J. Clin Invest., 106*, 643-53.

Shields, D. C. & Banik, N. L. (1998). Upregulation of calpain activity and expression in EAE: a putative role for calpain in demyelination. *Brain Res., 794*, 68-74.

Sibley, W. A., Bamford, C. R. & Clark, K. (1985). Clinical viral infections and MS. *Lancet I*, 1313-1315.

Silver, N. C., Tofts, P. S., Symms, M. R., Barker, G. J., Thompson, A. J. & Miller, D. H. (2001). Quantitative contrast-enhanced magnetic resonance imaging to evaluate blood-brain barrier integrity in MS: a preliminary study. *Mult. Scler., 7*, 75-82.

Simon, J. & Anzil, A. P. (1974). Immunohistological evidence of perivascular localization of basic protein in early development of EAE. *Acta Neuopath (Berl.), 27*, 33-42.

Smeltz, R. B., Wolf, N. A. & Swanborg, R. H. (1998). Delineation of two encephalitogenic myelin basic protein epitopes for DA rats. *J. Neuroimmunol., 87*, 43-48.

Snyder, D. S., Simonis, S., Uzman, B. G. & Whitaker, J. N. (1985). Rat neural tissue cathepsin D: ultrastructural immunocytochemistry. *J. Neurocytol., 14*, 579-96.

Stebbins, J. W., Jaffe, H. & Moeller, J. R. (1998). Characterization of myelin-associated glycoprotein proteolysis in the human CNS. *Neurochem Res., 23*, 1005-10.

Stover, J. F., Pleines, U. E., Morgan-Kossmann, M. C., Lowitzsch, K. & Kempski, O. S. (1997). Neurotransmitters in cerebrospinal fluid reflect pathological activity. *Eur. J. Clin. Invest., 27*, 1038-1043.

Stratton, C. W. & Sriram, S. (2003). Association of *Chlamydia pneumoniae* with CNS disease. *Microbe Infect., 5*, 1249-1253.

Suzuki, K. & Sasaki, Y. (1974). Studies on encephalitogen fragments of myelin basic protein. IV. Synthesis of glycine analogs of tryptophan containing fragments. *Chem. Pharm. Bull., 22*, 2181-2187.

Swanborg, R. H., Whittum-Hudson, J. A. & Hudson, A. P. (2003). Infectious agents of MS. *J. Neuroimmunol., 136*, 1-8.

Tejada-Simon, M. V., Zang, Y. C., Yang, D., Hong, J., Li, S., Singh, R. A. et al. (2000). Aberrant T cell responses to myelin antigens during clinical exacerbation in patients with MS. *Int. Immunol., 12*, 1641-50.

Tomizawa, K., He, X. P, Yamanaka, H., Shiosaka, S. & Yoshida, S. (1999). Injury inuces neuropsin mRNA in the CNS. *Brain Res., 824*, 308-11.

Toullet, F., Audibert, F., Voisin, G. A. & Chedid, L. (1977). Production d'orchiepididymite aspermatogenique autoimmune chez le cobaye, a l'aide de differents adjuvants hydrosolubles. *Ann Immunol. (Inst Pasteur), 128C*, 267-269.

Trotter, J. L., Perfrey, C. M., Trotter, A. L., Selvidge, J. A., Gushleff, K. C. & Mohanakumaar, T. (1998). T. cell recognition of myelin proteolipid protein and myelin proteolipid protein peptides in the peripheral blood of MS and control subjects. *J. Neuroimmunol, 84*, 172-8.

Tuohy, V. K., Lu., Z., Sobel, R. A., Laursen, R. A. & Lees, M. B. (1989). Identification of an encephalitogenic determinant of myelin proteolipid protein from SJl mice. *J. Immunol. 142*, 1523-1532.

Tuohy, V. K., Sobel, R. A. & Lees, M. B. (1988). Myelin proteolipid protein induced EAE. Variations of disease expression in defferent mice strains. *J. Immunol., 140*, 1868-73.

Ufret-Vincenty, R. I., Quigley. L., Tresser, N., Pak, S. H., Gado, A., Hausm N. S., Wucherpfennig, K. W. & Brocke, S. (1998). In vivo survival of viral antigen specific T cells that induce EAE. *J. Exp. Med., 188*, 1725-1737.

van Boxel-Dezaire, A. H. H., Hoff, S. C. J., van Oosten, B. W., Verweij, C. L., et al. (1999). Decreaed Interleukin-10 and Increased Interleukin-12p40 mRNA are associated with Disease activity and characterize different disease stages in MS. *Ann Neurol., 45*, 695-703.

Waksman, B. J., Adams, R. D. & Mansmann, H. C., Jr. (1957). Experimental study of diphtheritic polymeutitis in the rabbit and guinea pig. Immunologic and histologic observations. *J. Exp. Med, 105*, 591-614.

Waubert, E., Goodkin, D. E., Gee, L., Bacchetti, P., Sloan, R., et al. (1999). Serum MMP-9 and TIMP-1 levels are related to MRI activity in relapsing MS. *Neurology, 53*, 1397-1401.

Werner, P., Pitt, D. & Raine, C. S. (2001). MS: altered glutamate hetrostasis in lesions correlates with oligodendrocyte and axonal damage. *Ann. Neurol., 50*, 169-180.

Westall, F. C. (2006a). Molecular mimicry revisited: Gut bacteria and multiple sclerosis. *J. Clin. Microbiol., 44*, 2099-2105.

Westall, F. C. (2006b). Histoclinical variation in MS: heterogeneous proteolytic immunogenic processing. *Med. Hypoth., 66*, 566-569.

Westall, F. C. (2007). Abnormal hormonal control of gut hydrolytic enzymes causes autoimmune attack on the CNS by production of immune-mimic and adjuvant molecules: a comprehensive explanation for the induction of MS. *Med. Hypoth., 68*, 364-368.

Westall, F. C. (1977). Hyperacute allergic encephalomyelitis: a single determinant. *Immunol.Comm., 6*, 227-237.

Westall, F. C. (1978). High dose inhibition of the tryptophan peptide induced encephalitogenicity. *Immunol. Comm., 7*, 57-67.

Westall, F. C. (1974). Released myelin basic protein: the immunogenic factor? *Immunochem., 11,* 513-515.

Westall, F. C. (1972). Solid phase peptide synthesis as applied to EAE. Field, In: E. J., Bell. T. M. & Carnegie, P. R., (eds). *In Multiple Sclerosis: Progress in Research.* (72-79).Amsterdam, North-Holland, Amsterdam.

Westall, F. C., Hawkins, A., Ellison, G. W. & Myers, L. W. (1980). Abnormal glutamic acid metabolism in MS. *J. Neurol. Sci., 47*, 353-364.

Westall, F. C., Robinson, A. B., ,Caccam, J., Jackson, J. & Eylar, E. H. (1971). Essential chemical requirements for induction of allergic encephalomyelitis. *Nature, 229,* 22-24.

Westall, F. C. & Root-Bernstein, R. S. (1986). Cause and prevention of post-infectious and post-vaccinal neuropathies in light of a new theory of autoimmunity. *Lancet, II,* 251-253.

Westall, F. C. & Thompson, M. (1977a). Encephalitogenic region for the Lewis rat within the myelin basic protein. *Immunol. Comm., 6,* 13-21.

Westall, F. C. & Thompson, M. (1977b). Further definition of the encephalitogenic region for guinea pigs. *Immunol. Comm., 6,* 23-27.

Westall, F. C. & Thompson, M. (1978). An encephalitogenic region in rabbits. *Immunochem., 15,* 189-191.

Westall, F. C., Thompson, M. & Lennon, V. A. (1977). Hyperacute autoimmune encephalomyelitis induced by a synthetic autoantigen. *Nature, 269,* 425-427.

Westall, F. C., Thompson, M., Migliore-Samour, D. & Jolles, P. (1975). Induction of allergic encephalomyelitis using hydrosoluble mycobacterial fractions. *Eur. J. Immunol., 5,* 504-505.

Westall, F. C., Thompson, M., Migliore-Samour, D. & Jolles, P. (1974). Induction of EAE using hydrosoluble adjuvants and the enephalitogenic tryptophan peptide. *Immunol. Comm. 4,* 353-9.

Whitaker, J. N. (1997). Myelin encephalitogenic protein fragments in CSF of persons with MS. *Neurology, 27,* 911-20.

Wong, A. & Toth, I. (2001). Lipid, sugar and lipopolysaccharides based delivery systems. *Curr. Med. Chem., 8,* 1123-36.

Wucherpfennig, K. W. & Strominger, J. L. (1995). Molecular mimicry in T cell mediated auatoimmunity: viral peptides activate human T cell clones specific for MBP. *Cell, 80,* 695-705.

Yamanaka, H. He, X. P, Matsumoto, K., Shiosak, S. & Yoshida, S. (1999). Protease M/neurosin mRNA is expressed in mature oligodendrocytes. *Mol. Brain Res., 71,* 217-24.

Xaio, H., Banks, W. A., Niehoff, M. L. & Morley, J. E. (2001). Effects of LPS on the permeability of the blood-brain barrier to insulin. *Brain Research, 896,* 36-42.

Young, J. D., Tsuchiya, D., Geier, M., Geier, S., Westall, F. C., Thompson, M., Cyr, R., Ward, E. & Yurochko, F. (1974). The encephalitogenic dose-response in guinea pigs of the tryptophan region of myelin basic protein. *Immunol.Comm., 3,* 219-226.

Zamvil, S. S., Mitchell, D. J., Moore, A. C., Kitamura, K., Steinman, L. & Rothbars, J. B. (1986). T-cell epitope of the autoantigen myelin basic protein that induces encephalomyelitis. *Nature, 324,* 58-67.

Chapter 16

GENETIC CONTROL OF T CELL TOLERANCE AND SUSCEPTIBILITY TO AUTOIMMUNE DISEASE

Lydia Makaroff[1,*], *Michelle Linterman*[2,*] *and Adrian Liston*[3,*]

[1] Business and Decision Life Sciences, Brussels 1200, Belgium;
[2] Cambridge Institute for Medical Research, University of Cambridge, Cambridge, United Kingdom
[3] VIB and University of Leuven, Leuven 3000, Belgium

ABSTRACT

The majority of human autoimmune diseases have a complex aetiology with strong genetic and environmental components. The genetic component of disease susceptibility is generally highly polygenic, with multiple loci acting synergistically, and genetically heterogenous, with diverse sets of polymorphic loci capable of driving the same autoimmune reaction. The genetics of autoimmunity is further complicated by the division of genetic susceptibility into general autoimmune propensity polymorphisms and disease-specific polymorphisms. Despite the complexity of autoimmune genetics at the locus level, it appears that a limited number of conserved mechanistic pathways are affected by genetic polymorphisms. The conserved tolerance pathways subverted by autoimmune polymorphisms are being unravelled by the analysis of mouse models of autoimmunity. These models have identified three key fragile links in the T cell tolerance pathway - antigen presentation and the apoptotic response in the thymus, cis- and trans-acting peripheral suppression of autoreactive T cells, and the target organ response to autoimmunity.

THE GENETIC EPIDEMIOLOGY OF AUTOIMMUNE DISEASES

The common autoimmune diseases cluster within families, indicating a genetic basis for disease susceptibility. The genetic component of disease susceptibility, based on monozygotic twin concordance for disease, is around 20-50% for most prevalent autoimmune diseases

---

[*] All authors contributed equally. Address correspondence to adrian.liston@vib.be

(Table 1), indicating a strong additional influence of environmental and developmental factors in determining disease outcome.

Since autoimmune diseases share a common basic aetiology, that of inappropriate activation of the immune response towards self-antigens, it is not surprising that they also share common genetic components of susceptibility. There are three main lines of evidence supporting the existence of genetic factors that contribute towards general autoimmune disease susceptibility.

1. There is a large amount of clinical data that multiple autoimmune diseases cluster in the same patient population (Table 2). For example, patients with type 1 diabetes (T1D) have elevated risks of developing autoimmune thyroid disease (AITD) [8], Sjogren's syndrome [9] and Coeliac disease [10], among others. This may indicate a primary genetic defect predisposing the proband to multiple autoimmune diseases, or alternatively it may represent a genetic defect causing a single primary autoimmune disease that later catalyses multiple secondary autoimmune diseases.

2. Autoimmune diseases as a broad classification show tighter familial clustering than specific autoimmune diseases. Numerous studies have demonstrated that the first degree relatives of patients with a particular autoimmune disease have a greater risk of developing autoimmune conditions beyond that which the proband was effected with (Table 3). For example, the first degree relatives of T1D probands in Columbia have a 2.3% risk of developing T1D, but a 6% risk of developing an alternative autoimmune disease, giving an overall 8.3% risk of developing any autoimmune condition [16].

3. Genetic association studies have been performed for multiple common autoimmune diseases and several loci have been consistently associated with more than one autoimmune disease (Table 4). While ascertainment bias exists for many of these associations and some show little effect in the larger population, the clustering of association is striking. For example, polymorphisms in *IL2RA* have been associated with T1D [23], AITD [24], multiple sclerosis (MS) [25] and rheumatoid arthritis (RA) [26]. Likewise the *PTPN22* locus has been associated with T1D [26, 27], AITD [28], systemic lupus erythematosus (SLE) [29], RA [26, 30], and Crohn's disease [26]. *HLA* is more complicated, as the locus is consistently associated with autoimmune disease (in many cases as the strongest single genetic contributor) but different alleles are largely associated with specific diseases [31].

Table 1. Examples of disease incidence in autoimmune proband twins

	Disease risk for twin of proband			
	Monozygotic	Dizygotic	Population	Reference
Type 1 Diabetes	27.3%	3.8%	Finnish	[1]
Rheumatoid arthritis	15.4%	3.6%	British	[2]
Multiple sclerosis	24%	3%	Danish	[3]
Systemic Lupus erythematosus	24%	2%	American	[4]
Autoimmune thyroid disease - Graves' disease - Hashimoto's disease	 22% 37.5%	 0% 0%	 Danish Danish	 [5] [6]
Crohn's disease	50%	0%	Danish	[7]

Table 2. Examples of increased incidence of additional autoimmunity in patients with one autoimmune disease

	Incidence of additional autoimmunity (vs control population)	Population	Reference
Type 1 Diabetes	AITD (25% vs 8%) Sjogren's syndrome (18-55% vs 3-14%) Coeliac disease (1.6%)	Korean English French	[8] [9] [10]
Autoimmune thyroid disease	T1D (6.7%) Coeliac disease (3.3%)	Brazilian Italian	[11] [12]
Coeliac disease	AITD (20.5% vs 11.2%)	Italian	[12]
Addison's disease	AITD (21.7%) Vitiligo (9.6%) Sjogren's syndrome (2.4%) T1D (1.2%) Coeliac disease (1.2%)	Dutch	[13]
Multiple sclerosis	AITR (9.4% vs 1.9% in males)	Austrian	[14]
Juvenile arthritis	AITR (44%)	Bulgarian	[15]
Systemic lupus erythematosus	AITD (58%)	Bulgarian	[15]

Together these data indicate that the genetic component to autoimmune disease includes both general autoimmune susceptibility loci and organ-specific autoimmune susceptibility loci. In this model of the genetics of autoimmunity, general autoimmune susceptibility loci result in a susceptibility to immune tolerance failure and hence predispose the individual to developing a range of autoimmune diseases. By contrast, organ-specific autoimmune susceptibility loci direct the pathogenicity of immune tolerance failure towards a specific antigen group or anatomical location. This accounts for the existence of shared and unique gene associations in the mapping studies (Table 4). It also proposes an explanation for why autoimmune disease in general clusters in families (Table 3), yet the most common autoimmune disease manifestation in an autoimmune monozygotic twin pair is for both individuals to develop the same disease (Table 1).

Table 3. Examples of increased incidences of autoimmunity in families of autoimmune probands

	Autoimmune risk of family members (vs control population)	Population	Reference
Type 1 Diabetes	8.3% any autoimmune disease in first degree relatives (vs 2.5%)	Columbian	[16]
Sjogren's syndrome	7.3% any autoimmune disease in first degree relatives (vs 3.9%)	Columbian	[17]
Celiac disease	4.8% any autoimmune disease in first degree relatives (vs 0.85%)	Italian	[18]
Multiple Sclerosis	3.1% any autoimmune disease in siblings (vs 1.8%)	British	[19]
Juvenile rheumatoid arthritis	16.1% any autoimmune disease in 1st degree relatives (vs 4%)	American	[20]
Systemic lupus erythematosus	6.5% any autoimmune disease in offspring	American	[21]
Idiopathic inflammatory myopathies	21.9% any autoimmune disease in first degree relatives (vs 4.9%)	American	[22]

Table 4. Examples of gene associations in common autoimmune diseases

	OMIM	Unique locus associations	Unique locus associations in pathways shared with multiple autoimmune diseases	Locus associations shared with multiple autoimmune diseases	References
Type 1 Diabetes	222100	CLEC16A, ERBB3, INS	CD226	CTLA4, HLA, IFIH1, IL2RA, IL2RB, IL7RA, KIAA1109/TENR/IL2/IL21, PTPN2, PTPN22, SH2B3, SUMO4, VDR	[23, 26, 27, 32-35]
Rheumatoid arthritis	180300	KAZALD1, PADI4	GC, NFKBIL1, RUNX1	CTLA4, FCRL3, HLA, IL1B, IL2RA, IL2RB, IL18, IRF5, KIAA1109/TENR/IL2/IL21, MHC2TA, PTPN22, SH2D2A, SLC22A4, STAT4, SUMO4, TNFA	[26, 30, 32, 33, 36-46]
Multiple sclerosis	126200	MBP	CD58, LAG3, PRKCA, TCRβ	CD24, CD45, CTLA4, IL2RA, IL7RA, HLA, ICAM-1, IRF5, MHC2TA, SH2D2A	[25, 41, 47-58]
Systemic lupus erythematosus	152700	DNASE1, FCGR2A, FCGR2B, FCGR3A, TREX1	FASL	CD24, CTLA4, FCRL3, HLA, IL18, IRF5, PTPN22, STAT4, TNFA	[29, 36, 37, 59-68]
Autoimmune thyroid disease	275000 140300	PDS, TG, TSHR	CD40	CTLA4, FCRL3, HLA, IFIH1, IL2RA, PTPN22, SUMO4, VDR	[24, 28, 33, 34, 36, 69-72]
Crohn's disease	266600	ABCB1, ATG16L1, CARD15, DGL5, IRGM, NCF4, NKX2-3, MST1, PHOX2B		HLA, IL10, IL12B, IL23R, IRF5, PTPN2, PTPN22, SLC22A4, TNFA	[26, 73-81]

Recent advances in mouse models of autoimmunity have begun to unravel the mechanistic understanding of how genetic defects can contribute to both general autoimmune susceptibility and organ-specific autoimmune susceptibility. For the general autoimmune susceptibility mechanisms, the Non-obese diabetic (NOD) mouse strain has highlighted the potential role defects in thymic negative selection can play in allowing autoreactive T cell clones to enter the periphery. The *Foxp3* knockout mouse has demonstrated the importance of Foxp3$^+$ regulatory T cells in maintaining peripheral tolerance by *trans*-mediated suppression of autoreactive T cells, and the *sanroque* mutant mouse illustrates the requirement for autoreactive effector T cells to have innate restraints on activation. Each of these pathways represents likely mechanisms that are altered during human autoimmunity, with multiple minor effects acting synergistically to produce immune tolerance failure. In addition, *Aire* knockout mice have illustrated the manner in which organ-specific tolerance defects can occur through reduced thymic expression of the target antigen and NOD mice indicate the potential for organ-intrinsic defects in resistance to autoimmunity to play a role in susceptibility.

GENERALISED GENETIC DEFECTS IN CENTRAL TOLERANCE MECHANISMS

The first form of immunological tolerance to be experimentally established was the clonal deletion of T cells that recognise self-antigens with a high affinity during T cell differentiation [82]. This process of thymic negative selection relies on the differential 'wiring' of immature thymocytes compared to mature T cells, with strong interaction with MHC bound to self-peptide causing apoptosis through the upregulation of Bim [83, 84]. Despite the firm establishment of thymic negative selection as a key immune tolerance mechanism, until recently it was not considered a likely contributor to tolerance against organ-specific antigens and therefore a poor candidate for a defective mechanism during autoimmune disease. Even after the initial assumption that organ-specific genes were not present in the thymus was proven incorrect [85, 86], the efficiency of the negative selection process to act through trace quantities of proteins was not fully appreciated.

NOD mice are a well-established model of autoimmune diabetes. One of the interesting aspects of the NOD model is that NOD mice show the same general autoimmune susceptibility that is demonstrated by familial studies in human cohorts. NOD mice spontaneously develop multiple autoimmune disorders, sialitis and dacryoadenitis in addition to T1D, and are susceptible to additional autoimmune diseases when modified by experimental challenge or genetic alteration [87-97]. For example, replacement of the T1D MHC susceptibility allele, $H2^{g7}$, with $H2^{h4}$ prevents T1D but results in spontaneous AITD [92]. Susceptibility to multiple autoimmune diseases have been genetically mapped in NOD mice, with similar results to human studies - highly polygenic control of disease susceptibility with partially overlapping sets of loci involved.

The NOD mouse therefore represents a model where the mechanistic basis for a general genetic propensity to autoimmune disease can be unravelled. One of the promising candidates for such a broad mechanistic defect in immune tolerance is the resistance of NOD thymocytes to undergoing negative selection in response to self-antigen. This trait has been observed *in vitro* [98] and *in vivo* for both MHC class II-restricted [99] and MHC class I-restricted [100] T cells. The defect in negative selection is T cell-intrinsic and is observed at all stages of maturation with an approximately ten-fold reduction in the apoptotic response to a fixed amount of antigen presentation [99, 101, 102]. This resistance to negative selection has been mapped by us and others [101-103], and while there are differences in the genomic linkage patterns that can probably be attributed to the different models used, in each case prominent linkage was observed to regions known to contribute to autoimmune diabetes in NOD mice. The precise mechanism by which NOD thymocytes are resistant to negative selection has not yet been fully determined, however factors likely to play a role in the resistance are reduced levels of surface T cell receptor (TCR) expression during early stages of thymocyte maturation [103, 104], poor upregulation of the key apoptotic mediator Bim [101, 102] and a global defect in the initiation of the negative selection transcriptome [104].

Currently it is unknown whether an analogous genetic defect is present in human populations and the answer to this question probably awaits further elucidation of the mechanism of negative selection in thymocytes. There are, however, suggestions from a range of monogenic autoimmune disorders that central tolerance defects could contribute to autoimmune susceptibility in humans. These are the partial T cell immunodeficiencies, which can be caused by mutations in a range of genes including *RAG1, RAG2, DCLRE1C, IL7RA, RMRP, IL2RG, ADA, ZAP70* and *LIG4* [105-114]. Some of these genes are involved in TCR somatic recombination, some in TCR signalling, some in cytokine signalling and some in basic metabolic processes. The common thread, however, is that severe loss-of-function causes complete T cell immunodeficiency, while moderate loss-of-function causes partial T cell immunodeficiency with autoimmunity or immune dysregulation. A number of mouse models have recently been developed to mimic this partial T cell immunodeficiency, such as partial loss-of-function alleles of *Rag1* [115], *Rag2* [116] and *Zap70* [117].

An analysis of the genetic mechanism by which *Zap70* hypomorphic alleles can produce autoimmune outcomes was performed by crossing a minor loss-of-function allele ($Zap70^{mrd}$) to a severe loss-of-function allele ($Zap70^{mrt}$) to produce a mouse strain with Zap70 activity in the critical range ($Zap70^{mrd/mrt}$) [118]. The spontaneous development of immune dysregulation in these mice, but not in either parental strain, demonstrates that the crucial factor in the development of autoimmunity is the degree of impairment rather than the particular allelic variant involved. The immune dysregulation in these mice is intrinsic to effector T cells, indicating that the impact on negative selection is greater than the impact on effector T cell activation [118]. As a similar phenotype is observed in partial loss-of-function *Rag1* and *Rag2* mutant mice [115, 116], it is possible that a common causality is involved, suggesting that the level of T cell immunodeficiency is able to impact the efficiency of thymic negative selection.

The mechanism by which partial T cell immunodeficiency may alter the efficiency of thymic negative selection is just starting to be unravelled. Thymic micro-architecture depends on crosstalk between thymocytes and the epithelium using the lymphotoxin (LT) pathway [119, 120]. In mice where the LT pathway is crippled, the structure of the thymic epithelial cell network is disturbed, as is the expression of chemokines involved in the migration of thymocytes [120, 121]. These combined factors alter the efficiency of negative selection even without altering the thymic expression of the self-antigen involved [121]. It is therefore possible that partial immunodeficiency, by limiting the number of mature thymocytes and hence LT production, disrupts the normal thymic micro-architecture and reduces the efficiency of negative selection. Additional, or alternative, factors involved may be a restriction in the TCR repertoire of Foxp3$^+$ regulatory T cells or the increased activation potential of effector T cells due to the lymphopenic environment overriding intrinsic restraints on activation [122], tolerance mechanisms that are treated in more detail in following sections.

While these mouse studies were led by clues from monogenic autoimmune conditions, it is likely that minor levels of T cell immunodeficiency, insufficient to cause autoimmunity alone, are able to act in concert with additional genetic factors to result in autoimmunity. This hypothesis explains the association of a number of gene loci involved in determining the size of the T cell repertoire with common autoimmune diseases. For example, the gain-of-function

PTPN22 allele associated with T1D, RA, SLE, AITD and Crohn's disease and the *SH2D2A* allele associated with RA and MS (see Table 4) result in a reduction in TCR signalling [43, 123]. Interestingly, moderate loss-of-function alleles of *IL7RA* can precipitate autoimmunity due to partial T cell immunodeficiency [106] while an allele of *IL7RA* which likely gives a two-fold increase in soluble IL-7RA is associated with MS and T1D [34, 47]. Potentially, this allele contributes to autoimmune susceptibility by reducing effective IL-7 serum levels and creating a degree of T cell immunodeficiency. Therefore, in a variety of way genetic defects in the efficiency of negative selection are likely to be playing a role in human susceptibility to autoimmune disease.

GENERALISED GENETIC DEFECTS IN *TRANS*-ACTING PERIPHERAL TOLERANCE MECHANISMS

Research into another monogenic autoimmune disease, Immune dysregulation, Polyendocrinopathy, Enteropathy and X-linked syndrome (IPEX), has revealed a key mechanism of immunological tolerance. Both IPEX and the murine equivalent, Scurfy, are fatal multi-organ autoimmune syndromes caused by loss-of-function mutations in the gene *FOXP3/Foxp3*. The necessity of Foxp3 for immune tolerance is caused by the role of Foxp3 in coordinating the lineage differentiation of regulatory T cells (T_R) from the naïve T cell pool [124-126]. In the absence of Foxp3$^+$ T_R self-reactive T cells undergo uncontrolled activation and mediate autoimmunity [127]. It is thought that the majority of Foxp3$^+$ T_R are generated in the thymus as a consequence of moderate-affinity recognition of self-antigen [128-132]. However, Foxp3 can also be induced in the periphery under a number of different tolerogenic contexts [133-142]. Expression of Foxp3 results in the upregulation of a broad set of genes that confer T_R suppressor activity, proliferative capacity, metabolic fitness and suppression of alternative T cell lineages [143-145]. After commitment to the T_R lineage cells require antigen-specific stimulation in order to initiate their suppressive capacity [146].

As a crucial mediator of peripheral immune tolerance, T_R are a candidate for genetic impairment in the common autoimmune diseases. Genetic factors that reduce the commitment, homeostasis or function of Foxp3$^+$ T_R would lower the threshold for activation of autoreactive T cells. One of the known requirements for Foxp3$^+$ T_R is IL-2 signalling. Mice deficient in *Il2*, *Il2ra* and *Il2rb* show severe immunopathology due to a *trans*-acting (phenotypic dominant) immune tolerance mechanism [147-152]. In both *Il2* and *Il2ra* deficient mice Foxp3$^+$ cells are generated at lower levels in the thymus [153, 154]. In the periphery, T_R cells deprived of IL-2 signalling have a reduced metabolic fitness and proliferative capacity when in competition, but reach near-normal absolute numbers and are still able to suppress in *in vitro* assays and high affinity autoreactive T cells *in vivo* [153-155]. The IL-2-deprived T_R are not, however, efficient at suppressing low affinity autoreactive T cells *in vivo*, which are capable of undergoing proliferative expansion and driving autoimmune disease [154]. In NOD mice the *Il2* locus is variant and shows two-fold lower production of IL-2 [156]. This loci is linked to the susceptibility to T1D and enhanced proliferation of autoreactive T cells [157, 158]. Critically, the IL-2 pathway is also intimately connected with human autoimmunity, with loci associations between *IL2* and T1D and MS, *IL2RA* and T1D, RA, MS and AITD, and *IL2RB* and T1D and RA (Table 4). It is likely that these associations are limiting the supply of IL-2 to Foxp3$^+$ T$_R$ and thereby decreasing the regulatory suppression of low affinity autoreactive T cells. Partial immunodeficiency (described above) may also act to induce immunodeficiency by limiting the production of Foxp3$^+$ T$_R$ in the thymus, as successive waves of thymocyte maturation are required to upregulate the necessary cofactors for Foxp3 induction ([159] and AL, unpublished observations).

As well as the quantity of Foxp3$^+$ T$_R$, reductions in the suppressive capability of the cell type could lead to autoimmunity. Two mediators of *trans*-acting dominant tolerance, soluble CTLA4 (sCTLA4) and IL-10, are produced in abundance, but not exclusively, by T$_R$ and have suppressive properties [160]. Both loci have been associated with multiple autoimmune diseases, indicating a role in generalised tolerance mechanisms (Table 4). CTLA4 is a high affinity ligand for B7.1/B7.2, which can out-compete CD28 and produce negative signalling [161, 162]. A ligand-independent form of CTLA4 (liCTLA4) exists that probably acts to dampen basal T cell activation without B7.1/B7.2 stimulation [163]. In the NOD mouse, where the *Ctla4* locus is one of the strongest diabetogenic genomic regions [164], a splice variation decreases production of liCTLA4 and thus probably creates an effector T cell-intrinsic defect in tolerance (covered in greater detail below) [163]. Another form of CTLA4 can be produced which does not act in an effector T cell-intrinsic manner, sCTLA4. sCTLA4 in the serum can blockade available B7.1/B7.2, reducing the capacity of autoreactive T cells to become activated [165], and can also stimulate IDO production by dendritic cells, precipitating tryptophan metabolism and T cell suppression [166]. Recombinant sCTLA4 (CTLA4-Ig) is in use as a therapeutic for autoimmune diseases due to these properties [167]. It is therefore notable that the autoimmune susceptibility allele of CTLA4 associated with multiple diseases contains a splice variant that reduces the production of sCTLA4 [163]. Another immunomodulatory product, produced by Tr1 and T$_R$, is IL-10 [168, 169]. IL-10 is particularly important in maintaining T cell tolerance at the mucosal sites [170], and both *Il10*-deficient mice and mice with a Foxp3-specific abatement of IL-10 show immune dysregulation in the gut and lung [171]. The association of *IL10* promoter polymorphisms with autoimmune disease may therefore represent impairment in production of this tolerance mediator by T$_R$ and other regulatory cell types, including regulatory B cells [172, 173].

Defects in regulatory cell types beyond Foxp3$^+$ T$_R$ may also be involved in general susceptibility to autoimmunity. Invariant Natural Killer T (iNKT) cells, for example, have regulatory properties and can inhibit autoimmune disease in mouse models of MS (experimental autoimmune encephalomyelitis, EAE) and T1D [174, 175]. Both the EAE-prone SJL strain and the T1D-susceptible NOD strain have a numerical [176-179] and functional [176, 179, 180] defect in iNKT cells. In NOD mice the defect is caused by multiple loci, several of which colocalise with diabetogenic loci [181], and transfer of additional NKT cells inhibit autoimmunity [177, 182]. It is likely that a similar genetic contribution to autoimmune susceptibility occurs in humans, as T1D patients show reduced numbers of iNKT cells with reduced production of the effector cytokine IL-4 [183].

GENERALISED GENETIC DEFECTS IN *CIS*-ACTING EFFECTOR T CELL TOLERANCE MECHANISMS

Beyond the *trans*-acting tolerance mechanisms described above, effector T cells also have intrinsic *cis*-acting mechanisms that limit activation. One of the most important *cis*-acting tolerance mechanisms is the intrinsic maintenance of the quiescent naïve T cell state unless the cell is licensed to enter effector lineages. The association of multiple cytokine pathway genes with autoimmune disease, including *STAT4*, *TNFA*, *IL12B*, *IL23R*, *IL10* and *IFIH1* (Table 4), is likely to reflect subtle alterations in the ease with which a naïve autoreactive T cell is able to transition into a pathogenic effector cell. While different effector T cell lineages have been associated with different autoimmune diseases, here we concentrate on the mechanisms by which naïve T cells are normally restrained from inappropriately entering the T_H17 and T_{FH} lineages.

T_H17 cells are a newly described subset of $CD4^+$ T cells that secrete IL-17 and other pro-inflammatory cytokines [184]. Many of the roles previously ascribed to T_H1 cells during the pathogenisis of autoimmune mouse models such as EAE and Collagen-Induced Arthritis (CIA) respectively are now thought to be mediated by T_H17 cells as $Il17^{-/-}$ mice are resistant to EAE and CIA [185, 186]. Follicular B helper T cells (T_{FH}) are a subset of effector T cells distinct from T_H1, T_H2 and T_H17 lineages. Among their key characteristics they express CXC-chemokine receptor 5 (CXCR5), allowing them to respond to CXCL13 produced by follicular stromal cells and migrate to the follicles [187]. T_{FH} cells also express high levels of the Inducible T Co-Stimulator (ICOS) and IL-10, allowing them to provide B cell help once they have entered the follicle [188, 189]. Both T_H17 and T_{FH} cells are powerful immune mediators and therefore inappropriate entry of autoreactive T cells into the linage can predispose an individual to autoimmunity.

Generation of T_H17 cells is directed by a milieu of cytokines including IL-6, IL-21, IL-23 and TGFβ [190-194] turning on the T_H17 master regulator, RORγt [195]. Initially it was reported that differentiation of T_H17 cells required only TGFβ and IL-6, however it has since become apparent that T_H17 cells can be induced in the absence of IL-6 provided IL-21 is present. IL-6 initiates the STAT3-dependant production of IL-21, which, in conjunction with RORγt, allows the expression of the IL-23 receptor on the T cell surface [184]. It is essential to note that while TGFβ and IL-6 can drive the differentiation of T_H17 cells, it is only in the presence of IL-23 that these cells can express their full compliment of pro-inflammatory cytokines and become pathogenic [196]. IL-23-deficient mice do not develop EAE [197], while IL-23 over-expressing mice have an increased susceptibility to EAE [198]. It is therefore interesting that the *IL23R* locus is associated with ankylosing spondylitis [69], Crohn's disease [73] and psoriasis [199], while *IL12B* (a component of IL-23) is linked to psoriasis [199]. The linkage of allelic variations in *IL23R* and *IL12B* to multiple autoimmune diseases is highly suggestive of a genetic dysfunction in the normally tightly regulated process of T_H17 induction.

The role of T_{FH} cells in autoimmune disease is exemplified by studies of the *sanroque* mouse strain. The *sanroque* mouse recapitulates the hallmark features of the human autoimmune disorder SLE, including anti-nuclear antibodies with dsDNA specificities, focal proliferative glomerulonephritis with IgG-containing immune complex deposition, anaemia and autoimmune thrombocytopenia [200]. Interestingly this murine model also has aberrant expression of ICOS on all T cells, a cell-autonomous overrepresentation of T_{FH} and spontaneous formation of germinal centres. These characteristics are the result of homozygosity for a hypomorphic 'san' allele where a point mutation in the gene Roquin (*Rc3h1*) causes the methionine at position 199 to be substituted for arginine [200]. One of the key functions of Roquin is to restrict the expression of ICOS to effector T cells that have been legitimately licensed for activation.

ICOS is structurally and functionally related to CD28. Unlike CD28, which is constitutively expressed, ICOS expression is only upregulated on T cells after priming. Due to lack of ICOS on naïve T cells, priming of naïve T cells is controlled by the expression kinetics of the ligands for CD28, B7.1 and B7.2, which are limited to activated antigen presenting cells. This *trans* requirement ensures that only T cells responding to antigen presented by licensed dendritic cells are activated. After activation the expression of ICOS on T cells allows the primed T cell to proliferate independent of licensed dendritic cells, as the ICOS ligand is constitutively expressed on many different cell types. The repression of ICOS in naïve T cells therefore represents a *cis*-acting tolerance mechanism essential for the maintenance of tolerance, in particular entry into the T_{FH} lineage required for efficient germinal centre reactions. This intrinsic repression of ICOS is mediated by Roquin. Homozygosity of the *san* allele of *Roquin* causes naïve T cells to express ICOS and proliferate independent of licensing by dendritic cells, allowing the spontaneous formation of germinal centres [201]. The lupus-like phenotype in the *sanroque* mouse strain can be partially corrected by loss of one allele of *ICOS* [201], loss of *CD28* or loss of *Shd1a*, genes encoding three key molecules for T_{FH} formation and function (ML and C. Vinuesa unpublished data), indicating that the *cis*-acting tolerance system is composed of a number of molecules that contribute to a common pathway.

It is likely that defects in the same process occur in SLE patients. SLE is mediated by the production of anti-nuclear antibodies that deposit in immune complexes. The self-reactive immunoglobulins produced are of high affinity and have undergone class switching, indicating that they derive from within the germinal centre. As self-reactive B cells are normally excluded from the germinal centre, their participation in germinal centres in SLE patients represents a tolerance failure [202]. Within germinal centres T_{FH} cell help is essential for the maintenance of the reaction and selection of high affinity somatically mutated centrocytes prior to class switching. As ICOS over-expression has been linked to the pathogenesis of SLE [203], it appears that an unknown genetic defect in the Roquin-ICOS pathway allows the inappropriate commitment of naïve autoreactive T cells to the pathogenic T_{FH} lineage. As autoantibodies also contribute to other autoimmune diseases, once the genetic defects in this pathway have been determined they are likely to be found to contribute to multiple autoimmune diseases.

In addition to restricting entry into the effector lineages, another tolerance mechanism intrinsic to effector T cells is the limitation of the effector phase. The apoptosis of effector T cells at the end of the immune response is coordinated by Fas and Bim. These two apoptotic pathways are partially redundant, as demonstrated by the relative health of Bim and Fas knockouts on a pure B6 background. Double deficiency, however, results in increased survival of T cells following an immune response [204] causing severe autoimmunity [204-206]. Even the loss of a single *Bim* allele on the *lpr* (Fas mutant) background results in autoimmunity [205]. The relevance of this tolerance mechanism for human autoimmunity is demonstrated by the monogenic autoimmune disease ALPS. ALPS is a severe autoimmune disease caused by dysfunctions in FAS, FASL or the downstream mediators of apoptosis Caspase 8 and Caspase 10. ALPS patients characteristically develop lymphadenopathy and splenomegaly due to the failure of TCR-mediated apoptosis of mature T cells following activation [207]. There is strong evidence that this pathway is impaired in the common autoimmune diseases. Wu et al identified an SLE patient with mutations in *FASL* [62]. While this particular case may be a variant of typical ALPS [62], expression of FLIP, the inhibitor of the Fas pathway, is upregulated in T cells from SLE patients [208]. Similarly, T cells from RA patients have been documented to express elevated levels of Bcl-2 [209] and those from MS patients have increased Survivin expression [210], both anti-apoptotic proteins. Genetic abnormalities in the post-effector phase apoptotic process may therefore represent a mechanism of shared susceptibility to autoimmunity.

GENETIC DEFECTS CONTRIBUTING TO ORGAN-SPECIFIC AUTOIMMUNE DISEASE

Failures in organ-specific tolerance can occur in multiple ways. Factors outside the organ, such as the thymic presentation of organ-specific antigens, can modify the immune response altering negative selection and increasing self-reactive T cells. Alternatively, antigen expression or antigenicity within the target organ can be altered, increasing immune priming or otherwise bringing about attack by self-reactive T cells. Additionally, the organ itself can change in its structural and metabolic resilience to damage. It is likely that these and other pathways contribute to various human autoimmune diseases (Table 5).

Organ-Specific Genetic Defects in Immune Tolerance

Table 5. Potential mechanisms of organ-specific autoimmune disease susceptibility

Potential mechanism of organ-specific effect	Disease	Putative examples	References
Poor presentation of target antigen in the thymus	T1D Myasthenia gravis	*INS* *CHRNA1*	[211, 212] [213]
Altered production of non-protein target antigen	RA SLE	*PADI4* *TREX1, DNASE1*	[214] [64, 65]
Alteration of antigenicity of target antigen	AITD	*PDS*	[72]
Altered thymic/peripheral presentation of target antigen	T1D	*HLA*	[215]
Altered lymphocyte trafficking through the organ	Crohn's disease	*ATG16L1, IRGM*	[216, 217]
Impairment of the metabolic integrity of the organ	T1D	unknown	unpublished observations
Decreased ability to regenerate after insult	RA	*KAZALD1*	[26]

The generalised resistance to negative selection in the NOD mouse described above demonstrates that genetic defects in the negative selection process can increase susceptibility to autoimmune disease. The study of Autoimmune Polyendocrinopathy Syndrome type 1

(APS-1) has revealed that the expression of self-antigens in the thymic epithelium is a complex and exquisitely sensitive process, and represents a key fracture point in immune tolerance.

APS-1 is a monogenic autoimmune disease caused by homozygous mutations in the gene AIRE [218, 219]. Clinical manifestations of APS-1 include a variety of organ-specific autoimmune diseases, usually including hypoparathyroidism and primary adrenocortical failure, accompanied by chronic mucocutaneous candidiasis [220]. *Aire* deficient mice were developed as a model of APS-1, and also present with multi-organ autoimmunity [221, 222]. Expression of Aire is limited to epithelial cells in the thymic medulla and rare cells in secondary lymphoid organs [222-224], and the role of Aire in suppressing autoimmunity is mediated by the thymic stroma [221]. In the absence of Aire, medullary thymic epithelial cells lose the trace expression of ~500 organ-specific antigens such as insulin [221, 225]. While these transcripts had been previously dismissed as non-functional, in the absence of Aire-mediated activation of the insulin promoter a dramatic reduction was observed in the efficiency of the negative selection of autoreactive T cells [226, 227]. This defect directly contributes to an increase in the number of autoreactive T cells in the periphery and the incidence of autoimmune disease [227, 228].

The mechanism by which Aire regulates transcription of organ-specific genes remains an open question. The Aire protein has biochemical properties suggestive of transcription factor activity [229-233], and has been proposed to act directly upon target genes [234]. Alternatively, the quantity of Aire-dependent genes [221, 225] and the erratic expression patterns at the level of individual cells [235] suggest that Aire may function via intermediates, such as functional interaction with additional cofactors [236] or binding chromatin structures and recruiting transcriptional components [237, 238]. Aire also appears to have functions in thymic epithelial differentiation [235, 239], which may be integral or unrelated to its activity to activate transcription of peripheral antigens. It does, however, suggest an explanation for the previously orphan data that impaired negative selection is observed against target antigens with unchanged thymic expression profiles [240, 241]. With subtle alterations in thymic structure [235, 239] and late thymocyte development [242] thymic crosstalk between thymocytes and thymic epithelial cells is likely to be impaired [119, 120] and hence the generalised efficiency of negative selection reduced [121].

Of interest to the genetics of common polygenic autoimmunity, Aire deficiency has been shown to interact with the loci involved in common autoimmune diseases, with susceptibility loci altering the disease progression in APS-1 patients [243, 244] and *Aire*-deficient mice [240, 245]. Furthermore, several studies have demonstrated that the Aire pathway is sensitive to even small reductions in activity, with reduced expression of Aire causing a reduction in the expression of Aire-dependent antigens [228, 246] and hence negative selection towards those antigens [228]. This result alludes to the possibility that small changes in the thymic expression or presentation of individual antigens may contribute to autoimmune susceptibility in a disease-specific manner. Mouse model examples of this include the proteolipid protein splice variant found in SJL mice, which is expressed in the thymus in a version lacking the region $PLP^{116-151}$. SJL mice show an increased frequency of peripheral T cells autoreactive to $PLP^{139-151}$ and have an enhanced susceptibility to PLP-induced EAE [247]. Likewise, artificial heterozygous loss of the Myelin P0 protein is associated with increasing T cell autoimmunity towards this autoantigen [248].

Of the gene associations unique to particular autoimmune diseases (Table 4), a number are likely to contribute to autoimmune susceptibility via altered thymic expression. For example polymorphisms in the VNTR microsatellite of the insulin promoter are associated with T1D [211, 212]. The susceptibility alleles of the *INS* locus cause a 2-3 fold decrease in AIRE-dependent thymic expression of the insulin gene [211, 249] (Table 5). Another example is the gene *CHRNA1*, another organ-specific gene expressed in the thymus in an AIRE-dependent manner. Similar to *INS*, *CHRNA1* has allelic variants that reduce thymic expression of the antigen and are associated with autoimmunity directed against the self-antigen, in this case resulting in the autoimmune disease myasthenia gravis [213]. In both of these cases it is expected that the reduced thymic expression allows the escape of autoreactive T cell clones which can participate in autoimmune reactions, but only towards specific tissues (Table 5). Other putative gene variants in this category are myelin basic protein (*MBP*, associated with MS), thyroid stimulating hormone receptor (TSHR, associated with AITD) and thyroglobulin (TG, associated with AITD).

In each case the protein product is a major target antigen of the autoimmune disease, thus reduced thymic expression would predispose the individual to developing that specific autoimmune disease. Alternatively, the genes may be associated with heightened expression in the periphery, creating an imbalance between thymic and peripheral expression with the same functional outcome. A variant of this theme may be behind the association of the *PADI4* locus with RA [214] and the *TREX1* and *DNASE1* loci with SLE [64, 65]. While the protein products are not major target antigens of the disease, they are involved in the production of non-protein target antigens, with PADI4 producing peptidyl citrulline and TREX1 and DNASE1 producing DNA fragments (Table 5). Another example which illustrates the synergy between genetic and environmental factors is the association of the *PDS* locus with AITD [72]. The protein product of PDS, pendrin, is required for sulfation of thyroglobulin, which serves a role in thyroglobulin function and likely influences iodination of the protein (Table 5). Iodination of thyroglobulin, in turn, generates new epitopes [250] and increases its antigenicity, as the primary autoantibodies and autoreactive T cells in the NOD.H2^{h4} AITD mouse model recognise highly iodinated thyroglobulin with a higher affinity than weakly iodinated thyroglobulin [251]. An interesting explanation for this observation is the possibility that thymic production of thyroglobulin is limited to the uniodinated form, allowing T cells reactive to the iodinated form to bypass negative selection. Increased activity of PDS may therefore act in a similar manner to increased dietary iodine intake, which increases the risk of AITD in both NOD.H2^{h4} mice [251] and human populations [252].

In addition to the tolerogenic necessity of antigen expression, efficient antigen presentation also needs to take place. This requirement is the basis for the strong association of the *HLA* locus, especially the MHC class II genes within the locus, with autoimmune diseases. The *HLA* locus encodes, among other proteins, the HLA class I and class II molecules that present peptides to CD8 and CD4 T cells, respectively. For many autoimmune diseases *HLA* is the greatest genetic contributor, and variants of the class II *HLA-DR* and *-DQ* genes have been associated with a plethora of autoimmune diseases. However generally different alleles of *HLA* are associated with different autoimmune diseases, and *DQB1*, *DQA1*, and *DRB1* allelic variants have been identified which act as resistance alleles for one disease and susceptibility alleles for another. For example, the *HLA-DR2* haplotype is protective against T1D, yet predisposes towards MS and SLE [253]. Similarly in NOD mice the replacement of the $H2^{g7}$ allele with $H2^{h4}$ blocks the development of T1D but promotes

AITD [254]. This indicates that the tolerance defect that *HLA* variants represent is antigen-specific in nature, representing altered presentation of peptide subsets rather than generalised presentation issues (Table 5).

The main *HLA* allelic variations appear to alter the binding pocket of the MHC molecules and thus change the range of peptides that the protein is capable of presenting to T cells. Variants also act along a continuum to also alter the strength of the peptide-MHC interaction and the interaction between the peptide-MHC and TCR. Susceptibility-associated *HLA* variants may allow certain autoreactive T cell clones to escape tolerance mechanisms, while protection may occur by certain MHC molecules sequestering potentially autoimmunogenic peptides away from more dangerous MHC molecules. Two alternative mechanisms exist for the association of altered peptide presentation to autoimmunity – reduced thymic presentation of major target autoantigens for tolerogenic purposes and enhanced peripheral presentation of major target autoantigens.

A well studied variation associated with type 1 diabetes is the absence of an aspartic residue at position 57 of the HLA-DQ β protein (HLA-DQ8). When this amino acid is substituted with a serine, alanine or valine immunogenic insulin peptides have enhanced binding to HLA-DQ and may elicit an autoimmune response [215]. The NOD mouse also has a MHC Class II allele, $I-A^{g7}$, that contains a non-aspartic acid at position β57. In the NOD mouse this allele permits preferential binding to an alternative and larger set of peptides than MHC molecules with a β57 aspartic residue [255, 256]. Mouse transgenic studies have shown that the HLA-DQ8 can directly substitute for the diabetogenic role of $I-A^{g7}$, with an absence of negative selection of pancreas-specific T cell clones and an enhanced level of peripheral activation [257]. Another example is the association of *HLA-DR2* alleles with MS. The associated variants have an increased ability to display a dominant epitope of myelin basic protein (MBP) to CD4 T cells. Structural studies have indicated that there is a very weak interaction between the DR2-MBP peptide complex and the cognate TCR, which indicates that the mechanism of susceptibility is enhanced peripheral presentation of antigen to weakly-binding and promiscuous autoreactive T cells that escaped thymic negative selection [258, 259].

A particular case for genetic synergy can be made for the association of altered presentation of peptide and altered TCR signalling capacity. For example, in rheumatoid arthritis, some variants of class II HLA-DRB1 are biased towards recognising a cartilage-specific protein CII. When this allele is combined with the *PTPN22* allele that reduces the strength of TCR signalling there is a greatly compounded risk of developing disease [260]. These two mutations may combine to reduce the strength of TCR signalling during negative selection to allow the escape of autoreactive T cells from central tolerance and then have enhanced peripheral presentation to compensate for the reduced TCR signal strength and precipitate autoimmunity.

While most of the effects of the *HLA* locus are likely to be antigen-specific in nature, the *HLA* region also contains the *HLA-Cw* locus, encoding molecules that are recognised by NK cells. NK cells express both inhibitory and activating NIK receptors. The inhibitory receptors bind to HLA-Cw epitopes that are often absent on infected or cancerous cells. An imbalance between signals through the inhibitory and activating receptors of NK cells has been associated with autoimmune disease. Two of the activating receptors on NK cells, KIR2DS1 and KIR2DS2, are found in approximately 35% and 55% of European Americans, respectively [261]. The presence of an activating KIR is most detrimental when the patient also lacks ligands for an inhibitory KIR receptor that could otherwise dampen the NK response. For example, subjects were found to be most at risk for psoriatic arthritis if they carried the activating receptors KIR2DS1 and/or KIR2DS2 and also lacked the HLA-Cw group ligands for the inhibitory receptors KIR2DL1 or KIR2DL2/3 [261]. Furthermore, subjects that have NK cells expressing the inhibitory KIR2DL3 receptor along with target gut epithelial cells expressing the ligand HLA-Cw class 1 show a mild protective effect against ulcerative colitis, possibly due to the increased inhibition of NK cells in the gut [262]. The HLA locus may therefore also alter susceptibility to autoimmunity by generalised effects on the activation of an effector cell population.

The Contribution of Genetic Defects Intrinsic to the Target Organ on Autoimmunity

In the above scenarios the genetic predisposition to autoimmunity was modified by changes extrinsic to the target organ, reducing immune tolerance in a generalised or antigen-specific manner. However an additional mechanism is also likely to synergise with these immune tolerance-modifying genetic components, that of genetic variations that act intrinsic to the target organ itself. Target organ-intrinsic genetic defects could increase susceptibility to autoimmunity in a number of ways. For example, the expression or presentation of key target antigens within the organ and draining lymph nodes could be altered, promoting autoimmune attack. Alternatively, changes to the target organ could increase immune trafficking, raising the chances that the ignorance of autoreactive T cell clones will be broken. Another putative mechanism is developmental alterations in the functionality of the target organ altering the resistance of the constituting cells to apoptosis under low-grade apoptotic pressure. This area of research is still nascent; however there are a number of gene associations suggestive of these functions in Crohn's disease, diabetes, AITD, and rheumatoid arthritis.

Multiple gene associations unique to Crohn's disease are suggestive of increased leukocyte trafficking through the organ increasing the risk of precipitating an autoimmune reaction, including *ATG16L1, IRGM, MDR1, MST1, NCF4 and NKX-2.3* (Table 4). Both ATG16L1 and IRGM are involved in the elimination of bacterial infections from the gut [216, 217]. MST1 influences the movement and phagocytosis of resident peritoneal macrophages and NCF4 assists in the generation of antimicrobial reactive oxygen species [263, 264]. *MDR1* encodes Pgp-1, a protein pump that transports lipophilic compounds out of intestinal epithelial cells and is thought to have a protective role against potentially harmful microbial products. NKX-2.3 is a transcriptional regulator that is required for proper architecture of the small intestine, a change which likely weakens defences against infection. Changes in these genes which reduce the capacity of innate and structural defences may increase the reliance on adaptive immune defences, with the corresponding risk of autoimmunity (Table 5).

A number of defects in the target organ may also be operating during T1D. In the NOD mouse in addition to the known immune defects genes linked to pancreas-intrinsic defects have also been discovered. Lymphocyte infiltration of the pancreas appears to be assuaged by TRPV1, a sensory channel expressed by sensory neurons in beta-islets that is less active in NOD mice and is encoded by a polygenic gene within a known diabetogenic locus [265].

Another polymorphic gene within a diabetogenic locus is *TNFR2*. After infiltration occurs, the NOD islet cells display an intrinsic increase in susceptibility to destruction, possibly due to prolonged signalling through TNFR2 on beta islets [266]. We have also observed increased susceptibility of NOD β islets to non-autoimmune destruction due to metabolic stress (AL, unpublished observations). In human T1D there are not the gene association studies to clearly demonstrate a similar contribution of organ-intrinsic function. There are, however, epidemiologic studies which link T1D with the non-autoimmune type 2 diabetes (T2D). Fourteen percent of Finnish families with a T2D proband also have at least one member with T1D [267]. Ten percent of T2D patients later develop an autoimmune component to this disease [268-270]. Relatives of women who develop gestational diabetes, another syndrome due to metabolic defects of the pancreas [271], have an increased chance of developing both T1D [272] and T2D [273, 274]. Furthermore, progression of T1D children from sublinical to clinical disease is more rapid in individuals who are obese, and thus have a greater metabolic stress on their pancreas [275]. These data suggest that there is a genetic component to the metabolic fitness of the pancreas, and that genetic reductions in this fitness can enhance susceptibility to autoimmune diabetes (Table 5).

Other complicated gene associations with autoimmunity are *TG* and *TSHR* with AITD. As discussed above, since TG and TSHR are key target autoantigens in AITD, altered thymic expression may predispose an individual to anti-thyroid autoimmunity. However other possible explanations of the association exist with organ-intrinsic mechanisms. One possibility is that polymorphisms may result in increased antigen shedding from the organ, seeding higher levels of presentation in the draining lymph node [276]. Another putative mechanism is altered cellular stress due to reduced functionality. Loss-of-function allelic variants of *TG* have been associated with non-autoimmune hypothyroidism [277], raising the possibility that partial reduction in activity alleles exist which are sufficient for thyroid function but place the producing cells under increased metabolic stress.

Table 6. Lessons on T cell tolerance mechanisms from monogenic autoimmune diseases

Disease	OMIM	Causative gene(s)	Main mechanism of tolerance failure
Autoimmune Lymphoproliferative Syndrome (ALPS)	601859	*CASP8, CASP10, FAS, FASL*	Defect in the shutdown of effector T cell response
Autoimmune Polyendocrinopathy Syndrome Type 1 (APS1)	240300	*AIRE*	Defect in thymic presentation of organ-specific antigens
Immunodysregulation, polyendocrinopathy, and enteropathy, X-linked (IPEX)	304790	*FOXP3*	Defect in the production of regulatory T cells
Omenn Syndrome (OS) and related syndromes	603554 102700 606593 176947	*ADA, DCLRE1C, IL3RG, IL7RA, LIG4, RAG1, RAG2, RMRP, ZAP70*	Reduced effectiveness of tolerance mechanisms during partial T cell immunodeficiency

This functional stress may then result in failure under conditions of autoimmunity which would otherwise be subclinical, resulting in Hashimoto's disease. In the case of *TSHR* and Graves' disease, pathology results from autoantibodies to TSHR constitutively activating the receptor. Since polymorphisms exist which are known to result in non-autoimmune hyperthyroidism via increased activity [278], it is possible that partial gain-of-function alleles exist that are not sufficient to cause non-autoimmune hyperthyroidism but can trigger pathogenesis at lower levels of autoantibodies.

Another possible mechanism that could underlie organ-intrinsic defects is an inability for the organ to recover after immunological insult. A polymorphism in *KAZALD1* has been linked to rheumatoid arthritis [26]. As this gene is involved in tissue regeneration, it may be modifying the ability of the joints to heal after autoimmune attack, resulting in pathogenic damage being caused under lower levels of autoimmune pressure (Table 5).

CONCLUDING REMARKS

Autoimmune diseases constitute a diverse range of conditions caused by dysregulation of the adaptive immune system and the generation of T and B cell responses against the target organ. The genetic component of predisposition to autoimmune diseases is strong but complex, with most individual autoimmune diseases controlled in a polygenic manner with a high degree of genetic heterogeneity. Despite the complexity of autoimmune genetics, the common aetiology of the syndromes allows genetic lesions in immune tolerance pathways to contribute to multiple disorders. The few rare monogenic autoimmune conditions are enlightening as to the immune tolerance pathways that constitute the genetic weak points – defects in the negative selection of autoreactive T cells in the thymus, defects in *trans*-acting tolerance mechanisms in the periphery and defects in the *cis*-acting mechanisms restraining effector T cells (Table 6). Numerous genetic associations in the common autoimmune diseases (Table 4) indicate that while complete failure in a given mechanism is limited to the multi-organ monogenic syndromes, partial defects in these same mechanisms are likely to underlie polygenic autoimmunity. Layered on top of this complex interplay of defects in generalised immune tolerance are genetic defects that impair organ-specific immune tolerance pathways and the innate capacity of the target organ to withstand pathogenic onslaught (Table 5). The development of autoimmune disease is therefore a cumulative effect of partial and synergistic defects in multiple immune tolerance mechanisms being directed towards a specific target organ by additional organ-specific defects, heavily modified by environmental influences. The relatively limited number of pathways involved, as opposed to the large number of individual genes, increases the likelihood that targeted intervention to reinforce these pathways will result in effective blockade of autoimmunity.

ACKNOWLEDGMENTS

The authors would like to thank Chris Goodnow, Owen Siggs, Anselm Enders, Sylvie Lesage, Andrew Farr, Alexander Rudensky and Carola Vinuesa for many stimulating discussions on the genetic basis of autoimmunity. This article was originally printed in Genetic Predisposition to Disease in 2008.

REFERENCES

[1] Hyttinen, V., Kaprio, J., Kinnunen, L., Koskenvuo, M. & Tuomilehto, J. (2003). Genetic liability of type 1 diabetes and the onset age among 22,650 young Finnish twin pairs: a nationwide follow-up study. *Diabetes, 52*, 1052-1055.

[2] Silman, A. J., et al. (1993). Twin concordance rates for rheumatoid arthritis: results from a nationwide study. *Br J Rheumatol, 32*, 903-907.

[3] Hansen, T., et al. (2005). Concordance for multiple sclerosis in Danish twins: an update of a nationwide study. *Mult Scler, 11*, 504-510.

[4] Deapen, D., et al. (1992). A revised estimate of twin concordance in systemic lupus erythematosus. *Arthritis Rheum, 35*, 311-318.

[5] Brix, T. H., Christensen, K., Holm, N. V., Harvald, B. & Hegedus, L. (1998). A population-based study of Graves' disease in Danish twins. *Clin Endocrinol (Oxf), 48*, 397-400.

[6] Brix, T. H., Kyvik, K. O. & Hegedus, L. (2000). A population-based study of chronic autoimmune hypothyroidism in Danish twins. *J Clin Endocrinol Metab, 85*, 536-539.

[7] Orholm, M., Binder, V., Sorensen, T. I., Rasmussen, L. P. & Kyvik, K. O. (2000). Concordance of inflammatory bowel disease among Danish twins. Results of a nationwide study. *Scand J Gastroenterol, 35*, 1075-1081.

[8] Park, Y. S., Kim, T. W., Kim, W. B. & Cho, B. Y. (2000). Increased prevalence of autoimmune thyroid disease in patients with type 1 diabetes. *Korean J Intern Med, 15*, 202-210.

[9] Binder, A., Maddison, P. J., Skinner, P., Kurtz, A. & Isenberg, D. A. (1989). Sjogren's syndrome: association with type-1 diabetes mellitus. *Br J Rheumatol, 28*, 518-520.

[10] Poulain, C., Johanet, C., Delcroix, C., Levy-Marchal, C. & Tubiana-Rufi, N. (2007). Prevalence and clinical features of celiac disease in 950 children with type 1 diabetes in France. *Diabetes Metab, 33*, 453-458.

[11] Cruz, A. A., Akaishi, P. M., Vargas, M. A. & de Paula, S. A. (2007). Association between thyroid autoimmune dysfunction and non-thyroid autoimmune diseases. *Ophthal Plast Reconstr Surg, 23*, 104-108.

[12] Sategna-Guidetti, C., et al. (1998). Autoimmune thyroid diseases and coeliac disease. *Eur J Gastroenterol Hepatol, 10*, 927-931.

[13] Zelissen, P. M., Bast, E. J. & Croughs, R. J. (1995). Associated autoimmunity in Addison's disease. *J Autoimmun, 8*, 121-130.

[14] Niederwieser, G., et al. (2003). Prevalence of autoimmune thyroiditis and non-immune thyroid disease in multiple sclerosis. *J Neurol, 250*, 672-675.

[15] Mihailova, D., et al. (1999). Autoimmune thyroid disorders in juvenile chronic arthritis and systemic lupus erythematosus. *Adv Exp Med Biol, 455*, 55-60.

[16] Anaya, J. M., et al. (2006). Familial clustering of autoimmune diseases in patients with type 1 diabetes mellitus. *J Autoimmun, 26*, 208-214.

[17] Anaya, J. M., Tobon, G. J., Vega, P. & Castiblanco, J. (2006). Autoimmune disease aggregation in families with primary Sjogren's syndrome. *J Rheumatol, 33*, 2227-2234.

[18] Cataldo, F. & Marino, V. (2003). Increased prevalence of autoimmune diseases in first-degree relatives of patients with celiac disease. *J Pediatr Gastroenterol Nutr, 36*, 470-473.

[19] Broadley, S.A., Deans, J., Sawcer, S.J., Clayton, D. & Compston, D.A. Autoimmune disease in first-degree relatives of patients with multiple sclerosis. A UK survey. *Brain* 123 (Pt 6), 1102-1111 (2000).

[20] Prahalad, S., Shear, E. S., Thompson, S. D., Giannini, E. H. & Glass, D. N. (2002). Increased prevalence of familial autoimmunity in simplex and multiplex families with juvenile rheumatoid arthritis. *Arthritis Rheum* 46, 1851-1856.

[21] Martin, V., Lee, L. A., Askanase, A. D., Katholi, M. & Buyon, J. P. (2002). Long-term followup of children with neonatal lupus and their unaffected siblings. *Arthritis Rheum, 46*, 2377-2383.

[22] Ginn, L. R., et al. (1998). Familial autoimmunity in pedigrees of idiopathic inflammatory myopathy patients suggests common genetic risk factors for many autoimmune diseases. *Arthritis Rheum, 41*, 400-405.

[23] Vella, A., et al. (2005). Localization of a type 1 diabetes locus in the IL2RA/CD25 region by use of tag single-nucleotide polymorphisms. *Am J Hum Genet, 76*, 773-779.

[24] Brand, OJ., et al. (2007). Association of the interleukin-2 receptor alpha (IL-2Ralpha)/CD25 gene region with Graves' disease using a multilocus test and tag SNPs. *Clin Endocrinol (Oxf), 66*, 508-512.

[25] Hafler, DA., et al. (2007). Risk alleles for multiple sclerosis identified by a genomewide study. *N Engl J Med, 357*, 851-862.

[26] Wellcome Trust Case Control Consortium. Genome-wide association study of 14,000 cases of seven common diseases and 3,000 shared controls. *Nature, 447*, 661-678.

[27] Bottini, N., et al. (2004). A functional variant of lymphoid tyrosine phosphatase is associated with type I diabetes. *Nat Genet, 36*, 337-338.

[28] Velaga, M. R., et al. (2004). The codon 620 tryptophan allele of the lymphoid tyrosine phosphatase (LYP) gene is a major determinant of Graves' disease. *J Clin Endocrinol Metab, 89*, 5862-5865.

[29] Harley, J. B., et al. (2008). Genome-wide association scan in women with systemic lupus erythematosus identifies susceptibility variants in ITGAM, PXK, KIAA1542 and other loci. *Nat Genet, 40*, 204-210.

[30] Begovich, A. B., et al. (2004). A missense single-nucleotide polymorphism in a gene encoding a protein tyrosine phosphatase (PTPN22) is associated with rheumatoid arthritis. *Am J Hum Genet, 75*, 330-337.

[31] Thorsby, E. & Lie, B. A. (2005). HLA associated genetic predisposition to autoimmune diseases: Genes involved and possible mechanisms. *Transpl Immunol, 14*, 175-182.

[32] Zhernakova, A., et al. (2007). Novel association in chromosome 4q27 region with rheumatoid arthritis and confirmation of type 1 diabetes point to a general risk locus for autoimmune diseases. *Am J Hum Genet, 81*, 1284-1288.

[33] Tsurumaru, M., et al. (2006). Evidence for the role of small ubiquitin-like modifier 4 as a general autoimmunity locus in the Japanese population. *J Clin Endocrinol Metab, 91*, 3138-3143.

[34] Todd, J. A., et al. (2007). Robust associations of four new chromosome regions from genome-wide analyses of type 1 diabetes. *Nat Genet, 39*, 857-864.

[35] Motohashi, Y., et al. (2003). Vitamin D receptor gene polymorphism affects onset pattern of type 1 diabetes. *J Clin Endocrinol Metab, 88*, 3137-3140.

[36] Kochi, Y., et al. (2005). A functional variant in FCRL3, encoding Fc receptor-like 3, is associated with rheumatoid arthritis and several autoimmunities. *Nat Genet, 37*, 478-485.

[37] Remmers, E. F., et al. (2007). STAT4 and the risk of rheumatoid arthritis and systemic lupus erythematosus. *N Engl J Med, 357*, 977-986.

[38] Mulcahy, B., et al. (1996). Genetic variability in the tumor necrosis factor-lymphotoxin region influences susceptibility to rheumatoid arthritis. *Am J Hum Genet, 59*, 676-683.

[39] Tokuhiro, S., et al. (2003). An intronic SNP in a RUNX1 binding site of SLC22A4, encoding an organic cation transporter, is associated with rheumatoid arthritis. *Nat Genet, 35*, 341-348.

[40] Okamoto, K., et al. (2003). Identification of I kappa BL as the second major histocompatibility complex-linked susceptibility locus for rheumatoid arthritis. *Am J Hum Genet, 72*, 303-312.

[41] Swanberg, M., et al. (2005). MHC2TA is associated with differential MHC molecule expression and susceptibility to rheumatoid arthritis, multiple sclerosis and myocardial infarction. *Nat Genet, 37*, 486-494.

[42] Kurylowicz, A., Ramos-Lopez, E., Bednarczuk, T. & Badenhoop, K. (2006). Vitamin D-binding protein (DBP) gene polymorphism is associated with Graves' disease and the vitamin D status in a Polish population study. *Exp Clin Endocrinol Diabetes, 114*, 329-335.

[43] Smerdel, A., et al. (2004). Genetic association between juvenile rheumatoid arthritis and polymorphism in the SH2D2A gene. *Genes Immun, 5*, 310-312.

[44] Sigurdsson, S., et al. (2007). Association of a haplotype in the promoter region of the interferon regulatory factor 5 gene with rheumatoid arthritis. *Arthritis Rheum* 56, 2202-2210.

[45] You, C. G., et al. (2006). Association of interleukin-1 genetic polymorphisms with the risk of rheumatoid arthritis in Chinese population. *Clin Chem Lab Med, 45*, 968-971.

[46] Pawlik, A., et al. (2006). Interleukin-18 promoter polymorphism in patients with rheumatoid arthritis. *Tissue Antigens, 67*, 415-418.

[47] Gregory, S. G., et al. (2007). Interleukin 7 receptor alpha chain (IL7R) shows allelic and functional association with multiple sclerosis. *Nat Genet, 39*, 1083-1091.

[48] Teutsch, S. M., Booth, D. R., Bennetts, B. H., Heard, R. N. & Stewart, G. J. (2003). Identification of 11 novel and common single nucleotide polymorphisms in the interleukin-7 receptor-alpha gene and their associations with multiple sclerosis. *Eur J Hum Genet, 11*, 509-515.

[49] Zhang, Z., et al. (2005). Two genes encoding immune-regulatory molecules (LAG3 and IL7R) confer susceptibility to multiple sclerosis. *Genes Immun, 6*, 145-152.

[50] Jacobsen, M., et al., (2000). A point mutation in PTPRC is associated with the development of multiple sclerosis. *Nat Genet, 26*, 495-499.

[51] Zhou, Q., et al. (2003). CD24 is a genetic modifier for risk and progression of multiple sclerosis. *Proc Natl Acad Sci U S A, 100*, 15041-15046.

[52] Tienari, P. J., Wikstrom, J., Sajantila, A., Palo, J. & Peltonen, L. (1992). Genetic susceptibility to multiple sclerosis linked to myelin basic protein gene. *Lancet, 340*, 987-991.

[53] Harbo, H. F., Celius, E. G., Vartdal, F. & Spurkland, A. (1999). CTLA4 promoter and exon 1 dimorphisms in multiple sclerosis. *Tissue Antigens, 53*, 106-110.

[54] Dai, K. Z., et al. (2001). The T cell regulator gene SH2D2A contributes to the genetic susceptibility of multiple sclerosis. *Genes Immun, 2*, 263-268.

[55] Mycko, M. P., Kwinkowski, M., Tronczynska, E., Szymanska, B. & Selmaj, K. W. (1998). Multiple sclerosis: the increased frequency of the ICAM-1 exon 6 gene point mutation genetic type K469. *Ann Neurol, 44*, 70-75.

[56] Kristjansdottir, G., et al. (2008). Interferon Regulatory Factor 5 (IRF5) Gene Variants are Associated with Multiple Sclerosis in Three Distinct Populations. *J Med Genet*.

[57] Hockertz, M. K., Paty, D. W. & Beall, S. S. (1998). Susceptibility to relapsing-progressive multiple sclerosis is associated with inheritance of genes linked to the variable region of the TcR beta locus: use of affected family-based controls. *Am J Hum Genet, 62*, 373-385.

[58] Saarela, J., et al. (2006). PRKCA and multiple sclerosis: association in two independent populations. *PLoS Genet, 2*, e42.

[59] Graham, R. R., et al. (2007). Three functional variants of IFN regulatory factor 5 (IRF5) define risk and protective haplotypes for human lupus. *Proc Natl Acad Sci U S A, 104*, 6758-6763.

[60] Gaffney, P. M., et al. (1998). A genome-wide search for susceptibility genes in human systemic lupus erythematosus sib-pair families. *Proc Natl Acad Sci U S A, 95*, 14875-14879.

[61] Lee, Y. H., Harley, J. B. & Nath, S. K. (2005). CTLA-4 polymorphisms and systemic lupus erythematosus (SLE): a meta-analysis. *Hum Genet, 116*, 361-367.

[62] Wu, J., et al. (1996). Fas ligand mutation in a patient with systemic lupus erythematosus and lymphoproliferative disease. *J Clin Invest, 98*, 1107-1113.

[63] Kyogoku, C., et al. (2002). Fcgamma receptor gene polymorphisms in Japanese patients with systemic lupus erythematosus: contribution of FCGR2B to genetic susceptibility. *Arthritis Rheum, 46*, 1242-1254.

[64] Shin, H. D., et al. (2004). Common DNase I polymorphism associated with autoantibody production among systemic lupus erythematosus patients. *Hum Mol Genet, 13*, 2343-2350.

[65] Lee-Kirsch, M. A., et al. (2007). Mutations in the gene encoding the 3'-5' DNA exonuclease TREX1 are associated with systemic lupus erythematosus. *Nat Genet, 39*, 1065-1067.

[66] Wang, L., et al. (2007). A dinucleotide deletion in CD24 confers protection against autoimmune diseases. *PLoS Genet, 3*, e49.

[67] Ye, D., et al. (2006). A novel single-nucleotide polymorphism of the Fcgamma receptor IIIa gene is associated with genetic susceptibility to systemic lupus erythematosus in Chinese populations: a family-based association study. *Clin Exp Dermatol* 31, 553-557.

[68] Lin, Y. J., et al. (2008). A/C polymorphism in the interleukin-18 coding region among Taiwanese systemic lupus erythematosus patients. *Lupus, 17*, 124-127.

[69] Burton, P. R., et al. (2007). Association scan of 14,500 nonsynonymous SNPs in four diseases identifies autoimmunity variants. *Nat Genet, 39*, 1329-1337.

[70] Jacobson, E. M. & Tomer, Y. (2007). The genetic basis of thyroid autoimmunity. *Thyroid, 17*, 949-961.

[71] Ban, Y., Taniyama, M. & Ban, Y. (2000). Vitamin D receptor gene polymorphism is associated with Graves' disease in the Japanese population. *J Clin Endocrinol Metab, 85*, 4639-4643.

[72] Hadj Kacem, H., et al. (2003). PDS is a new susceptibility gene to autoimmune thyroid diseases: association and linkage study. *J Clin Endocrinol Metab, 88*, 2274-2280.

[73] Duerr, R. H., et al. (2006)A genome-wide association study identifies IL23R as an inflammatory bowel disease gene. *Science, 314*, 1461-1463.

[74] Hampe, J., et al. (2007). A genome-wide association scan of nonsynonymous SNPs identifies a susceptibility variant for Crohn disease in ATG16L1. *Nat Genet, 39*, 207-211.

[75] Brant, S. R., et al. (2003). MDR1 Ala893 polymorphism is associated with inflammatory bowel disease. *Am J Hum Genet, 73*, 1282-1292.

[76] Fowler, E. V., et al. (2005). TNFalpha and IL10 SNPs act together to predict disease behaviour in Crohn's disease. *J Med Genet, 42*, 523-528.

[77] Parkes, M., et al. (2007). Sequence variants in the autophagy gene IRGM and multiple other replicating loci contribute to Crohn's disease susceptibility. *Nat Genet, 39*, 830-832.

[78] Peltekova, V. D., et al. (2004). Functional variants of OCTN cation transporter genes are associated with Crohn disease. *Nat Genet, 36*, 471-475.

[79] Urcelay, E., et al. (2006). MDR1 gene: susceptibility in Spanish Crohn's disease and ulcerative colitis patients. *Inflamm Bowel Dis, 12*, 33-37.

[80] Dideberg, V., et al. (2007). An insertion-deletion polymorphism in the interferon regulatory Factor 5 (IRF5) gene confers risk of inflammatory bowel diseases. *Hum Mol Genet, 16*, 3008-3016.

[81] Stoll, M., et al. (2004). Genetic variation in DLG5 is associated with inflammatory bowel disease. *Nat Genet, 36*, 476-480.

[82] Kappler, J. W., Roehm, N. & Marrack, P. (1987). T cell tolerance by clonal elimination in the thymus. *Cell, 49*, 273-280.

[83] Villunger, A., et al. (2004). Negative selection of semimature CD4(+)8(-)HSA+ thymocytes requires the BH3-only protein Bim but is independent of death receptor signaling. *Proc Natl Acad Sci U S A 101*, 7052-7057 Epub 2004 Apr 7026.

[84] Bouillet, P., et al. (2002). BH3-only Bcl-2 family member Bim is required for apoptosis of autoreactive thymocytes. *Nature, 415*, 922-926.

[85] Hanahan, D. (1998). Peripheral-antigen-expressing cells in thymic medulla: factors in self-tolerance and autoimmunity. *Curr Opin Immunol, 10*, 656-662.

[86] Kyewski, B., Derbinski, J., Gotter, J. & Klein, L. (2002). Promiscuous gene expression and central T-cell tolerance: more than meets the eye. *Trends Immunol 23*, 364-371.

[87] Wicker, L. S., Todd, J. A. & Peterson, L. B. (1995). Genetic control of autoimmune diabetes in the NOD mouse. *Annu Rev Immunol, 13*, 179-200.

[88] Baker, D., Rosenwasser, O. A., O'Neill, J. K. & Turk, J. L. (1995). Genetic analysis of experimental allergic encephalomyelitis in mice. *J Immunol, 155*, 4046-4051.

[89] Oldenborg, P. A., Gresham, H. D., Chen, Y., Izui, S. & Lindberg, F. P. (2002). Lethal autoimmune hemolytic anemia in CD47-deficient nonobese diabetic (NOD) mice. *Blood, 99*, 3500-3504.

[90] Boulard, O., et al. (2002). Genetic analysis of autoimmune sialadenitis in nonobese diabetic mice: a major susceptibility region on chromosome 1. *J Immunol, 168*, 4192-4201.

[91] Zaccone, P., et al. (2002). Autoimmune thyroid disease induced by thyroglobulin and lipopolysaccharide is inhibited by soluble TNF receptor type I. *Eur J Immunol, 32*, 1021-1028.

[92] Braley-Mullen, H., Sharp, G. C., Medling, B. & Tang, H. (1999). Spontaneous autoimmune thyroiditis in NOD.H-2h4 mice. *J Autoimmun, 12*, 157-165.

[93] Rivero, V. E., Cailleau, C., Depiante-Depaoli, M., Riera, C. M. & Carnaud, C. (1998). Non-obese diabetic (NOD) mice are genetically susceptible to experimental autoimmune prostatitis (EAP). *J Autoimmun, 11*, 603-610.

[94] Takahashi, M., et al. (1997). High incidence of autoimmune dacryoadenitis in male non-obese diabetic (NOD) mice depending on sex steroid. *Clin Exp Immunol, 109*, 555-561.

[95] Ridgway, W. M., Fasso, M., Lanctot, A., Garvey, C. & Fathman, C. G. (1996). Breaking self-tolerance in nonobese diabetic mice. *J Exp Med, 183*, 1657-1662..

[96] Baxter, A. G., et al. (1994). Mycobacteria precipitate an SLE-like syndrome in diabetes-prone NOD mice. *Immunology, 83*, 227-231.

[97] Vyse, T. J. & Todd, J. A. (1996). Genetic analysis of autoimmune disease. *Cell 85*, 311-318.

[98] Kishimoto, H. & Sprent, J. (2001). A defect in central tolerance in NOD mice. *Nat Immunol, 2*, 1025-1031..

[99] Lesage, S., et al. (2002). Failure to censor forbidden clone of CD4 T cells in autoimmune diabetes. *J Exp Med, 196*, 1175-1188.

[100] Choisy-Rossi, C. M., Holl, T. M., Pierce, M. A., Chapman, H. D. & Serreze, D. V. (2004). Enhanced pathogenicity of diabetogenic T cells escaping a non-MHC gene-controlled near death experience. *J Immunol, 173*, 3791-3800.

[101] Liston, A., et al. (2004). Generalised resistance to thymic deletion in the NOD mouse: a polygenic trait characterized by defective induction of Bim. *Immunity, 21*, 817-830.

[102] Zucchelli, S., et al. (2005). Defective central tolerance induction in NOD mice: genomics and genetics. *Immunity, 22*, 385-396.

[103] Serreze, D. V., et al. (2008). Through Regulation of TCR Expression Levels, an Idd7 Region Gene(s) Interactively Contributes to the Impaired Thymic Deletion of Autoreactive Diabetogenic CD8+ T Cells in Nonobese Diabetic Mice. *J Immunol, 180*, 3250-3259.

[104] Liston, A., et al. (2007). Impairment of organ-specific T cell negative selection by diabetes susceptibility genes: genomic analysis by mRNA profiling. *Genome Biol, 8*, R12.

[105] Roifman, C. M., Gu, Y. & Cohen, A. (2006). Mutations in the RNA component of RNase mitochondrial RNA processing might cause Omenn syndrome. *J Allergy Clin Immunol, 117*, 897-903.

[106] Giliani, S., et al. (2006). Omenn syndrome in an infant with IL7RA gene mutation. *J Pediatr, 148*, 272-274.

[107] Shibata, F., et al. (2007). Skin infiltration of CD56(bright) CD16(-) natural killer cells in a case of X-SCID with Omenn syndrome-like manifestations. *Eur J Haematol, 79*, 81-85.

[108] Santagata, S., Villa, A., Sobacchi, C., Cortes, P. & Vezzoni, P. (2000). The genetic and biochemical basis of Omenn syndrome. *Immunol Rev, 178*, 64-74.

[109] Aleman, K., Noordzij, J. G., de Groot, R., van Dongen, J. J. & Hartwig, N. G. (2001). Reviewing Omenn syndrome. *Eur J Pediatr, 160*, 718-725.

[110] Enders, A., et al. (2006). A severe form of human combined immunodeficiency due to mutations in DNA ligase IV. *J Immunol, 176*, 5060-5068.

[111] Toyabe, S., Watanabe, A., Harada, W., Karasawa, T. & Uchiyama, M. (2001). Specific immunoglobulin E responses in ZAP-70-deficient patients are mediated by Syk-dependent T-cell receptor signalling. *Immunology, 103*, 164-171.

[112] Shovlin, C. L., et al. (1993). Adult presentation of adenosine deaminase deficiency. *Lancet, 341*, 1471.

[113] Hirschhorn, R., Yang, D. R., Israni, A., Huie, M. L. & Ownby, D. R. (1994). Somatic mosaicism for a newly identified splice-site mutation in a patient with adenosine deaminase-deficient immunodeficiency and spontaneous clinical recovery. *Am J Hum Genet, 55*, 59-68.

[114] Hirschhorn, R., et al. (1996). Spontaneous in vivo reversion to normal of an inherited mutation in a patient with adenosine deaminase deficiency. *Nat Genet, 13*, 290-295.

[115] Khiong, K., et al. (2007). Homeostatically proliferating CD4 T cells are involved in the pathogenesis of an Omenn syndrome murine model. *J Clin Invest, 117*, 1270-1281.

[116] Marrella, V., et al. (2007). A hypomorphic R229Q Rag2 mouse mutant recapitulates human Omenn syndrome. *J Clin Invest, 117*, 1260-1269.

[117] Sakaguchi, N., et al. (2003). Altered thymic T-cell selection due to a mutation of the ZAP-70 gene causes autoimmune arthritis in mice. *Nature, 426*, 454-460.

[118] Siggs, O. M., et al. (2007). Opposing Function of the T Cell Receptor Kinase ZAP-70 in Immunity and Tolerance Differentially Titrate in Response to Nucleotide Substitutions. *Immunity, 27*, 912-926.

[119] Venanzi, E. S., Gray, D. H., Benoist, C. & Mathis, D. (2007). Lymphotoxin pathway and Aire influences on thymic medullary epithelial cells are unconnected. *J Immunol 179*, 5693-5700.

[120] Gray, D. H., et al. (2005). Controlling the thymic microenvironment. *Curr Opin Immunol, 17*, 137-143.

[121] Zhu, M., Chin, R. K., Tumanov, A. V., Liu, X. & Fu, Y. X. (2007). Lymphotoxin receptor is required for the migration and selection of autoreactive T cells in thymic medulla. *J Immunol, 179*, 8069-8075.

[122] Fazekas de St Groth, B. (2001). DCs and peripheral T cell tolerance. *Semin Immunol, 13*, 311-322.

[123] Vang, T., et al. (2005). Autoimmune-associated lymphoid tyrosine phosphatase is a gain-of-function variant. *Nat Genet, 37*, 1317-1319.

[124] Hori, S., Nomura, T. & Sakaguchi, S. (2003). Control of regulatory T cell development by the transcription factor Foxp3. *Science, 299*, 1057-1061.

[125] Fontenot, J. D., Gavin, M. A. & Rudensky, A. Y. (2003). Foxp3 programs the development and function of CD4+CD25+ regulatory T cells. *Nat Immunol, 4*, 330-336.

[126] Khattri, R., Cox, T., Yasayko, S. A. & Ramsdell, F. (2003). An essential role for Scurfin in CD4+CD25+ T regulatory cells. *Nat Immunol, 4*, 337-342.

[127] Kim, J. M., Rasmussen, J. P. & Rudensky, A. Y. (2007). Regulatory T cells prevent catastrophic autoimmunity throughout the lifespan of mice. *Nat Immunol 8*, 191-197.

[128] Jordan, M. S., et al. (2001). Thymic selection of CD4+CD25+ regulatory T cells induced by an agonist self-peptide. *Nat Immunol, 2*, 301-306.

[129] Kawahata, K., et al. (2002). Generation of CD4(+)CD25(+) regulatory T cells from autoreactive T cells simultaneously with their negative selection in the thymus and from nonautoreactive T cells by endogenous TCR expression. *J Immunol, 168*, 4399-4405.

[130] Lohr, J., Knoechel, B., Jiang, S., Sharpe, A. H. & Abbas, A. K. (2003). The inhibitory function of B7 costimulators in T cell responses to foreign and self-antigens. *Nat Immunol, 4*, 664-669.

[131] Hsieh, C. S., et al. (2004). Recognition of the Peripheral Self by Naturally Arising CD25(+) CD4(+) T Cell Receptors. *Immunity, 21*, 267-277.

[132] Pacholczyk, R., Ignatowicz, H., Kraj, P. & Ignatowicz, L. (2006). Origin and T cell receptor diversity of Foxp3+CD4+CD25+ T cells. *Immunity, 25*, 249-259.

[133] Kretschmer, K., et al. (2005). Inducing and expanding regulatory T cell populations by foreign antigen. *Nat Immunol, 6*, 1219-1227.

[134] Bruder, D., et al. (2005). On the edge of autoimmunity: T-cell stimulation by steady-state dendritic cells prevents autoimmune diabetes. *Diabetes, 54*, 3395-3401.

[135] Chen, W., et al. (2003). Conversion of peripheral CD4+CD25- naive T cells to CD4+CD25+ regulatory T cells by TGF-beta induction of transcription factor Foxp3. *J Exp Med, 198*, 1875-1886.

[136] Fu, S., et al. (2004). TGF-beta induces Foxp3 + T-regulatory cells from CD4 + CD25 - precursors. *Am J Transplant, 4*, 1614-1627.

[137] Fantini, M. C., et al. (2004). Cutting edge: TGF-beta induces a regulatory phenotype in CD4+CD25- T cells through Foxp3 induction and down-regulation of Smad7. *J Immunol, 172*, 5149-5153.

[138] Kim, J. M. & Rudensky, A. (2006). The role of the transcription factor Foxp3 in the development of regulatory T cells. *Immunol Rev, 212*, 86-98.

[139] Peng, Y., Laouar, Y., Li, M. O., Green, E. A. & Flavell, R. A. (2004). TGF-beta regulates in vivo expansion of Foxp3-expressing CD4+CD25+ regulatory T cells responsible for protection against diabetes. *Proc Natl Acad Sci U S A 101*, 4572-4577 Epub 2004 Mar 4518.

[140] Park, H. B., Paik, D. J., Jang, E., Hong, S. & Youn, J. (2004). Acquisition of anergic and suppressive activities in transforming growth factor-beta-costimulated CD4+CD25- T cells. *Int Immunol, 16*, 1203-1213 Epub 2004 Jul 1205.

[141] Verhasselt, V., et al. (2004). Induction of FOXP3-expressing regulatory CD4pos T cells by human mature autologous dendritic cells. *Eur J Immunol, 34*, 762-772.

[142] Polanczyk, M. J., et al. (2004). Cutting edge: estrogen drives expansion of the CD4+CD25+ regulatory T cell compartment. *J Immunol, 173*, 2227-2230.

[143] Zheng, Y., et al. (2007). Genome-wide analysis of Foxp3 target genes in developing and mature regulatory T cells. *Nature, 445*, 936-940.

[144] Gavin, M. A., et al. (2007). Foxp3-dependent programme of regulatory T-cell differentiation. *Nature*.

[145] Williams, L. M. & Rudensky, A. Y. (2007). Maintenance of the Foxp3-dependent developmental program in mature regulatory T cells requires continued expression of Foxp3. *Nat Immunol, 8*, 277-284.

[146] Takahashi, T., et al. (1998). Immunologic self-tolerance maintained by CD25+CD4+ naturally anergic and suppressive T cells: induction of autoimmune disease by breaking their anergic/suppressive state. *Int Immunol, 10*, 1969-1980.

[147] Kramer, S., Schimpl, A. & Hunig, T. (1995). Immunopathology of interleukin (IL) 2-deficient mice: thymus dependence and suppression by thymus-dependent cells with an intact IL-2 gene. *J Exp Med, 182*, 1769-1776.

[148] Almeida, A. R., Legrand, N., Papiernik, M. & Freitas, A. A. (2002). Homeostasis of peripheral CD4+ T cells: IL-2R alpha and IL-2 shape a population of regulatory cells that controls CD4+ T cell numbers. *J Immunol, 169*, 4850-4860.

[149] Suzuki, H., Zhou, Y. W., Kato, M., Mak, T. W. & Nakashima, I. (1999). Normal regulatory alpha/beta T cells effectively eliminate abnormally activated T cells lacking the interleukin 2 receptor beta in vivo. *J Exp Med, 190*, 1561-1572.

[150] Sadlack, B., et al. (1993). Ulcerative colitis-like disease in mice with a disrupted interleukin-2 gene. *Cell, 75*, 253-261.

[151] Suzuki, H., et al. (1995). Deregulated T cell activation and autoimmunity in mice lacking interleukin-2 receptor beta. *Science 268*, 1472-1476.

[152] Willerford, D. M., et al. (1995). Interleukin-2 receptor alpha chain regulates the size and content of the peripheral lymphoid compartment. *Immunity, 3*, 521-530.

[153] Fontenot, J. D., Rasmussen, J. P., Gavin, M. A. & Rudensky, A. Y. (2005). A function for interleukin 2 in Foxp3-expressing regulatory T cells. *Nat Immunol, 6*, 1142-1151.

[154] Liston, A., Siggs, O. M. & Goodnow, C. C. (2007). Tracing the action of IL-2 in tolerance to islet-specific antigen. *Immunol Cell Biol, 85*, 338-342.

[155] Antony, P. A., et al. (2006). Interleukin-2-dependent mechanisms of tolerance and immunity in vivo. *J Immunol, 176*, 5255-5266.

[156] Yamanouchi, J., et al. (2007). Interleukin-2 gene variation impairs regulatory T cell function and causes autoimmunity. *Nat Genet*.

[157] Podolin, P. L., et al. (2000). Differential glycosylation of interleukin 2, the molecular basis for the NOD Idd3 type 1 diabetes gene? *Cytokine, 12*, 477-482.

[158] Martinez, X., et al. (2005). CD8+ T cell tolerance in nonobese diabetic mice is restored by insulin-dependent diabetes resistance alleles. *J Immunol, 175*, 1677-1685.

[159] Fontenot, J. D., Dooley, J. L., Farr, A. G. & Rudensky, A. Y. (2005). Developmental regulation of Foxp3 expression during ontogeny. *J Exp Med, 202*, 901-906.

[160] Gough, S. C., Walker, L. S. & Sansom, D. M. (2005). CTLA4 gene polymorphism and autoimmunity. *Immunol Rev, 204*, 102-115.

[161] Krummel, M. F. & Allison, J. P. (1996). CTLA-4 engagement inhibits IL-2 accumulation and cell cycle progression upon activation of resting T cells. *J Exp Med, 183*, 2533-2540.

[162] Walunas, T. L., Bakker, C. Y. & Bluestone, J. A. (1996). CTLA-4 ligation blocks CD28-dependent T cell activation. *J Exp Med, 183*, 2541-2550.

[163] Ueda, H., et al. (2003). Association of the T-cell regulatory gene CTLA4 with susceptibility to autoimmune disease. *Nature, 423*, 506-511.

[164] Hill, N. J., et al. (2000). NOD Idd5 locus controls insulitis and diabetes and overlaps the orthologous CTLA4/IDDM12 and NRAMP1 loci in humans. *Diabetes 49*, 1744-1747..

[165] Oaks, M.K., et al. A native soluble form of CTLA-4. *Cell Immunol 201*, 144-153 (2000).

[166] Grohmann, U., et al. CTLA-4-Ig regulates tryptophan catabolism in vivo. *Nat Immunol 3*, 1097-1101 (2002).

[167] Chitale, S. & Moots, R. Abatacept: the first T lymphocyte co-stimulation modulator, for the treatment of rheumatoid arthritis. *Expert Opin Biol Ther 8*, 115-122 (2008).

[168] Wu, K., Bi, Y., Sun, K. & Wang, C. (2007). IL-10-producing type 1 regulatory T cells and allergy. *Cell Mol Immunol, 4*, 269-275.

[169] Maynard, C. L., et al. (2007). Regulatory T cells expressing interleukin 10 develop from Foxp3+ and Foxp3- precursor cells in the absence of interleukin 10. *Nat Immunol, 8*, 931-941.

[170] Davidson, N. J., et al. (1996). T helper cell 1-type CD4+ T cells, but not B cells, mediate colitis in interleukin 10-deficient mice. *J Exp Med, 184*, 241-251.

[171] Rubtsov, Y. P., et al. (2008). IL-10 produced by regulatory T cells contributes to their suppressor function by limiting inflammation at environmental interfaces. *Immunity, 28*, 546-558.

[172] Mizoguchi, A. & Bhan, A. K. (2006). A case for regulatory B cells. *J Immunol 176*, 705-710.

[173] Fillatreau, S., Sweenie, C. H., McGeachy, M. J., Gray, D. & Anderton, S. M. (2002). B cells regulate autoimmunity by provision of IL-10. *Nat Immunol, 3*, 944-950.

[174] Singh, A. K., et al. (2001). Natural killer T cell activation protects mice against experimental autoimmune encephalomyelitis. *J Exp Med, 194*, 1801-1811.

[175] Sharif, S., et al. (2001). Activation of natural killer T cells by alpha-galactosylceramide treatment prevents the onset and recurrence of autoimmune Type 1 diabetes. *Nat Med, 7*, 1057-1062.

[176] Yoshimoto, T., Bendelac, A., Hu-Li, J. & Paul, W. E. (1995). Defective IgE production by SJL mice is linked to the absence of CD4+, NK1.1+ T cells that promptly produce interleukin 4. *Proc Natl Acad Sci U S A, 92*, 11931-11934.

[177] Baxter, A. G., Kinder, S. J., Hammond, K. J., Scollay, R. & Godfrey, D. I. (1997). Association between alphabetaTCR+CD4-CD8- T-cell deficiency and IDDM in NOD/Lt mice. *Diabetes, 46*, 572-582.

[178] Godfrey, D. I., Kinder, S. J., Silvera, P. & Baxter, A. G. (1997). Flow cytometric study of T cell development in NOD mice reveals a deficiency in alphabetaTCR+CDR-CD8- thymocytes. *J Autoimmun, 10*, 279-285.

[179] Gombert, J. M., et al. (1996). Early quantitative and functional deficiency of NK1+-like thymocytes in the NOD mouse. *Eur J Immunol, 26*, 2989-2998.

[180] Poulton, L. D., et al. (2001). Cytometric and functional analyses of NK and NKT cell deficiencies in NOD mice. *Int Immunol 13*, 887-896.

[181] Esteban, L. M., et al. (2003). Genetic control of NKT cell numbers maps to major diabetes and lupus loci. *J Immunol, 171*, 2873-2878.

[182] Hammond, K. J., et al. (1998). alpha/beta-T cell receptor (TCR)+CD4-CD8- (NKT) thymocytes prevent insulin-dependent diabetes mellitus in nonobese diabetic (NOD)/Lt mice by the influence of interleukin (IL)-4 and/or IL-10. *J Exp Med, 187*, 1047-1056.

[183] Wilson, S. B., et al. (1998). Extreme Th1 bias of invariant Valpha24JalphaQ T cells in type 1 diabetes. *Nature, 391*, 177-181.

[184] Ivanov, II, Zhou, L. & Littman, D. R. (2007). Transcriptional regulation of Th17 cell differentiation. *Semin Immunol, 19*, 409-417.

[185] Nakae, S., Nambu, A., Sudo, K. & Iwakura, Y. (2003). Suppression of immune induction of collagen-induced arthritis in IL-17-deficient mice. *J Immunol, 171,* 6173-6177.

[186] Komiyama, Y., et al. (2006). IL-17 plays an important role in the development of experimental autoimmune encephalomyelitis. *J Immunol, 177,* 566-573.

[187] Hutloff, A., et al. (1999). ICOS is an inducible T-cell co-stimulator structurally and functionally related to CD28. *Nature, 397,* 263-266.

[188] Mak, T. W., et al. (2003). Costimulation through the inducible costimulator ligand is essential for both T helper and B cell functions in T cell-dependent B cell responses. *Nat Immunol, 4,* 765-772.

[189] Rousset, F., et al. (1992). Interleukin 10 is a potent growth and differentiation factor for activated human B lymphocytes. *Proc Natl Acad Sci U S A, 89,* 1890-1893.

[190] Nurieva, R., et al. (2007). Essential autocrine regulation by IL-21 in the generation of inflammatory T cells. *Nature, 448,* 480-483.

[191] Korn, T., et al. (2007). IL-21 initiates an alternative pathway to induce proinflammatory T(H)17 cells. *Nature, 448,* 484-487.

[192] Zhou, L., et al. (2007). IL-6 programs T(H)-17 cell differentiation by promoting sequential engagement of the IL-21 and IL-23 pathways. *Nat Immunol 8,* 967-974.

[193] Bettelli, E., et al. (2006). Reciprocal developmental pathways for the generation of pathogenic effector TH17 and regulatory T cells. *Nature, 441,* 235-238.

[194] Mangan, P.R., et al. Transforming growth factor-beta induces development of the T(H)17 lineage. *Nature, 441,* 231-234.

[195] Ivanov, II et al. (2006). The orphan nuclear receptor RORgammat directs the differentiation program of proinflammatory IL-17+ T helper cells. *Cell, 126,* 1121-1133.

[196] McGeachy, M. J., et al. (2007). TGF-beta and IL-6 drive the production of IL-17 and IL-10 by T cells and restrain T(H)-17 cell-mediated pathology. *Nat Immunol, 8,* 1390-1397.

[197] Langrish, C. L., et al. (2005). IL-23 drives a pathogenic T cell population that induces autoimmune inflammation. *J Exp Med, 201,* 233-240.

[198] Cua, D. J., et al. (2003). Interleukin-23 rather than interleukin-12 is the critical cytokine for autoimmune inflammation of the brain. *Nature, 421,* 744-748.

[199] Cargill, M., et al. (2007). A large-scale genetic association study confirms IL12B and leads to the identification of IL23R as psoriasis-risk genes. *Am J Hum Genet, 80,* 273-290.

[200] Vinuesa, C. G., et al. (2005). A RING-type ubiquitin ligase family member required to repress follicular helper T cells and autoimmunity. *Nature, 435,* 452-458.

[201] Yu, D., et al. (2008). Roquin represses autoimmunity by limiting inducible T-cell co-stimulator messenger RNA. *Nature, 451,* 1022.

[202] Cappione, A., 3rd et al. (2005). Germinal center exclusion of autoreactive B cells is defective in human systemic lupus erythematosus. *J Clin Invest, 115,* 3205-3216.

[203] Hutloff, A., et al. (2004). Involvement of inducible costimulator in the exaggerated memory B cell and plasma cell generation in systemic lupus erythematosus. *Arthritis Rheum, 50,* 3211-3220.

[204] Weant, A. E., et al. (2008). Apoptosis regulators bim and fas function concurrently to control autoimmunity and CD8(+) T cell contraction. *Immunity, 28,* 218-230.

[205] Hughes, P. D., et al. (2008). Apoptosis regulators fas and bim cooperate in shutdown of chronic immune responses and prevention of autoimmunity. *Immunity, 28*, 197-205.

[206] Hutcheson, J., et al. (2008). Combined Deficiency of Proapoptotic Regulators Bim and Fas Results in the Early Onset of Systemic Autoimmunity. *Immunity, 28*, 206-217.

[207] Fisher, G. H., et al. (1995). Dominant interfering Fas gene mutations impair apoptosis in a human autoimmune lymphoproliferative syndrome. *Cell, 81*, 935-946.

[208] Xu, L., Zhang, L., Yi, Y., Kang, H. K. & Datta, S. K. (2004). Human lupus T cells resist inactivation and escape death by upregulating COX-2. *Nat Med, 10*, 411-415.

[209] Schirmer, M., Vallejo, A. N., Weyand, C. M. & Goronzy, J. J. (1998). Resistance to apoptosis and elevated expression of Bcl-2 in clonally expanded CD4+CD28- T cells from rheumatoid arthritis patients. *J Immunol, 161*, 1018-1025.

[210] Sharief, M. K. & Semra, Y. K. (2001). Heightened expression of survivin in activated T lymphocytes from patients with multiple sclerosis. *J Neuroimmunol, 119*, 358-364.

[211] Vafiadis, P., et al. (1997). Insulin expression in human thymus is modulated by INS VNTR alleles at the IDDM2 locus. *Nat Genet, 15*, 289-292.

[212] Pugliese, A., et al. (1997). The insulin gene is transcribed in the human thymus and transcription levels correlated with allelic variation at the INS VNTR-IDDM2 susceptibility locus for type 1 diabetes. *Nat Genet, 15*, 293-297.

[213] Giraud, M., et al. (2007). An IRF8-binding promoter variant and AIRE control CHRNA1 promiscuous expression in thymus. *Nature, 448*, 934-937.

[214] Yamada, R. & Yamamoto, K. (2007). Mechanisms of disease: genetics of rheumatoid arthritis--ethnic differences in disease-associated genes. *Nat Clin Pract Rheumatol, 3*, 644-650.

[215] Faas, S. & Trucco, M. (1994). The genes influencing the susceptibility to IDDM in humans. *J Endocrinol Invest, 17*, 477-495.

[216] Rioux, J. D., et al. (2007). Genome-wide association study identifies new susceptibility loci for Crohn disease and implicates autophagy in disease pathogenesis. *Nat Genet, 39*, 596-604.

[217] Singh, S. B., Davis, A. S., Taylor, G. A. & Deretic, V. (2006). Human IRGM induces autophagy to eliminate intracellular mycobacteria. *Science, 313*, 1438-1441.

[218] Nagamine, K., et al. (1997). Positional cloning of the APECED gene. *Nat Genet, 17*, 393-398.

[219] The Finnish-German APECED Consortium. An autoimmune disease, APECED, caused by mutations in a novel gene featuring two PHD-type zinc-finger domains. *Nat Genet 17*, 399-403, 1997.

[220] Betterle, C., Greggio, N. A. & Volpato, M. (1998). Autoimmune polyglandular syndrome type 1. *J Clin Endocrinol Metab, 83*, 1049-1055.

[221] Anderson, M. S., et al. (2002). Projection of an Immunological Self-Shadow Within the Thymus by the Aire Protein. *Science, 298*, 1395-1401.

[222] Ramsey, C., et al. (2002). Aire deficient mice develop multiple features of APECED phenotype and show altered immune response. *Hum Mol Genet, 11*, 397-409.

[223] Heino, M., et al. (1999). Autoimmune regulator is expressed in the cells regulating immune tolerance in thymus medulla. *Biochem Biophys Res Commun, 257*, 821-825.

[224] Kogawa, K., et al. (2002). Expression of AIRE gene in peripheral monocyte/dendritic cell lineage. *Immunol Lett, 80*, 195-198.

[225] Derbinski, J., et al. (2005). Promiscuous gene expression in thymic epithelial cells is regulated at multiple levels. *J Exp Med, 202*, 33-45.
[226] Liston, A., Lesage, S., Wilson, J., Peltonen, L. & Goodnow, C. C. (2003). Aire regulates negative selection of organ-specific T cells. *Nat Immunol, 4*, 350-354.
[227] DeVoss, J., et al. (2006). Spontaneous autoimmunity prevented by thymic expression of a single self-antigen. *J Exp Med, 203*, 2727-2735.
[228] Liston, A., et al. (2004). Gene dosage limiting role of Aire in thymic expression, clonal deletion and organ-specific autoimmunity. *J Exp Med, 200*, 1015-1026.
[229] Heino, M., et al. (2000). RNA and protein expression of the murine autoimmune regulator gene (Aire) in normal, RelB-deficient and in NOD mouse. *Eur J Immunol, 30*, 1884-1893..
[230] Rinderle, C., Christensen, H. M., Schweiger, S., Lehrach, H. & Yaspo, M. L. (1999). AIRE encodes a nuclear protein co-localizing with cytoskeletal filaments: altered subcellular distribution of mutants lacking the PHD zinc fingers. *Hum Mol Genet, 8*, 277-290.
[231] Pitkanen, J., et al. (2000). The autoimmune regulator protein has transcriptional transactivating properties and interacts with the common coactivator CREB-binding protein. *J Biol Chem, 275*, 16802-16809.
[232] Kumar, P. G., et al. (2001). The autoimmune regulator (AIRE) is a DNA-binding protein. *J Biol Chem, 276*, 41357-41364.
[233] Bjorses, P., et al. (2000). Mutations in the AIRE gene: effects on subcellular location and transactivation function of the autoimmune polyendocrinopathy-candidiasis-ectodermal dystrophy protein. *Am J Hum Genet, 66*, 378-392.
[234] Ruan, Q. G., et al. (2007). The autoimmune regulator directly controls the expression of genes critical for thymic epithelial function. *J Immunol, 178*, 7173-7180.
[235] Gillard, G. O. & Farr, A. G. (2006). Features of medullary thymic epithelium implicate postnatal development in maintaining epithelial heterogeneity and tissue-restricted antigen expression. *J Immunol, 176*, 5815-5824.
[236] Ilmarinen, T., et al. (2008). Functional interaction of AIRE with PIAS1 in transcriptional regulation. *Mol Immunol, 45*, 1847-1862.
[237] Org, T., et al. (2008). The autoimmune regulator PHD finger binds to non-methylated histone H3K4 to activate gene expression. *EMBO Rep.*
[238] Tao, Y., et al. (2006). AIRE recruits multiple transcriptional components to specific genomic regions through tethering to nuclear matrix. *Mol Immunol, 43*, 335-345.
[239] Gillard, G. O., Dooley, J., Erickson, M., Peltonen, L. & Farr, A. G. (2007). Aire-dependent alterations in medullary thymic epithelium indicate a role for Aire in thymic epithelial differentiation. *J Immunol, 178*, 3007-3015.
[240] Kuroda, N., et al. (2005). Development of autoimmunity against transcriptionally unrepressed target antigen in the thymus of Aire-deficient mice. *J Immunol, 174*, 1862-1870.
[241] Anderson, M. S., (2005). et al. The cellular mechanism of Aire control of T cell tolerance. *Immunity, 23*, 227-239.
[242] Li, J., et al. (2007). Developmental pathway of CD4+CD8- medullary thymocytes during mouse ontogeny and its defect in Aire-/- mice. *Proc Natl Acad Sci U S A, 104*, 18175-18180.

[243] Halonen, M., et al. (2002). AIRE mutations and human leukocyte antigen genotypes as determinants of the autoimmune polyendocrinopathy-candidiasis-ectodermal dystrophy phenotype. *J Clin Endocrinol Metab, 87*, 2568-2574.

[244] Kogawa, K., et al. (2002). Distinct clinical phenotype and immunoreactivity in Japanese siblings with autoimmune polyglandular syndrome type 1 (APS-1) associated with compound heterozygous novel AIRE gene mutations. *Clin Immunol 103*, 277-283.

[245] Jiang, W., Anderson, M. S., Bronson, R., Mathis, D. & Benoist, C. (2005). Modifier loci condition autoimmunity provoked by Aire deficiency. *J Exp Med, 202*, 805-815.

[246] Kont, V., et al. (2008). Modulation of Aire regulates the expression of tissue-restricted antigens. *Mol Immunol, 45*, 25-33.

[247] Anderson, A. C., et al. (2000). High frequency of autoreactive myelin proteolipid protein-specific T cells in the periphery of naive mice: mechanisms of selection of the self-reactive repertoire. *J Exp Med, 191*, 761-770.

[248] Miyamoto, K., Miyake, S., Schachner, M. & Yamamura, T. (2003). Heterozygous null mutation of myelin P0 protein enhances susceptibility to autoimmune neuritis targeting P0 peptide. *Eur J Immunol, 33*, 656-665.

[249] Taubert, R., Schwendemann, J. & Kyewski, B. (2007). Highly variable expression of tissue-restricted self-antigens in human thymus: implications for self-tolerance and autoimmunity. *Eur J Immunol, 37*, 838-848.

[250] Saboori, A. M., Rose, N. R., Bresler, H. S., Vladut-Talor, M. & Burek, C. L. (1998). Iodination of human thyroglobulin (Tg) alters its immunoreactivity. I. Iodination alters multiple epitopes of human Tg. *Clin Exp Immunol, 113*, 297-302.

[251] Barin, J. G., Talor, M. V., Sharma, R. B., Rose, N. R. & Burek, C. L. (2005). Iodination of murine thyroglobulin enhances autoimmune reactivity in the NOD.H2 mouse. *Clin Exp Immunol, 142*, 251-259.

[252] Laurberg, P., et al. (1998). Iodine intake and the pattern of thyroid disorders: a comparative epidemiological study of thyroid abnormalities in the elderly in Iceland and in Jutland, Denmark. *J Clin Endocrinol Metab, 83*, 765-769.

[253] Brand, O., Gough, S. & Heward, J. (2005). HLA, CTLA-4 and PTPN22: the shared genetic master-key to autoimmunity? *Expert Reviews in Molecular Medicine 7*, 1-15.

[254] Wicker, L. S. (1997). Major histocompatibility complex-linked control of autoimmunity. *J Exp Med, 186*, 973-975.

[255] Corper, A. L., et al. (2000). A structural framework for deciphering the link between I-Ag7 and autoimmune diabetes. *Science, 288*, 505-511.

[256] Stratmann, T., et al. (2000). The I-Ag7 MHC class II molecule linked to murine diabetes is a promiscuous peptide binder. *J Immunol, 165*, 3214-3225.

[257] Wen, L., Wong, F. S., Sherwin, R. & Mora, C. (2002). Human DQ8 can substitute for murine I-Ag7 in the selection of diabetogenic T cells restricted to I-Ag7. *J Immunol, 168*, 3635-3640.

[258] Li, Y., et al. (2005). Structure of a human autoimmune TCR bound to a myelin basic protein self-peptide and a multiple sclerosis-associated MHC class II molecule. *Embo J, 24*, 2968-2979.

[259] Maynard, J., et al. (2005). Structure of an autoimmune T cell receptor complexed with class II peptide-MHC: insights into MHC bias and antigen specificity. *Immunity, 22*, 81-92.

[260] Burkhardt, H., et al. (2006). Association between protein tyrosine phosphatase 22 variant R620W in conjunction with the HLA-DRB1 shared epitope and humoral autoimmunity to an immunodominant epitope of cartilage-specific type II collagen in early rheumatoid arthritis. *Arthritis Rheum, 54*, 82-89.

[261] Nelson, G. W., et al. (2004). Cutting Edge: Heterozygote Advantage in Autoimmune Disease: Hierarchy of Protection/Susceptibility Conferred by HLA and Killer Ig-Like Receptor Combinations in Psoriatic Arthritis. *J Immunol, 173*, 4273-4276.

[262] Jones, D. C., et al. (2006). Killer Ig-like receptor (KIR) genotype and HLA ligand combinations in ulcerative colitis susceptibility. *Genes Immun, 7*, 576.

[263] Ellson, C. D., et al. (2006). Neutrophils from p40phox-/- mice exhibit severe defects in NADPH oxidase regulation and oxidant-dependent bacterial killing. *J Exp Med, 203*, 1927-1937.

[264] Suh, C. I., et al. (2006). The phosphoinositide-binding protein p40phox activates the NADPH oxidase during FcgammaIIA receptor-induced phagocytosis. *J Exp Med, 203*, 1915-1925.

[265] Razavi, R., et al. (2006). TRPV1(+) sensory neurons control beta cell stress and islet inflammation in autoimmune diabetes. *Cell, 127*, 1123-1135.

[266] Hill, N. J., et al. (2007). Resistance of the target islet tissue to autoimmune destruction contributes to genetic susceptibility in Type 1 diabetes. *Biol Direct, 2*, 5.

[267] Li, H., et al. (2001). Possible human leukocyte antigen-mediated genetic interaction between type 1 and type 2 Diabetes. *J Clin Endocrinol Metab, 86*, 574-582.

[268] Schernthaner, G., et al. (2001). Progress in the characterization of slowly progressive autoimmune diabetes in adult patients (LADA or type 1.5 diabetes). *Exp Clin Endocrinol Diabetes* 109 Suppl, *2*, S94-108.

[269] Palmer, J. P., Hampe, C. S., Chiu, H., Goel, A. & Brooks-Worrell, B. M. (2005). Is latent autoimmune diabetes in adults distinct from type 1 diabetes or just type 1 diabetes at an older age? *Diabetes* 54 Suppl, *2*, S62-67.

[270] Turner, R., et al. (1997). UKPDS 25: autoantibodies to islet-cell cytoplasm and glutamic acid decarboxylase for prediction of insulin requirement in type 2 diabetes. UK Prospective Diabetes Study Group. *Lancet, 350*, 1288-1293.

[271] Watanabe, R. M., et al. (2007). Genetics of gestational diabetes mellitus and type 2 diabetes. *Diabetes Care,* 30 Suppl, *2*, S134-140.

[272] Dorner, G., Plagemann, A. & Reinagel, H. (1987). Familial diabetes aggregation in type I diabetics: gestational diabetes an apparent risk factor for increased diabetes susceptibility in the offspring. *Exp Clin Endocrinol, 89*, 84-90.

[273] McLellan, J. A., et al. (1995). Prevalence of diabetes mellitus and impaired glucose tolerance in parents of women with gestational diabetes. *Diabetologia, 38*, 693-698.

[274] Martin, A. O., Simpson, J. L., Ober, C. & Freinkel, N. (1985). Frequency of diabetes mellitus in mothers of probands with gestational diabetes: possible maternal influence on the predisposition to gestational diabetes. *Am J Obstet Gynecol, 151*, 471-475.

[275] Kibirige, M., Metcalf, B., Renuka, R. & Wilkin, T. J. (2003). Testing the accelerator hypothesis: the relationship between body mass and age at diagnosis of type 1 diabetes. *Diabetes Care, 26*, 2865-2870.

[276] Dechairo, B. M., et al. (2005). Association of the TSHR gene with Graves' disease: the first disease specific locus. *Eur J Hum Genet, 13*, 1223-1230.

[277] Targovnik, H. M., et al. (1995). A 138-nucleotide deletion in the thyroglobulin ribonucleic acid messenger in a congenital goiter with defective thyroglobulin synthesis. *J Clin Endocrinol Metab, 80*, 3356-3360.

[278] de Roux, N., et al. (1996). A neomutation of the thyroid-stimulating hormone receptor in a severe neonatal hyperthyroidism. *J Clin Endocrinol Metab, 81*, 2023-2026.

INDEX

A

abnormalities, 413, 433
acceleration, 150
acetaminophen, 149
acetate, 3, 36, 117, 118
acetic acid, 385
acetylcholinesterase, 17
acid, 3, 6, 7, 18, 36, 38, 57, 60, 62, 78, 82, 93, 98, 104, 116, 118, 133, 155, 185, 193, 203, 234, 237, 258, 259, 260, 264, 315, 355, 357, 361, 363, 366, 378, 384, 385, 387, 388, 390, 391, 395, 397, 402, 416, 434, 435
acidic, 37, 38, 42, 53, 62, 65, 67, 76
acidosis, 136
ACL, 293, 294
acne, 279, 280, 286
acne vulgaris, 286
acquired immunodeficiency syndrome, 90
ACR, 211, 216, 219, 222
actin, xiii, 360, 361, 362, 403
action potential, xi, 329, 332, 334, 336
activators, 307, 314, 387
active centers, 18, 36, 76, 77
active site, 17, 18, 36, 78, 97, 393
acute, viii, ix, 134, 147, 161, 207, 209, 210, 211, 215, 218, 219, 220, 221, 222, 234, 253, 255, 259, 263, 265, 266, 267, 269, 270, 272, 273, 274, 276, 278, 300, 311, 345, 350, 367, 370, 371, 376, 383, 385, 387, 389, 392, 395
acute confusional state, 210, 211, 222
acute kidney injury, 255
acute rejection, 161
acute renal failure, 147, 253, 255, 263
acute tubular necrosis, 259
ADA, 408, 418, 434
adalimumab, 287
Adams, 154, 164, 192, 194, 199, 326, 376, 401
adaptive immune system, 177, 184, 419

adenosine, 77, 426
adenosine deaminase, 426
adenovirus, 242
adhesion, 109, 153, 206, 260, 309, 355, 357, 388, 393, 395
adhesion properties, 206
adjunctive therapy, 141
administration, 20, 32, 87, 130, 131, 135, 139, 145, 151, 188, 200, 220, 221, 229, 235, 238, 239, 245, 246, 249, 279, 285
adolescents, 145, 147, 149
ADP, 40
adult, viii, x, xii, 107, 131, 148, 150, 187, 200, 204, 205, 235, 241, 243, 246, 258, 294, 301, 303, 304, 305, 306, 307, 310, 311, 312, 313, 314, 315, 322, 349, 350, 351, 400, 434
adult population, 258
adult stem cells, 235, 300
adulthood, 168, 306
adults, ix, 111, 147, 148, 163, 251, 266, 269, 272, 330, 434
adverse event, 132, 134, 137, 139
African-American, 145, 150
age, x, xi, xii, 4, 13, 21, 22, 23, 25, 26, 28, 29, 93, 113, 134, 139, 146, 175, 176, 180, 218, 234, 252, 271, 272, 289, 291, 292, 295, 330, 331, 341, 369, 370, 383, 397, 420, 431, 434
agent, 83, 111, 133, 135, 148, 149, 151, 221, 260, 279, 282, 391
agents, ix, xii, 16, 86, 87, 92, 129, 131, 136, 137, 142, 144, 150, 168, 221, 260, 265, 280, 307, 324, 337, 369, 385, 394, 401
aggregation, 87, 420, 434
AIDS, 10, 15, 17, 19, 35, 38, 55, 56, 72, 81, 82, 86, 88, 112, 278, 280, 283, 284, 285, 287, 288
alanine, 15, 377, 381, 392, 396, 416
alanine aminotransferase, 15
albumin, 55, 254, 258
aldosterone, 141
algorithm, 342, 344, 345, 346

alkaline, 6, 49, 61, 62, 65, 67, 71, 102, 103
alkaline phosphatase, 6, 102
allele, 142, 169, 189, 407, 408, 409, 410, 412, 415, 416, 421
alleles, 170, 185, 195, 207, 234, 404, 408, 409, 415, 416, 418, 421, 428, 431
allergic reaction, 138
allergy, 249, 285, 429
allogeneic, 203, 234, 289, 290, 293, 295, 297, 298, 299, 300, 301
allograft, viii, 107, 143, 144, 145, 146, 163, 239, 242, 243, 247
allograft survival, 143, 145, 146, 239, 242
allografts, 206, 291, 299
alopecia, ix, 21, 251, 279, 280, 281, 282, 286
alopecia areata, 279, 281, 282, 286
alpha, 109, 194, 197, 204, 226, 246, 278, 285, 286, 287, 288, 307, 313, 314, 315, 364, 377, 378, 386, 387, 399, 421, 422, 428, 429
alpha blocker, 287
alpha interferon, 278
alpha-galactosylceramide, 429
altered peptide ligand, 237, 245, 365
alternative, viii, 86, 132, 133, 167, 205, 216, 235, 299, 304, 357, 404, 408, 409, 416, 430
alters, 175, 309, 377, 433
Alzheimer disease, 87, 92
amaurosis, 222
amaurosis fugax, 222
amino, xii, 36, 38, 57, 77, 78, 185, 203, 237, 315, 357, 366, 369, 370, 381, 396, 416
amino acid, xii, 36, 38, 57, 77, 78, 185, 203, 237, 357, 366, 369, 370, 381, 396, 416
amino acids, xii, 77, 357, 369, 370, 381, 396
amplitude, 332, 335, 336
Amsterdam, 105, 402
amygdala, 304, 312
amylase, 19, 21, 22, 23, 24, 30, 33, 36, 43, 62, 63, 77, 83, 100
amyloid, 4, 87, 92
anaemia, 134, 159, 411
analog, 2, 98, 237, 400
anatomy, 321, 325, 392
anemia, 129, 136, 158, 259
Anemia, 136, 263
angiogenesis, 242
angiography, 143, 218, 228
angiotensin converting enzyme, 136
angiotensin II, 141
angiotensin-converting enzyme, 129
animal models, 11, 215, 263, 359
animal studies, 134, 221

animals, 3, 4, 16, 18, 19, 20, 21, 22, 24, 25, 26, 28, 29, 31, 32, 41, 42, 43, 45, 69, 81, 173, 294, 371
Animals, 391
ankylosis, 321
antagonist, 225, 337
anti-apoptotic, 242, 413
anti-atherogenic, 145
anti-bacterial, 258
antibiotics, 324
Antibodies, 1, 12, 16, 89, 90, 92, 95, 96, 97, 100, 101, 108, 109, 153, 155, 236, 278
anticardiolipin, 93, 143, 225, 226, 262
anticoagulant, 253
anticoagulation, 141, 143, 222
anticonvulsants, 152, 220
antidepressants, 220, 324
antigen presenting cells, 237, 412
antigenicity, 361, 413, 415
antigen-presenting cell, 10, 193, 202, 203, 236, 244, 383
Antigens, 191, 201, 237, 238, 422
anti-HIV, 87
antihypertensive drugs, 148
antiidiotypic, vii, 1, 4, 16, 17, 18, 76, 97
anti-inflammatory agents, 324
antimalarial drugs, 135
antimalarials, 135
antinuclear antibodies, 10, 18, 94, 109, 110, 151
Antiphospholipid, 5, 157, 162, 215, 219, 225, 226, 262
antiphospholipid antibodies, 143, 157, 211, 214, 216, 218, 222, 223, 231, 262
antiphospholipid syndrome, 5, 129, 130, 150, 156, 225, 230, 231, 253
APC, 173, 174, 175, 181, 184, 194, 203, 244, 247
APCs, 175, 177, 179, 396
aPL, 140, 143, 146, 147, 222
aplastic anemia, 294
apoptosis, 10, 18, 19, 20, 21, 28, 30, 31, 32, 33, 76, 77, 80, 99, 109, 110, 119, 153, 154, 172, 173, 174, 176, 178, 183, 187, 192, 201, 202, 310, 315, 407, 412, 417, 424, 431
apoptotic, xiii, 10, 76, 110, 154, 173, 184, 185, 203, 205, 239, 403, 407, 412, 417
apoptotic cells, 76, 110, 154, 184, 203
apoptotic pathway, 412
aqueous humor, 280
aqueous solution, 351, 352, 353, 363, 375, 376, 377, 393
ARB, 129
arc plasma, 68
arginine, 91, 381, 392, 412
arrhythmias, 152, 269

arterial hypertension, 131
arthritis, xi, 35, 44, 179, 198, 278, 280, 281, 317, 318, 320, 322, 323, 325, 327, 404, 405, 406, 416, 417, 419, 420, 421, 422, 426, 429, 430, 431, 434
articular cartilage, 319
aseptic, 220, 223
aseptic meningitis, 220
Asia, ix, 265, 267
Asian, 133
aspartate, 15, 215, 220, 225
aspiration, 294, 295, 301
assessment, 128, 214, 262, 298, 319, 321
associations, 404, 405, 406, 409, 415, 417, 418, 419, 421, 422
asthma, vii, 1, 2, 3, 15, 17, 35, 36, 37, 56, 57, 69, 79, 105
astrocyte, 304, 312
astrocytes, 304, 306, 309, 315, 387
astroglial, 309, 395
asymptomatic, 112, 147, 150, 218, 234, 254
atherosclerosis, x, 58, 131, 150, 252, 260, 277, 285, 295
atherosclerotic plaque, 163, 301
ATP, xi, 3, 21, 22, 23, 36, 39, 40, 45, 53, 54, 58, 60, 61, 62, 64, 76, 329
ATPase, 19, 21, 22, 23, 24, 25, 28, 30, 31, 33, 36, 53, 77, 82, 83, 335, 337
atrophy, xii, 120, 121, 127, 214, 218, 221, 224, 226, 230, 267, 326, 333, 341, 342, 343, 346
autoantibodies, vii, 1, 20, 89, 92, 93, 94, 96, 97, 102, 103, 104, 105, 108, 109, 110, 151, 153, 154, 174, 179, 180, 184, 188, 214, 216, 221, 225, 234, 240, 252, 253, 259, 263, 412, 415, 418, 434
autoantibody, 89, 93, 96, 101, 102, 103, 110, 154, 180, 197, 238, 240, 361, 423
autoantigens, xii, 11, 15, 77, 110, 179, 236, 237, 238, 245, 246, 349, 354, 355, 359, 364, 416, 418
autocrine, 307, 430
autoimmune disorders, 15, 248, 407, 408
autoimmune hemolytic anemia, 424
autoimmune hepatitis, 10
autoimmune polymorphisms, xiii, 403
autoimmune responses, 174, 178, 188
autologous bone, 297
autologous bone marrow transplant, 297
autonomic nervous system, ix, 265, 269
autophagy, 424, 431
autopsy, 214, 266, 294, 321
autoreactive T cells, xiii, 110, 173, 174, 175, 177, 179, 180, 184, 403, 406, 409, 410, 411, 412, 414, 415, 416, 419, 426, 427
autosomal recessive, 174

availability, 86, 108, 169, 171, 178, 218, 321, 380, 389
avascular necrosis, 320, 327
avian flu, 280
axon, xi, 14, 37, 309, 329, 331, 337, 350
axonal, ix, xi, xii, 220, 224, 265, 266, 267, 268, 270, 271, 272, 273, 274, 275, 276, 329, 332, 337, 344, 345, 347, 349, 350, 360, 401
axonal degeneration, ix, 220, 265, 266, 270, 271, 273
axons, xii, 80, 266, 271, 331, 337, 349, 350
Azathioprine, 134, 158, 221, 260

B

B cell, viii, 5, 11, 34, 93, 94, 95, 100, 110, 112, 137, 138, 149, 159, 160, 168, 173, 176, 177, 178, 179, 180, 181, 197, 198, 199, 208, 244, 253, 304, 305, 306, 307, 371, 387, 410, 411, 412, 419, 429, 430
B cell activating factor, 178
B cells, 5, 11, 34, 94, 95, 110, 112, 137, 138, 149, 160, 173, 176, 177, 178, 179, 180, 181, 197, 198, 244, 253, 304, 305, 306, 307, 387, 410, 412, 429, 430
B lymphocytes, 15, 34, 177, 186, 197, 199, 244, 360, 430
bacteria, 14, 20, 30, 35, 60, 279, 280, 323, 379, 381, 382, 383, 385, 389, 390, 401
bacterial, 4, 14, 16, 17, 19, 32, 35, 45, 67, 69, 76, 77, 81, 82, 83, 87, 91, 96, 104, 132, 135, 138, 198, 200, 216, 237, 258, 327, 375, 376, 383, 385, 394, 417, 434
bacterial cells, 81
bacterial infection, 4, 14, 17, 32, 35, 45, 69, 76, 81, 83, 91, 96, 132, 200, 383, 417
bacterium, 266, 381
BAFF, 178, 198
barrier, 111, 215, 225, 304, 383, 385, 387, 399, 400, 402
basement membrane, 110, 111, 116, 117, 118, 125, 126, 253
B-cell, 11, 14, 34, 35, 84, 86, 95, 100, 104, 137, 138, 139, 159, 199, 222, 236, 388
B-cell lymphoma, 222
B-cells, 11, 14, 84, 222, 236
Bcl-2, 173, 192, 413, 424, 431
bell-shaped, 65, 67, 69
beneficial effect, 134, 135, 139, 221
benefits, 169, 281
Best Practice, 143
beta, 417, 423, 427, 428, 429, 430, 434
beta cell, ix, 201, 233, 234, 235, 236, 237, 239, 240, 242, 244, 434
Beta cell, 236, 241
BFU-E, 24, 26, 31, 32, 33, 34, 88

BH3, 192, 424
bias, 210, 309, 404, 429, 433
biceps, 267, 330
biceps brachii, 3305
Bim, 173, 192, 407, 408, 412, 424, 425, 431
binding, 2, 3, 6, 7, 11, 16, 36, 40, 77, 82, 86, 89, 100, 104, 108, 109, 112, 119, 136, 153, 154, 155, 173, 176, 184, 187, 195, 237, 258, 259, 264, 309, 352, 354, 355, 357, 364, 366, 367, 399, 414, 416, 422, 431, 432, 434
biocatalysts, 79
biochemical, 414, 425
biochemistry, 94, 102, 154
biodegradable, 249
biologic agents, viii, 107
biological activity, 280
biological markers, 108
biological processes, 168
biological systems, 168
biomarker, 79, 84, 105, 255, 259, 263
biomarkers, 216, 255, 259, 260, 261, 263, 264
biomaterials, 249
biopsies, ix, 128, 251, 258, 259
biopsy, viii, 107, 113, 114, 123, 127, 128, 129, 130, 131, 144, 147, 148, 156, 252, 254, 258, 259, 260
biosynthesis, 99
biotechnological, 4, 104
biotechnology, 88, 242, 243, 281
birds, 304, 312
birefringence, 342, 347
birth, 81, 284, 383
Bisphosphonate, 327
bladder, ix, 12, 13, 14, 251, 269, 275
blocks, 337, 415, 428
blood flow, 218, 219, 228
blood glucose, 234
blood plasma, 68
blood pressure, 130, 132, 141, 148, 253, 269
blood transfusion, 145
blood transfusions, 145
blood vessels, 125, 305, 370
blood-brain barrier, 215, 225, 304, 383, 387, 399, 400, 402
bloodstream, 19
B-lymphocytes, 30
body image, 149
body mass, 434
body temperature, 331
bonds, 57, 62, 77, 91
bone marrow, vii, x, 1, 4, 24, 26, 27, 28, 30, 31, 32, 33, 34, 42, 77, 79, 80, 112, 178, 186, 188, 204, 206, 207, 249, 289, 290, 292, 293, 294, 295, 296, 297, 298, 299, 300, 301, 302, 322, 323

bone marrow aspiration, 294
bone marrow transplant, 112, 188, 206, 289, 297, 298, 299, 300, 301
bovine, 18, 46, 55, 88, 356, 363, 365, 367, 399
bowel, 269, 275, 420, 424
brain, xi, 11, 12, 13, 14, 80, 83, 87, 174, 196, 210, 214, 218, 219, 220, 221, 225, 226, 227, 228, 230, 285, 303, 304, 307, 308, 309, 312, 313, 314, 361, 363, 370, 389, 392, 393, 394, 395, 397, 398, 400, 430
brain abnormalities, 214
brain damage, 218, 219, 230
brain injury, 218, 307, 308, 309, 312, 395
brain stem, 12, 13, 14
Brazil, 209, 273, 317
Brazilian, 392, 405
breakdown, 170, 180, 284, 383, 400
breast cancer, 293, 300
brevis, 332, 334, 335
British, 404, 405
bronchial asthma, 2, 15, 79
bronchial tree, 34
Brussels, 403
buccal mucosa, 320
buffer, 3, 40, 41, 46, 47, 53
bulbar, 268, 275
bypass, 333, 415

C

Ca^{2+}, 52, 66, 69, 70, 72, 73, 75, 360, 361
calcium, 131, 144, 217, 332
calmodulin, 352, 360, 361, 364, 365
Campylobacter jejuni, ix, 265, 266, 270, 272, 273, 274, 275
cancer, 138, 181, 262, 293, 294, 295, 300, 301, 302
cancer cells, 293, 301
cancerous cells, 186, 187, 416
candidates, 143, 147, 407
candidiasis, 414, 432, 433
capacity, 409, 410, 416, 417
capillary, 111, 116, 117, 118, 124, 125, 252, 367
carbohydrate, 11, 62, 63, 358, 359, 367, 379
carboxylic, 39
carcinogenic, 81, 87
carcinoma, 293, 300, 310, 315
CARD15, 406
cardiac arrhythmia, 152
cardiomyopathy, 176
cardiopulmonary, 114, 333
cardiopulmonary bypass, 333
cardiovascular disease, 108, 145, 252
Cardiovascular disease, 143
cardiovascular risk, 141, 145

carpal tunnel syndrome, 335, 336, 337, 339
carrier, 139, 155, 388
cartilage, 319, 321, 322, 416, 434
casein, 17, 37, 54, 55, 56, 57, 60, 61, 67, 72, 77, 78, 105
caspase, 387, 394
castration, 375, 376, 380, 393, 395
catabolism, 104, 185, 203, 429
catalysis, 3, 4, 35, 36, 44, 78, 89, 91, 101
catalytic activity, vii, 1, 3, 16, 18, 19, 21, 35, 36, 37, 54, 75, 76, 82, 83, 86, 89, 92, 97, 103, 105, 358
catalytic properties, 2, 37, 39, 47, 78, 79, 103, 104
Caucasian, 133, 142, 161
CD28, 410, 412, 428, 430, 431
CD4, 411, 415, 416, 424, 425, 426, 427, 428, 429, 431, 432
CD40, 406
CD45, 406
CD8+, 5, 113, 201, 236, 239, 244, 247, 293, 425, 428
cDNA, 245
CDR, 429
Celiac disease, 405
cell adhesion, 206, 355, 357, 398
cell body, 305
cell cycle, 176, 315, 428
cell death, 109, 110, 112, 173, 176, 201, 207, 315, 388, 395, 398
cell differentiation, 196, 197, 204, 207, 307, 315, 407, 427, 429, 430
cell division, 235, 309
cell fate, x, 303, 304
cell fusion, 299
cell growth, 109
cell invasion, 385
cell line, 155, 169, 196, 243, 279, 293, 391, 393, 409, 411, 431
cell lines, 169, 279, 391, 393
cell organization, 305
cell surface, 11, 41, 82, 95, 102, 108, 154, 411
cell transplantation, 241, 300, 301
cellulose, 36, 37, 40, 41, 46, 47, 52, 53, 70, 71, 79
central nervous system, viii, x, 5, 10, 108, 209, 210, 218, 222, 223, 225, 226, 227, 228, 229, 230, 231, 281, 303, 304, 309, 312, 313, 337, 363, 364, 367, 369, 370, 383, 400
centromere, 93
cerebellum, 14
cerebral blood flow, 218, 219, 228
cerebral cortex, 315, 390
cerebral ischemia, 215, 314
cerebral palsy, 333
cerebral venous thrombosis, 215, 222

cerebrospinal fluid, 11, 84, 103, 215, 216, 225, 226, 280, 392, 396, 397, 398, 399, 400
cerebrovascular, 211, 215, 333
cerebrovascular accident, 215
cerebrovascular disease, 211, 333
cerebrovascular diseases, 333
ceruloplasmin, 258
CFA, 188, 391
CFU-GM, 24, 26, 32, 33, 34, 88
Chagas disease, 96
chemical agents, 240, 280
chemical engineering, 89
chemical reactions, 2, 16, 44
chemoattractant, 258, 263, 314
chemokine, 196, 260, 263, 264, 309, 310, 312, 314, 315, 397, 411
chemokine receptor, 312, 314, 397, 411
chemokines, x, 14, 187, 205, 247, 263, 264, 303, 304, 307, 309, 310, 311, 408
chemotherapy, 300, 301
childhood, xii, 112, 147, 149, 163, 164, 165, 240, 263, 341
children, 112, 131, 143, 147, 148, 149, 150, 155, 163, 164, 165, 222, 229, 246, 258, 263, 266, 269, 272, 418, 420, 421
China, ix, 265, 266, 268, 269, 270, 271, 272, 273
Chinese, 422, 423
chloroform, 61
cholinesterase, 97
chromatin, 112, 119, 180, 305, 414
chromatography, 3, 37, 40, 41, 46, 47, 52, 53, 54, 71, 72, 79, 87, 384
chromosome, 170, 180, 183, 189, 208, 421, 424
chromosomes, 183
chronic, 414, 420, 431
chronic disease, 126, 136, 152, 284, 285
chronic diseases, 152, 285
chronic illness, 330
chronic kidney disease (CKD), 259
chronic pain, 319, 324, 326
chymotrypsin, 56, 57
CIA, 411
cilia, 305, 313
circulation, 34, 82, 110, 111, 112, 137, 176, 235
cis, xiii, 403, 411, 412, 419
CKD, 259
class switching, 412
classes, 65, 76, 112, 116, 128, 252, 254, 255, 259, 260
classical, 2, 49, 59, 169, 170, 189, 190, 203, 266, 385
classification, ix, 114, 128, 148, 156, 163, 206, 210, 222, 251, 252, 254, 255, 259, 262, 274, 319, 320, 343, 404

claustrophobia, 322
cleavage, 10, 18, 21, 44, 50, 57, 58, 59, 60, 69, 70, 71, 72, 78, 83, 90, 106, 109, 153, 358
clinical, 404, 418, 420, 426, 433
clinical approach, 229
clinical assessment, 342
clinical diagnosis, 214, 321
clinical examination, 319
clinical oncology, 86, 92
clinical presentation, 95, 114, 147, 229, 252
clinical symptoms, 169, 219, 321
clinical syndrome, 284
clinical trial, 87, 135, 138, 156, 228, 235, 236, 237, 238, 239, 240, 255, 260, 278, 282, 283, 330, 337
clinical trials, 87, 135, 138, 156, 235, 236, 237, 238, 240, 255, 278, 330, 337
clinics, x, 249, 277, 345
clones, 406, 415, 416, 417
cloning, 11, 84, 90, 205, 360, 431
cluster analysis, 6, 7, 8, 9, 14
CNS, viii, xii, 95, 114, 196, 207, 209, 210, 211, 212, 214, 215, 216, 217, 218, 219, 220, 221, 222, 228, 306, 349, 350, 351, 354, 360, 363, 365, 367, 369, 370, 371, 372, 380, 383, 384, 385, 386, 387, 389, 392, 393, 394, 395, 396, 397, 399, 400, 401
Co, 68, 72, 73, 89, 90, 102, 263, 296, 411, 420
cofactors, 2, 70, 75, 78, 410, 414
cognition, 220
cognitive dysfunction, 215, 218, 221, 222, 224
cognitive function, 214, 224, 226, 327
cognitive impairment, 214, 218, 230
cohort, 13, 134, 135, 152, 157, 158, 216, 223, 225, 252, 258, 259
colitis, 417, 424, 428, 429, 434
Collaboration, 190, 315
collagen, 253, 263, 430, 434
collateral, 271
colon, 293, 294, 300, 301
colon cancer, 293, 294, 301
colonization, 313
colony-stimulating factor, 315
common findings, xii, 341
communication, 37, 45, 57, 69, 72, 77, 79, 283, 309, 327, 386
complement, 5, 14, 86, 108, 111, 114, 121, 124, 125, 136, 138, 139, 142, 149, 150, 156, 159, 184, 203, 216, 221, 240, 252, 254, 255, 259, 367
complement components, 114, 203, 221, 254, 255
complement system, 14
complete remission, 129, 130, 133, 138, 255
complexity, xiii, 403, 419
compliance, 129, 130, 145, 147, 148, 149
complications, ix, 108, 134, 136, 138, 140, 143, 145, 150, 152, 233, 235, 240, 246, 253, 261, 262, 281, 282, 318
components, xii, 10, 15, 16, 30, 35, 59, 74, 81, 114, 169, 203, 221, 254, 255, 321, 350, 351, 355, 385, 387, 403, 404, 414, 417, 432
composition, 34, 50, 117, 155, 288, 355, 384, 389
compounds, 10, 19, 62, 81, 87, 130, 383, 385, 388, 417
computed tomography, 219, 227, 228, 321, 326
concentration, 5, 6, 15, 21, 22, 29, 31, 40, 43, 45, 46, 47, 48, 49, 50, 55, 67, 69, 71, 73, 74, 75, 78, 80, 84, 85, 86, 122, 125, 150, 215, 237, 294, 383, 388, 389
conditioning, 140, 293, 300, 313
conduction, ix, xi, xii, 135, 265, 266, 270, 271, 273, 276, 329, 330, 331, 332, 334, 335, 337, 338, 339, 349
conduction block, xi, 271, 329, 330, 331, 332, 334, 337, 338, 339
confidence, 26, 28, 29, 234, 345
confidence interval, 26, 28, 29, 345
conformational states, 362
congestive heart failure, 281
connective tissue, 10, 18, 94, 318, 320
consensus, 149, 156, 157, 210, 261, 357
control group, 30, 113, 146, 344, 345
controlled, 412, 419, 425
controlled studies, 128, 220, 221
controlled trials, 131, 133, 138, 148, 221
conversion, 41, 184, 234, 259
cornea, 342
corneal transplant, 280, 283, 287
coronavirus, 95
corpus callosum, 218, 226, 305, 390
correlation, ix, 5, 6, 7, 8, 9, 11, 12, 13, 14, 15, 59, 78, 82, 83, 85, 88, 93, 115, 116, 136, 138, 148, 153, 251, 342, 366, 386, 387, 395
correlation coefficient, 6, 8, 11, 13, 14, 15, 88
correlations, 8, 11, 13, 14, 15, 21, 155, 163, 331, 386
cortex, 225, 260, 312, 314, 322, 331, 390
corticosteroid therapy, 128, 143, 147, 220, 323
corticosteroids, 108, 109, 129, 130, 131, 132, 134, 135, 137, 139, 140, 144, 147, 149, 150, 151, 211, 219, 220, 221, 222, 228, 229, 261, 323, 324, 327
costimulatory molecules, 247
COX-2, 431
cranial nerve, 266, 268, 274
craniofacial bone, 320
CRC, 106
creatinine, 6, 122, 125, 129, 132, 133, 138, 139, 140, 142, 148, 150, 253, 259
CREB, 432

crescentic glomerulonephritis, 147, 263
cross-linking, 139
cross-sectional study, 210, 386
crosstalk, 248, 408, 414
crystal structure, 36, 351, 354, 355, 356, 358, 359, 360, 361
crystal structures, 351, 360
crystalline, 124
CSF, 11, 80, 140, 187, 215, 216, 310, 311, 315, 383, 385, 387, 388, 389, 397, 399, 402
CT, 218, 219, 321, 324, 326
CT scan, 324
352, 354, 358, 364
C-terminus, 352, 358, 380
CXC, 309, 411
CXC chemokines, 309
cyclophosphamide, 129, 133, 134, 136, 137, 138, 139, 140, 157, 158, 159, 160, 161, 220, 221, 228, 229, 230, 260
cyclosporine, 141, 144, 145, 146, 158, 159, 161, 162, 164
Cyclosporine A, 134, 159
cysteine, 110, 309, 357
Cysteine, 390
cysteine proteases, 110
cysteine residues, 309
cystine, 388, 393
cytokine, x, 109, 172, 176, 177, 178, 185, 187, 188, 189, 192, 196, 197, 198, 236, 238, 239, 242, 245, 246, 263, 277, 278, 279, 280, 281, 282, 284, 285, 286, 309, 408, 410, 411, 430
cytokines, x, xi, 14, 108, 153, 174, 176, 177, 178, 179, 184, 187, 188, 196, 198, 207, 216, 226, 234, 236, 247, 248, 259, 277, 278, 279, 280, 283, 284, 285, 286, 303, 304, 307, 309, 310, 311, 313, 314, 319, 331, 387, 393, 394, 411
cytomegalovirus, 280
cytometry, 99
cytopenias, 137, 139
cytoplasm, 112, 116, 305, 307, 434
cytoplasmic membrane, 305
cytoplasmic tail, 357
cytotoxic, vii, viii, 1, 4, 80, 92, 94, 107, 128, 131, 144, 157, 176, 183, 187, 236, 241, 253, 307, 323
cytotoxic agents, 131, 144
cytotoxicity, 80, 188, 205, 206

D

dacryoadenitis, 407, 425
database, 146, 162, 345
death, 108, 109, 110, 112, 132, 134, 143, 154, 157, 173, 176, 187, 201, 207, 252, 285, 315, 323, 388, 395, 398, 424, 425, 431

deaths, 83, 132, 140
decompression, 324, 327
defects, viii, 21, 96, 99, 136, 168, 172, 173, 174, 175, 176, 180, 181, 184, 185, 200, 203, 292, 295, 297, 324, 406, 407, 408, 409, 411, 412, 413, 417, 419, 434
defense, 35, 87, 92, 208, 307
deficiency, 104, 136, 176, 193, 194, 200, 202, 203, 298, 412, 414, 426, 429, 433
deficit, 20, 79, 88, 330
deficits, 219, 268
definition, xii, 255, 263, 330, 369, 375, 402
degradation, 44, 69, 79, 84, 87, 103, 105, 319, 385
degrading, 17, 19, 62, 76, 87, 396
degree, 404, 405, 408, 409, 419, 420, 421
dehydrogenase, 133
delivery, 19, 20, 23, 24, 25, 26, 27, 28, 29, 30, 32, 33, 34, 86, 235, 239, 402
dementia, 222, 227
demographic factors, 108
demyelinating disease, 10, 95, 281, 337, 389
demyelination, xii, 11, 331, 334, 335, 337, 341, 366, 369, 394, 395, 399, 400
demyelinization, 14
dentate gyrus, 306, 314
depolarization, xi, 329
deposition, 110, 111, 252, 253, 411
deposits, 110, 111, 114, 116, 117, 118, 120, 121, 122, 123, 124, 125, 126, 128, 154, 155, 253, 254, 256, 257, 258
depression, xi, 131, 149, 215, 285, 306, 326, 329, 330, 337
depressive disorder, 324
deprivation, 175
derivatives, 36, 392, 394
dermatology, 248
dermatomyositis, 333
destruction, 10, 14, 195, 235, 236, 239, 240, 252, 319, 322, 323, 418, 434
detection, 3, 17, 22, 82, 83, 94, 100, 108, 136, 150, 165, 218, 234, 344, 347
detoxification, 81, 87
developed countries, 190
developmental factors, 404
deviation, 176
dexamethasone, 230
Diabetes, 404, 405, 406, 420, 422, 427, 428, 429, 434
diabetes mellitus, 131, 143, 240, 244, 248, 297, 420, 429, 434
diabetic, 406, 424, 425, 428, 429
diabetic nephropathy, 259
diabetic neuropathy, 332, 338

diabetic patients, 189, 208, 234, 236, 237, 238
diagnostic criteria, 269, 274, 326
dialysis, 69, 72, 73, 77, 108, 140, 142, 143, 144, 147, 150, 161, 162, 285, 288
dietary iodine, 415
differential diagnosis, 218, 268
dilated cardiomyopathy, 195
dinucleotides, 69, 77
diode laser, 343
dipeptides, 392, 397
disabilities, xi, 317, 385
disability, 211, 214, 224, 267, 269, 270, 330, 350
disabled, x, 265, 267, 271
discriminant analysis, 347
discrimination, 173
disease activity, 109, 128, 129, 130, 137, 140, 144, 147, 149, 151, 152, 153, 161, 163, 211, 216, 218, 261, 263, 264, 387, 393, 394, 395, 396, 399
disease gene, 424
disease model, 185
disease progression, 14, 175, 177, 179, 181, 188, 189, 414
disease-free survival, 140
Disease-specific, 15
disequilibrium, 95, 169, 170
disorder, ix, xi, 20, 21, 80, 87, 99, 212, 224, 230, 251, 252, 284, 297, 317, 355, 411
distribution, 24, 54, 116, 120, 199, 318, 322, 356, 390, 432
disulfide, 357, 365
diversity, 4, 35, 36, 37, 38, 43, 53, 54, 55, 59, 65, 68, 69, 70, 72, 78, 79, 101, 105, 196, 202, 427
division, xii, 8, 12, 13, 235, 309, 403
DNA ligase, 426
DNase, 2, 17, 18, 19, 20, 21, 22, 23, 24, 25, 28, 30, 31, 32, 33, 35, 36, 37, 39, 40, 41, 42, 43, 44, 45, 46, 47, 51, 52, 53, 54, 58, 59, 60, 65, 66, 69, 70, 71, 76, 77, 78, 79, 80, 82, 83, 84, 85, 97, 98, 104, 153, 423
donor, x, 60, 61, 62, 63, 142, 144, 146, 161, 234, 289, 290, 291, 292, 293, 298, 299, 300, 301
donors, 3, 4, 5, 8, 10, 11, 13, 19, 33, 44, 48, 55, 58, 68, 82, 83, 90, 142, 146, 161, 163, 234, 290, 291
dopamine, 313, 337
dosage, 141, 149, 193, 237, 432
double-blind trial, 287
down-regulation, 160, 427
Drosophila, 169, 190
drug addict, 86
drug addiction, 86
drug delivery, 235
drug interaction, 151
drug targets, 190
drug-induced, 151, 152, 165
drug-induced lupus, 151, 152, 165
drugs, 4, 105, 132, 135, 137, 145, 148, 151, 157, 217, 235, 323, 385
duodenum, 235
duplication, 199
duration, ix, 4, 55, 67, 93, 129, 130, 138, 141, 149, 151, 218, 251, 260, 334, 335
DWI, 218
dysregulation, 20, 181, 193, 244, 408, 409, 410, 419

E

EAE, xii, 179, 185, 196, 354, 363, 369, 370, 371, 372, 373, 374, 375, 376, 377, 378, 379, 382, 384, 385, 389, 390, 391, 392, 394, 395, 396, 397, 398, 399, 400, 401, 402, 410, 411, 414
ECM, 387
economic status, 108
edema, 281, 283
EDSS, 12, 13, 282
Egypt, 107, 164
electrocardiogram, 143
electromyography, 330
electron, 81, 114, 117, 124, 125, 126, 258, 305, 307, 351, 353
electron microscopy, 114, 125, 126, 258, 305, 307, 351, 353
electrophoresis, 38, 65, 88, 367
ELISA, 83, 114
embryology, 168
embryonic stem, 235, 242, 243, 310, 315
embryonic stem cells, 235, 242, 243, 310, 315
emission, 68, 219, 227, 228
emotional, 319, 324
emphysema, 292, 295, 299
employment, 3, 214, 224
employment status, 214, 224
encephalitis, 15, 88, 96, 333
encephalomyelitis, xii, 87, 95, 179, 203, 207, 333, 354, 364, 365, 369, 370, 393, 394, 395, 396, 397, 398, 401, 402, 410, 424, 429, 430
encephalopathy, 333
encoding, 109, 196, 206, 313, 412, 416, 421, 422, 423
endocarditis, 216
endocrine, x, 168, 234, 242, 243, 277, 331
endocytosis, 238
endoderm, 242, 243
endogenous, 427
endogenous progenitors, 241
endothelial cell, 109, 116, 125, 153, 226, 252, 264
endothelial cells, 109, 116, 125, 153, 264
endothelium, 252, 387, 393

end-stage kidney disease, 255
end-stage renal disease, 132, 152, 153, 161
engagement, 196, 198, 428, 430
England, 159, 242, 266, 278
engraftment, 242, 290, 301
environment, xi, 188, 190, 235, 341, 351, 362, 408
environmental, xii, 403, 404, 415, 419, 429
environmental factors, 171, 190, 350, 415
environmental influences, 419
enzymatic, 3, 17, 19, 20, 29, 39, 40, 42, 49, 67, 71, 79, 87, 358
enzymatic activity, 3, 17, 39, 358
enzyme inhibitors, 129, 141
enzyme-linked immunosorbent assay, 10
enzymes, vii, 1, 2, 3, 14, 17, 18, 19, 37, 39, 41, 42, 44, 52, 56, 58, 60, 61, 62, 63, 64, 65, 86, 87, 88, 89, 104, 106, 185, 205, 384, 401
eosinophils, 119, 126
epidemiologic studies, 418
epidemiological, 433
epidemiology, xii, 273, 369, 403
epidermolysis bullosa, 284, 288
epithelial cell, 121, 173, 192, 279, 286, 292, 408, 414, 417, 426, 432
epithelial cells, 121, 173, 192, 292, 414, 417, 426, 432
epithelium, 20, 82, 252, 300, 344, 408, 414, 432
epitope, 11, 191, 225, 245, 352, 354, 356, 358, 359, 361, 362, 365, 366, 367, 392, 396, 398, 399, 402, 416, 434
epitopes, 77, 86, 87, 112, 266, 355, 357, 358, 359, 371, 392, 396, 400, 415, 416, 433
Epstein-Barr virus, 270
ER, 223
erosion, 322
erysipelas, 35
erythematous, 262
erythrocyte, 112, 159
erythrocytes, 185
erythroid, 88
erythropoietin, 159, 316
Escherichia coli, 104
ester, 341, 346
esterase, 21, 36, 101
esterases, 89
esters, 2, 62, 91
ethnic groups, ix, 171, 225, 251
ethnicity, 108, 150, 252
etiologic factor, 319
etiology, 10, 210, 211, 214, 219, 259, 318, 319, 324, 326, 332, 359, 399
euglycemia, 234, 236, 238
eukaryotic cell, 133

Euro, 132, 157, 158
evidence, 404, 413
evoked potential, 346
evolution, viii, 2, 81, 107, 152, 157, 253, 394
examinations, 210, 216, 325, 330
excitability, 267, 338
excitotoxicity, 310
exclusion, 215, 216, 430
excretion, 129, 138, 141
executive function, 214
executive functions, 214
exercise, 143, 330, 331, 332, 335
exocrine, 100, 234, 241
exonuclease, 58, 423
experimental allergic encephalomyelitis, 424
experimental autoimmune encephalomyelitis, 95, 179, 207, 354, 365, 410, 429, 430
exposure, 10, 77, 112, 135, 154, 309, 311, 389
extracellular matrix, 385
extrinsic, 417
eye, 235, 283, 287, 342, 343, 344, 424
eyes, 174, 283, 322, 342, 344, 345, 346, 347

F

facial pain, 318, 326
facial palsy, 268
factor VII, 2, 4, 87, 90, 92
factor VIII, 2, 4, 87, 90, 92
failure, ix, xi, 5, 140, 143, 144, 145, 255, 263, 265, 266, 268, 270, 271, 273, 290, 329, 330, 331, 335, 405, 406, 412, 413, 414, 418, 419
false positive, 171
familial, 404, 407, 421
family, xii, 93, 111, 151, 173, 178, 180, 184, 187, 188, 192, 194, 196, 201, 205, 206, 309, 341, 351, 356, 357, 361, 363, 365, 385, 387, 405, 423, 424, 430
family members, xii, 341, 357, 405
Fas, 20, 99, 110, 154, 203, 205, 242, 412, 423, 431
FAS, 413, 418
FasL, 242
fatigue, xi, 211, 214, 329, 330, 331, 332, 333, 337, 338
females, 19, 20, 22, 23, 24, 25, 26, 27, 28, 29, 30, 31, 32, 33, 34, 319, 350
fetal, 151, 158, 204, 315
fetal growth, 151
fiber, 330, 342, 346, 347, 348
fibers, 331, 335, 338, 346
fibrils, xii, 341
fibroblasts, 243, 393
fibrogenesis, 263
fibrosarcoma, 293

fibrosis, 120, 121, 126, 127, 259, 260
fibrous tissue, 322
filtration, 3, 128, 252
Finland, 95, 349, 360, 363
first degree relative, 404, 405
flare, 114, 128, 129, 136, 139, 142, 160, 255, 258, 259, 260
flow, 42, 99, 102, 218, 230
fluid, 11, 84, 103, 215, 216, 225, 226, 263, 280, 318, 322, 323, 324, 385, 392, 396, 397, 398, 399, 400
focal adhesion kinase, 260
follicular, 411, 430
Food and Drug Administration, 337
Ford, 194, 224, 397, 399
forebrain, 313, 316
fracture, 321, 414
fragmentation, 6, 7, 9, 13, 80, 322
France, 162, 167, 420
free radicals, 319
frontal lobe, 390
functional aspects, 362
fundus, 343, 344, 346
fusion, 240, 299, 309
fusion proteins, 240
FVIII, 87

G

GABAergic, 314
gadolinium, 282, 385
Galileo, 312
Gamma, 155
ganglion, xii, 314, 341, 342, 344, 345, 398
gangliosides, ix, 62, 225, 265, 266, 350
gas chromatograph, 384
gastric, 67, 295
gastrointestinal, 112, 136, 149
G-CSF, 140, 310, 311, 315
gender, 150, 151, 287, 319
gender differences, 287, 319
gene expression, 153, 169, 170, 196, 225, 263, 284, 313, 424, 432
gene promoter, 235
gene therapy, 248
gene transfer, 242
generation, vii, 1, 2, 4, 16, 19, 20, 43, 86, 97, 151, 172, 175, 177, 183, 185, 201, 202, 242, 309, 314, 417, 419, 430
genes, xii, 109, 161, 168, 169, 170, 171, 172, 180, 183, 186, 187, 189, 190, 197, 199, 341, 407, 408, 409, 411, 412, 414, 415, 417, 419, 422, 423, 424, 425, 427, 430, 431, 432

genetic, xii, 403, 404, 405, 406, 407, 408, 409, 410, 411, 412, 413, 415, 416, 417, 418, 419, 421, 422, 423, 425, 430, 433, 434
genetic alteration, 407
genetic defect, 175, 404, 406, 407, 408, 409, 411, 412, 413, 417, 419
genetic factors, 10, 168, 172, 404, 408
genetic information, 190
genetic traits, 168, 170
genetics, xii, 168, 169, 171, 172, 186, 190, 191, 193, 203, 403, 405, 414, 419, 425, 431
genome, viii, 111, 112, 167, 168, 169, 170, 171, 177, 188, 190, 191, 367, 421, 423, 424
genomic, 169, 407, 410, 425, 432
genomic regions, 410, 432
genomics, 367, 425
genotype, 169, 170, 172, 191, 397, 434
genotypes, 171, 433
Germany, 349
gestational diabetes, 418, 434
gland, 80, 86, 100
glass, 108
glaucoma, 341, 342, 344, 345, 346, 347
glia, xii, 312, 313, 349
glial, xii, 220, 304, 309, 311, 341, 350
glial cells, 304, 350
glioblastoma, 313
gliosis, 388
globulin, 155, 230
glomerulonephritis, 20, 109, 111, 121, 122, 138, 144, 151, 153, 154, 156, 157, 160, 165, 203, 252, 254, 256, 257, 258, 261, 262, 297, 393, 411
glomerulopathy, 125, 156
glomerulus, 110, 119, 121, 127
GLP-1, 242
glucoamylase, 62, 63, 64
glucocorticoids, 132
glucose, ix, 131, 233, 234, 235, 240, 434
glucose tolerance, 434
glucoside, 64
glutamate, 225, 240, 310, 311, 381, 388, 393, 395, 401
glutamate decarboxylase, 240
glutamic acid, 234, 237, 388, 402, 434
glutamine, 381
glycemia, 242
glycine, 41, 79, 377, 381, 401
glycoconjugates, 106
glycogen, 57
glycol, 139
glycoprotein, 11, 95, 106, 180, 205, 258, 260, 357, 360, 361, 362, 364, 365, 366, 367, 372, 384, 392, 395, 396, 397, 398, 400

Glycoprotein, 354, 357
glycoproteins, 11, 260, 309, 363, 365, 366, 370, 395
glycosylated, 287, 359
glycosylation, 194, 260, 366, 428
GM-CSF, 187, 310, 311, 315
gold standard, viii, 128, 130, 209, 210, 216
gouty arthritis, 322
grafts, 144, 202, 242, 283, 300
graft-versus-host disease, 293, 300
gram-negative bacteria, 383
gram-positive bacteria, 379, 382
granulocyte, 200, 315
granzyme, 110, 187
growth, 109, 131, 151, 153, 203, 234, 249, 263, 264, 292, 294, 301, 307, 309, 310, 314, 315, 386, 388, 427, 430
growth factor, 153, 203, 234, 249, 263, 264, 307, 310, 315, 386, 388, 427, 430
growth factors, 234, 310
Guangzhou, 154
guidance, ix, 87, 251, 321
guidelines, 143, 149, 162, 216
Guillain-Barre syndrome, 230, 338, 339, 355, 362, 363, 367
Guillain-Barré syndrome, xi, xii, 213, 266, 272, 273, 274, 275, 276, 329, 330, 333, 349, 350
Guinea, 372, 373, 374, 377, 378, 379, 391
gut, 34, 381, 382, 383, 384, 385, 389, 392, 401, 410, 417

H

H. pylori, 4, 17, 87, 92
H1N1, 280
H_2, 433
HA, 262, 313
hair follicle, 287
hairy cell leukemia, 204
half-life, 86
handicapped, 330
hands, 267, 321, 325, 326
haplotype, 415, 422
haplotypes, 171, 187, 423
harm, ix, 151, 251
harmful, 417
Harvard, 107
head injury, 333
headache, viii, 209, 210, 221, 222, 318, 325
health, x, 21, 60, 214, 277, 281, 284, 362, 412
heart, 132, 151, 152, 165, 224, 283, 291
heart disease, 132
heart failure, 165, 281
heart rate, 151
heat, 237, 246, 324, 332
heat shock protein, 237, 332
Hedgehog signaling, 313
height, 343, 346
Helicobacter pylori, 17, 97
helper cells, 236, 430
hematologic, 149
hematological, 5, 108, 293
hematopoietic, vii, 1, 4, 16, 21, 24, 34, 42, 77, 79, 80, 88, 96, 160, 186, 201, 297, 298, 299, 300, 306, 315
hematopoietic cells, 298
hematopoietic precursors, 186
hematopoietic stem cell, vii, 1, 4, 16, 21, 24, 34, 42, 77, 79, 80, 88, 96, 160, 297, 298, 299, 300
Hematopoietic stem cell, 160
hematopoietic stem cells, vii, 1, 4, 16, 21, 24, 34, 42, 77, 79, 80, 88, 96, 297, 298, 299
hematoxylin-eosin, 116
hematuria, 115, 125, 128, 147, 148, 150, 160, 252, 255
hemodialysis, 161, 285
hemoglobin, 9, 136, 254
hemolytic anemia, 424
hemolytic uremic syndrome, 120
hemophilia, 2, 90, 92
hemorrhage, 214, 217, 218
hepatitis, 10, 15, 16, 17, 19, 35, 45, 58, 59, 69, 82, 83, 102
hepatitis a, 10, 17
Hepatitis B, 48, 216, 382
hepatocyte, 299
hepatocyte-like, 299
hepatocytes, 292
herpes, 14, 16, 282
heterogeneity, vii, 1, 47, 50, 76, 101, 169, 419, 432
heterogeneous, 8, 41, 50, 67, 76, 171, 184, 188, 210, 401
high affinity receptors, 309
high blood pressure, 165
high resolution, 321
high risk, 143, 234
hippocampal, 214, 218
hippocampus, 304, 306
Hispanic, 133, 252
histochemistry, 102
histological, ix, xii, 131, 144, 148, 150, 155, 251, 252, 254, 369, 385, 389
histology, ix, xii, 134, 163, 196, 223, 251, 259, 369, 388, 389
histone, 10, 110, 112, 151, 155, 432
histoplasmosis, 138

HIV, 2, 15, 17, 37, 38, 54, 55, 56, 57, 67, 69, 78, 81, 82, 86, 87, 90, 92, 103, 106, 138, 216, 280, 283, 284, 315
HIV infection, 15, 81
HIV-1, 17, 55, 56, 90, 106, 315
HLA, xi, 151, 161, 170, 171, 191, 205, 207, 234, 341, 361, 363, 364, 366, 396, 404, 406, 413, 415, 416, 421, 433, 434
HLA-B, 205, 207
Holland, 105, 402
homeostasis, ix, x, 194, 233, 277, 278, 284, 409
homogeneity, 3, 68
homogenous, 14, 215
homology, 111, 206, 351, 357, 366, 367, 395
homozygosity, 412
Hong Kong, 154, 158
hormonal control, 384, 392, 401
host, 83, 112, 173, 237, 290, 292, 293, 298, 300, 376, 397
hostile environment, 235
HRP, 45, 65, 73, 81
HSC, x, 24, 26, 30, 31, 32, 33, 34, 289, 294, 296
HSP60, 237
human adult stem cells, 300
human brain, 220, 300, 312, 366, 367
human condition, 168
human embryonic stem cells, 242, 243
human genome, 170, 171, 367
Human Genome Project, viii, 167
human leukocyte antigen, 433, 434
human milk, 2, 17, 36, 37, 39, 44, 45, 53, 54, 55, 56, 57, 58, 60, 61, 62, 63, 64, 65, 67, 69, 82, 97, 98, 99, 105, 106
human subjects, 397
humans, 3, 16, 17, 18, 19, 20, 22, 30, 35, 36, 42, 43, 45, 60, 69, 76, 80, 81, 82, 83, 86, 90, 106, 112, 168, 169, 170, 172, 174, 175, 176, 186, 187, 195, 236, 240, 246, 248, 290, 293, 294, 304, 381, 392, 398, 408, 410, 428, 431
humoral immunity, 197
hyaline, 116, 117, 120, 124, 127, 322
hybridoma, 21
hydrolases, 62, 77
hydrolysis, 3, 18, 20, 21, 22, 23, 25, 35, 36, 37, 38, 39, 40, 41, 42, 43, 45, 46, 47, 48, 49, 50, 51, 53, 55, 56, 57, 58, 59, 62, 64, 65, 66, 67, 69, 71, 72, 76, 77, 78, 79, 82, 89, 90, 91, 92, 96, 98, 100, 101, 102, 103
hydrolyzed, 35, 36, 40, 41, 42, 45, 47, 50, 57, 58, 60, 62, 64
hydrophobic, 357
hydrophobicity, 351
hyperactivity, 180

hyperbolic, 47, 73
hypergammaglobulinemia, 20
hyperglycemia, ix, 233, 235
hyperhidrosis, 269
hyperlipidemia, 131, 132, 141
hyperplasia, 134, 320
hypertension, viii, 5, 108, 122, 124, 125, 126, 130, 131, 132, 134, 135, 141, 143, 151, 152, 161, 209, 210, 216, 218, 219, 220, 227, 253
Hypertension, 115, 147, 161, 165, 217
hyperthyroidism, 419, 435
hypertrophy, 143
hypomorphic, 408, 412, 426
hypoparathyroidism, 414
hypoperfusion, 221
hypoplasia, 320
hypothesis, 34, 78, 111, 180, 187, 196, 214, 241, 312, 388, 408, 434
hypothyroidism, 99, 418, 420

I

IAP, 200
iatrogenic, 147
IBM, x, 289, 290, 291, 292, 293, 294, 295, 296, 299
ICAM, 109, 387, 392, 396, 406, 423
ICD, 176
identification, viii, 167, 168, 169, 171, 172, 174, 183, 186, 220, 254, 325, 346, 362, 430
idiopathic, 124, 125, 141, 149, 151, 152, 276, 297, 421
idiopathic thrombocytopenic purpura, 297
IFN, 176, 178, 183, 187, 188, 189, 196, 197, 201, 202, 278, 279, 280, 281, 282, 283, 284, 285, 286, 287, 288, 307, 309, 311, 314, 423
IgE, 5, 429
IGF, 307, 309, 311, 314
IGF-1, 307, 309, 311, 314
IL-1, 109, 172, 175, 176, 177, 179, 185, 186, 188, 196, 197, 198, 208, 236, 238, 242, 282, 285, 307, 309, 386, 387, 396, 410, 411, 429, 430
IL-10, 175, 176, 179, 185, 188, 198, 236, 238, 242, 282, 386, 410, 411, 429, 430
IL-13, 188
IL-15, 186, 208, 396
IL-17, 172, 176, 196, 411, 430
IL-2, 112, 174, 175, 176, 177, 194, 196, 197, 205, 208, 236, 286, 409, 411, 421, 428, 430
IL-21, 177, 194, 196, 197, 411, 430
IL-4, 176, 279, 307, 309, 311, 314, 410
IL-6, 109, 153, 176, 196, 215, 226, 259, 263, 282, 309, 311, 397, 399, 411, 430
IL-8, 109, 176
images, 17, 97, 218, 343

imaging, xi, xii, 218, 219, 224, 226, 227, 228, 298, 317, 321, 322, 323, 324, 325, 326, 342, 343, 344, 347, 369, 385, 395, 400
imaging modalities, xi, 317, 321
immature cell, 186
immune activation, 182
immune cells, 176, 181, 236, 239, 304, 307, 308, 384, 387, 389
immune function, ix, 181, 233, 237, 240
immune reaction, 32
immune regulation, 174, 177, 198
immune response, 2, 15, 16, 18, 76, 81, 87, 93, 99, 108, 110, 136, 168, 173, 175, 177, 178, 181, 184, 187, 190, 203, 237, 245, 246, 307, 309, 350, 375, 387, 394, 404, 412, 413, 431
immune system, vii, viii, x, xii, 1, 2, 5, 8, 10, 14, 16, 17, 18, 19, 21, 31, 32, 33, 34, 37, 38, 40, 42, 67, 76, 77, 81, 82, 86, 87, 96, 140, 168, 177, 181, 184, 190, 204, 235, 236, 238, 239, 284, 286, 303, 304, 341, 351, 381, 382, 384, 389, 419
immunity, 4, 10, 81, 82, 87, 92, 100, 105, 181, 187, 202, 203, 205, 206, 240, 247, 248, 365, 428
immunization, 14, 16, 17, 18, 20, 21, 23, 24, 30, 31, 42, 43, 45, 54, 77, 78, 80, 89, 104, 279, 395
immunocompromised, 112, 138
immunocytes, 34
immunocytochemistry, 307, 400
immunodeficiency, 408, 410, 418, 426
immunofluorescence, 114, 117, 121, 126, 258
immunogen, 41, 42, 46, 47, 372, 375, 376, 379, 380, 381, 382, 383, 391
immunogenicity, 18, 86
immunoglobulin, 81, 91, 92, 98, 99, 103, 108, 109, 110, 114, 136, 139, 160, 177, 197, 205, 206, 207, 221, 230, 244, 245, 276, 286, 363, 366, 387, 426
immunoglobulin G, 91, 92, 110
immunoglobulin superfamily, 207, 363
immunoglobulins, 5, 96, 98, 101, 103, 121, 124, 125, 129, 252, 412
immunological, xii, 4, 5, 8, 10, 14, 80, 83, 85, 108, 113, 145, 155, 160, 163, 170, 192, 309, 310, 311, 369, 372, 383, 385, 395, 407, 409, 419
immunology, viii, xii, 107, 192, 193, 194, 203, 210, 240, 241, 244, 245, 246, 247, 248, 286, 313, 369
immunomodulation, 246
immunomodulatory, 260, 410
immunomodulatory agent, 260
immunopathogenesis, 11, 95, 193
immunopathology, 93, 198, 286, 397, 409
immunoregulation, 4, 14, 84, 236
immunostimulant, 375, 376
immunosuppression, 131, 138, 143, 144, 145, 146, 147, 160, 164, 221, 222, 236, 238, 239, 240, 247

immunosuppressive, ix, 80, 86, 108, 111, 113, 124, 125, 128, 131, 135, 136, 137, 138, 140, 141, 142, 143, 145, 150, 152, 157, 158, 185, 211, 221, 236, 241, 242, 251, 260, 261, 288
immunosuppressive agent, 142, 150
immunosuppressive drugs, 137, 138, 145, 152, 158, 211, 221, 242
immunosuppressive therapies, ix, 137, 251, 260, 261
immunosurveillance, 186, 187
immunotherapy, x, 87, 140, 199, 237, 238, 249, 277, 284
Immunotherapy, 137, 286
impaired glucose tolerance, 434
impulse conduction, 337, 338
in situ, 3, 194, 220
in vitro, 3, 59, 199, 207, 208, 238, 239, 242, 247, 263, 284, 286, 297, 298, 306, 310, 315, 316, 358, 407, 409
in vivo, 86, 112, 155, 182, 185, 194, 197, 198, 199, 200, 201, 204, 208, 235, 247, 284, 297, 298, 304, 316, 338, 342, 351, 358, 388, 407, 409, 426, 427, 428, 429
inactive, 18, 19, 35, 36, 39, 42, 43, 62, 69, 71, 110, 121, 123, 129, 141, 142, 220, 256, 257, 373, 377, 388
incidence, xi, 18, 19, 21, 82, 114, 138, 148, 150, 152, 163, 164, 185, 186, 189, 190, 208, 223, 236, 237, 252, 253, 266, 268, 272, 273, 324, 341, 374, 404, 405, 414, 425
incubation, 37, 38, 44, 45, 52, 56, 60, 61, 62, 70, 71, 72
independence, 238
India, 223, 268
indication, 159, 234
indicators, 8, 15, 22, 86, 169, 276, 395
indices, 4, 5, 8, 10, 14, 21, 22, 23, 25, 26, 27, 28, 29, 32, 33, 34, 80, 83, 85, 127, 254, 259, 347
indirect effect, 178
individual character, 145
individual characteristics, 145
individual differences, 343
inducer, 80, 279, 284, 375
infarction, 214, 292, 422
infection, ix, xii, 15, 16, 17, 32, 35, 44, 81, 83, 96, 111, 112, 113, 130, 135, 136, 137, 149, 150, 155, 184, 197, 200, 204, 208, 216, 220, 251, 260, 266, 270, 272, 273, 274, 276, 280, 282, 322, 323, 341, 381, 390, 391, 417
infections, viii, xi, 5, 14, 15, 16, 35, 45, 77, 81, 82, 83, 95, 112, 133, 136, 138, 143, 145, 163, 173, 177, 183, 188, 202, 204, 209, 210, 223, 252, 276, 280, 281, 307, 317, 323, 333, 350, 383, 390, 393, 400, 417

infectious, ix, 16, 44, 77, 81, 83, 112, 113, 215, 265, 307, 323, 375, 402
infectious disease, 44, 77, 81, 113
infectious diseases, 44, 77, 81, 113
infertility, ix, 251, 260
Infiltration, 234
inflammation, x, xi, 10, 14, 111, 124, 127, 131, 168, 173, 175, 179, 182, 184, 187, 188, 196, 201, 234, 239, 241, 252, 253, 259, 263, 267, 277, 281, 283, 284, 307, 317, 322, 385, 387, 390, 429, 430, 434
inflammatory bowel disease, 420, 424
inflammatory cells, 108, 111, 307
inflammatory demyelination, 366
inflammatory disease, 230, 318
inflammatory mediators, 214, 267
inflammatory response, viii, 107, 111, 176, 183, 187, 252, 383, 392, 397
inflammatory responses, 176, 183, 383
infliximab, 287
influenza, ix, 14, 16, 136, 197, 265, 270
information technology, 263
infusions, 137, 138, 220, 300
inheritance, 423
inherited, xii, 349, 359, 426
inhibition, 38, 111, 154, 161, 176, 177, 196, 237, 260, 360, 366, 383, 402, 417
inhibitor, 38, 80, 129, 176, 365, 387, 399, 413
inhibitors, 37, 38, 87, 110, 129, 135, 136, 141, 283, 385, 394, 396
inhibitory, 180, 187, 188, 199, 206, 207, 235, 307, 314, 315, 316, 416, 427
initiation, xii, 110, 128, 142, 148, 189, 244, 330, 369, 375, 384, 389, 408
injection, 19, 110, 188, 230, 284, 290, 293, 295, 297, 298, 299, 321, 370, 371, 373, 375, 394, 395, 398
injections, 327, 370
injuries, 319
injury, xii, 110, 111, 126, 128, 156, 215, 228, 252, 253, 254, 255, 258, 307, 309, 319, 321, 333, 349, 390, 395, 399
innate capacity, 419
inorganic, 61, 103, 104
iNOS, 110, 111, 185, 242
INS, 170, 406, 413, 415, 431
insulin, ix, 170, 175, 233, 234, 235, 236, 237, 238, 240, 242, 243, 244, 245, 246, 297, 307, 402, 414, 415, 416, 428, 429, 431, 434
insulin-like growth factor, 307
insulin-producing cells, 242, 243
integration, 10, 81, 190, 331
integrin, 182, 260, 264
integrity, 205, 220, 400, 413

interaction, 2, 43, 68, 75, 100, 173, 175, 190, 205, 222, 247, 314, 350, 352, 356, 360, 364, 376, 380, 407, 414, 416, 432, 434
interactions, xii, 16, 75, 90, 93, 99, 110, 238, 239, 248, 260, 307, 313, 349, 352, 354, 355, 358, 360, 377
intercellular adhesion molecule, 109, 388
interface, 21, 36, 89
interference, 195, 203, 286
interferon, 178, 183, 197, 201, 202, 206, 207, 264, 278, 279, 283, 285, 286, 287, 288, 307, 388, 393, 422, 424
interferon (IFN), 178
interferon gamma, 207, 307, 393
interferons, 197, 279, 280
interleukin, 139, 153, 192, 196, 197, 198, 207, 215, 226, 287, 307, 309, 315, 386, 387, 421, 422, 423, 428, 429, 430
interleukin-1, 153, 192, 196, 207, 307, 309, 386, 387, 422, 423, 430
Interleukin-1, 196, 248, 387, 394, 395, 401, 422
interleukin-17, 192
interleukin-2, 197, 421, 428
interleukin-6, 153, 196, 226, 287, 309, 315, 388
interleukin-8, 153
interneurons, 305, 314
interstitial, 34, 114, 119, 120, 121, 126, 133, 263
interval, 177, 183, 189
intervention, xi, 85, 234, 323, 324, 329, 337, 419
intestine, 417
intracranial, 214, 322
intramuscularly, 282, 284
intravenous, 110, 129, 131, 138, 140, 148, 157, 158, 160, 164, 220, 221, 229, 230, 276, 290, 295, 298
intravenously, 294
intrinsic, 3, 18, 21, 35, 36, 69, 72, 79, 81, 101, 175, 407, 408, 410, 411, 412, 417, 418, 419
invasive, 138
inversion, 218, 227
inversion recovery, 218, 227
investigative, 248
iodine, 415
Iodine, 433
ion channels, 332
ions, 6, 39, 45, 52, 54, 55, 58, 59, 60, 68, 69, 70, 71, 72, 74, 75, 76, 77, 78, 79, 101, 103, 104
iron, 185, 204, 258, 259, 263
irritability, 374
IS, 274, 338
ischemia, 215, 217, 218, 314
ischemic, 219, 222, 400
ischemic stroke, 222
Islam, 315

islet isolation, 235
islet transplantation, 234, 235, 240, 241
isoelectric point, 37
isoforms, 259, 351, 357, 362
isolation, 204, 235, 399
isomers, 351, 367
isoniazid, 152
isotope, 81
Italy, 272, 341
IVIg, 139, 221

J

JAMA, 152, 190
Japan, ix, 265, 266, 268, 269, 270, 271, 272, 273, 289, 296, 329
Japanese, 267, 270, 271, 283, 421, 423, 433
jaw, 268, 318, 319, 320
jejunum, 235
JNK, 310, 315
joint pain, 281, 323, 325, 326
joints, 210, 318, 321, 322, 323, 419
Jordan, 208, 244, 427
Jun, 192, 310, 315
Jung, 203, 224
juvenile rheumatoid arthritis, 207, 421, 422

K

K^+, xi, 329, 335, 337, 338
kainic acid, 390
kappa, 97, 201, 249, 422
kappa B, 201, 422
keratinocytes, 110
kidney, 31, 34, 108, 109, 112, 128, 133, 136, 140, 142, 144, 147, 150, 152, 160, 161, 162, 173, 210, 235, 252, 255, 258, 259, 262, 285, 295
kidney dialysis, 285
kidney transplant, 108, 142, 147, 161, 162
kidney transplantation, 108, 142, 147, 161, 162
kidneys, 109, 110, 143, 146, 283
killer cells, 205, 207, 208, 425
killing, 168, 187, 188, 205, 434
kinase, 19, 53, 54, 60, 61, 82, 99, 200, 243, 307, 309, 314, 315, 357, 367
Kinase, 426
kinase activity, 53, 54, 61, 99
kinases, 60, 61
kinetic parameters, 79
kinetic studies, 104
kinetics, 47, 48, 86, 412
knockout, 169, 279, 406
Korean, 405, 420

L

L1, 61, 62
L2, 61, 62
LA, 224, 234, 253, 261, 263
lactating, 19, 20, 22, 23, 24, 27, 28, 30, 32, 33, 34
lactation, 20, 21, 22, 23, 24, 26, 27, 30, 32, 33, 34, 98, 151
Lactobacillus, 382
large-scale, 430
laser, 342, 343, 346, 347
latency, xii, 112, 335, 336, 341
LDL, x, 277
learning, 215, 225, 306
lectin, 136, 206
left ventricular, 143
leptin, 309
leucocyte, 153
leukaemia, 300, 315
leukemia, 186, 204, 238, 293, 307, 316
leukemias, 294
leukocyte, 120, 184, 200, 236, 247, 252, 258, 287, 393, 417, 433, 434
Leukocyte, 127, 170, 263, 312
leukocytes, 104, 116, 184, 205, 221, 387, 393, 397
leukocytic cells, 370
LIF, 307, 309, 311, 314
life expectancy, 129
ligand, 20, 36, 99, 160, 175, 182, 189, 195, 200, 203, 207, 245, 315, 352, 365, 410, 412, 417, 423, 430, 434
ligands, xii, 187, 188, 189, 205, 206, 237, 349, 351, 358, 412, 417
likelihood, 172, 419
limb weakness, 266
limitation, viii, 135, 167, 171, 234, 318, 324, 382, 412
linear, 43, 45, 70, 73, 78, 85, 102, 116, 218, 395
linkage, 97, 98, 168, 169, 170, 171, 172, 183, 191, 357, 365, 407, 411, 424
links, xiii, 262, 403
lipid, 19, 53, 54, 60, 61, 82, 136, 164, 247, 350, 353, 355, 356, 361, 362
Lipid, 99, 367, 402
lipid kinase, 53, 54, 61
lipids, 16, 60, 61, 62, 82, 99, 106, 148, 164, 390
lipophilic, 417
lipopolysaccharide, 394, 425
lipopolysaccharides, 383, 385, 402
lipoprotein, 164, 371, 372, 384
Lipoprotein, 372
liver, 205, 259, 264, 283, 290, 293, 295, 299, 301, 302

L-lactide, 249
localization, 356, 366, 397, 400
location, xii, 239, 342, 349, 369, 381, 389, 405, 432
locus, viii, xiii, 167, 170, 175, 176, 180, 194, 195, 196, 204, 234, 403, 404, 406, 409, 410, 411, 415, 416, 417, 421, 422, 423, 428, 431, 434
LOD, 170, 180
London, 326, 400
long period, x, 277
longitudinal studies, 388
longitudinal study, 224, 226, 346, 385, 388
long-term potentiation, 225
low molecular weight, 398
low risk, 140, 168, 170
low-dose aspirin, 141
LPS, 402
luciferase, 112
lumen, 116, 118
lung, 5, 290, 291, 294, 295, 299, 410
lupus anticoagulant, 225, 253, 262
lupus erythematosus, viii, ix, 101, 102, 108, 151, 152, 153, 161, 163, 164, 165, 209, 210, 223, 224, 226, 228, 251, 252, 263, 318, 322, 325, 326, 404, 405, 406, 420, 421, 422, 423, 430
luteinizing hormone, 393
lymph, 20, 27, 28, 31, 33, 182, 194, 238, 239, 247, 298, 413, 417, 418
lymph node, 27, 28, 31, 33, 182, 194, 238, 239, 247, 417, 418
lymphadenopathy, 20, 413
lymphocyte, vii, 1, 21, 27, 28, 30, 31, 32, 33, 34, 42, 77, 119, 133, 143, 151, 164, 165, 186, 204, 222, 244, 260, 293, 300, 301, 413, 429
lymphocytes, 15, 27, 31, 33, 34, 42, 116, 119, 126, 133, 144, 151, 170, 174, 175, 177, 186, 187, 197, 199, 204, 222, 244, 253, 284, 286, 304, 308, 309, 360, 372, 397, 430, 431
lymphoid, 20, 34, 173, 175, 182, 186, 199, 200, 201, 204, 414, 421, 426, 428
lymphoid cells, 34
lymphoid organs, 20, 173, 175, 199, 200, 414
lymphoid tissue, 34
lymphokine-activated killer, 205
lymphoma, 205, 206, 222, 281
lysine, 392
lysis, 86, 206
lysosomal enzymes, 205
lysozyme, 55

M

M.O., 427
mAb, 244
macrophage, 185, 204, 207, 310, 315

macrophages, viii, xii, 14, 26, 81, 126, 168, 173, 176, 179, 184, 185, 186, 188, 202, 203, 207, 279, 287, 304, 341, 417
magnesium, 104
magnetic, xi, xii, 214, 218, 219, 224, 226, 227, 228, 282, 317, 321, 323, 325, 326, 334, 335, 338, 342, 369, 376, 377, 385, 395, 400
magnetic resonance, xi, xii, 214, 218, 219, 224, 226, 227, 228, 282, 317, 321, 323, 325, 326, 342, 369, 385, 395, 400
magnetic resonance imaging, xi, xii, 218, 219, 224, 226, 227, 317, 321, 323, 325, 326, 342, 369, 385, 395, 400
Magnetic Resonance Imaging, 219, 326
magnetic resonance scanning, 227
magnetic resonance spectroscopy, 214, 228
magnetization, 227
magnetization transfer imaging, 227
main line, 11, 404
maintenance, ix, 130, 131, 132, 133, 134, 135, 142, 145, 148, 149, 158, 159, 175, 176, 180, 184, 199, 201, 228, 251, 260, 290, 307, 316, 411, 412
major histocompatibility complex, 201, 206, 290, 313, 422
Major Histocompatibility Complex, 170
males, 22, 23, 24, 25, 26, 27, 28, 29, 30, 31, 32, 33, 152, 319, 405
malignancy, 137, 143, 252
malignant, 293, 294, 295, 301, 320
malignant tumors, 293, 294
mammals, 4, 33, 36, 41, 43, 76, 77, 79, 80, 81, 83, 304, 312, 370, 385
management, viii, xi, 107, 108, 128, 129, 136, 156, 157, 160, 228, 229, 261, 273, 317, 322, 323, 324, 325
mandible, 318, 320
mandibular, 318, 324, 327
MAPK, 309, 314
marrow, vii, x, 1, 4, 24, 26, 27, 28, 29, 30, 31, 32, 33, 34, 42, 77, 79, 80, 178, 186, 204, 206, 207, 249, 289, 290, 291, 292, 293, 294, 295, 297, 298, 299, 300, 301, 302, 322, 323
Maryland, 223, 277, 311
masticatory, 318, 319, 324, 325
maternal, 34, 150, 434
matrix, 114, 115, 116, 226, 252, 256, 260, 385, 394, 396, 398, 399, 432
matrix metalloproteinase, 226, 385, 394, 396, 398, 399
maturation, 174, 177, 178, 186, 187, 188, 189, 202, 205, 238, 407, 410
maxillary, 323, 327

MBP, 13, 14, 37, 38, 44, 54, 56, 57, 67, 72, 78, 79, 82, 84, 87, 88, 95, 350, 351, 352, 353, 354, 362, 365, 370, 371, 372, 373, 374, 378, 379, 384, 389, 391, 393, 395, 398, 402, 406, 415, 416
MCP, 258, 263, 310, 311, 313, 315
MCP-1, 258, 263, 310, 311, 313, 315
measurement, 110, 345, 347
measures, 128, 136, 170, 263, 337
mechanical ventilation, 268, 275
median, 133, 138, 141, 271, 332, 335, 336
mediators, 10, 14, 86, 108, 110, 184, 214, 247, 267, 304, 309, 310, 311, 410, 411, 413
medication, 137, 138, 149, 151, 152, 337
medications, 128, 137, 211, 220
medulla, 390, 414, 424, 426, 431
medulla oblongata, 390
membranes, xii, 116, 349, 354, 356, 361, 393
membranoproliferative glomerulonephritis, 124
membranous glomerulonephritis, 254, 258
membranous nephropathy, 111, 113, 125, 141, 144, 158, 161
memory, 20, 32, 34, 177, 198, 214, 215, 218, 224, 225, 304, 306, 430
memory deficits, 215
memory formation, 304
men, 149, 207, 287, 319, 331, 370
Mendel, 361, 363, 370, 371, 396, 398
meningitis, 15, 35, 45, 138, 211, 212, 333
meningoencephalitis, 215
menstrual cycle, 325
mesangial cells, 116, 252, 263
mesenchymal stem cell, x, 289, 295
mesenchymal stem cell (MSC), x, 289
mesoderm, 243
messenger RNA, 264, 399, 430
meta-analysis, 158, 225, 423
metabolic, viii, ix, 14, 136, 141, 144, 209, 210, 216, 220, 233, 318, 385, 408, 409, 413, 418
metabolism, 219, 246, 285, 361, 382, 385, 402, 410
metabolites, 151, 185, 220
metal content, 69
metal ions, 45, 54, 55, 60, 68, 69, 71, 72, 73, 75, 76, 77, 78, 79, 103, 104
metalloproteinase, 215, 393, 397, 398
metalloproteinases, 385, 394, 396, 399
metals, 68, 69, 72, 73, 75, 77, 78
metastatic, 293, 300
methanol, 61
methionine, 412
Methotrexate, 151
methylprednisolone, 131, 137, 157, 158, 220, 228, 229, 230

Mg^{2+}, 39, 45, 52, 58, 59, 66, 69, 70, 71, 72, 73, 75, 76
MHC, 170, 173, 174, 175, 177, 182, 183, 187, 188, 189, 191, 197, 199, 205, 238, 245, 290, 364, 407, 415, 416, 422, 425, 433
micelles, 365
microbial, 104, 350, 375, 417
Microbial, 16
microenvironment, 203, 426
microglia, 304, 306, 307, 308, 309, 313, 387
microglial, 307, 313
microglial cells, 307
microorganism, xii, 369, 380, 381
microorganisms, 20, 96, 371, 384, 389
microscopy, 114, 115, 116, 117, 121, 125, 126, 253, 258, 305, 307, 351, 353
microspheres, 239, 249
microtubule, 345
microtubules, 305, 364
microvascular, 80
microvasculature, 215
migration, xi, 247, 260, 303, 307, 309, 310, 311, 312, 313, 314, 315, 320, 341, 408, 426
milk, 2, 17, 19, 20, 30, 32, 34, 36, 37, 39, 40, 44, 45, 53, 54, 55, 56, 57, 58, 60, 61, 62, 63, 64, 65, 67, 69, 72, 76, 82, 97, 98, 99, 100, 105, 106
mimicry, 16, 17, 96, 97, 273, 360, 363, 367, 401, 402
mineralized, 321
Ministry of Education, 296
MIP, 187, 263
mitochondria, 305
mitochondrial, 59, 333, 425
mitogen, 27, 29, 31, 307, 309, 314
mitogen activated protein kinase, 307
mitogen-activated protein kinase, 309, 314
mitogenic, 375
ML, 223, 229, 338, 412
MMP, 385, 386, 387, 388, 390, 401
MMP-2, 387
MMP-3, 386, 387
MMP-9, 385, 388, 390, 401
MMPs, 385, 386, 387
mobility, 65, 320
modalities, xi, 317, 321, 323
modality, 321, 323, 324
modeling, 21, 353, 366
models, xiii, 11, 100, 110, 168, 169, 172, 183, 185, 188, 215, 236, 239, 263, 347, 359, 367, 393, 403, 406, 407, 408, 410, 411
modulation, 181, 184, 186, 190, 208, 307
Mofetil, 133, 164
MOG, 354, 355, 360, 371, 384, 396
moieties, 62, 358, 359, 360

molar ratio, 371
molecular mass, 55, 57
molecular mechanisms, 20, 32, 193, 245, 304
molecular mimicry, 16, 266, 350, 381, 382
molecular weight, 105, 398
molecules, x, xii, 2, 18, 75, 76, 77, 86, 109, 139, 153, 173, 175, 177, 179, 182, 183, 184, 187, 188, 200, 205, 207, 222, 238, 245, 247, 266, 303, 309, 349, 350, 351, 352, 353, 354, 360, 363, 369, 380, 382, 383, 385, 388, 395, 401, 412, 415, 416, 422
monoclonal, 2, 3, 11, 17, 21, 36, 39, 40, 42, 43, 47, 50, 58, 68, 72, 73, 76, 77, 78, 79, 86, 87, 93, 97, 103, 137, 222, 240, 243, 244, 278, 281, 286, 288, 355, 362, 363
monoclonal antibodies, 36, 240, 278, 281, 288
Monoclonal antibodies, 102, 285
monoclonal antibody, 78, 93, 137, 222, 243, 244, 281, 286, 355
monocyte, 119, 182, 185, 263, 431
monocyte chemoattractant protein, 263
monocytes, 116, 119, 121, 126, 176, 179, 184, 253, 263, 309, 387, 393
monogenic, 408, 409, 412, 414, 418, 419
monolayer, 305, 306, 353
monomeric, 63, 395
mononeuritis multiplex, 211
mononuclear cell, xii, 110, 116, 196, 286, 341, 387, 396, 399, 400
mononuclear cells, 110, 116, 196, 286, 387, 396, 399, 400
mononucleotides, 40, 69, 76
Monozygotic, 404
mood, viii, 209, 210, 211, 220
mood disorder, viii, 209, 210, 211
morbidity, viii, 107, 108, 143, 145, 147, 150, 224
morphology, 102, 256, 307, 335, 343
morphometric, 342
mortality, viii, 107, 108, 130, 135, 136, 140, 143, 145, 146, 147, 150, 162, 211, 224, 252, 261, 374
Moscow, 89, 90, 91, 93, 94, 95, 96, 97, 98, 99, 100, 102, 103, 104
mothers, 19, 20, 30, 32, 37, 39, 53, 56, 58, 72, 98, 99, 434
motion, 318, 320, 322, 324
mouse model, xiii, 76, 100, 169, 172, 175, 236, 237, 263, 403, 406, 408, 410, 411, 415
mouth, 319, 321
movement, 318, 321, 324, 417
MRI, xii, 214, 215, 218, 219, 222, 227, 228, 282, 321, 322, 369, 385, 394, 397, 400, 401
mRNA, 109, 112, 154, 259, 260, 264, 302, 357, 386, 387, 388, 394, 396, 400, 401, 402, 425
MRS, 220, 222, 224

MSC, x, 289, 292, 296
multiple factors, 331
multiple myeloma, 2, 80, 105
multiplicity, viii, 2
multipotent, 234, 309, 311
multipotential, 306, 307, 314
murine model, 110, 174, 183, 411, 426
murine models, 110, 183
muscle, xi, 266, 267, 274, 302, 322, 324, 329, 330, 331, 332, 334, 335, 336
muscle contraction, xi, 329
muscle relaxant, 324
muscle strength, xi, 329, 331
muscle weakness, 266, 267, 274, 330
muscles, 318, 320, 324, 325
musculoskeletal, 165, 318
mutagen, 169
mutagenesis, 3, 42, 91, 104, 190
mutagenic, 81, 87
mutant, 168, 406, 408, 412, 426
mutation, 20, 153, 175, 412, 422, 423, 425, 426, 433
mutations, 99, 109, 169, 174, 175, 193, 359, 408, 409, 413, 414, 416, 426, 431, 433
MV, 314
myasthenia gravis, 10, 188, 221, 333, 335, 415
Myasthenia Gravis, 211
myasthenic syndrome, 333, 335
mycobacteria, 431
Mycobacterium, 185, 280, 376, 379
Mycophenolate, 111, 133, 154, 158, 161, 163, 164, 221
Mycophenolate mofetil, 111, 154, 158, 163, 164, 221
myelin antigens, 361, 384, 389, 396, 399, 401
myelin basic protein, 13, 17, 37, 88, 90, 95, 101, 103, 105, 350, 361, 362, 363, 364, 365, 366, 367, 370, 376, 377, 379, 381, 384, 390, 391, 393, 398, 399, 400, 401, 402, 415, 416, 422, 433
myelin oligodendrocyte glycoprotein, 11, 95, 361, 392, 395, 396, 397, 398
myelination, 349, 367, 393
myeloid, 201
myocardial infarction, 292, 422
myocarditis, 19, 32
myoclonus, 333
myopathies, 333, 405
myopathy, 143, 421
Myotonic dystrophy, 333

N

NA, 229, 272, 274, 425
Na^+, xi, 329, 335, 337, 338
NAA, 220
NAc, 377

N-acety, 62, 64, 220, 273, 378, 390, 396
NaCl, 40, 41, 46, 47, 53, 55, 58, 59, 71, 79
NADH, 65, 81
Nash, 338
nation, xi, 341
National Academy of Sciences, 204, 243, 245, 246
National Institutes of Health, 131
native population, xi, 341
natural, vii, 1, 2, 3, 4, 17, 18, 20, 35, 44, 60, 81, 86, 88, 91, 96, 109, 142, 174, 188, 190, 204, 205, 206, 207, 208, 223, 253, 290, 297, 326, 425, 429
natural killer, 204, 205, 206, 207, 208, 253, 425, 429
natural killer cell, 204, 205, 206, 207, 208, 253, 425
Natural Killer cell, 183, 186
natural selection, 91, 190
natural selection processes, 190
necrosis, 80, 118, 119, 120, 121, 122, 123, 126, 127, 131, 132, 135, 178, 215, 223, 246, 259, 278, 285, 286, 287, 288, 307, 313, 315, 320, 323, 324, 327, 386, 387, 388, 393, 395, 399, 422
negative regulatory, 195
negative selection, 173, 174, 177, 181, 193, 200, 406, 407, 408, 409, 413, 414, 415, 416, 419, 425, 427, 432
neocortex, 304, 312
neonatal, 100, 186, 421, 435
neonates, 81, 82
neoplastic, 320, 375
nephritic syndrome, 262
,
nephrologist, 142, 150
nephropathy, 111, 125, 130, 147, 157, 159, 160, 161, 163, 253, 262
nephrosis, 139, 141
nephrotic syndrome, 115, 122, 124, 140, 145, 147, 149, 150, 253
nephrotoxic, 259
nephrotoxicity, 134, 135
nerve, xi, xii, 267, 268, 271, 275, 276, 292, 315, 329, 331, 332, 333, 334, 335, 336, 338, 339, 341, 342, 343, 346, 347, 348, 349, 350, 360, 361, 362, 363, 366, 367
nerve cells, 292
nerve conduction failure, xi, 329
nerve fibers, 338, 346
nerve growth factor, 315
nerves, ix, 265, 266, 268, 269, 336, 350, 397
nervous system, xii, 211, 218, 219, 223, 225, 226, 229, 230, 235, 304, 306, 312, 349, 350, 359, 370, 389, 400
network, 16, 96, 162, 259, 263, 305, 408
neural network, 259
neural stem cell, x, 303, 304, 312, 313, 314, 315, 316

neural stem cells, x, 303, 304, 312, 313, 315, 316
neural stem/progenitor cell, 313, 315
neural tissue, 14, 400
neuritis, 344, 345, 356, 365, 366, 367, 395, 433
neurobiology, 312
neuroblasts, 305
neurodegenerative, 14, 312
neurodegenerative disorders, 312
neuroectoderm, 243
neurofilament, 315, 364
neurogenesis, x, 303, 304, 307, 309, 310, 311, 312, 313, 314, 315
neurogenic, xi, 303, 305, 310, 320
Neurogenic, 306
neuroimaging, ix, 209, 210, 216, 218
neurological deficit, 330
neurological disease, 221, 330, 331, 332, 392, 399
neurological disorder, xii, 215, 280, 337, 349, 350
neuronal cells, 11, 220
neuronal loss, 220
neuronal migration, 313
neurons, xii, 168, 207, 214, 220, 279, 300, 304, 306, 307, 310, 311, 312, 313, 314, 315, 349, 366, 417, 434
Neuropathic pain, 267
neuropathological, 215, 224, 272
neuropathy, ix, 211, 213, 265, 266, 267, 270, 272, 273, 274, 275, 276, 332, 334, 335, 338, 346, 359, 362, 366
neuroprotection, 310
neuropsychiatric disorders, 215
neurotoxicity, 87, 141
neurotransmitters, 304
neurotrophic, 307, 309, 316
neutralization, 87, 280
neutrophil, 119, 200
neutrophils, 8, 9, 26, 119, 126, 127, 153, 176, 309
New England, x, 277, 288
New York, iv, 89, 90, 100, 104, 105, 195, 228, 241, 242, 243, 248, 284, 325, 329, 363, 394
New Zealand, 199
NFI, 345
NFkB, 239
NHL, 138
Ni, 68, 72, 73, 92, 98, 314
NIH, 131, 132, 133, 134, 140
nitric oxide, 110, 153, 154, 185, 203, 260, 279, 398
nitric oxide (NO), 110
nitric oxide synthase, 153, 154, 185, 203, 260, 398
nitrogen, 108, 110
NK cells, viii, 168, 186, 187, 188, 189, 204, 205, 207, 208, 309, 416
NMDA, 215, 225, 310, 315, 337, 398

NMDA receptors, 310
N-methyl-D-aspartate, 215
NMR, 351, 362, 365, 366, 377, 378, 393, 394, 398
NO, 14, 110, 111, 185, 279, 388
NO synthase, 388
nociceptive, 267
nodes, 27, 28, 29, 271, 417
non-invasive, 235
non-myeloablative, 140
non-obese diabetic, 192, 208, 392, 425
normal conditions, 238
normal distribution, 24
normal stem cell, x, 289
normalization, 221, 230
North America, 162, 249
NSAIDs, 151
NSC, x, 303, 304, 307, 309, 311
NSCs, xi, 303, 304, 310, 311
N-terminal, 309, 310, 365
nuclear, 5, 16, 76, 109, 110, 113, 119, 153, 168, 239, 249, 299, 376, 377, 411, 412, 430, 432
nuclear magnetic resonance, 376, 377
nuclease, 18, 19, 22, 43, 54, 58, 69, 80, 82, 83, 98
nuclei, 108, 119, 153, 305
nucleic acid, vii, 1, 4, 18, 19, 20, 35, 42, 46, 80, 82, 98
nucleoli, 305
nucleolus, 93
nucleophilicity, 77
nucleoprotein, vii, 1
nucleosome, 110, 112, 155
nucleosomes, 108, 110, 154, 155, 261
nucleotide sequence, 113
nucleotides, 2, 4, 39, 45, 98, 133
nucleus, 80, 112, 151, 307, 312

O

obese, 236, 406, 418, 425
observations, 16, 21, 32, 65, 81, 111, 164, 188, 219, 266, 297, 327, 389, 401, 410, 413, 418
obstruction, 275
occlusion, 214, 253, 319, 322
OCT, 342, 343, 344, 345
odds ratio, viii, 167, 170
oil, 375, 376, 377, 394
olfaction, 304, 305
olfactory, 304, 305, 310, 313
olfactory bulb, 304, 305, 310, 313
oligodendrocytes, 11, 168, 304, 305, 309, 311, 313, 350, 389, 390, 395, 398, 400, 402
oligomeric, 36, 43, 62, 360, 364
oligonucleotides, 40, 44, 51, 58, 69, 198, 239, 249
oligosaccharide, 61, 64

oligosaccharides, 21, 62, 63, 105, 106
Oncogenic stress, 204
ophthalmologist, xi, 341
ophthalmoplegia, 268
ophthalmoscopy, 342
optic disc, 342, 343, 344, 345, 346
optic nerve, xii, 341, 342, 343, 347, 348
optic neuritis, 229, 342, 344, 345, 347, 370, 399
Optical Coherence Tomography, 343, 344
Optical Coherence Tomography (OCT), 343, 344
oral, 19, 32, 129, 131, 132, 134, 135, 138, 140, 148, 149, 157, 220, 228, 235, 246, 325, 326
orchitis, 375, 395
organ, x, xiii, 10, 15, 27, 112, 140, 150, 162, 173, 175, 176, 190, 193, 211, 231, 245, 246, 247, 277, 289, 291, 294, 295, 296, 304, 403, 405, 406, 407, 409, 413, 414, 415, 417, 418, 419, 425, 432
organic, 219, 326, 422
organism, xii, 16, 35, 168, 279, 280, 324, 369, 381
orthopedic surgeon, 319
osteochondritis dissecans, 327
osteocytes, 292
osteomyelitis, 327
osteoporosis, x, 131, 132, 143, 144, 289, 291, 292, 295, 298, 299
oxidation, 4, 65, 67, 73, 74, 75, 87, 92, 101
oxidative, 77, 81, 153
oxidative reaction, 77
oxygen, 81, 87, 103, 108, 110, 304, 417

P

PA, 3, 36, 38, 55, 56, 57, 61, 62, 63, 64, 88, 230, 233, 272, 273, 274, 276, 327, 338, 339, 347, 387
pain, xi, 138, 214, 267, 274, 281, 284, 317, 318, 319, 320, 321, 323, 324, 325, 326, 331
PAN, 126
pancreas, 64, 174, 234, 239, 240, 241, 242, 291, 416, 417
pancreatic, ix, 17, 18, 40, 48, 51, 52, 60, 97, 104, 168, 177, 182, 188, 196, 208, 233, 234, 240, 241, 242, 243, 299
pancreatic islet, 196, 208, 234, 242, 299
pannus formation, 319
paradoxical, 310, 311
paralysis, 266, 272, 370
parameter, 12, 13, 344, 345
parasite, 16
parasympathetic, 268
parenchyma, 383, 392
parenchymal, 304
parenchymal infiltration, 304
Paris, 94, 96
Parkinson, x, 217, 277, 285, 333

particles, 79, 111, 322, 361
PAS stain, 123
patents, 278, 281, 282
pathogenesis, vii, viii, x, 1, 2, 4, 10, 11, 15, 20, 37, 80, 81, 84, 95, 105, 108, 109, 110, 112, 171, 182, 185, 222, 225, 244, 258, 259, 274, 277, 279, 280, 282, 285, 312, 330, 363, 365, 366, 367, 393, 395, 399, 412, 419, 426, 431
pathogenic, ix, 15, 20, 108, 109, 110, 153, 173, 179, 180, 185, 188, 214, 233, 244, 246, 254, 381, 411, 412, 419, 430
pathogens, 16, 86, 87, 106, 173, 184, 185, 190, 204, 381
pathology, vii, xi, 1, 5, 8, 10, 12, 13, 14, 21, 22, 23, 30, 43, 44, 55, 58, 77, 80, 83, 85, 86, 90, 100, 114, 128, 139, 152, 163, 164, 174, 193, 222, 240, 252, 254, 259, 262, 278, 280, 313, 317, 318, 321, 323, 341, 383, 388, 418, 430
pathophysiological mechanisms, 151, 331, 345
pathophysiology, ix, xi, 79, 265, 266, 271, 273, 329, 337, 367
pathways, viii, xii, xiii, 19, 35, 91, 103, 107, 109, 167, 170, 172, 175, 176, 177, 178, 190, 195, 196, 204, 247, 315, 341, 385, 403, 406, 412, 413, 419, 430
pattern recognition, 179
PC12 cells, 310, 315
PE, 225, 262, 263, 264, 326
pediatric, viii, 107, 148, 150, 162, 163, 164, 165, 258, 263
pediatric patients, viii, 107
Peptide, 194, 237, 366, 374, 379, 382
peptide bonds, 57, 77
peptides, vii, xii, 1, 2, 35, 57, 79, 84, 105, 110, 170, 173, 237, 245, 249, 351, 360, 362, 363, 367, 369, 371, 372, 373, 375, 377, 381, 389, 396, 398, 399, 401, 402, 415, 416
perfusion, 218, 221, 294, 295, 297, 301
periodontal disease, 320
Peripheral, 140, 174, 176, 194, 211, 331, 333, 355, 384, 386, 394, 424, 427
peripheral blood, 96, 102, 140, 205, 286, 294, 397, 401
peripheral blood mononuclear cell, 286
peripheral nerve, 266, 331, 332, 360, 361, 362, 363, 366, 367, 398
peripheral nervous system, xi, xii, 15, 210, 213, 329, 337, 349, 351, 355
peripheral neuropathy, 221, 355
peritoneal, 143, 161, 417
perivascular cuffing, 389
personal communication, 37, 45, 57, 67, 69, 72, 73, 77, 79, 283, 386

personality, 319
pertussis, 99, 367, 370, 376, 378, 379, 391
PET, 219
PG, 272, 327, 347
pH, 3, 40, 41, 45, 46, 53, 59, 60, 65, 66, 67, 68, 70, 76, 79
pH values, 65, 66, 67, 68
phage, 3, 79, 101
phagocyte, 247
phagocytosis, 184, 185, 239, 249, 314, 417, 434
pharmaceutical, 337, 383, 385
pharmaceutical industry, 383, 385
pharynx, 268
phenol, 65, 81
phenotype, 20, 100, 169, 172, 174, 175, 182, 183, 186, 189, 196, 309, 408, 412, 427, 431, 433
phenotypes, viii, 151, 168, 169, 177, 181, 183, 184, 186
phenotypic, 182, 183, 186, 409
phenylalanine, 381
Philadelphia, 262, 326, 327
philosophy, 148
phone, 329
phosphatases, 39, 40, 58, 76
phosphate, 40, 58, 59, 60, 61, 63, 76, 103, 104
phosphates, 358, 361
phosphodiesterase, 358, 361, 363, 364, 365, 366, 367
phospholipids, 19, 32, 41, 98, 214
phosphorylates, 61
phosphorylation, 61, 62, 98, 357, 364
Phosphorylation, 82, 98, 99, 309
photographs, 342
photon, 219, 227, 228
physicians, 137, 282, 325, 330, 337
Physicians, 255
physicochemical, 79
physicochemical methods, 79
physiological, xi, 92, 105, 240, 303, 304, 306, 331, 360, 385
physiology, 249
pI, 50, 351
pigs, 370, 371, 373, 376, 379, 392, 394, 399, 402
pilot study, 159, 160, 161, 228, 347
plaque, 279, 286
plaques, xii, 11, 83, 280, 307, 341, 350, 358
plasma, 34, 68, 93, 96, 100, 112, 119, 122, 125, 126, 148, 150, 177, 179, 197, 225, 253, 260, 276, 284, 358, 360, 387, 388, 393, 394, 399, 430
plasma cells, 34, 96, 100, 112, 119, 126, 179, 253
plasma membrane, 225, 358, 360, 393
plasmapheresis, 120, 129, 135, 159, 221, 230, 276
plasmid, 40, 43, 44, 46, 58, 59, 70, 102, 112
plasminogen, 387, 394, 399

plasticity, 198, 302, 312
platelets, 8
play, vii, xi, 1, 15, 35, 79, 80, 81, 82, 109, 168, 175, 177, 178, 179, 181, 183, 184, 187, 188, 190, 290, 303, 305, 306, 341, 360, 406, 407
PLP, 414
pluripotency, 243, 315
PMSF, 37, 38
point mutation, 169, 412, 422, 423
polarization, 187, 279, 342
polarized light, 342, 345
polyacrylamide, 88
polyarticular, 318, 322
polyethylene, 139
polygenic, xii, 192, 403, 407, 414, 417, 419, 425
polymerization, 361
polymorphism, 189, 361, 362, 419, 421, 422, 423, 424, 428
polymorphisms, xii, 169, 170, 176, 193, 287, 403, 404, 410, 415, 418, 421, 422, 423
polymorphonuclear, 121, 153, 393
polymyositis, 15, 19, 32
polynucleotide, 58
polyomavirus, 155
polypeptide, 101, 309
polypeptides, 57, 387
polysaccharide, 19, 53, 54, 58, 60, 61, 62, 63, 64, 80, 82, 99
polysaccharides, vii, 1, 2, 4, 16, 17, 19, 20, 35, 41, 60, 61, 62, 63, 64, 82, 99, 385
poor, ix, x, 86, 116, 144, 145, 148, 149, 157, 164, 189, 211, 251, 253, 262, 264, 265, 266, 270, 271, 300, 322, 330, 345, 376, 407, 408
population, xi, 16, 99, 111, 113, 134, 137, 169, 170, 171, 174, 182, 184, 186, 187, 188, 199, 210, 215, 218, 219, 222, 224, 236, 238, 240, 244, 258, 273, 281, 304, 306, 341, 392, 404, 405, 417, 420, 421, 422, 423, 428, 430
population size, 236, 238
portal vein, 293, 298
positive correlation, 5, 8, 14
positive feedback, 304
post-hoc analysis, 133
postmortem, 342
postsynaptic, 337
post-translational, 352, 363
post-translational modifications, 352, 363
prebiotics, 106
precipitation, 3, 74
precursor cells, 241, 314, 429
predictors, 128, 129, 140, 150, 161, 223, 270, 275
predisposing factors, 136, 319

prednisone, 131, 138, 140, 148, 149, 157, 158, 160, 161, 164, 220
Prednisone, 151
preference, 58, 72, 381
prefrontal cortex, 225, 331
pregnancy, 19, 20, 21, 23, 24, 26, 27, 30, 32, 33, 98, 112, 113, 129, 134, 135, 150, 151, 158, 165
pregnant, 19, 22, 23, 24, 26, 27, 28, 30, 31, 32, 33, 34, 99, 113
pregnant women, 19, 30, 99, 113
preoperative screening, 143
press, 138, 160, 263, 301, 347, 363, 365
pressure, 130, 132, 141, 148, 165, 253, 269, 325, 417, 419
presynaptic, 337
prevention, 131, 135, 160, 165, 172, 173, 175, 176, 184, 186, 229, 239, 260, 366, 402, 431
preventive, 249
primate, 304
primates, 312, 313
priming, 188, 201, 202, 248, 412, 413
probability, 140, 148, 170, 234, 347, 375
proband, 404, 418
probands, 404, 405, 434
procoagulant, 87
progenitor cells, 207, 234, 301, 314, 315
progenitors, 24, 26, 30, 31, 34, 100, 186, 204, 234, 305, 306, 307, 309, 310, 311, 314, 316
prognosis, viii, ix, x, 107, 108, 114, 115, 120, 122, 126, 152, 156, 214, 223, 226, 251, 252, 253, 255, 260, 261, 262, 265, 266, 270, 271, 272, 275, 276, 323, 330, 395
prognostic factors, 163, 214, 276, 330
prognostic value, 276
program, 204, 281, 296, 324, 427, 430
progressive, 423, 434
proinflammatory, 192, 285, 314, 430
promoter, 235, 315, 410, 414, 415, 422, 431
promoter region, 422
propagation, 307
prophylactic, 87, 109, 143
prophylaxis, 144
prostaglandin, 258
prostatitis, 425
protease inhibitors, 37
proteases, 3, 37, 38, 55, 56, 57, 67, 72, 76, 77, 87, 89, 104, 389
protection, 10, 81, 82, 130, 183, 190, 238, 416, 423, 427
protective role, 20, 81, 417
protein binding, 112
protein family, 355
protein kinase C, 357

protein sequence, 78, 351
protein structure, 360
proteinase, 56, 57, 393
Proteinases, 104
Proteins, 361, 373, 378, 379, 382
proteinuria, 21, 22, 23, 24, 27, 29, 30, 31, 34, 52, 115, 122, 124, 125, 128, 129, 130, 132, 134, 135, 137, 139, 141, 147, 148, 161, 252, 254, 255, 259, 261
proteolipid protein, 350, 370, 392, 394, 395, 399, 401, 414, 433
proteolysis, 384, 400
proteomics, 263
protocol, 131, 132, 141
protocols, 148, 235, 238, 255
pruritus, 138
pseudo, 43
Pseudomonas, 382
psoriasis, 279, 280, 281, 282, 286, 411, 430
Psoriasis, 282, 286, 287
psoriatic, 286, 322, 417
psoriatic arthritis, 286, 322, 417
psychiatric disorder, 224
psychiatric illness, 217
psychological stress, 217
psychological stressors, 217
psychosis, 210, 211, 215, 220, 221, 222, 225, 226, 228, 230
psychosocial stress, 327
psychosomatic, 327
pulse, 131, 134, 149, 157, 158, 159, 220, 228, 229, 230, 260
pulses, 131, 132, 133, 137, 148, 149
purification, 3, 4, 68, 72, 301, 365
pyramidal, 12, 13, 14
pyrophosphate, 104

Q

qualitative differences, 254, 297
quality of life, 147, 211, 330, 331, 337
Quebec, 167
quinidine, 151, 152

R

RAC, 272, 274, 276
race, 93, 146
radiation, 291, 293
radiography, 321, 322
radioisotope, 323
radiological, 323
radionuclides, 86
radiopaque, 321

radiopaque contrast, 321
radiopaque contrast dye, 321
random, 10, 94, 172
range, 22, 23, 24, 37, 42, 44, 45, 48, 49, 51, 53, 57, 60, 65, 67, 69, 83, 122, 148, 168, 169, 237, 253, 280, 320, 324, 331, 351, 405, 408, 416, 419
RANTES, 187
rapidly progressive glomerulonephritis, 147
RAS, 332
rat, 36, 45, 54, 68, 77, 101, 133, 188, 207, 241, 242, 300, 304, 312, 313, 314, 315, 361, 362, 366, 371, 372, 373, 379, 392, 393, 395, 397, 400, 402
RDA, 52, 71
reaction rate, 3, 44, 53, 67, 78
reaction rate constants, 53
reaction time, 62
reactive arthritis, 35, 45
reactive nitrogen, 108
reactive oxygen, 81, 87, 110, 304, 417
reactive oxygen species, 81, 87, 110, 304, 417
reactive oxygen species (ROS), 110
reactivity, 41, 89, 109, 190, 237, 361, 396, 400, 433
reagents, 86, 87
real time, 343
recall, 218
receptors, x, 82, 136, 179, 184, 186, 187, 188, 189, 197, 198, 204, 206, 207, 215, 244, 263, 277, 283, 309, 310, 312, 314, 337, 383, 388, 416
recognition, xi, 2, 10, 11, 57, 100, 104, 110, 168, 173, 175, 177, 179, 187, 205, 206, 229, 237, 245, 247, 268, 329, 332, 363, 401, 409
recombination, 171, 172, 408
recovery, x, 80, 142, 144, 150, 239, 255, 265, 266, 267, 270, 271, 272, 275, 276, 310, 330, 334, 426
recruiting, 414
recurrence, viii, 107, 129, 131, 140, 144, 145, 146, 147, 162, 240, 290, 429
recycling, 185, 204
red blood cell, 254
red blood cells, 254
redness, 323
reduction, 407, 409, 414, 418
reflectivity, 344
reflexes, 266, 267, 270, 272, 274
refractory, 133, 135, 140, 149, 157, 158, 159, 160, 164, 221, 231
regeneration, x, xii, 137, 234, 236, 239, 241, 267, 271, 289, 291, 292, 296, 309, 349, 360, 419
regression analysis, 343
regular, 116, 380
regulation, 82, 109, 110, 160, 174, 175, 176, 177, 179, 180, 186, 193, 198, 206, 207, 222, 246, 247, 310, 314, 315, 360, 427, 428, 429, 430, 432, 434

regulator gene, 423, 432
regulators, 174, 238, 248, 281, 309, 310, 311, 430, 431
rejection, x, 150, 161, 205, 235, 243, 247, 277, 280, 283, 287, 291, 294
relapse, 113, 132, 133, 134, 138, 140, 141, 263, 382, 385, 387, 388, 397
relapses, 95, 153, 369, 382, 385, 397
relapsing-remitting multiple sclerosis, 95
relationship, 78, 113, 186, 215, 223, 224, 271, 272, 273, 274, 326, 393, 395, 434
relationships, 8, 10, 24, 30, 85, 104, 397, 400
relatives, 186, 240, 404, 405, 420, 421
relaxation, 44, 70
relevance, xi, 168, 211, 219, 225, 231, 286, 303, 312, 361, 412
remission, ix, 11, 84, 85, 111, 129, 130, 131, 132, 133, 134, 138, 141, 149, 150, 159, 185, 243, 251, 260, 284, 293
remodeling, 319
remyelination, 11, 95
renal cell carcinoma, 293, 300
renal disease, 108, 109, 110, 113, 114, 127, 128, 131, 132, 139, 145, 147, 148, 150, 151, 152, 153, 154, 155, 156, 157, 161, 164, 252, 253, 255, 263, 285
Renal disease, 156
renal dysfunction, 122, 133, 139, 144, 150
renal failure, viii, 107, 126, 135, 140, 144, 146, 147, 148, 161, 255, 285, 288
renal function, 113, 129, 130, 131, 132, 133, 134, 135, 140, 142, 144, 147, 148, 150, 158, 255
renal replacement therapy, 136, 147
repair, 11, 300, 301, 304
reparation, 52, 65
replication, 155, 171, 185, 234, 253, 283
reproduction, 158, 171
residues, 35, 36, 38, 57, 62, 78, 86, 237, 309, 351, 356, 357, 358, 363, 375, 381
resilience, 413
resistance, 183, 185, 192, 194, 200, 204, 206, 393, 407, 413, 415, 417, 425, 428
resolution, 271, 321, 344, 351, 356, 360, 365
respiratory, 79, 81, 112, 268, 275
respiratory failure, 268, 275
responsiveness, 31, 178, 204, 206, 236, 237, 239
retardation, 131, 342, 345, 347
retention, 3, 269, 275
reticular activating system, 332
retinal pigment epithelium, 344
retinoic acid, 315
retroviruses, 283, 312
revascularization, 143
reverse transcriptase, 2, 17, 54, 55, 56, 81, 82, 87

rewards, 191
Reynolds, 243
RF, 5, 6, 7, 9, 88, 261
rheumatic, 10, 93, 94, 160, 164, 286, 320, 326
rheumatic diseases, 10, 93, 94, 160, 286, 326
rheumatic fever, 320
rheumatoid arthritis, x, 2, 5, 10, 17, 56, 90, 170, 222, 223, 277, 278, 280, 281, 282, 285, 286, 287, 288, 318, 320, 404, 405, 416, 417, 419, 420, 421, 422, 429, 431, 434
rheumatoid factor, 5, 6, 8, 88
rheumatologist, 142
ribonucleic acid, 435
ribosomal, 10, 94, 215, 225
ribosomal RNA, 10, 94
ribosomes, 214, 305
risk factors, 129, 130, 139, 141, 142, 143, 145, 157, 211, 226, 323, 421
risks, 137, 148, 281, 404
rituximab, 137, 138, 149, 159, 160, 181, 220, 222, 231, 236
Rituximab, 137, 222, 230, 260
RNA, 2, 3, 4, 10, 15, 16, 17, 18, 35, 36, 37, 39, 40, 41, 42, 45, 46, 47, 48, 54, 59, 60, 67, 69, 71, 72, 76, 78, 79, 80, 82, 90, 93, 94, 97, 98, 101, 102, 103, 180, 195, 199, 203, 260, 387, 425, 430, 432
RNA processing, 425
rodent, 305, 306, 307
rubella, 280
rubella virus, 280
Russia, 1, 283
Russian, 1, 88, 100, 101
Russian Academy of Sciences, 1, 88

S

safety, viii, 107, 135, 139, 149, 221, 235, 237, 239, 245
saline, 294, 373, 391, 393, 395
Salmonella, 16, 96, 185, 327, 382
sample, 141, 156, 171
Schwann cells, 350, 355, 366
scleroderma, 93, 320
sclerosis, xi, xii, 10, 13, 95, 120, 126, 127, 280, 282, 297, 322, 333, 341, 342, 345, 363, 369, 404, 405, 406, 420, 421, 422, 423, 431, 433
scores, 170, 211, 214, 218, 331
SCs, 16, 290, 294
SDS, 3, 36, 38, 55, 56, 57, 61, 63, 88
search, 173, 365, 391, 423
searching, 128, 381
seborrheic dermatitis, 282
secondary progressive multiple sclerosis, 287
secrete, 176, 178, 183, 187, 396, 411

secretin, 242
secretion, 175, 179, 184, 235, 386
sediment, 126, 128, 129, 138, 216, 255, 259, 260
seeding, 112, 298, 299, 418
seizures, 210, 211, 215, 219, 222, 231, 374
selectivity, 102
Self, 165, 427, 431
self-antigens, 109, 170, 173, 174, 178, 180, 181, 184, 247, 252, 404, 407, 414, 427, 433
self-renewal, 307, 309, 311, 314
senescence, 291
senile, 292, 298, 299
sensation, 221, 331
sensitivity, 17, 82, 120, 170, 180, 215, 255, 258, 259, 260, 285, 346
sensitization, 186, 370, 399
sensory symptoms, 267
separation, 3, 36, 37, 43, 55, 111
sepsis, 80, 83, 91
sequelae, 330
series, 144, 149, 227, 326, 343, 372
serine, 37, 38, 72, 76, 86, 381, 387, 400, 416
serology, 142, 164
serotonergic, 331
serotonin, 375, 383, 385, 399
Serotonin, 382, 399
serum albumin, 17, 18, 55, 56, 88, 138, 141, 148
serum erythropoietin, 159
SES, 108
severity, 5, 108, 113, 116, 127, 128, 129, 134, 150, 154, 176, 180, 188, 219, 220, 254, 255, 270, 319, 326, 338
sex, 4, 93, 113, 146, 252, 330, 425
sex steroid, 425
shape, 344, 345, 346, 347, 352, 428
shock, 3, 32, 37, 237, 246, 332
sialic acid, 62, 82, 357, 363, 366
siblings, 405, 421, 433
side effects, 131, 134, 138, 149, 287
sign, 8, 14, 80, 183, 319
signal transduction, 82, 260, 264
signaling, x, 196, 198, 242, 243, 260, 303, 307, 309, 311, 314, 315, 316, 424
signaling pathway, x, 303, 307, 309, 311
signaling pathways, x, 303, 307, 309, 311
signalling, 105, 110, 169, 176, 178, 179, 180, 187, 314, 367, 408, 409, 410, 416, 418, 426
signals, 175, 181, 195, 197, 238, 247, 416
signs, viii, xi, 5, 19, 22, 82, 112, 128, 209, 210, 214, 317, 318, 321, 322, 325, 326, 330, 338, 341, 370, 374, 387, 389
silver, 3, 116, 125
similarity, 12, 13, 16, 31, 34, 275

simulation, 365
single nucleotide polymorphism, 169, 422
single photon emission computerized tomography, 228
single-nucleotide polymorphism, 421, 423
sites, 57, 77, 78, 79, 103, 111, 153, 154, 180, 184, 187, 352, 364, 367, 371, 392, 399, 410
Sjogren, 10, 94, 179, 320, 404, 405, 420
skin, 4, 135, 138, 174, 210, 269, 279, 280, 283, 284, 286, 288, 291, 301, 327
skin diseases, 288, 327
SLAM, 137, 180
sleep, 284, 331, 333, 375, 398
sleep disorders, 333
small intestine, 417
small vessel disease, 218
SNP, 169, 422
SNPs, 169, 171, 183, 421, 423, 424
social life, xi, 329, 330
social support, 350
socioeconomic, 145, 261
socioeconomic conditions, 145
socioeconomic status, 261
sodium, 62, 160, 217, 327
software, 8, 343, 344, 345
solid tumors, 293
somatic cell, 243
somatic cells, 243
somatic mutations, 109
sorbents, 43, 53
species, 81, 87, 108, 110, 304, 312, 351, 370, 371, 372, 375, 376, 379, 381, 392, 417
specific surface, 11
specificity, 3, 39, 47, 57, 58, 59, 60, 61, 65, 67, 72, 73, 76, 78, 79, 81, 83, 86, 89, 91, 93, 100, 101, 102, 113, 174, 177, 187, 205, 210, 215, 237, 239, 245, 252, 255, 258, 259, 260, 346, 375, 387, 389, 398, 433
SPECT, 219, 221, 228
spectroscopy, 220, 228, 357, 367, 393
spectrum, 148, 221, 224, 252, 272, 389
sphincter, 272, 275
sphingolipids, 105
spinal cord, 230, 362, 367, 376, 390, 395, 399, 400
spleen, 27, 28, 30, 31, 32, 33, 34, 77, 181, 182, 199, 200, 293
splenomegaly, 413
sprouting, 271, 349
SRD, 131
St. Louis, 155
stability, 3, 14, 37, 72, 76, 155
stabilization, 91, 144, 196, 214, 324

stages, vii, x, 1, 21, 83, 99, 168, 205, 207, 277, 323, 394, 401, 407
standard deviation, 25, 38, 343
standardization, 210
staphylococci, 35, 45
Staphylococcus aureus, 35
statistical analysis, 12, 13
status epilepticus, 314
steady state, 182, 200, 201
Stem cell, 235, 242, 243, 302
stem cell lines, 243
stem cell transplantation, 132, 140, 149, 157, 160, 297
stem cells, vii, x, 1, 4, 16, 21, 24, 31, 34, 42, 77, 79, 80, 88, 96, 137, 140, 235, 242, 243, 289, 290, 292, 294, 295, 297, 298, 299, 300, 303, 304, 310, 312, 313, 314, 315, 316
Stem cells, 235, 242, 243
steroid, viii, 107, 128, 143, 148, 221, 425
steroids, 138, 144, 148, 164, 260, 399
Stieltjes, 90
Stochastic, 197
strain, 174, 176, 183, 188, 279, 370, 406, 408, 410, 411, 412
strains, 18, 21, 113, 155, 168, 169, 172, 174, 176, 180, 185, 187, 189, 198, 206, 208, 376, 401
strategies, 3, 141, 169, 214, 234, 237, 238, 240, 248, 294
strength, xi, 133, 173, 329, 331, 344, 416
streptococci, 286
stress, ix, 14, 136, 204, 233, 324, 418, 434
stroke, viii, 162, 209, 210, 215, 218, 220, 222, 315, 331
stroma, 194, 300, 414
stromal, 175, 290, 291, 292, 298, 314, 411
stromal cell-derived factor-1, 314
stromal cells, 175, 290, 291, 292, 298, 411
strong interaction, 407
structural changes, 72
structural knowledge, 350
structural protein, 366
subacute, 11, 218
sub-cellular, 432
subgranular zone, x, 303, 304
subgroups, 6, 7, 8, 9, 10, 11, 12, 13, 14, 15, 345
substances, 86, 304, 332, 375
substantia nigra, 304, 312, 313
substrates, 3, 17, 19, 36, 39, 42, 43, 45, 47, 50, 53, 55, 57, 58, 59, 60, 61, 67, 68, 69, 76, 77, 82, 358
subventricular zone, x, 303, 304, 305, 313, 314, 315
success rate, 294
suffering, 172, 175, 284, 290, 319
Sun, 100, 101, 153, 194, 243, 429

superimposition, 319, 321
superiority, 133
superoxide, 36, 75, 81, 87, 110
superoxide dismutase, 36, 75, 81, 87
supplements, 131
supply, 323, 410
suppression, xiii, 30, 32, 33, 34, 77, 150, 178, 185, 203, 235, 240, 282, 292, 391, 399, 403, 406, 409, 410, 428
suppressor, 242, 290, 297, 380, 409, 429
suppressor cells, 290
supramaximal, xi, 329
surgical, 35, 45, 323, 324
surgical intervention, 324
surrogates, 236, 240
surveillance, 151, 162, 205
survival, ix, x, 108, 133, 135, 140, 143, 145, 146, 150, 157, 159, 161, 163, 164, 173, 177, 178, 182, 190, 239, 242, 249, 251, 252, 260, 293, 303, 304, 307, 309, 310, 311, 315, 401, 412
survival rate, 135, 145, 252, 293
survivors, xi, 271, 329
susceptibility genes, 170, 171, 172, 423, 425
SV40, 111
SVZ, 304, 305, 307, 310, 311, 313, 314
swelling, 284, 322, 323
switching, 31, 34, 197, 412
Switzerland, 281
symmetry, 320
symptom, 217, 267, 268, 269, 318, 319, 324, 326, 330
symptoms, xi, 14, 21, 22, 26, 37, 150, 151, 152, 169, 214, 216, 218, 219, 220, 221, 228, 267, 269, 270, 317, 318, 319, 321, 322, 324, 325, 326, 331, 370, 371, 388
synapses, 207
synchronization, 159
synergistic, 419
synovial fluid, 280, 318, 324
synovial membrane, 318
synthesis, x, 35, 86, 87, 92, 99, 263, 277, 282, 284, 285, 394, 400, 402, 435
synthetic oligopeptides, 399
Systemic Lupus Erythematosus, 108, 111, 142, 156, 163, 209, 317, 322, 324, 327

T

T lymphocyte, 172, 173, 175, 185, 429, 431
T lymphocytes, 172, 173, 175, 185, 431
T regulatory cells, 248, 259, 426
tacrolimus, 129, 135, 141, 145, 146, 159, 161
Taiwan, 272

targets, viii, 11, 94, 108, 110, 130, 167, 177, 186, 187, 190, 237, 247, 288, 354, 367
T-cell, 424, 426, 427, 428, 429, 430
T-cell receptor, 398, 426
TCR, 20, 173, 175, 181, 194, 207, 236, 237, 238, 244, 364, 407, 408, 409, 413, 416, 425, 427, 429, 433
telencephalon, 304
temperature, 15, 284, 331, 338
temporal, 113, 312, 318, 334, 335, 342, 343, 344, 390
temporomandibular disorders, 325, 326
TGF, 174, 184, 185, 193, 203, 242, 244, 248, 411, 427, 430
Th cells, 236, 279
Thai, 163, 165, 262
thalamus, 331
thallium, 143
T-helper cell, 236, 237
therapeutic, 410
therapeutic agents, 92
therapeutic approaches, 170, 181, 182
therapeutic targets, viii, 167, 177, 186, 288
therapeutics, 86, 237, 248
thermal stability, 3, 76
thermodynamic, 45
Thomson, 243, 248
threatening, viii, 209, 210
three-dimensional, 59, 343
threshold, 171, 173, 176, 258, 325, 336, 344, 409
thrombocytopenia, 134, 158, 411
thrombocytopenic purpura, 120, 224
thromboembolic, 157
thromboembolism, 139
thrombosis, viii, 5, 80, 107, 135, 143, 145, 146, 161, 215, 222, 226, 229, 253, 262
thrombotic, 120, 143, 146, 156, 222, 224, 253
thrombus, 120
thymocytes, 173, 174, 175, 181, 192, 200, 407, 408, 414, 424, 429, 432
thymus, xiii, 27, 28, 30, 31, 32, 33, 34, 112, 173, 174, 175, 177, 192, 200, 309, 398, 403, 407, 409, 413, 414, 415, 419, 424, 427, 428, 431, 432, 433
thyroglobulin, 5, 6, 8, 15, 17, 56, 78, 80, 83, 85, 96, 415, 425, 433, 435
thyroid, 5, 15, 80, 85, 94, 96, 99, 404, 405, 406, 415, 418, 420, 423, 424, 425, 433, 435
thyroid gland, 15, 80, 85
thyroid stimulating hormone, 415
thyroiditis, 2, 5, 10, 15, 17, 19, 20, 32, 35, 48, 56, 59, 69, 80, 82, 85, 88, 94, 96, 99, 102, 105, 172, 174, 192, 420, 425
thyrotoxicosis, 99

thyrotropic hormone, 84, 85
thyroxin, 85
tight junction, 385
TIMP, 386, 397, 401
TIMP-1, 386, 397, 401
TIMPS, 385
TLR, 179, 198
TLR9, 198
T-lymphocytes, 286
TM, 224, 228
TNF, 109, 129, 139, 153, 176, 178, 187, 205, 259, 278, 279, 280, 281, 282, 283, 285, 287, 307, 309, 310, 311, 313, 386, 387, 396, 425
TNF-alpha, 109, 285, 287
TNF-α, 278, 307, 309, 310, 311
toxic, 14, 60, 81, 86, 87, 144, 151, 242, 252, 279
toxic effect, 144, 242, 279
toxicities, 137
toxicity, viii, 107, 129, 130, 131, 132, 134, 139, 149, 157, 260
toxin, 367
TPO, 94
trabecular bone, 291, 292, 323
training programs, 214
traits, 168, 169, 183, 190
trans, xiii, 403, 406, 409, 410, 411, 412, 419
transcript, 59
transcriptase, 2, 17, 54, 55, 56, 81, 82, 87
transcription, 111, 155, 174, 182, 186, 193, 234, 239, 249, 259, 385, 414, 426, 427, 431
transcription factor, 155, 174, 182, 186, 193, 234, 239, 249, 259, 414, 426, 427
transcription factors, 155, 182, 186, 234
transcriptional, 414, 417, 432
transcripts, 239, 367, 414
transducer, 309
transfer, 61, 82, 172, 183, 202, 218, 227, 242, 246, 299, 356, 410
transferrin, 258
transformation, 128, 148, 295
transforming growth factor, 153, 203, 263, 388, 427
transgenic, 169, 197, 242, 363, 416
transgenic mice, 197, 363
transgenic mouse, 197
transient ischemic attack, 222
transition, vii, 1, 2, 15, 16, 17, 19, 21, 25, 31, 32, 33, 43, 44, 81, 89, 98, 241, 411
translocation, 180, 199, 239
transmembrane, 351, 354, 357, 359
transmission, xi, 105, 112, 329, 331, 338
transplant, 112, 138, 140, 142, 143, 144, 145, 146, 162, 248, 280, 283, 287, 296, 300
transplant recipients, 143, 145, 162

transplantation, x, 108, 132, 140, 142, 143, 144, 145, 146, 147, 149, 150, 157, 158, 160, 161, 162, 163, 188, 206, 234, 235, 236, 240, 241, 242, 247, 248, 283, 288, 289, 296, 297, 298, 299, 300, 301
transport, 182, 204, 385
trauma, 320, 322, 323, 350, 360
treatment methods, 183
Tregs, 174, 175, 177, 181, 184, 238, 244
trial, 132, 133, 134, 135, 137, 138, 139, 140, 157, 158, 159, 160, 161, 221, 228, 229, 238, 239, 246, 260, 282, 283, 287, 337, 338, 392
Trichoderma viride, 64
triggers, 201, 207, 309, 315, 385
Trp, 373, 378, 400
trypsin, 56, 57, 393, 400
tryptophan, 185, 370, 371, 372, 373, 376, 377, 379, 380, 381, 382, 385, 392, 401, 402, 410, 421, 429
Tryptophan, 373, 374, 382
TSA, 174, 175
tuberculosis, 281, 376
tubular, 114, 120, 121, 125, 126, 133, 252, 253, 254, 259
tumor, 168, 202, 203, 205, 206, 215, 278, 285, 286, 287, 288, 292, 293, 300, 301, 307, 313, 387, 388, 393, 395, 422
tumor cells, 168, 202, 205
tumor growth, 292, 294
tumor necrosis factor, 215, 278, 285, 286, 287, 288, 307, 313, 387, 393, 395, 422
tumors, 218, 220, 293, 294
tumour, 80, 82, 178, 186, 187, 188, 206
tumours, 183, 186, 187
turnover, 43, 83, 184, 389
type 1 diabetes, ix, 168, 175, 191, 192, 194, 195, 197, 203, 233, 234, 235, 236, 237, 238, 240, 241, 244, 245, 246, 248, 280, 404, 416, 420, 421, 428, 429, 431, 434
type 2 diabetes, 418, 434
tyrosine, 187, 200, 367, 421, 426, 434

U

ubiquitin, 421, 430
UK, 421, 434
ULBPs, 205
ulcerative colitis, 170, 322, 417, 424, 434
ultrasound, 151, 321, 326
uncertainty, 234, 269
unemployment, 211, 214
uniform, x, 121, 254, 255, 265, 270
United Kingdom, 403
United States, 146, 204, 243, 245, 246, 280
universe, 286, 350
urease, 4, 17, 87, 92

uric acid, 6
urinalysis, 128, 148
urinary, 12, 13, 113, 126, 128, 129, 138, 141, 147, 262, 263, 264, 269, 292, 382, 385
urinary bladder, 12, 13
urinary retention, 269
urinary tract, 262
urine, 6, 21, 22, 25, 29, 31, 66, 83, 112, 128, 129, 138, 155, 204, 216, 254, 255, 259, 260, 263, 327, 370, 382, 385, 398, 426

V

vaccination, 136, 181, 356
vaccinations, 136
vaccine, 87, 136, 249, 391, 393
Valencia, 264, 303
validation, 170, 263, 347
values, 6, 7, 8, 9, 11, 12, 13, 22, 23, 33, 42, 43, 44, 45, 46, 47, 48, 49, 50, 51, 53, 54, 55, 65, 66, 67, 68, 69, 129, 170, 258, 259, 331, 345, 351, 386, 388
valvular heart disease, 132
variability, 188, 210, 342, 347, 379, 388, 422
variable, 423, 433
variables, 223, 252, 330, 343, 386
variance, 384, 388, 389
variation, 169, 170, 171, 193, 234, 401, 410, 416, 424, 428, 431
vascular cell adhesion molecule, 398
vascular risk factors, 130, 141
vasculitis, 5, 114, 126, 135, 214, 224, 228, 253, 333
vasoactive intestinal peptide, 15, 88, 89, 103, 105
vasoactive intestinal polypeptide, 101
vasomotor, 268, 269
VCAM, 109, 388, 398
VDR, 406
VEGF, 242
vein, 109, 253, 262, 293, 298
velocity, 330, 335
ventricular zone, 312
vessels, 125, 126, 214, 218, 253, 285, 305, 342, 370
VIP, 2, 3, 15, 17, 35, 37, 56, 57, 78, 79, 83, 88
viral diseases, 2, 10, 15, 17, 19, 35, 39, 44, 56, 58, 59, 80, 82
viral hepatitis, 10, 17, 35, 82, 83, 102
viral infection, 15, 17, 83, 111, 112, 113, 135, 155, 183, 197, 208, 280, 400
viremia, 112, 113, 155
virus, xii, 57, 81, 102, 111, 112, 155, 197, 206, 270, 280, 282, 283, 341, 350, 390, 395, 396, 398
virus infection, 112, 155, 197, 280, 350
virus replication, 155, 283
viruses, 10, 14, 16, 20, 30, 60, 155, 279, 283, 381

visible, 21, 22, 23, 29, 30, 31, 65, 67, 83, 256, 343, 344
vision, xi, 341, 370
visual acuity, 283
visual field, 342, 346, 347
visualization, 218
vitamin D, 131, 144, 422

W

warfarin, 229
water, 4, 77, 92, 101, 103, 285, 394
weak interaction, 416
weakness, xi, 266, 269, 274, 329, 330, 370
well-being, 151, 284
western countries, ix, 265, 266, 271, 272
Western countries, 270
white matter, 218, 220, 227, 312, 387, 395, 400
WHO, 114, 115, 140, 147, 148, 163, 254, 259
WHO classification, 163, 254
Wistar rats, 36, 45, 55, 65, 67, 73, 78, 81, 101, 104
WM, 219, 220, 224, 227, 228

women, xi, 19, 30, 32, 34, 57, 98, 99, 107, 113, 134, 145, 146, 162, 165, 319, 331, 341, 370, 418, 421, 434
World Health Organization, 108, 156
World Health Organization (WHO), 108

X

xenografts, 206, 242
X-linked, 193, 409, 418
X-ray crystallography, 357

Y

Y chromosome, 180
yeast, 48, 60, 103, 104
yield, 216, 235, 358
young adults, 266, 269, 272
young women, 134, 162

Z

ZAP-70, 426
zinc, 193, 260, 354, 357, 364, 431, 432
Zn, 68, 72, 73, 75